Medical Marriage *meets the needs of a market eager to understand more about the complementary therapies whilst providing a way in which there can be a healthy partnership between the orthodox and the more holistic medicines. Importance is given to patient self-responsibility so that they may become an active member of the multidisciplinary health team.*

In a concise and easy to comprehend manner, the reader is able to make more informed choices and hence to create a better relationship with all those involved in optimal health.

— **Dr Christine Page** MB MS MRCGP DCH DRCOG MFHom

I have been most impressed by the work that Dr Cornelia Featherstone has done in this excellent book. Not only is she the person to judge the present situation in so many countries of the world... but she has gone deeply into all the disciplines... The book is so well worth reading as it gives an overall picture of what is happening and is also very realistic and to the point.

— **Jan de Vries** DHOMed DOMRO NDMRN DAc MBAcA

This is a warm, wonderful, thorough and above all honest exploration of a new medical dimension which is emerging out of mutually respectful teamwork between orthodox and complementary health care professionals... The messages which this book offers should be read – and above all applied – by every health care professional.

— **Leon Chaitow** ND DO
Consultant osteopath and naturopath
Marylebone Health Centre (NHS), London

D1495180

Fifteen years ago Paul Starr predicted a "Social Transformation of American Medicine." His prophecy has come through but not only in America. A marked change is taking place in the very fabric of society's approach to medical care. One of the most socialised systems in the world, that of New Zealand, has been turned on its ear. Major changes are taking place in every country in the world.

Medical Marriage: The New Partnership Between Orthodox and Complementary Medicine *provides a road map to the social transformation of medicine taking place throughout the world.*

— ***Dr C Norman Shealy*** MD PhD
Founder of the Shealy Institute for Comprehensive Health Care
Founding President, American Holistic Medical Association
Research & Clinical Professor of Psychology, Forest Institute of Professional Psychology

Essential reading for all those interested in the field of alternative health, Medical Marriage *presents a dynamic and healthy perspective on the evolving relationship between orthodox and complementary medicine.*

— ***Caroline Myss*** PhD
Co-author of *The Creation of Health*
Author of *Anatomy of the Spirit*

...it is important that patients do take responsibility for their own health and furthermore it is important that doctors adopt a more co-operative and less pedagogic attitude to their patients and health care in general... so much of the book is excellent common sense, clearly written and a superb blueprint for the future.

— ***Dr G T Lewith*** MA DM MRCP MRCGP
Honorary Visiting Clinical Senior Lecturer, Southampton University

MEDICAL MARRIAGE

MEDICAL MARRIAGE

*The New Partnership Between Orthodox
and Complementary Medicine*

Dr Cornelia Featherstone

&

Lori Forsyth

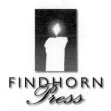

FINDHORN
Press

First published 1997

ISBN 1–899171–16–9

British Library Cataloguing-in-Publication Data.
A catalogue record for this book is available from the British Library.

Cover design and book layout by David Gregson.
Printed on environment-friendly paper.
Printed and bound by J W Arrowsmith Ltd., Bristol, England.

Published by
Findhorn Press
The Park, Findhorn, Forres IV36 0TZ, Scotland
tel +44 (0)1309 690582 • fax 690036
email thierry@findhorn.org
http://www.gaia.org/findhornpress/

To our children, Kevin and Sophie.
May this book further co-operation, respect
and understanding, thereby making a positive
difference in the world you inherit.

Contents

Part 1 The Concept

Part 2 A–Z of Complementary Therapies

Part 3 Essays

Acknowledgments

We would like to acknowledge everyone who contributed to the production of this book, most importantly our partners, Alan and Bruce, and our young children. They loved and supported us despite our antisocial schedules and preoccupation over the last two years.

Wholehearted thanks are due to the writers who contributed to Parts 2 and 3 for without them this book would never have come into being. They were patient and flexible, accommodating the changes that evolved as the concept of the book became clearer. Many editorial decisions were required to create a cohesive whole from the sum of many parts. At times these affected the personal expressiveness of the writers' original work. We are very grateful for the good grace with which these alterations were accepted.

We also want to express our thanks to the team at Findhorn Press: Thierry Bogliolo for his faith in the concept of the book and his steadfast support in its unfolding process; editorial input from Lynn Barton was invaluable as was the working relationship with David Gregson, the designer, whose calm and approachable manner nourished us when the project seemed altogether too big; while without Karin Bogliolo's professionalism in marketing and PR, this book would never have found its way to the public.

Authors' Introduction

This book and the process of its coming together is an excellent expression of co-operation. The co-authors' partnership was enriched by the fact that one of us is a medical doctor and the other is a complementary practitioner, each with a profound understanding of the holistic paradigm and its applications and a great respect for the contributions of orthodox medicine which saved our respective lives in life-threatening conditions. We were amused that during the intense process of completing this book, we made use of various different approaches to keep us functioning, including stress release techniques, meditation and fresh air as well as taking paracetamol and lying down with a hot water bottle! This exemplifies multidisciplinary co-operation at its best.

Cornelia Featherstone

I became a doctor because, as a child, I had been a mis-treated patient. From the age of four, I was very ill for several days every month with no doctor being able to find out what was wrong. They suggested various syndromes, removed my appendix, and in the end concluded that I was making it all up. I was in fact suffering from renal colic attacks which persisted for six years before a diagnosis was eventually reached: hydronephrosis – pressure damage to the kidney due to compression of the ureter. By that time my left kidney was irreversibly damaged and had to be removed. It was the opinion of the surgeon who performed the operation that another colic attack could well have resulted in life-threatening complications due to rupture of the damaged organ. This experience led me to take the decision to become a doctor so I could prevent other children from having to endure what I had undergone. In particular, I was adamant that no person in pain should ever have to suffer the humiliation of having their symptoms disbelieved and dismissed as attention-seeking behaviour.

In due course, I joined medical school at Ulm University which was pioneering psychosomatic medicine in Germany. It provided students with a broader outlook than most traditional schools and offered optional introductory courses in acupuncture, homoeopathy and patient-centred care based on the work of Carl Rogers.

When attending the acupuncture course, I was impressed and daunted at the same time. I realised that to do any justice to this system I would have to study it at least as long as I was studying Western medicine and I would have to practise it on a daily basis to become accomplished in all its complexities and applications. I had the same reaction to the homoeopathy course.

It was then that I was first attracted by the idea of working in a team of experts where each was a specialist in their own discipline, providing patients with access to other powerful forms of healing without having to be the one to provide them all. Since that time I have pursued the ideal of multi-disciplinary co-operation, an ideal which I have termed, Medical Marriage.

Lori Forsyth

I was a complementary therapist for whom there was no overlap with orthodoxy until I became ill with ulcerative colitis and had to be hospitalised. I insisted on being admitted to the Homoeopathic Hospital in London, where homoeopathy is used by medically trained doctors alongside traditional methods of treatment. I was given homoeopathic treatment, but it was unsuccessful in arresting my condition and my health continued to deteriorate. The doctors painstakingly explained to me why I should start taking drugs. I refused, becoming more entrenched in my position as I became weaker and lost full grip of my faculties to reason and make sensible choices. No one pressured me. After seven weeks, during which they monitored me carefully, I was given a four pint blood transfusion as my blood count was getting dangerously low. When I awoke the next morning, I was immediately aware of two changes. One, I was warm again. Two, I could think coherently, and saw at once the futility of maintaining my position, which might lead to my death if I continued to abide by it. I began a drug regimen and within a fortnight was well enough to leave hospital, although because of my inflexibility in the face of reason, I was so weak that I left in a wheelchair and took nearly two years to convalesce back to full health.

This experience was clearly dramatic and altered my outlook on life and health. I saw that there was a place for Western medicine in our society and that there are times when taking drugs is the only way to save lives. I appreciated how caring and genuine the doctors had been in wanting the best for me, and discovered that, far from steam-rollering me, they had respected my wishes, even beyond, perhaps, a point that was sensible.

Therefore, Medical Marriage is a concept which is close to my heart. Working as a complementary therapist, I do not want or need a full grounding in medical procedures, but feel enormously relieved knowing there is a supportive doctor whom I can contact if I am having difficulty with a patient or am concerned for their physical or mental health in any way. As a back-up to my own work, I find the co-operative support invaluable.

Implementing the Vision

For the last two years we have been working together in a multidisciplinary team at HealthWorks, the Forres Centre for Holistic Health Care where we are exploring ways to implement the concept of Medical Marriage.

Apart from the practice, we are involved in educational work which includes a series of annual conferences entitled 'Holistic Health Care for the 21st Century' hosted by the Findhorn Foundation. In lectures and presentations to the general public and professional colleagues, we aim to nurture the evolution of a better health care system.

With reference to this book we invite any complementary practitioner, who feels that they have a contribution to make to the project, to send us a manuscript. We intend to revise and expand the present edition in due course.

Cornelia Featherstone & Lori Forsyth
HealthWorks
5 Bank Lane
Forres IV36 0NU
Scotland

March 1997

How to Use the Book

Part One

The first section of this book introduces the concept of Medical Marriage and discusses its implications for health care and disease care.

Part Two

The second section of this book contains chapters on more than 60 different complementary therapies.

◆ These chapters provide a basic introduction to the various therapies and each contains information which can broadly be divided into three main categories:

◆ information about the historical and theoretical base of the therapy;

◆ an explanation of how the therapy is practised;

◆ detailed information about a specific application of the technique, either in the form of case histories, or exemplifying treatment procedures in relation to a specific condition.

At the end of each chapter are:

◆ the author's biographical details;

◆ references supporting information given in the text;

◆ a list of recommended further reading;

◆ a resource section containing relevant addresses of professional bodies and training institutions.

Each chapter is written by a practitioner of that discipline. The compilers approached people known to them to write the contributions, with the view that someone who is working on a daily basis with the therapy or modality is in the best position to convey a sense of what it is, rather than a professional writer, who may not be immersed in the discipline. The contributors are passionate about their unique contribution to health care and this personal involvement pervades each chapter.

This is not an exhaustive listing of therapies practised in the West, but comprises a good representation of that which is available.

Having considered all the different options in orthodox and complementary medicine, we acknowledge that we are not in a position to declare any of the options as irrelevant or ineffective. We always know of someone who has benefited at some time, be it from chemotherapy or from a meditation technique. There is validity in every approach. Our conclusion is that we need to carry everything with us for the development of an integrated health care system at this stage.

We have included chapters about therapies which we would not necessarily choose to make use of ourselves, accepting that for different people they may provide the perfect solution. This openness to others being different from ourselves and having different needs of which we may not necessarily be the best judge, is crucial to the ability to be truly effective as gatekeeper, care co-ordinator or simply informed adviser to another person.

For example, the chapter on the 'Medical Assistance Program' (MAP) may seem strange or unlikely to be of significant value. However, for one of our friends, it has provided the perfect solution.

At this time in her life she was nervous and withdrawn. She found talking intensely stressful and said it was because she was unable to find words to describe how she felt. She was very aware of her feelings but unable to verbalise them. She was given information about the MAP technique and decided to try it. Several months later she was using the technique regularly and with good results. She was more relaxed, more confident and found it empowering to have a tool which she could use whenever she needed, which did not cost her money and did not cause her stress, but afforded her significant relief when necessary. She was stronger in herself and more able to verbalise her thoughts and feelings.

Each therapy will have its staunch supporters who can provide anecdotal evidence as to its efficacy. In the spirit of co-operation, the main point is to stay open and not judge with the rational mind, through filters of our own projections and preferences. Every therapy has its place in the overall scheme of health care. Matching the patient to the appropriate practitioner requires a basic knowledge of the contents of a wide range of therapies, and a network of reliable and suitably trained therapists to refer them to, or, at the very least, information on how to find a therapist via a professional register or equivalent.

Part Three

The third section of this book contains essays on specific topics of interest. It expands on health-focused care with a description of the Peckham Experiment, preconceptual care (Foresight Programme) and thoughts on integrating death in health care. The essay 'A Future Scenario' reports on a danger potentially inherent in Western medicine. We have included this alarming account to highlight the urgent need for change in health care.

Other esssays explore practical aspects essential for the integration of complementary therapies in health care: 'Principles and Terminology' attempts to define the terms used to create a common ground of understanding; 'Choosing a Practitioner' gives guidelines for questions to pose when entering a therapeutic contract; 'Who Should Practise Complementary Therapies: The Take-Over Debate' discusses the different possibilities for the involvement of medical staff in providing complementary therapies; 'Educating Complementary Therapists' looks at how the education system can adapt to the phenomenon of complementary therapies; 'Research in Holistic Medicine' makes suggestions for research methodology fostering the reflective practitioner; and 'Complementary Medicine and the Law' debates the issue of self-regulation versus statutory regulation.

The Leaf ♣

This symbol in the margin indicates that something mentioned in the text can be expanded on by turning to the chapter listed.

What This Book is Not

This book does not give a list of symptoms or conditions and how they can be treated. The case reports in each chapter merely exemplify each particular treatment approach. Our policy not to include suggestions for treatment supports the paradigm of holistic health care which is patient-centred rather than disease-centred.

Disclaimer

The authors do not present any part of this work, directly or indirectly, for the diagnosis or prescription of any disease or condition. Many of the therapies described are not yet scientifically endorsed. People who use the book, or receive any of the therapies described, take responsibility for consulting the health professional of their choice regarding all matters pertaining to their health. The authors and publisher expressly disclaim information from this responsibility for any adverse effects resulting from your use of the information contained in this book.

Part 1 | The Concept

Modern medical science, with its biochemistry, X-rays, and biopsies, is a marvellous triumph of our technological prowess, yet it is representative of a worldview that has fragmented mind and body, the individual and society, spirit and landscape.

— F David Peat

Reprinted by permission of Fourth Estate Ltd from *Blackfoot Physics* by F David Peat ©1994

Medical Marriage

Medical Marriage is the concept of an integrated health care system where doctors work hand in hand with practitioners of complementary therapies. Through the meeting of two very different paradigms – the so-called reductionist and the holistic – a new way of operating can develop and the best of both worlds may become available to everyone: the doctor, the complementary practitioner and the patient.

Arguments for Change

Patients are already using both orthodox and complementary medicine for their health care: 30% of people have used complementary therapies with a great degree of satisfaction and would use them again in the future.[1] This can lead to fragmentation of care which does not allow for the highest quality of health care. Now the time is right for the professionals to honour the lead that has been taken by those they are endeavouring to serve. Professionals from the complementary and orthodox fields have to engage in a concerted effort to provide patients with the integrated care they want.

Modern medicine has made tremendous progress in the treatment of certain conditions. Its contribution to increased life quality of many individuals is invaluable. However, the general level of health of the population has not increased to a degree that might be expected considering the enormous efforts which sustain modern health care systems.

A Future Scenario

The treatment modalities currently available to doctors, namely allopathic drugs and surgery, have proven to be dangerous through their side effects and of dubious benefit in the long term in many cases. There is a long list of iatrogenic conditions caused by medical interventions.

Complementary therapies, on the other hand, use treatment modalities which are less invasive and appear to be effective much of the time. In order to provide these to the patient, doctors do not have to study them in depth or practise all the complementary therapies themselves. They do, however, need to know enough to be able to make referrals and co-operate as colleagues.

Medical Marriage promotes a model of equal partnership between doctors and complementary practitioners who are skilled and experienced in their own field of specialisation. Respecting each other's unique contribution to health care, communicating openly, thus educating and supporting each other on a personal level, and doing what is best for each patient is the ideal of multidisciplinary co-operation.

For this integration to occur, openness, trust, non-defensiveness and respect on all sides are required. Doctors and complementary practitioners have to recognise and honour the part each plays in ensuring the overall well-being of the patient and the community. It is important for this integration to occur slowly to allow a synthesis of the two approaches to emerge, so that the best in each is preserved to create a viable model of health care for the twenty-first century.

Who Stands to Gain from This Model?

The patients are the most obvious beneficiaries. Their interest in a new form of health care is already evidenced by the enormous increase in popularity of complementary therapies. In a model of multidisciplinary co-operation they do not have to feel torn in their loyalties or be secretive about seeing a complementary practitioner. They can expect their health care professionals to co-operate and communicate to provide the best care for them in all circumstances, enhancing each other's skills and contributions. Education empowers patients to take an active role in their own care which emphasises life quality and self-responsibility.

Doctors benefit from an increased range of therapeutic interventions available for patient care which carry fewer side effects and improve patients' quality of life, as well as engaging patients in their own care. The complementary therapies offer elements of care which are difficult to provide in a busy surgery with seven-minute appointments – namely time, attention, caring touch and consideration of all aspects of the patient's life. This frees the doctor to give more time and attention to those cases which require their specialist help. The stress in doctors' working lives can therefore be dramatically reduced as they are no longer expected to provide the magic cure in all cases.

Complementary practitioners have the opportunity to expand their practice to cater for a broader spectrum of cases, making their work more varied, challenging and relevant to society. Through multidisciplinary co-operation the professions stand to gain acceptance and validation. They have access to more resources, not only financial, but more importantly to academic support and research opportunities which are essential for the further development of their disciplines. Complementary practitioners are included as partners in the patient's care and therefore have the backup of the established medical system (with 24-hour cover, specialists' care and in-patient facilities).

Core Elements for Medical Marriage

The following premises are essential for the concept of integrated health care:

◆ In Medical Marriage the principles of holism are understood, embraced and applied in practice. Patients are treated as whole people, taking into account their physical, emotional and mental health. They are seen as a product of their family, social and cultural context, as well as their natural environment. The whole spectrum of approaches to health care, complementary and orthodox, are offered for the patient to choose from. The relationship aspect of the therapeutic interaction is of high import. Practitioners' dedication to their own health is a crucial aspect of the equation.

◆ Health and wellness are the focus of health care and the treatment of disease is only one small aspect of that. Rather than concentrating on the removal of symptoms the health care professionals support patients in helping themselves to increase their life quality. Education is a major tool to facilitate health enhancement. Life quality is more important than quantity – in the form of longevity; death becomes an integral part of the life process.

◆ Patients are in charge of their own care. People have the right to take responsibility for their lives as much as they want to, and they have the right to receive all the information they need in order to do that. They are the experts in their own lives and being a patient is only a minor and hopefully temporary role.

◆ In disease care the least harmful intervention has to be provided first. Only if that fails to solve the problem are more invasive treatments justified. This means in most cases that complementary modalities should be applied first with the technology of orthodox medicine being a back-up or last resort.

◆ Multidisciplinary co-operation is the strategy which best provides this effectively and safely. This means a team consisting of a medical doctor and complementary practitioners of various disciplines working together within a framework of clear communication and respectful co-operation for the optimal care of the patient.

◆ Education is the core for understanding. In the same way as doctors have an understanding of the many different aspects of contemporary medicine everyone working within the model of Medical Marriage needs to have a basic knowledge of the theory, practice and application of the wide range of complementary therapies.

The Application of Holism in Health Care

The Two Paradigms

The reductionist paradigm, on which contemporary medical thinking has been based, is attributed to Newton and Descartes. Their contribution to civilisation has influenced the philosophy and science of the last three centuries as well as medicine and psychology. The Cartesian/Newtonian system leads to a world view which is analytical and reductionist. It arrives at an understanding of the whole by looking at ever smaller parts. The body is seen as a machine; illness is the breakdown of this machine; the function of health care is to repair or replace parts.

Reductionism is the tendency to look for and focus on the parts of things and to group these parts into categories. Once this happens, things tend to seem to exist independently – a malfunction is seen affecting only a specific organ system or tissue, a drug may be thought of as affecting electrochemical activities of only certain cells, diseases sometimes seem to almost stand alone.[2]

Modern Western science categorises, objectifies and seeks the right answer. 'Right' can be only one truth, which results in 'either/or' thinking. One point of view or solution is better than the other and therefore superior. Once the right way has been decided, action is necessitated (activism). This leads to interventions to align what has been found with what is thought to be right. Just-in-case interventions are sanctioned because of projected future threats (future-time orientation). This science focuses on the presenting condition captured and frozen in a static form. If something cannot be seen, observed or measured with the five senses and the instruments available within the scientific context, it does not exist.

Holism looks at the person as a whole, recognising that individuals are unique and deserve to be allowed all their different expressions. Holism does not find one truth but allows different perspectives, which leads to 'both/and' thinking. One point of view or solution is not better than, but complements, the other. An aim in itself within the holistic paradigm, is simply to 'be' and observe the movement of the process rather than manipulate it (presentism). Reality is never static but ever changing. Present-time orientation is to be in the moment. Even if something cannot be seen or perceived, the possibility is accepted that it exists at a different level of reality, as beliefs determine what we are able to observe, and the limitation may be in our heads, not outside.

Reductionist	Holistic
categorising process	individualising process
objectification	personification
either/or thinking	both/and thinking
hierarchical approach	co-operative approach
opposition	complementarity
activism	presentism
future-time orientation	present-time orientation
focus on state	focus on movement
'seeing is believing'	'believing is seeing'

Table 1: Opposing characteristics of the reductionist and holistic paradigms[3]

Pasteur and Koch, 200 years after Newton, demonstrated that germs cause disease. When penicillin was found, giving doctors a 'weapon' against these disease–causing agents, the biomedical model was complete, creating medicine as a war where experts, with ever more potent interventions, battle valiantly against disease.

This model leads to many 'just-in-case' interventions. The world is perceived as a hostile environment which needs to be fought and conquered. Arguments of having to be on the safe side, of protecting innocent victims, lead to interventions which are potentially harmful when there is not even a problem present. This is compounded by the increasing tendencies towards defensive medical practice.

Defensive medical practice can be defined as:

> *...ordering treatments, tests and procedures for the purpose of protecting the doctor from criticism rather than diagnosing or treating the patient.*[4]

Defensive medicine has some positive aspects, such as taking more detailed notes in the patient's records, giving more detailed information to the patient or taking more time to establish a stronger rapport with the patient, but this mainly stems from concern that the patient may sue if anything goes wrong.[5] With fear at its back, this type of medical help also involves increased referral rates, follow-up and diagnostic testing, which puts the patient at risk of over-intervention, that is receiving unnecessary tests and treatments with all the potential risks and side effects, and does not do much to improve authentic rapport with the doctor.

The Current Change in Emphasis

The dominance of this archetype, however, has never been total. There have always been those within Western medicine who spoke of the art in caring for the sick, the consideration for the individual, and the relevance of the soul in illness and health. Very often this point of view was heard in the caring professions, especially in nursing. This is the voice which has found reinforcement in the last two decades outwith the recognised medical system through complementary therapies becoming known and established.

Now the two paradigms are increasingly being looked at side by side, and the benefits of both are being evaluated. The choice does not have to be 'either/or' but can be 'both/and', with health professionals learning to assess when it is appropriate to deduce knowledge of the whole by looking at the parts, and categorising, and when it serves better to observe the whole process and accept the individualised approach.

For this to occur, everyone needs to have sufficient information to make clear decisions. Health professionals from both sides need to know and understand the options. In practice, this involves doctors and other medically trained professionals becoming aware of the complementary therapies and what they have to offer. It also involves complementary therapists, who already know (because they have been brought up in the Western medical system) what medicine offers, appreciating the benefits of medical interventions in appropriate situations.

Suspicion and hostility arise generally from lack of understanding and holding entrenched positions. Dualism and polarity reactions are a result of reductionist thinking from which everyone suffers, whether choosing to work in the world of holism or remaining within orthodox structures. In upholding the ideal of Medical Marriage, understanding and acceptance are the keys to co-operation. Understanding is born of education and information coupled with willingness and openness. For this reason it is worthwhile spelling out the principles of the new paradigm in detail.

The Principles of Holism

Holistic care involves:

> *Responding to the person as a whole (body, mind and spirit) within the context of their environment (family, culture and ecology);*

> *A willingness to use a wide range of interventions, from drugs and surgery to meditation and diet;*

> *An emphasis on a more participatory relationship between doctor and patient;*

> *An awareness of the impact of the 'health' of the practitioner on the patient (physician, heal thyself).*[6]

Holism addresses all aspects of the human being: body, mind, psyche and spirit

A human being cannot be defined by only one level of existence; each one needs to be taken into account as all affect and are affected by one another. The interconnection of these levels is recognised, and holistic practitioners strive to address all these aspects when relating to a patient. The knowledge that one level is influenced through others opens possibilities for many different approaches to care. For example, a physical complaint can be addressed on the physical level, but this is not the only avenue available. A practitioner may choose not to act at all on the physical but to work with the emotional or mental level instead. This has been widely recognised in recent years, with counselling being observed as an effective form of treatment in stress related conditions.

Often a combination of approaches on different levels increases the effect of intervention dramatically; giving some immediate relief and improving the general life quality for the patient, as well as helping with the presenting problem. For example, a patient with asthma and eczema may need to be prescribed an inhaler and cortisone cream for emergency use and for peace of mind, but this will not address the underlying issues of their symptoms. Diet may help in the longer term and at times even provide a full cure. Stress management skills may reduce some causative factors, and will be of more significance if the patient also receives some counselling or therapy which addresses childhood emotional distortions and traumas. Inherited factors are also often a contributory influence in these symptoms and these can be counteracted with homoeopathic remedies.

Holism implies the willingness to use a wide range of care modalities

As in the previous example, holistic health care takes advantage of the full spectrum of orthodox and complementary medicine. This allows practitioner and patient together to make the best choice for the individual situation.

Many GPs have felt increasingly reluctant to prescribe drugs to all patients, especially those for whom they know drug therapy will have little or no beneficial effect on the patient's life quality in the long run. However, the alternative, in most cases, is simply to send the patient home with no help, which is also unacceptable. Within a holistic model, especially that of multidisciplinary co-operation, a GP can make use of the complementary therapies, which have fewer (if any) side effects, which care for the patient with positive input and attention and in offering 'listening' services, and which are therefore particularly suited to dealing with patients who suffer from chronic or stress related diseases and conditions. In this scenario, orthodox treatments (drugs or surgery) become the backup, or last resort treatment, if the complementary health care is unable to relieve the symptoms.

Relationship-centred care is essential to holism

The partnership between practitioner and patient is crucial to the healing process and cannot be separated from the treatment given.

> *Practitioners' relationships with their patients, their patients' communities, and other health care practitioners are central to health care and are the vehicle for putting into action a paradigm of health that integrates caring, healing and community.*[7]

The practitioner/patient relationship is pivotal for the well-being of the patient, as well as for that of the practitioner. For the patients, positive rapport ensures compliance to the agreed treatment regimen, a sense of empowerment and active involvement in their care and the trust that they can go to the practitioner whenever they feel the need. This trust engenders openness and sharing of intimate details, which will help patients to gain insight into the complex connections regarding their health as the practitioner assesses the relevant implications for care.

In the 1960s Michael Balint, a psychiatrist in London, asked questions regarding the one 'drug' applied most and studied the least: the doctor.[8] He studied the actions and interactions of this 'drug' and its side effects, positive and negative. He requested that doctors become more conscious of the effect they have on patients and more skilled in putting this to best use. Following his work, Balint-groups sprang up which were attended by doctors and psychotherapists who used the peer group to review cases and reflect upon their own contribution to the case.

Recent studies show that the patient relationship is one of the main sources of stress in doctors' lives.[9] Within the holistic model, attending to this relationship with skill and care can turn the source of stress into a source of nourishment and inspiration. Further exploration of how the practitioner can help to create such positive rapport is essential. Education plays a major role here. Supervision, especially peer supervision, is another important tool which practitioners can use to reflect on their own part in the relationship and to expand their skills in communication and rapport building.

The relationship with the patient's community includes the patient's close family and friends, as well as the larger community. This ideal scenario makes health care an integral part of everybody's daily life. All aspects of health care, health enhancement, health education and promotion, as well as health and safety are relevant, and disease care is available and accessible when needed. The relationship with the community has been formulated as one of the core values for the medical profession for the twenty-first century.[10] This value applies to all health care professionals whether they work in the field of mainstream medicine or in the complementary field.

A mutually respectful relationship with other health care professionals is a crucial element in providing patients with a co-ordinated service and cohesive health care.

Holistic means that the practitioners' own health and healing processes are relevant to their work

'Healer heal thyself' reflects the need for an openness to change and development in practitioners. As they grow and evolve with their work, their own healing can continue to unfold. This asks a high level of personal integrity. Health care professionals need to be willing to practise themselves what they ask from their patients: self-responsibility and self-care.

Health and Wellness as the Focus of Health Care

It would seem obvious, when looking at a model for a health care system, to consider health. However, medical training until now has tended to focus on pathologies and its treatments rather than on health.

The World Health Organisation has defined health as:

> *Not the mere absence of symptoms or infirmities but a state of physical, psychological, spiritual and social well-being.*

In the public health sector, much thought and action is influenced by this definition but in the practice of medicine it seems to remain a theoretical concept. The daily work of doctors is dominated by finding a diagnosis for the presenting symptoms and taking measures to treat the condition. While the aim is essentially to reduce suffering, and is therefore commendable, it is the experience of many doctors that the system is not as effective as it should be. Often patients' symptoms may clear up, but are replaced by other symptoms, sooner or later. Then the doctor is challenged to go on handing out more drugs, often quite a cocktail, not knowing what else to do. In cases of long-term chronic illness this approach can become particularly disheartening. All doctors know 'heart sink' patients whom they dread to see – yet again – as they feel unable to offer any significant help and this is stressful and demoralising.

Medical practice can become much lighter and more inspiring if the focus turns to health, wellness and life quality. Stress management, lifestyle changes, improved social interactions, insight into behavioural or emotional patterns which aggravate or maintain the illness and, above all, increased self-care can all make a tremendous difference to patients' lives. With these tools used as an integrated approach to health care, all patients can be supported, no matter how severely ill or chronically debilitated they are, to improve their life quality. Doctors can then feel their contribution as valid and real, while patients feel empowered and in charge of their health care.

To implement such an integration, the shift has to take place from a disease-centred approach to a health-focused approach to health care. In addition to studying pathology, medical students need to study that which constitutes health, so they can measure people's present situation and assess their progress as time goes by. Health is less easy to define than illness, but it is more than absence of symptoms.

Working Definitions of Health

Many attempts have been made to define a yardstick of optimum health. The challenge is that health cannot be defined by objective standards but rather through subjective experiences and processes. This is reflected in the following definitions.

*Bioenergetic Analysis
Naturopathy*

> *We are coming to understand health not as the absence of disease, but rather the process by which individuals maintain their sense of coherence (i.e., sense that life is comprehensible, manageable, and meaningful) and ability to function in the face of changes in themselves and their relationship with their environment.*[11]

In the first half of the twentieth century there was an inspiring research project into factors which foster health, called the Peckham Experiment. It resulted in some guidelines which can be summed up as:

Building Health

> *Health is the ability to respond to all life situations in a way that increases capability, responsibility, autonomy, spontaneity and joy.*

These definitions acknowledge that changes and challenges in life have an essential role in human development as they potentially increase skills and expertise, as well as broadening a person's world view. Capability expands, for instance, when constructive coping mechanisms or self-care skills are learned. Autonomy results from increased self-awareness and self-esteem finding the strength within to utilise available resources. With a widened awareness of health and the interconnectedness of their well-being with that of others and their surroundings, people assume more responsibility for their own lives and take on a more responsible role in striving for the integrity of society and the natural environment. Spontaneity comes with the freedom and empowerment of people taking full responsibility and trusting their own capabilities. All this leads to the appreciation of the role they can play in the world. Joy comes from many things, small and big, especially when people are in touch with their own strength and the beauty and perfection all around them.

The value of these definitions of health is that they give specific qualities which can be observed by the health care practitioner as well as by the patient. They make it possible to assess the degree of health present and to decide which strategy can move the patient towards greater health. The question can be asked: will this particular step/treatment/intervention increase the sense of coherence and ability to function of the patient? Will it expand the person's capability, spontaneity and joy?

These definitions can also be applied in situations of chronic illness. Someone can be intensely physically ill, with cancer for example, yet if their spirit is soaring and

Integrating Death into Healthcare

they are taking steps to assist humanity's progress, then they are dealing with life in a most healthy and creative way. It can even apply to the last stage of life – death – for at a certain point in each person's life, the healthiest option is to die.

An important aspect which must not be overlooked is that health is a process, a dynamic rather than an absolute state.

Psychosynthesis

> *Health is not a static condition achieved once and for all, but a dynamic on-going process of change. It is interwoven with all the elements of well-being, and depends on the integration of physical, emotional and spiritual levels of consciousness.*[12]

If health becomes a standardised norm, it is never achievable and leads to a tyranny of health much like the tyranny of youth – an ideal which is always out of reach. As people are all different from one another, applying any norm is disrespectful of their individual expression. This has been seen in the tyranny of the 'perfect body', which has led directly to society's collusion with conditions such as anorexia or bulimia. This can be illustrated in the case of a young woman who had been a stocky teenager. She lost a lot of weight in her twenties which led to severe health problems, including gastro-intestinal ulcers, amenorrhoea and immune deficiencies. For two years she presented symptoms bordering on anorexia. She eventually recovered her health with the help of various complementary therapists who enabled her to recognise the pathological patterns she had been exhibiting. Now in her thirties, she condemns the social sanctioning and the praise – even from her family and close friends – which she received for being fashionably thin, when in fact she was destroying her health and well-being.

Health therefore has to be tailored to the individual. Life quality is more relevant than absence of symptoms or longevity. The quality of each interaction, including that of the caring relationship, is where health is being expressed and experienced moment by moment.

The 'Health Doctor'

In implementing a positive definition of health, health care professionals are able to shift their attention from disease care to health-focused care. The expansion of health becomes the objective – the reduction or cure of symptoms are almost incidental.

In this scenario, they have the opportunity to become 'health doctors' which requires different skills and brings with it its own rewards. Health doctors will provide services to benefit people in all different situations in life. They can give:

- nutritional advice;
- help create strategies for active living which provide exercise in the daily routines;
- offer stress management skills;
- advice on child rearing;
- guidance on relationship challenges and so on.

The recommendations they make to their patients on positive living may include:

- taking up a hobby which provides physical activity and social interaction;
- attending a yoga class;
- learning a new style of cooking;
- expanding the range of healthy options when shopping for food;
- entering an evening class for intellectual stimulation or expanding career options;
- having regular bodywork sessions to deal with stress-related physical tensions;
- exploring new ways of expressing creativity;
- engaging in counselling to release old patterns of limiting interaction and improve communication skills with partners or children.

The Health Overhaul

Health doctors will recommend that their patients have a regular annual 'health overhaul' to review the present state of health on all different levels, to confirm what works well and to introduce new goals of health enhancement. A possible format for the health overhaul is for the patient to fill in an extensive questionnaire covering all medical information, family history, social background, lifestyle, and the functioning of their different physical organs or systems. Before any future overhaul they will reflect on any changes which have occurred, and use a shorter questionnaire to assess their present situation. In the consultation, apart from the physical examination and some laboratory tests, the doctor and patient will reflect together on the following areas: diet; exercise; emotional, social, spiritual and work life; and creativity, as well as family and intimate relationships. Future goals are discussed and concrete steps towards achieving them agreed.

Health overhauls are particularly relevant at specific crossroads in life:

Preconceptual Care

- preconception
- antenatal
- early childhood
- weaning
- entering school
- puberty
- family planning
- menopause/middle age
- retirement and old age

These particular stages are opportunities to evolve and monitor strategies for health enhancement in an individual's life.

The relationship between the health doctor and the patient takes the best from the old-fashioned family doctor who knew everyone in the extended family and could provide care from birth to death bed. Family doctors were companions on their patients' life paths, advisers to be at hand when their expertise was required. However, the new health doctors will not be 'experts' who disempower patients but partners interested in empowering patients to take increasing responsibility for their lives.

Moves in the Right Direction

While fully embracing a holistic attitude towards disease may be some way distant for much of the medical profession, steps have been made for some time towards expanding medicine beyond disease care. Vaccination programmes, which are promoted by the NHS, are an example of an attempt at disease prevention rather than cure. Screening programmes for cancer are not preventative as such, but may enable disease to be detected and treated earlier, which potentially increases the chances for a better outcome. Health promotion educates the public and has been shown to contribute to increased general awareness.[13] Health protection includes legal measures, regulations, health policies and voluntary codes of practice used in the workplace to stop people from being harmed.

But while health care today may be increasing its focus on these preventative and educational measures, the concept of health enhancement is still missing. One of the motivating factors which may lead the NHS towards adopting the major shift in emphasis that is needed, is desperation to find a way of reducing the ever spiralling cost of health care.

Health Enhancement

Health enhancement is the care that is relevant in everyone's daily life. No matter what people's current state of health, there is always some measure that can be taken that will increase their quality of life. This applies as much to the chronically ill as to those who are blessed with physical fitness and a strong constitution. Health enhancement requires education which goes much further than that which is currently on offer. It provides the individual with information and basic skills such as nutritional awareness, dealing with emotions, social and communication skills and stress management. The health doctor's primary role is the fostering of empowerment and motivation for self-care.

Currently health education has achieved general public awareness of health hazards, such as smoking and alcohol and the links between diet, exercise and common disease. However, studies have shown that this knowledge is not matched by action.[14]

Choosing health is still not a high priority in our society – neither for individuals nor for the collective.

What will allow healthy choices to become easy choices? An individual needs motivation, positive reinforcement and inspiring examples. The Peckham Experiment demonstrated some of the resources which facilitate the nurturing of health:

Building Health

> *The health doctor, just like the sickness doctor, needs tools, but they are of a very different kind – the gymnasium, the swimming pool, the cafeteria and so on. It is natural that the instruments for health should be varied because health covers a very wide field and includes physical, mental, social and even economic life.*[15]

The participants in the Peckham Experiment found company in their striving for health and well-being. Social norms were formed which sanctioned and reinforced positive healthy choices.

Strategies for Implementing Positive Health Care

Too often health gets taken for granted until it fails. Illness calls attention to the precious nature of health and spurs the commitment to foster and nurture it. It is in this situation that a practitioner focusing on health enhancement can make a great difference. With a 'captive audience' the disease care necessary is provided for relief or cure and then the issue of health restoration and maintenance can be addressed. Patients are often grateful to hear what they can do to ensure that illness does not recur. This is an opportunity to instigate changes in attitude and behaviour in a sustainable way. The health care professional then becomes the companion and resource of information and support for health enhancement. This way practitioner and patient become partners in positive health care.

The following points are important in applying this ideal:

◆ focusing on the areas of strength;
◆ determining small manageable next steps;
◆ monitoring progress and offering ongoing encouragement.

Focusing on the areas of good health and affirming patients in what they are already doing well is a cornerstone of the partnership. It is important to find out where their strengths lie, whether it is a good exercise routine, a sensible diet, positive relationships or a strong spiritual connection. This may require detective work on the part of the doctor, as many people take for granted their strengths and only mention their difficulties. However, affirming a person's strengths and encouraging them to take pride in what they are doing well is a strong foundation for further progress.

From these points of strength, options can be explored to find small, manageable steps leading to improved health, which can be sustained on a long-term basis. This may be a change in diet from using refined carbohydrates to using whole foods. If, for example, a person who uses a lot of refined produce starts to use brown rice instead of white, their health gain may be considerable as long as they manage to sustain that change and expand on it. Similarly someone who decides to cycle to work instead of driving may experience increased sensations of well-being over a period of time. Aspirations for dramatic changes are not encouraged, as experience shows that high ideals may not be achieved and the benefit of good intention is lost. Potential damage may be done as people become less confident in their ability to change or even become cynical about healthy choices.

Monitoring the progress is crucial, as individuals need a point of review and continuing support. Without this the intentions may well be smothered by daily routines and the all too common resistance to change. These points of review are also an opportunity to continue education and broaden the options for healthy choices. This ongoing relationship with the 'health doctor' ensures that the changes can be sustained and expanded upon. For the patient this becomes a success story of ever increasing self-empowerment, confidence and improved life quality. For the health care practitioner it is the guarantee of high job satisfaction.

The Economics of Health Enhancement

Remuneration for service makes health care professionals reliant on ill health for income. A built-in conflict of interest may prevent them from working to make themselves redundant.

In the old Chinese system, doctors were only paid by those individuals in their community who they had enabled to remain healthy. This ensured that they were mainly preoccupied with health care rather than disease care. The National Health Service in Britain in its purest essence is not that different, as the tax payers contribute only as long as they are fit enough to work. However, contributions to National Insurance are so far removed from the contributor, as well as from the health care provider, that the immediacy and therefore the power of the Chinese tradition is lost. The greatest power lies in the relationship between the individual who makes the payment and the attending health care professional. For people to invest in their own health – by paying for it – is often a crucial part of taking responsibility for their own care. This is the argument for private health care, as it empowers patients and puts them in charge of the contract with the health care professional. Private health care may be a solution in an affluent society, as a health enhancement contract, but for disease care in a society where there are people who would not be able to afford appropriate care, it is a source of social injustice and deprivation. For this reason it cannot be advocated even though the education and self-empowerment value of it is considerable.

A system needs to be developed which will provide the best of both worlds:

◆ the necessary care provision free at the point of delivery;

◆ the immediacy and empowerment of a private contribution or subscription scheme.

In an intentional community with a population of 500, an experimental private subscription scheme was implemented and surveyed after three years. Even though it was a middle class, affluent community with a theoretical knowledge of health issues, less than 20% of the population joined the scheme and the main usage of the services provided was when health failed.[16] This demonstrates what an enormous effort it will take to shift general consciousness from disease care to health care. This is a task truly deserving of considerable and concerted effort for the next century.

Self-Responsibility of the Patient

People have the right to take responsibility for their lives as much as they want to, and they have the right to receive all the information they need in order to do that. They are the experts in their own lives and being a patient is only a minor and hopefully temporary role.

The word 'patient' implies patience and passivity. However, since other terms such as client, customer, consumer and user also have drawbacks and seem unsuitable, the word 'patient' has been retained throughout much of this text, with an awareness of its limitations and without supporting its passive connotations. It is important for health care professionals always to stay conscious of the fact that a person is much more than a patient. People have complex lives beyond the limited role of receiving health care, where they are required on a daily basis to make decisions affecting their life and well-being. Since they manage to fulfil these demands in all other areas of their lives, they can be considered competent to do the same in relation to their health.

Self-responsible patients are fully informed about their health and their options for health enhancement and disease care, when needed. They feel empowered to ask all the questions they need before making a decision. They use the experts as a source of information and support. They will not tolerate a therapeutic relationship where they feel patronised or ignored but will seek out the health care professionals who are willing to co-operate with them as partners. They do not try to replace the experts but they utilise their expertise to enhance their own discretion. A parallel would be to listen to the opinion of a car dealer but to make the final choice oneself of which car to buy.

To achieve this vision of the self-responsible patient, both patients and health care professionals have to evolve beyond their current roles. The implications of this evolution affect all areas of our society – right back to the school curricula which would be required to provide the relevant knowledge and empowerment to pupils.

The Present Situation

As a consequence of the reductionist model, old-style doctors have all the power and the responsibility, while patients suffer from disempowerment and feel like helpless victims. The science of medicine has become an enormous maze of technical terms, which is a language unto itself and completely removed from the patient. The doctor has become the omnipotent life saviour who needs to be blindly trusted. This may attribute to them prestige and power but also responsibilities which are, at times, inhumanely demanding and stressful.[17] In turn, the system has created passive patients who require health experts to rescue them when they get sick. This disenfranchisement has a profound effect on patients' ability to take responsibility for their own health. If they are seen as playing no part in the creation of their disease processes, then they cannot contribute significantly to their own health or healing processes. They become victims of intangible or unknown outer causes, living in a hostile universe which is out to get them.

Patients are, however, becoming increasingly less patient. Many want more information and often more involvement in their health care. This new development has found its expression in the various patient's charters which have been drawn up in the UK in the last few years.[18] These emphasise the right of information, choice and care with respect for the whole person. It is important that these charters have been written. More important still is that the values represented will affect the daily care provided and that patients will find support and empowerment for being active partners in their own health care, for making informed choices about interventions and taking active steps to improve their health with self-care.

In a state of illness or weakness, people are often not in touch with personal power and confidence. It depends very much on the attitude of the attending health care professional how fast they regain their sense of autonomy and self-responsibility, or whether their sense of helplessness is reinforced. Health care professionals who are interested in partnership with patients will provide as much information and choice as possible. They will support patients to make up their own minds, giving them time and space, and possibly the opportunity to talk it over with somebody else.

In the early stages of patients' self-responsibility they may need a considerable amount of support from the experts, but the long-term goal is for them to achieve autonomy. This is a process during which the individual patient determines the pace. Reclaiming self-responsibility is an essential aspect of the healing process.

Challenges to Self-Responsibility

The ideal of integrated health care asks a lot from patients: the willingness to become active partners in their health care and to make healthy choices in their lives, which does not always come easily, but in the longer term produces a win/win situation for both patient and health care professional.

The following scenario exemplifies the implications of the self-responsible patient:

> Every person holds their own 'health book'. It contains all the information regarding their medical history, treatments received, health assessments and experts reports. During any contact with a health professional, notes will be entered in the book, as well as examination results. At any time the person may add comments and observations, which may include disagreement with the experts' picture. Their health records are their personal property and responsibility.

This is a long way off from the present situation – until recently the folder containing patient notes had printed on it the words 'Not to be Read by the Patient'. Many patients are not ready to take this step towards self-responsibility as Cornelia discovered in her practice when she tried to introduce the health book. She found that patients would forget to bring it to the consultation. She had conceived the idea during a visit to Papua New Guinea where she observed villagers bringing their own health records to the monthly clinics, a system which seemed to work well. It is interesting to note that it worked in Papua New Guinea, where there has been no health system before, whereas in Britain patients have been so disempowered by the existing system that they find it hard to take up the reins even when offered them. It is not that British people are incapable of keeping records – all car owners produce MOT and insurance certificates each year when they apply for their car tax – it is simply that we are not programmed to take the same responsibility for our health.

Society shapes medicine, as well as medicine influencing the values and paradigms of society. People do not necessarily want to implement the changes required to improve their health and well-being. It is not only 'the system' which feeds drugs to the patients but in many cases the patients themselves who want the 'quick fix' – the antibiotics, painkillers, or antidepressants to remove symptoms.

The Concept of Victim Consciousness

Victimisation is one of the most powerful pathogens in our society and is highly contagious. It creates disease on a physical as much as on an emotional level. People are victim to many things: their social class, their parents, their biology, their economic reality, their life experiences. Illness happens to them – they are struck down by it. In the position of victim they do not have the power and resources to contribute to the solution, to help themselves or to improve their life quality. They have to suffer ill fate, give themselves over to the hands of experts to get fixed and if the experts cannot help, they are hopeless and doomed to a limited and unhappy life.

On the larger scale victim consciousness creates 'disease' in a society in the form of dependencies and expectations that one will be provided for, which further suppresses individual initiative and creativity. Globally it causes the utter deprivation of whole countries dependent on foreign aid, which never can give back what they lost in the first place: sovereignty, pride and an intact social and natural environment.

'Creating Your Own Reality'

Within the holistic view of self-responsibility has evolved the concept that 'we create our own reality' – a maxim which provides a clear antidote to victim consciousness. It can be a source of great empowerment and liberation for individuals to view themselves as directors as well as actors in life's play. Acknowledging the director's role is often a great step towards healing and happiness.

There is, however, the possibility that distortions of this concept are applied to illness. Such distortions stem from an oversimplification and can lead to an unkind and uncompassionate attitude towards illness, in the sense of 'you have caused this yourself', 'it is your fault', or 'what have you done wrong to manifest this?' 'You have created this' in its simplified form is cruel and separating. Tempered with understanding and compassion it becomes an enlightening alternative to the reductionist paradigm.

Only when illness is considered as a result of a person's history and life circumstances and an expression of a soul's journey through human incarnation, can any judgement on disease be withheld and people be supported in a loving and compassionate way, as well as encouraged to do what they can to empower themselves, make changes in their lives and adopt habits of increasing self-care. The concept of the self-responsible person is a very important step to self-empowerment and is essential in many people's healing process.

A Personal Experience

This incident illustrates the negative potential of the old paradigm and highlights possible new ways forward with co-operation and respect on all sides.

Cornelia was 36 weeks pregnant when she went for a routine check-up with the hospital consultant. She and her husband were planning a home birth. In the previous consultation at 15 weeks, the consultant made it clear he was unhappy about Cornelia being exposed to the risks of birth in circumstances where he could not provide the help he has at his fingertips in the hospital. However, he was willing to let them have their way 'provided that everything was okay'.

The trip to the second appointment was stressful. Having left a bit late, they got stuck in traffic and Cornelia's husband was late to deliver an important document to the solicitors before they got to the hospital. It is little wonder that on examination the obstetrician found that Cornelia's blood pressure had increased since the previous check. It was now 140/95. He said that she should stay in for observation, as 'the only important thing is that you have the baby, isn't it?' Cornelia found herself bobbing her head up and down, agreeing with him. She omitted to tell him that the measured BP was what she had quite frequently before the pregnancy, or that they had been stressed prior to the appointment. Even the husband and the birth attendant, who was with them, were struck by the authority of the consultant's words and agreed to his plan.

In the event, the consultant changed his mind and agreed that they could go back home, have the community midwife measure the blood pressure again and only if it was the same in three days should Cornelia be admitted. Once they were home and thinking straight again, they were amazed that they had agreed to his proposal at all. They set about recovering their original vision, shaking off the fear and disempowerment with which they had been infected by both the doctor and the system.

In retrospect they realised how much they had been hypnotised by the certitude of the consultant. In his presence, Cornelia had not only lost her wits but also had delegated to the expert the power to decide what had to happen. It was a sobering experience for her, that even with all her background knowledge as a medical doctor and with the reinforcement of husband and birth attendant, she couldn't resist the mesmerisation of the fear concept and the 'just-in-case' provision.

The community midwife attending to their pregnancy helped them to reclaim their power by holding the perspective that birth was a physiological process of which any healthy woman is capable, without the need for holding onto the worst case scenario. Cornelia's blood pressure complied, and they proceeded with their original birth plan, holding, of course, an awareness of the risks involved, but without being dominated by it. The birth went smoothly and was attended by the midwife. The GP, who was also present, took a back-seat role, in fact she ended up taking photographs of the birth, which they had been keen to document.

New Strategies for Disease Care

First Do No Harm

In disease care the least harmful intervention has to be provided first. Only if that fails to solve the problem are more invasive treatments justified. This means, in many cases, that complementary modalities should be applied first with the technology of orthodox medicine being used as a back-up when needed.

There will always be conditions which need to be treated with orthodox interventions in the first instance, e.g. insulin dependent diabetes, severe asthma, epilepsy and severe infections to name a few. As efficacy must be the other deciding factor in choice of treatment, there are cases where orthodox intervention has to be given preference. For example, while complementary medical intervention for Hodgkin's disease may be far less harmful than chemotherapy, the cure rate of chemotherapy is high if provided early, thereby justifying its use.

The shift in health care towards an integration of complementary therapies with modern medicine will take place over a period of time. It has to be based on sound scientific evidence to be acceptable and applied in a broad medical context.

The paramount objective of health care is the provision of the best treatment for the patient in any given situation. Knowledge of and an open mind towards the whole spectrum of interventions including complementary approaches are essential for optimal patient care.

Arguments for Complementary Therapies as Treatment of Preference

Side Effects

The vast majority of complaints brought to a GP are minor ailments and chronic diseases. In both cases the armamentarium of contemporary Western medicine may not be very suitable. Many interventions produce side effects and do not address the underlying cause of the presenting problem, therefore not offering long-term solutions. These conditions, however, fall in the domain of complementary therapies which empirically have helped many people and for which demand is increasing dramatically. Complementary therapies have fewer (if any) side effects and should therefore be offered to the patient as the first option for treatment if suitable. Modern medicine then becomes the back-up option, to be used if less interventionist approaches fail to address the problem.

At the moment this is reversed, with complementary therapies being used often as a last resort after everything else has failed. It is the growing vision of many patients, as well as health care practitioners, to turn this situation around.

Patient Empowerment

Patients who are helped by complementary medicine experience an enhanced sense of self-empowerment, receive education and learn skills which they can use in future to improve their general health as well as deal with the presenting problem.

Economics

Apart from serving the patient, this strategy also has the advantage of reducing the use of orthodox medicine, with benefits all around. The increase in the cost of health care currently puts an ever greater burden on society and is confronting those in authority with uncomfortable questions as to what to spend the money on.

For example, what should £50,000 be spent on?

> 2000 people can be counselled to help them stop smoking;
> 200 babies can be vaccinated, who currently miss out;
> 60 people can be removed from the waiting list for hernia operations;
> 40 people who are dying can be nursed at home;
> 15 hip replacements can be performed;
> 3 elderly people can be cared for in a nursing home for one year; or
> 2 liver transplants can be given to patients who otherwise would die.[19]

Somebody somewhere has to make impossible choices which will cost lives.

The integration of complementary therapies in health care could potentially form the basis for a financially sustainable future. There is presently a debate as to whether using complementary therapies, particularly in primary care, may be more cost-effective. However, evidence to support this argument has yet to be forthcoming. Besides comparing the cost-effectiveness of both orthodox and complementary forms of treatment, the necessary long-term prospective studies will have to take into consideration the educational impact of complementary therapies, such as health-conscious lifestyle, self-care and personal responsibility, which may well reduce demand on expert services.

Pressures on Medical Staff

The staff providing medical care benefit from the strategy of using complementary therapies as the first line of treatment, for two primary reasons. Offering medication with potentially dangerous side effects is a great responsibility, leading to personal stress which contributes to the high rate of suicides, addictions and depression amongst doctors.[20] Having available a variety of less invasive treatments lightens their burden. The second benefit is that they are under less demand and therefore can give more quality time and attention to those patients who actually need their expertise. They can spend more time attending to severe acute situations, emergencies, crises and conditions where medical or surgical interventions are required.

The Role of Disease

Another reason for complementary therapies to be employed as a new strategy for disease care is that, being based on holistic principles, they virtually all embrace the concept that, within the process of health, disease has an important role to play in the evolution of the individual and, indeed, of humanity as a whole.

Physical symptoms indicate dis-ease within the human organism. It is not just the body; the person may be emotionally imbalanced, mentally confused, socially isolated or spiritually disconnected and undernourished. The physical symptom is a messenger for any of these underlying causative factors.

The way a person responds to life's challenges determines their health. If people are assisted or educated to be able to integrate challenges in a way that increases their capabilities, responsibility, autonomy, spontaneity and joy, they are more likely to grow into self-confident, flexible and loving individuals with ever increasing emotional, mental and social skills as well as a strong spiritual connection.

If, however, people lack assistance and education, they may develop sub-optimal coping mechanisms in relation to challenges, reacting with depression, rigidity of mind, addictions, and/or withdrawing either socially or from their source of spiritual nourishment. This can lead to somatisation, that is physical symptoms.

Considering the illness process in this way, it is obvious how 'our biography becomes our biology'.[21] People start to identify with their traumas or illnesses rather than seeing themselves as a person with a large array of qualities and levels of being, who happens to have an illness or to have experienced a trauma in the past. If individuals reduce themselves to a small segment of their being in this way, they debilitate and disempower themselves further, which can contribute to and exacerbate the disease process, leading to a career of ill-health and unhappiness.

The widely held holistic principle that everything happens for a purpose and is an opportunity for growth and expansion of consciousness can restore individuals to a position of power in their own lives. The challenge of disease can then become a turning point in their development and can facilitate health.

Naturopathy

In some circumstances disease is actually a positive process of evolution. Childhood illnesses are postulated to provide the immune system with challenges which trigger its maturation and ability to contend with the demands of a stimulating environment.[22] To illustrate this, the following case from Cornelia's practice is of a small child who made a leap in his emotional development through a measles infection.

John was two and a half years old when he contracted measles. He was a socially outgoing, alert little boy with a quick mind. His parents had consciously decided not to vaccinate him against measles or any other childhood illness and were therefore prepared to nurse him through this challenge. As he was their first child, they understandably had anxieties and insecurities. I was in the fortunate position to visit them almost every day throughout the illness and give them support and reassurance. For most of a week they had sleepless nights with a crying and fretful toddler who was very withdrawn, yet demanding at the same time. When his temperature was too high they lowered it with compresses and by sponging him down, encouraged his intake of fluids and gave him what little food he wanted. The atmosphere in the house was subdued. The curtains were drawn, the parents were tired and exhausted yet willing to persevere.

Then on the fifth morning I came into their home and everything had changed. The curtains were open, the mother received me with a big smile and the father reported that the fever had broken in the early hours of the morning and they had all slept well after that. When they woke up, John had clear eyes and a smile, went over to his father and said 'I love you, Daddy' – a concept which up to then had not been part of his awareness. The parents enthusiastically agreed 'that this made it all worth it'. John is now almost six years old. He has had most childhood illnesses in an easy and uncomplicated way. He is very healthy and the parents can trust his strong constitution even in times of greater challenge such as prolonged periods of travelling to the other side of the world.

'Love your disease – it's keeping you healthy.'[23] This aphorism encapsulates the concept that disease plays further positive roles such as those of balancing and harmonising a person's system on all levels and also of education and personal growth. Examples from the authors' own lives illustrate this:

Cornelia has suffered for many years from regular migraines which have served as her teacher, leading her into the exploration of many different therapies in an attempt to free herself from them. This has been a journey of health enhancement and self-empowerment. It has taught her about the nature of pain which has made her more understanding and empathetic with her patients. While the pains and the underlying reasons have shifted as she learned the lessons and integrated the messages into her life, the migraines still persist and she now sees their role as creating the balancing factor in her busy life as they force her to retreat into quiet and relaxation every so often. In time she hopes that she will learn to balance her energy in a way that does not require this painful symptom to recur.

Seen in this way it is possible to say that symptoms are a sign of health, of the ability of the organism to balance itself, an expression of the innate integrity and wisdom of the physical body.

One of Lori's symptoms has been interpersonal rather than physical. She found herself sharing a house with a woman friend who seemed to be her polar opposite. This led them to intense conflict and Lori found herself taking up ever more extreme positions in the polarity to a degree that denied a large part of her own personal expression and creativity. In the polarity she was the hard, fiery, ambitious, active one while her friend was the soft, Earthmother type, who found fulfilment in the routine tasks of a housewife. Over time they both recognised the classic archetypes of feminine and masculine, or yin/yang, roles with which they were identifying and saw how each was balancing out the other's need – however painful their partnership. To internalise this balance, they consciously embraced the opposite mode of being within themselves. Lori rediscovered her love of knitting and householding while her friend moved to a town and got a job. This allowed them to disentangle from their relationship distortions and be more whole in themselves.

Health care professionals faced with patients in situations like this would find their role to be one of education, assistance, and facilitation – enabling patients to undergo their process of growth with minimum pain and anguish. The professionals have to read the message being delivered by the symptom or the behaviour and help individual patients to understand for themselves and integrate, in their own time and in their own way, the aspects which the dis-ease is carrying for them. The symptom or dis-ease is not the enemy to be vanquished but a process to be worked through as individuals unfold their potential.

There is also the spiritual perspective which considers the person's life as a soul's journey through incarnation. From this point of view disease cannot be judged as good or bad but only be observed as an expression of evolution. One very moving and impressive example is the transformational nature of the life-threatening disease of AIDS.[24] Many sufferers have expressed their gratitude to the disease as it had led them to search for meaning in their lives and to come to a place of spiritual connection and serenity unknown to them before.

This understanding brings humility to health care as the carer learns to accept and respect the individual's journey and personal expression of their evolution.

The same humility applies when working with people in the dying process. When trusting in the innate wisdom of a person's transition, death no longer has to be feared or prevented but facilitated and witnessed. Death need not be the enemy which has to be fought at all cost.

The Practitioner's Evolution

Practitioners' personal life paths allows them to reach this state of humility as they tackle each challenge in ways that increases their capability, spontaneity, autonomy, responsibility and joy. In expanding their own health they apply the learning inherent in integrating illness to their work with patients, becoming more authentic, compassionate and empathetic. As they become less fearful of illness and death, they experience less need to take action – for the sake of taking action – in their patients' care. They can educate and assist their patients in integrating and maximising the benefits of a difficult situation, as illness and death are part of the learning process from which they themselves have benefited.

Some of the lessons the authors have learned from their own personal experiences of illness are:

◆ there are no easy answers – following a particularly healthy lifestyle does not guarantee freedom from illness at all times. Health is not the reward for good behaviour;

◆ illness is not 'bad', wellness is not 'good' – the state of a person's physical body is not the measure of a person's value or indication of their spiritual alignment;

◆ illness is the great equaliser – no one, no matter how rich, educated or enlightened is immune to illness;

◆ to respect deeply the suffering that people have to endure in life and to honour their resilience and fortitude. Human beings are extraordinary survivors;

◆ to be grateful for the privilege of witnessing so many people's life paths and to learn vicariously through their lessons;

◆ to trust in a greater purpose behind all suffering – experiencing that positive outcomes emerge from seemingly unbearable situations.

What Kind of Help Really Helps

The most powerful way of helping a person in a state of illness is to be fully present for them, not to judge their state and not to impose theories and assumptions on their process. Following a patient's inner process and unfoldment as they gain insight into the context, cause and purpose of their situation, offering them support, providing validation as well as information and suggesting positive choices is the best a practitioner can do. Any approach which provokes separation between patient and practitioner will compound the patient's loneliness and isolation: do not ask, 'What did you do to draw this to yourself?' with the implied judgement that they did something wrong but ask, 'How are you using this condition?' or 'What are you learning from it?', which will facilitate connection.[25]

Multidisciplinary Co-operation

Multidisciplinary co-operation is the ideal expression of Medical Marriage, where doctors and complementary practitioners work together as a team, providing care, support, health and welfare for patients, practitioners and doctors alike. It is the best guarantee for excellence, efficiency and safety of care provision, allowing for ongoing education, peer supervision and self-reflection – the cornerstones of good practice.

To refer patients to another health care professional – if that practitioner will be better suited to help them to improve their health – is the only ethical thing to do. Structures of professional relationships and communication need to be established which will allow access and movement across the boundaries of orthodox and complementary medicine. This has to become the norm within modern health care systems if patients are to be provided with the support they clearly want.

When patients hear about multidisciplinary co-operation for the first time, their reaction is often, 'It's about time!' It seems obvious to most people that co-operation is the best way to serve patients. However, from within the confines of whichever paradigm a practitioner operates, it may seem like an uneasy marriage. Historically the two health care systems have developed in opposing camps and often disrespect has dominated the relationship.

The vision of Medical Marriage asserts that all parties will benefit from a mutually respectful co-operation and integration of health care models. Each system can compensate for the weaknesses in the other. For example, holism is concerned with psychosomatic conditions and prides itself on treating the mind and spirit. How often does the body in fact come last, leaving people without relief from their symptoms, or in danger of having potentially serious symptoms overlooked? Medically trained professionals, on the other hand, have an extensive knowledge of body systems and pathologies, which allows them to address physical problems, but the mind and spirit may be ignored in the overriding desire to alleviate symptoms.

A medical specialist can intervene in the most dire situations, providing, for instance, a liver transplant to save a life. The GP is a generalist with broad-based clinical experience and the ability to co-ordinate care with all specialists. Similarly, complementary practitioners have access to a body of knowledge largely unavailable to medically trained professionals. Partnership is the obvious way to provide the best care for patients, with the option for practitioners to refer patients on to the specialist who is most suited to addressing the presenting problems.

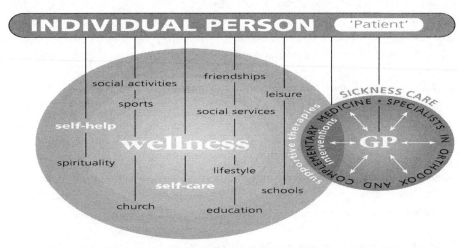

Fig.1: The model of integrated health care, as proposed by the working group on multidisciplinary co-operation at the Medical Marriage conference 1996 at Findhorn

The Contribution of Complementary Medicine

The many different complementary approaches offer a wide variety of treatment options, which allows flexibility and diversity to tailor patients' health care to their own preferences. The complementary approaches are often very gentle and work with the person's own body wisdom, facilitating the self-healing of which it is capable.

The practitioners of complementary therapies place high emphasis on patient contact and allow long consultation times, which give the patient the feeling of being listened to and respected. Physical touch is often used, which apart from the specific therapeutic effect also gives comfort and induces relaxation.

Complementary therapies are engaged in health enhancement, as they offer tools and services which are very useful for stress management. It seems perfectly normal for someone undergoing some stressful situation to go and have a massage when they would not dream of going to their GP, who would have nothing to offer in such a case. Complementary therapies will bring people into a health centre who are not ill. One does not have to have symptoms to seek treatment from a complementary therapist.

Complementary therapies are in the transition zone between disease care and health enhancement. Someone who has been ill may use complementary therapies – alongside or instead of orthodox treatment – to assist their return to full health, and continue, perhaps less frequently, the same treatments once they are better. The complementary therapy is used ongoingly as a preventative measure or for health enhancement.

Complementary therapies at times can offer an explanation for a presenting problem when orthodox medicine is not able to find a clinical diagnosis. This can give reassurance as well as providing a means of addressing the problem therapeutically. For example, a woman with a herpes lesion on her upper lip would have been given orthodox medical treatment to suppress the symptom. However, a homoeopath, on questioning the woman, noted that she had suffered from genital herpes 20 years previously, which had been suppressed at the time with drug treatment. The assessment in this case was entirely favourable for, in the homoeopathic model, the lesion was a recurrence of an old symptom in a milder form, indicating that the woman's body was throwing off the old suppressive drug treatment and was now processing the herpes virus. It indicated that she was in excellent health, and the remedy given was simply to speed up the process, so the lesion disappeared within three days, without, from a homoeopathic viewpoint, the body being compromised by suppressive drug treatment.

Homoeopathy

The Benefit for Complementary Practitioners

One of the benefits of Medical Marriage to practitioners in the complementary field is the potential increase in professional choice, as they are able to work within the mainstream system as well as outwith it. In mainstream medicine, they are available for patients with complaints which, in the present structure, they may not often see, but for whom their modality may be very effective. This applies in particular to problems experienced by deprived sectors of the population.

Another benefit to practitioners would concern the back-up of medical care: not only is it available as an emergency measure but the practitioner can be assured that they can call on a doctor to get a medical point of view on their patient's situation. Should medical care become necessary for the patient, it will be given in a way that respects and integrates the contribution of complementary care.

Research in Holistic Medicine

With the rapprochement of the two health care systems, complementary practitioners gain access to research resources which will advance the academic understanding of the different disciplines and further their acceptance and validation.

The Contribution of Contemporary Medicine

For a health care system which integrates the holistic paradigm, the role of contemporary medicine needs to be redefined. Even if complementary therapies become the first line of treatment in many cases, there is no suggestion within the model of Medical Marriage that contemporary medicine should be relegated to playing second fiddle. It obviously has a valid and essential part to play in the overall scheme of health care. This is most clear in cases where orthodox intervention is called for: in accidents and emergencies; when surgical intervention is needed; in the replacement of body parts or functions (for example insulin dependent diabetes); and when chemical drug treatment is the only successful avenue.

Contemporary medicine's role in diagnosis remains crucial, ensuring that a serious condition is not overlooked and appropriate treatment is not delayed. Most of the complementary modalities do not diagnose; some professional associations actually impose in their code of practice on the practitioner that they refrain from making a diagnosis.[26] Others, such as homoeopathy or traditional Chinese medicine, have a frame of reference for diagnosis which is foreign or unknown to many people. Medical diagnosis provides the background information necessary for the patient to decide on which health care approach they want to choose; a doctor's clinical judgement can assist them in creating a coherent treatment plan.

The importance of the family doctor – who is a partner to the patient in their health care – is greater than ever. With more information and options available, patients want the reassurance of one health care professional who can hold the overview of their care and give unbiased advice, who knows them well, is familiar with all the different aspects of their lives, who ideally knows their living circumstances and the other members of their family and is connected with all the specialist practitioners who have to be drawn in when needed. That practitioner has to have the breadth of clinical experience which allows them to accompany the patient in all life situations – from birth to death and everything in between. The GP is trained and suited to this role in a way that a complementary practitioner cannot be.

The curriculum for the future GP has to be extended to include the theory and basic practice of complementary therapies and most importantly the skills of relationship-centred care.[27]

The knowledge orthodox practitioners possess is extensive and one of the foundation stones of the multidisciplinary partnership. While some complementary therapists have a good grounding in anatomy and physiology, others have less. In the same way that doctors do not need to learn all complementary therapies to which they want to have access for their patients, neither do complementary therapists need to study pathology and pharmacology, etc. to the same depth a doctor has; they simply need to be willing to work together in partnership.

The medical profession has much to teach complementary therapists in the way of cross-discipline communication. Historically they co-operate and communicate as best they can via letters and phone-calls, keeping one another informed of their specialist treatments, a process which few complementary therapists have adopted at this point.

Benefits for the Doctor

Multidisciplinary co-operation offers relief to doctors from one of the biggest burdens within orthodox medicine. Doctors often reach a point of helplessness, particularly with patients with chronic disease, with stress-induced symptoms or with terminal illness when orthodox medicine has little to offer. This helplessness gets compounded by the expectations of both patient and doctor that the doctor should know how to help. The phrase 'You can't just do nothing' or 'Doctor, you have to do something' is a burden under which doctors labour. In many instances, for the sake of taking action – of doing something rather than nothing – this leads to a prescription being written, which serves no one in the long run.

In a multidisciplinary team, doctors can draw on supportive therapies which will not necessarily cure the symptom but will allow patients to cope better with their situation. They can work together with practitioners who have a completely different approach to health care and who therefore do not feel the same limitations. In holistic health care the focus can be on the improvement of health and life quality whatever the presenting problem. This can be achieved through lifestyle modulation, improved diet, nutritional supplementation, exercise, stress management or through support in the form of massage, relaxation or counselling. The patients play a more active role in their self-care. They are active partners with the health care professionals and determine, to a large degree, the different components of their care plan. All of this reduces stress and increases job satisfaction for the doctor, while providing the patient with safe, effective treatments and follow-up supervision.

The Role of the Doctor

There are two different roles attributed to doctors in the model of multidisciplinary co-operation. One is that of the specialist, such as a gynaecologist or an oncologist, who provides expert care much as they do today. The other is the role of the general practitioner which, in Medical Marriage, will be considerably expanded. Co-operating GPs have to embrace the holistic paradigm in health care, engage in a new relationship with patients and have a foundation knowledge of complementary therapies. They can then act as both gatekeeper and care co-ordinator for their patients.

The Gatekeeper

As gatekeeper in primary health care, GPs assess patients' needs and help them in making decisions regarding the next steps in their health care. This entails advice being given on the theoretical and practical background of the different orthodox and complementary modalities and knowing which approaches are appropriate choices in a given condition. Doctors working within multidisciplinary teams will naturally be very familiar with the disciplines practised by their colleagues while also needing to be aware of additional complementary practitioners in the local area.

Gatekeepers require the skills of clinical judgement as they meticulously collect relevant information, draw the appropriate conclusions and conscientiously communicate with the specialist practitioners to whom they are referring patients. They have to be able to create rapport with the patients; to be sensitive to their individual requirements; to provide information as diverse as pathophysiology and contact addresses of self-help organisations; to discuss options and give time for patients to reach their own decisions. The task of the gatekeeper is complete once patients have reached a decision regarding their next steps.

The Care Co-ordinator

The care co-ordinator fulfils the function of the gatekeeper and, beyond that, stays in touch with patients' progress. In situations where a patient sees several practitioners concurrently, patient and care co-ordinator meet on a regular basis to review progress. It is important to assess whether all necessary aspects are covered and the best combination of modalities is being used. The role of the care co-ordinator is to make suggestions from the perspective of the outside observer who may see things in a more detached way.

A case report by Cornelia, acting as care co-ordinator:

Jane, 34 years old, was suffering from severe respiratory problems due to sarcoidosis. She had had extensive diagnostic investigations and was on systemic steroids as well as inhalers. Clinically she was still unwell and her lung capacity and spirometry were severely reduced. The specialists were recommending more invasive treatments, such as laser surgery. She felt disempowered and violated by the medical establishment and wrote: 'How can I protect myself from being an 'interesting case' for the medical world?'

She wanted to explore complementary approaches to improve her symptoms and work with the emotional trauma caused by the condition and the medical interventions. She also wanted to unravel any emotional or thought patterns which might have caused the illness or be perpetuating it.

Through the first consultations with the case co-ordinator she had access to the specialist's reports and discussed them in detail; she also evaluated the complementary therapies she was receiving; and established a positive co-operative relationship with a new GP.

The following health care professionals were involved in her care:

> *consultant in thoracic medicine*
> *general practitioner*
> *medical doctor in the role of case co-ordinator*
> *classical homoeopath*
> *bodyworker – using biodynamic massage*
> *spiritual healer and psychic.*

The consultant in thoracic medicine wanted to repeat some of the earlier investigations to monitor the development. The patient was very frightened of the procedures. After expressing her fears and making sure she had friends and support available for the time of the hospitalisation, she agreed to co-operate with the specialist's recommendation for further assessment and treatment. This assessment showed no improvement under high doses of systemic steroid. Having come to the end of the therapeutic line, the consultant suggested a trial with azathioprin but offered little hope that it would have positive results. At this point he was able to support her when she asked to have the steroids reduced as she wanted to try classical homoeopathy. He continued to monitor her and, in co-operation with the GP, gradually reduced the steroids over time, ensuring that the lung function did not deteriorate any further.

In the following 15 months her clinical situation improved steadily and she now feels more in charge and satisfied with her care. She continues treatments with the homoeopath and sees the GP regularly.

This case demonstrates the value of the care co-ordinator being an advocate for the patient. Co-operation ensues once all different health care professionals involved are confident that the contribution they are making in the care for the patient is respected.

The Requirements of Working in Multidisciplinary Co-operation

Establishing co-operation across the boundaries of different paradigms is not easy as those involved are lacking even the basics of a shared language and understanding of each other's ways of working. Working together with colleagues who have the same training and therefore speak the same language and operate under the same paradigm is difficult enough. There is tremendous complexity within modern Western medicine and also enormous variety within complementary therapies. Co-operation under these circumstances cannot be taken for granted. It needs focused attention and requires the development of structures which facilitate the co-operation. The training of the different health care professions will have to expand to include enough information about the other disciplines that an understanding and common language can be developed.

At present the expectation is that the health care professionals in mainstream medicine co-operate and communicate with each other for the benefit of the patient. In reality this communication is sometimes effective but very often not. Patients complain that surgeons and physicians do not talk to each other but use their treatments parallel as if one does not affect the other. It is generally accepted, for example, that the difference in culture between general medicine and surgery hampers communication.

Holistic health care can only be provided if the professionals involved in a patient's care communicate with each other clearly and know enough about each other's work to assess what respective contribution each can make to the care of the patient. The communication structures which would best serve that co-operation have yet to be evolved since the only system operating on a large scale at present involves letters exchanged by doctors, hospitals and specialists. It is a frequent experience that this system does not work as well as it could. In the complementary field, letter writing is a little practised art and it would be helpful if practitioners would establish the routine of using this tool for co-operation.

Co-operation is easiest when colleagues know one another personally, having worked together in the past, creating a shared history. They then know and respect each other as professionals and as people; they are familiar with each other's area of expertise and methods of work, and what their strengths and weaknesses are. Personal rapport makes co-operation a positive and nourishing experience for all involved. Respect for other practitioners means accepting them as health care professionals who are doing their best and are contributing to the patients' care to the best of their abilities. In reality, there are very few 'bad' practitioners – either in the complementary or in the orthodox field. All practitioners are human and therefore have their limitations and weaknesses. It makes co-operation that much easier if all are aware of these without making them barriers to professional co-operation. Personal relationships are the best safeguard for assessing the competence of a fellow practitioner and for establishing co-operation which benefits the patients.

Co-operation will require individuals to open their minds and increase their knowledge of each other's work, world view and culture. This can be an exciting exploration and truly enlightening for all concerned.

Conferences, seminars and exhibitions will help health care professionals from all fields to meet one another, establishing trust and confidence which are essential for co-operation.

Case Conferences

Case conference meetings in multidisciplinary health care provide three major benefits:

◆ new perspectives on a patient's care;

◆ regular updating on the care of patients seen by more than one practitioner;

◆ personal and professional support for the practitioners.

When health care professionals from different backgrounds come together to discuss a patient's case, in the best scenario the perfect health care strategy can be identified and offered to the patient. While the reality in mainstream medicine can be that case conferences are a lifeless chore, they remain the most effective and immediate way to share information about patients.

A multidisciplinary case conference brings together a group of health carers with different perspectives applying themselves to the patient's story, highlighting considerations and making observations which were not previously thought of. In the dynamics of a well functioning group, so-called group wisdom can occur, which is more than the sum of the expertise of the individuals present. In such cases there is great potential for service to the patient.

The multidisciplinary perspective allows greater understanding of the presenting situation. This is particularly so when practitioners of different paradigms are included in the team. Some presenting situations are not easily understood with a Western world view, whereas an understanding from the Eastern paradigm, for instance traditional Chinese medicine, might allow a cohesive picture to emerge, as in the following example:

A man suffered two minor injuries in a fortnight: one a cut on his left index finger requiring six stitches, the other a fall which caused strain in his left shoulder. Within the Ayurvedic system, the index finger and shoulder both relate to the heart chakra, so these minor accidents suggested stress affecting matters of the heart. When questioned further, it emerged that the patient was about to divorce his wife of 25 years, and his children were about to leave home. He was not expressing his feelings about these intense changes. In addition, within the polarity therapy framework, the heart chakra relates to the air element; when asked about his life, the patient said he felt as if a hurricane was sweeping through it. His mind was employing symbolic images relating to air and his body was demonstrating symptoms which, if left without intervention to relieve his emotional stress, might have created serious physical problems.

Supervision

Case discussion in a group of health carers can, in addition, provide individual practitioners with supervision for their work. Supervision is a concept which is essential in health care. All practitioners should have a period of time after they complete their training when they work under the supervision of a more experienced colleague. This allows them to apply and expand the knowledge they acquired during their training. They gain confidence and acquire experience at the same time. Later in professional life not everybody has the opportunity of regular supervision. When a practitioner can talk freely about difficult cases or interactions with patients which did not feel positive, there is much learning to be gained and stress can be managed before it builds up. Conversely, practitioners can receive nourishment and inspiration when they share a 'good' case, where the relationship with the patient is working well and the treatment is successful.

There are basically two kinds of supervision. Technical supervision occurs when a more experienced practitioner of the same discipline is present. Peer supervision can be helpful in many areas of professional conduct, and can include practitioners with differing training backgrounds. Many questions arising in a case do not have to do with the technique of the modality used but with the practitioner-patient relationship, with ethical or organisational questions of professional practice. In fact, practitioners of other modalities may be able to bring in perspectives which would not have been thought of if only colleagues from the same disciplines were part of the discussion.

Supervision is the best guarantee for high standards of professional practice, good service to the patients and increased job satisfaction.

The Joys of Fruitful Team Work

Synergy means that the whole is more than the sum of the parts. In a synergistic team all partners are respected for their unique contribution. The more different aspects are represented in the team, the more colourful and enriching the co-operation can be. The synergy which can come about from such a pooling of information and perspective can be truly uplifting for all involved. People who are part of a well-functioning team are able to work more effectively, be accessible to patients without the threat of burn-out, and maybe take more professional risks leading to better results – knowing that positive team co-operation is available to give them personal, as well as professional, support.

To create a well-functioning team takes dedication and the attention of each individual in the group. Time needs to be allocated to nourish the bonds between members, to enhance the personal connections and to address any conflicts which may occur at a personal level, as well as through conflicts in the different roles within the team. From the individual, a dedication to personal development, as well as the willingness to contribute constructively to the collective are essential. Group dynamics is a relatively new science of how to harness the potential of such teams. It gives clear guidelines on how to nourish the collective and the individual within the collective.

Aspirations such as seeing beyond the personality, fully owning one's feelings and always speaking in 'I' statements – rather than in a generalised form, which can cause lack of clarity or avoidance – are useful in creating a cohesive group. Positive skills such as active listening and giving someone full attention when they are speaking will ensure effective communication and a feeling of safety and acceptance in the group. The group bonding will be nourished by social events and celebrations, and at other times by shared silence or group meditation. Inviting a group facilitator into the group during times of conflict or change can be productive in allowing the process to unfold more gracefully.

Challenges to Co-operation

It would not be realistic only to sing the praise of multidisciplinary teamwork without addressing the challenges it poses both personally and professionally. There are many hurdles in attitude, behaviour and expectations to be overcome, as in any relationship, if the ideal of Medical Marriage is to be attained.

Disrespect

Historically, the orthodox and 'alternative' health care systems have existed in uneasy tandem, each at least partially ignorant of the other and at worst mutually hostile and denigrating. Doctors often considered alternatives as quackery and a waste of money; irrelevant for health care, if not dangerous. In 1986 the BMA published a report on alternative medicine and predicted that it was a fad which would pass – it was nothing with which doctors need concern themselves.[28] Complementary practitioners fuelled the polarity by judging the orthodox medical system as the source of all patients' problems. Possibly as a response to not feeling respected by the doctors, many developed an attitude of disrespect for the medical profession and its role in health care.

The burden of the original culture difference is still relevant when exploring the question of professional co-operation. Simple and small issues such as dress code can, in many cases, influence whether confidence and rapport can be established.

Righteousness and Judgements

Righteousness in both camps – orthodox and complementary – is a hindrance which is considerable. It may reflect on the individuality of the people who choose to become health care professionals, that there is a pervading feeling that one's own discipline is the best (and perhaps the only) approach; that what anyone else is doing is suspicious, or less effective. These attitudes, although they often stem from a deep sense of care and compassion for patients and a desire to provide the best treatment, are, however, detrimental to positive professional relationships and support the ongoing illusion of separate camps.

The list of judgements or prejudices gets fed by many different aspects – professional training, the media, individual experiences – some of which are firsthand and many secondhand or hearsay. To maintain a positive attitude of co-operation, it is important to search for a balance, to consider that there are at least two sides to any story. In an ideal world, people would be able to listen to both sides, have understanding and compassion for both and reach their own assessment with an openness of both mind and heart.

Complementary therapies as professions are young and immature, with much of the arrogance that goes with youth and zeal. The medical profession, on the other hand, is moving towards maturity, and there is a notable lessening of the arrogance, an increased willingness to accept limitations, to change and grow and develop in new areas of understanding without overlooking others on the way. Co-operation from both sides fosters humility.

Misunderstanding

This point is illustrated by a personal experience from Cornelia's student days.

As a young medical student I was very judgmental about doctors who were creating what I perceived to be an inhumane health care system. I considered them uncaring, hungry for prestige and money, interested only in their career, obedient to orders from superiors and managers who were even further removed from the patient, and not willing to stand up for their patients' interest. I lumped all doctors together in one category. They were the ones who should do it 'right' and yet did it 'wrong'; because I was still a student, they were the 'faceless enemy'.[29] When I came to the point in my training when I actually worked alongside them, they started to have faces, becoming human beings with their own history, aspirations and dreams, limitations and pressures. They were not perfect by any means, but they were not all wrong either. Most of them were trying, doing their best, and sometimes they managed to achieve their aspirations though often they did not. It was important for me to know the difficult demands they were under, to see the conflicting interests, to watch the individuals struggling to get their priorities right. I observed some colleagues becoming numb under the pressures and losing contact with their inspiration and beliefs. They were generally not nourished by the work they were doing, suffered from depression and anxiety, and many were in the process of being burned out. Some would leave the job, others would stay on, out of touch with themselves and with the people around them, persevering because they could not think of anything better to do with their lives. I have seen the same happening in many other health care professions. Understanding what was happening to them entirely altered my righteous perspective.

Insecurity

Another stumbling block to co-operation and expansiveness is insecurity amongst practitioners. It is not considered professional to admit lack of knowledge or competence. Not many health care professionals feel safe or confident enough to own up to their insecurities and fears, despite the fact that everybody has them. Many are forced to hide behind a smokescreen of arrogance, mysteriousness, pretence or non-involvement. Having to maintain the image of the expert who knows everything can create one of the greatest stresses in their lives. On a professional level, this particular aspect has a dangerous side effect: it can cause practitioners not to recognise and be open about the limits of their competence. Given a positive, nourishing and accepting environment of multidisciplinary co-operation, many would be more than happy to admit that they do not know everything, and would have ways, through referral to other practitioners, of still helping patients.

Fear

Patients unwittingly slow the process of co-operation through fear and expectation of lack of acceptance. A considerable percentage (in the region of 30–40%) will not consent to having their GP informed if they consult a complementary practitioner, as they are afraid that the GP would not be supportive, that they would be ridiculed or labelled a difficult patient.[30] There are certainly some GPs who are not open to the idea that complementary therapies have a role to play in health care. However, there are many more who are exploring the possibilities for a wider choice in health care for their patients. Younger doctors especially are open-minded and keen to expand their knowledge in complementary therapies. This has been shown in many studies over the last ten years.[31] Therefore it is important to encourage patients to give their GP credit for being able and willing to support them in receiving the health care they want. In any case the more patients tell their GP that they are using complementary therapies, the more the GP will be inclined to become supportive of it – or at least wake up to the realisation that it is something that patients in their community want. From being a theoretical idea which is discussed in scientific papers, it might become real and tangible for them.[32]

Legal and Ethical Considerations

Legal and ethical considerations are one of the most prominent arguments which prevent doctors from considering co-operation with complementary practitioners. Referring to another practitioner can be considered to be delegation of duties and implies that the doctor remains responsible for the care of the patient.

> *The [General Medical] Council recognises and welcomes the growing contribution made to health care by nurses and other persons who have been trained to perform specialised functions, and it has no desire to either restrain the delegation to such persons of treatment or procedures falling within the proper scope of their skills... But a doctor who delegates treatment or other procedure must be satisfied that the person to whom they are delegated is competent to carry them out. It is also important that the doctor should retain ultimate responsibility for the management of these patients because only the doctor has received the necessary training to undertake this responsibility.*[34]

This guideline poses two major questions which have been debated a great deal in all the health care professions:

◆ What defines the competence of a person to carry out treatment or procedures and how can a doctor assess the competence of a practitioner of a discipline with which they are not familiar? Is it enough that they know the kind of training the practitioner had?

◆ How can doctors retain responsibility for the management of the patient if they refer them on to a practitioner who uses a different framework of treatment which the doctor cannot fully understand? The practitioner of, for instance, acupuncture cannot be bound by a doctor's assessment of what is necessary or not, especially if the doctor does not have the same training as the practitioner. Retaining responsibility then becomes an empty phrase for the doctor.

If the practitioner using the complementary discipline is also medically qualified, then the referral causes no official ethical difficulty. The Professions Supplementary to Medicine Act 1960 specifies the paramedical professions to which doctors can refer without legal or ethical problems. These include chiropodists, occupational therapists and physiotherapists. Other professions can be added to that list by the Privy Council, provided both Houses of Parliament agree. Some complementary disciplines may be willing to consider being added to that list if permitted. Others may well feel that the identification of being a profession supplementary to medicine would compromise their contribution to health care.

Complementary Medicine and the Law

Self-regulation of the professional bodies of complementary therapies is another avenue. As the General Medical Council does for medical doctors, the professions define their own code of ethics and conduct, implement a complaints procedure and hold a register of qualified practitioners. Guidelines for employment of complementary practitioners in the NHS were drawn up in 1995 and request qualification, registration and professional insurance.[34]

NHS Treatment vs Private Treatment

One of the basic differences between orthodox and complementary medicine in the UK at present is that orthodox medicine is provided under the National Health Service and is therefore free at the point of delivery while complementary medicine has almost exclusively developed in the field of private medicine.

While there are many arguments for and against private health care for the patient, a challenge to co-operation between practitioners may be the fact that complementary practitioners work privately and therefore many earn less than doctors or other health care professionals within the NHS. This may put pressure on them, and may cause a conflict of interests, making them reluctant to refer on a patient.

It certainly makes complementary therapies less accessible to the population with a lower income. This leads to an air of exclusiveness around complementary medicine as it is mainly used by the educated middle class.

Research and Resources

Another great hurdle for complementary therapies is the request that they prove themselves in scientific evaluations for efficacy and effectiveness before the medical profession will consider co-operation, or health care providers contemplate purchasing services. Because complementary medicine was for so long left to the alternative field or subculture, the resources for such research have not been available. Resources are lacking not only in funding but also in academic emphasis in the training of the practitioners and the structural set-up of the training institutions. Complementary medicine in the last 30 years has been geared towards clinical work with patients. Only recently is there an awareness of the need for research, which requires a new outlook and methodology in its application to disciplines which operate under the holistic paradigm.

Research in Holistic Medicine

Education – the Core for Understanding

Education is the core for understanding between the professions. In the same way as doctors have an understanding of the many different aspects of contemporary medicine, everyone working within the model of Medical Marriage needs to have a basic knowledge of the theory, practice and application of the wide range of complementary therapies.

> *Studies... indicate a persistent trend among doctors of a desire for more information on more non-conventional therapies.*[35]

> *... However it is important to distinguish here between training to practise and more general raising of awareness of basic principles and application of various techniques.... Doctors need to know more about non-conventional therapies not only for appropriate delegation of care, but also in their role as trusted advisors to their patients.*[36]

> *The key element for both the doctor and the therapist is understanding the different spheres of influence in which they operate. It is, therefore, necessary to consider actions which can be taken to improve communications and understanding between physicians and non-conventional practitioners in order to safeguard patients' health.*[37]

Fulfilling these recommendations was one of the primary motivations for this book. The need for education applies, of course, to complementary therapists as much as to doctors.

References

1   D M Eisenberg, et al., *Unconventional Medicine in the United States: prevalence, costs and patterns of use*, N Eng J Med, 1993; 328: 246-52.

      S J Fulder; R E Munro, *Complementary medicine in the UK: patients, practitioners, and consultations*, Lancet, *1985*; 2: 542-5.

      M Emslie; M Campbell; K Walker, *Complementary therapies in a local health care setting*, Compl. Therapies in Med, 1996; 4: 39-42.

2   Claire Monod Cassidy, *Unravelling the ball of strings: reality, paradigms, and the study of alternative medicine*, Advances: The Journal of Mind-Body Health, 1994; 10: 1, p9.

3   ibid. p11.

4   J S McQuade, *The medical malpractice crisis-reflections on the alleged causes and proposed cure*, J Royal Soc Med, (1991); 84: 408-11.

5   N Summerton, *Positive and negative factors in defensive medicine: a questionnaire study of general practitioners.* BMJ (1995), 310: 27-9.

6   Patrick Pietroni, *Holistic medicine: new lessons to be learned*, The Practitioner, 22 Oct 1987; Vol 231, p1386-90.

7   C P Tresolini and the Pew-Fetzer Task Force, *Health Professions Education and Relationship-Centred Care*, Pew Health Professions Commission, 1994.

8   M Balint, *The Doctor, His Patient and the Illness*, Pitman Medical, 1973.

9   Patient demands fuel GP stress, *Medical Monitor*, 10 Jan 1996; p11-2.

10   BMA, GMC, Joint Consultants Committee, Committee of Postgrad. Deans, Council of Deans of UK Med. Schools and Faculties, Conference of Medical Royal Colleges and their Faculties in the UK, Core Values for the Medical Profession in the 21st Century, BMA, 1994, p10.

11   A Antonovsky, *Unraveling the Mystery of Health: How People Manage Stress and Stay Well*, Jossey-Brass, 1987.

12   Diana Whitmore, *Psychosynthesis Counselling in Action*, Sage, 1994.

13   Highland Health Board, *Lifestyle survey 1991 – agenda for action*, Inverness, 1991.

14   ibid.

15   Lucy Crocker, *The Peckham Experiment*, Scottish Academy Press, 1985.

16   David Ponka, *A survey of attitudes towards health and the Community Health Scheme within the Findhorn Foundation Community*, Findhorn, 1996.

17   R P Chaplan, *Stress, anxiety, and depression in hospital consultants, general practitioners, and senior health service managers*, BMJ, Vol 309, 12 Nov 1994; p1261-63.

      British Medical Association, *Stress and the medical profession*, BMA 1992.

      Julie Coulson, *Doctors under stress*, BMA News Review, April 1996.

18   *The Patient's Charter*, NHS in Scotland, Scottish Office, 1991.

      A Charter for England – The Patient's Charter and You, Department of Health, 1995.

      Citizen's Charter, Patient's Charter for Wales, 1995.

      Code of Practice on Openness, NHS in Scotland – Management Executive, Scottish Office, 1995.

19   Source of this list: Shropshire Health Authority, (HC 288-1, Ev p 356).

20   R P Chaplan, *Stress, Anxiety, and depression in hospital consultants*, general practitioners, and senior health service managers, BMJ, Vol 309, 12 Nov 1994, p 1261-63.

21   Caroline Myss, *Why People Don't Heal*, Sounds True Audio, 1994.

22   Michaela Glöckler, Wolfgang Goebel, *A Guide to Child Health*, Anthroposophic Press, 1990.

23   John Harrison, *Love Your Disease Its Keeping You Healthy*, Angus & Robertson, 1984.

      Thorwald Dethlefsen, Rüdiger Dahlke, *The Healing Power of Illness – The Meaning of Symptoms and How to Interpret Them*, Element, Shaftsbury, 1990.

24   Norm Shealy, Caroline Myss, *AIDS: Passageway to Transformation*, Stillpoint, 1987.

      Oscar Moore, *A Matter of Life and Sex*, Penguin, 1996.

25   Ken Wilber, *Grace and Grit – Spirituality and healing in the life and death of Treya Killam Wilber*, 1993; p251-5.

26   examples are: the *Code of Practice and Ethics of The Scottish Institute of Reflexology*, and the *Code of Ethics of the National Federation of Spirtual Healers*.

27   C P Tresolini and the Pew-Fetzer Task Force, *Health Professions Education and Relationship-Centred Care*, Pew Health Professions Commission, 1994.

28   British Medical Association, *BMA board of science working party on alternative therapy*, BMA Publications, May 1986.

29   Sam Keen, *Faces of the Enemy*, HarperCollins, 1991.

30   unpublished survey in Dr Cornelia Featherstone's practice, April 1995.

31   D T Reilly and M A Taylor, *Young doctors' views on alternative medicine*, BMJ, 1983; 287: 337-9.

32   R Wharton and G Lewith, *Complementary medicine and the general practitioner*, BMJ, 292 (1986), 1, 498-500.

E and P Anderson, *General practitioners and alternative medicine*, JRCGP, 37 (1987) 52-5.

C Budd; B Fisher; D Parrinder; L Price, *A model of co-operation between complementary and allopathic medicine in a primary care setting*, BJGP, (1990) 40, 376-8.

P Pietroni, *Beyond the boundaries: relationship between general practice and complementary medicine*, BMJ, 1992; 305: 564-6.

33   GMC, *Professional conduct and discipline: fitness to practice*, 1992; p17.

34   Anne Hayes, *Guidelines for Employment of Complementary Therapists in the NHS*, West Yorkshire Health Authority, 1995

35   David T Reilly, *Young doctors' views on alternative medicine*, BMJ 287 (1983), 337-9.

36   BMA, *Complementary Medicine – New Apporaches to Good Practice*, Oxford Universtity Press, 1993; p48-9.

37   ibid. p48.

Further Reading

Adams, Patch, *Gesundheit!*, Healing Arts Press, VT, 1993.

BMA, *Complementary Medicine – New Approaches to Good Practice*, BMA, 1993.

Capra, Fritjof, *The Turning Point*, Simon & Schuster, 1982.

Lucy, Crocker, *The Peckham Experiment*, Scottish Academy Press, 1985.

Goldberg, Burton et al., *Alternative Medicine: The Definitive Guide*, Future Medicine Publ., 1994.

Goleman, Daniel; Gurin, Joel, *Mind/Body Medicine, How to Use Your Mind for Better Health*, Consumer Reports Books, 1993.

Hawkins, Peter; Shohet, Robin, *Supervision in the Helping Professions*, Open University Press, 1990.

Kilpatrick, Joseph; Danzinger, Sanford, *Better Than Money Can Buy – the New Volunteers*, Innersearch Publishing, 1996.

Lannoye, Paul, *European report on the status of non-conventional medicine*, The Natural Medicine Society, 1996.

Lerner, Michael, *Choices in Healing: Integrating the Best of Conventional and Complementary Approaches to Cancer*, MIT Press, 1994.

Maher, G., *Start a Career in Complementary Medicine*, Tackmart, 1992.

Melchart, D., Wagner, H. (eds), *Naturheilverfahren – Grundlagen einer Autoregulativen Medizin*, Schattauer, 1993.

Myss, Caroline, *Anatomy of the Spirit*, Random House, 1996.

Nehring, Julia; Hill, Robert, *The Blackthorn Garden Project – Community Care in the Context of Primary Care*, The Sainsbury Centre for Mental Health, 1995.

Pearse, Innes, *The Quality of Life*, Scottish Academy Press, 1979.

Pietroni, Patrick, *The Greening of Medicine*, Victor Gollancz, 1990.

Pietroni, Patrick and Christopher (eds), *Innovation in Community Care and Primary Health – The Marylebone Experiment*, Churchill Livingstone, 1996.

Robinson, Jane, *The Alternative and Complementary Health Compendium*, Millenium Profiles, 1996.

Shealy, Norm; Caroline Myss, *The Creation of Health*, Stillpoint, 1988.

Stone, Julie; Matthew, Joan, *Complementary Therapy and the Law*, Oxford University Press, 1996.

Widdicombe, C., *Group Meetings that Work*, St Pauls, 1994.

Alternative Medicine: Expanding Medical Horizons. A report to the National Institutes of Health on alternative medical systems and practices in the United States. US Government Printing Office, 1992.

Audio Tapes

Myss, Caroline, *Why People Don't Heal*, Sounds True Audio, 1994.

Myss, Caroline, *Energy Anatomy: The Science of Personal Power*, Spirituality and Health, Sounds True Audio, 1996.

Journals

Chaitow, Leon (ed), *Journal of Bodywork and Movement Therapies*, Churchill Livingstone.

Dossey, Larry (ed), *Alternative Therapies in Health and Medicine*, InnoVision Communications.

Goodman, Sandra, *Health: State-of-the-art – research at the cutting edge of complementary medicine*, Health Research

Lewith, George (ed), *Complementary Therapies in Medicine*, Churchill Livingstone.

McTaggart, Lynne, *What Doctors Don't Tell You*, Wallace Press.

——, *PROOF!*, Wallace Press.

Pietroni, Patrick (ed), *Journal of Interprofessional Care*, Carfax.

Rankin-Box, Denise (ed), *Complementary Therapies in Nursing and Midwifery*, Churchill Livingstone.

Tyrrell, Ivan; Winbolt, Barry, *The Therapist*, The European Therapy Studies Institute.

Articles and Publications

Bishop, M., *A Medical Marriage – a quiet revolution,* International Journal of Alternative and Complementary Medicine, June 1992, 19-26.

Bishop, M., *A Medical Marriage – the revolution continues,* International Journal of Alternative and Complementary Medicine, December 1992, 17-24.

Booth, B., *Complementary Therapy,* Nursing Times/Macmillan, 1993.

Ernst, Edzard, *Complementary medicine–doing more good than harm?,* British Journal of General Practice, 1996; 46: 403, 60-1.

Gordziejko, Tessa, *Complementary Therapies and the NHS – Added Value?* Huddersfield: West Yorkshire Health Authority, March 1994.

Pietroni, P. C., *Beyond the boundaries: relationship between general practice and complementary medicine,* BMJ, 1992; 305: 564-6.

Pietroni, Patrick, *Holistic medicine: new lessons to be learned,* The Practitioner, 1987; 231: 1386-90.

Reilly, D. T., *Young doctors' views on alternative medicine,* BMJ, 1983; 287: 337-9.

Richardson, J., *Complementary therapies in the NHS: a service evaluation of the first year of an outpatient service in a local disctrict general hospital,* Health Services Research and Evaluation Unit, The Lewisham Hospital NHS Trust, 1995.

Smith, Iain, *Clinical effectiveness needs to be more than pin money,* Health Service Journal, 25 Jan 1996, 24-5.

Smith I., *Commissioning complementary medicine,* BMJ, 1995; 310: 1151-2.

Stone, Julie, *Complements slips,* Health Service Journal, 25 Jan 1996, 26-7.

Anon., *Beyond the fringe: incorporating complementary therapies within the NHS,* Medical Law Monitor, May 1996, 8-11.

Complementary therapies – who benefits? report from the Nursing Times conference, October 1995.

The Peckham health centre experiment – its potential and lessons for Sheffield Workshop report, April 1993.

Anderson, E.; Anderson, P., *General practitioners and alternative medicine,* Journal of the Royal College of General Practitioners, 1987; 37: 52-5.

Budd, C.; Fisher, B.; Parrinder, D.; Price, L, *A model of co-operation between complementary and allopadlic medicine in a primary care,* British Journal of General Practice, 1990; 40: 376-8.

Eisenberg, D. M.; Kessler, R. C.; Foster, C.; Norlock, F. E.; Calkins, D. R.; Delbanco, T. L., *Unconventional medicine in the United States: prevalence, costs and pattern of use,* N Engl J Med, 1993; 328: 246-52.

Emslie, M.; Campbell, M.; Walker, K., *Complementary therapies in a local health care setting. Part 1: Is there real public demand?,* Complementary Therapies in Medicine, 1996; 4: 39-42.

Fulder, S. J.; Munro, R. E., *Complementary medicine in the United Kingdom: patients, practitioners and consultations,* Lancet, 1985; 542-5.

Fisher P.; Ward A., *Complementary medicine in Europe,* BMJ, 1994; 309: 107-11.

Fitter, Mike; Buchanan, Jo, *The integration of alternative approaches to health,* conference report, Sheffield, 1995.

Himmel W.; Schulte M.; Kochen M., *Complementary Medicine: Are patients' expectations being met by their general practitioners?* Br J Gen Pract, 1993; 43: 232-5.

Hooper, J.; Ruddlesden, J.; Heyes, A.; Ash, S.; Styan, S., *Introducing independent complementary therapists into GP practices in Huddersfield and Dewsbury. Evaluation Report,* West Yorkshire Health Authority, Huddersfield, 1996.

Hudson-Allez, G., *Issues of confidentiality for a counsellor in general practice,* CMS News, The Journal of the Counselling in Medical Settings, a division of the British Association for Counselling, 1995, 44, 8-9.

Lewith, George (ed), *Competence and Validation,* Complementary Therapies in Medicine, 1995; 3: 1, 1-64

Long, A. F.; Brettle, A.; Mercer, G., *Searching the literature on the efficacy and effectiveness of complementary therapies,* A report by the Yorkshire Collaborating Centre for Health Service Research, Nuffield Institute for Health, University of Leeds, 1995.

Long, A. F.; Mercer, G., *Reviewing the state of the evidence on efficacy and effectiveness of complementary therapies,* A report by the Yorkshire Collaborating Centre for Health Service Research, Nuffield Institute for Health, University of Leeds, 1995.

Melchart, D.; Worku, F.; Linde, K.; Wagner, H., *The university project Münchener Modell for the integration of naturopathy into research and teaching at the Ludwig-Maximilian University in Munich,* Complementary Therapies in Medicine, 1994; 2: 147-53.

Mercer, G.; Long, A. F.; Smith I., *Researching and evaluating complementary therapies: the state of the debate,* A report by the Yorkshire Collaborating Centre for Health Service Research, Nuffield Institute for Health, University of Leeds, 1995.

Pal, Badal; Morris, Julie, *Rheumatologists and complementary medicine,* Rheumatology in Practice, 1996, 18-20.

Reason, P.; Chase, H. D.; Desser, A.; Melhuish, C.; Morrison, S.; Peters, D.; Wallstein, D.; Webber, V., *Towards a clinical framework for collaboration between general and complementary practitioners: discussion paper,* J R Soc Med, 1992; 85: 161-4.

Reilly, D.; Taylor, M. A.; Beattie, N. G. M.; Campbell. J. H.; McSharry, C.; Aitchison, T. C.; Carter, R.; Stevenson, R. D., *Is evidence for homoeopathy reproducible?,* Lancet, 1994; 344: 1601-6.

Reilly, David; Taylor, Morag, *Developing integrated medicine – Report of the RCCM Fellowship in Complementary Medicine,* The University of Glasgow 1987-1990, Complementary Therapies in Medicine; 1993; 1: suppl. 1, p 1-50.

Tresolini, CP and the Pew-Fetzer Task Force, *Health Professions Education and Relationship-Centred Care*, Pew Health Professions Commission, 1994.

Wharton, R.; Lewith, G., *Complementary medicine and the general practitioner*, BMJ, 1986; 292: 1498-1500.

Wilson, B.; Goodwin, N.; Grimshaw, JM; Blumer, H.; Durno, D.; Wilson, H.; Williams, AM, *Complementary therapies in a local health care setting. Part 2: An experiment in bringing complementary therapies into local NHS commissioning. The Grampian concensus development conference*, Complementary Therapies in Medicine, 1996; 4: 118-23.

BMA., GMC., Joint Consultants Committee, Committee of Postgrad. Deans, Council of Deans of UK Med. Schools and Faculties, Conference of Medical Royal Colleges and their Faculties in the UK, *Core Values for the Medical Profession in the 21st Century*, BMA, 1994.

GMC., *Professional Conduct and Discipline: Fitness to Practise*, GMC, 1992.

GMC., *Duties of a Doctor*, GMC, 1995.

Grampian Health Board, *Complementary Therapies – Health Development Review Aberdeen*, Grampian Health Board, 1994.

Healthwatch Grampian, *Report of a Survey on Complementary Therapies*, by Grampian Local Health Council, 1993.

Highland Health Board, *Lifestyle survey 1991 – agenda for action*, Highland Health Board, 1991.

Which?, *Healthy Choices*, November 1995, 8-13

Part 2 | A–Z of Complementary Therapies

Acupuncture
by Tom Williams

Theoretical Background

Of all the treatment protocols associated with Chinese medicine, there is no doubt that the best known in the West is acupuncture. The image of needles being inserted into various locations in the body – often with no apparent relationship to the presenting problem – is what springs to the mind of most Westerners when they think of the medicine practised by the Chinese. It seems strange, illogical, yet the benefits of acupuncture are there for all to see. For over 3000 years the Chinese have been developing and using this therapy to treat the full range of physical, mental and spiritual problems that appear to afflict humankind. In the last thirty years or so, as acupuncture has been introduced and become established in the West, the benefits have been enjoyed by countless Westerners and the therapeutic effects have stood up to the most rigorous of Western scientific research protocols. Acupuncture works, and more and more people, both lay and professional, want to know more about it and experience its therapeutic benefits at first hand.

Traditional Chinese
Medicine

Acupuncture works by influencing the patient's 'vital energy' flow, or *qi* (also spelled *ki* or *chi*), through the stimulation of this energy flow as a result of the insertion of very fine needles into the areas of qi concentration. These areas are called meridians and are sometimes referred to as channels. On a model or a chart of the acupuncture meridians, they appear as discrete distribution lines running all over the body, parallel to the networks of arteries, veins and capillaries that carry our blood supply round the body. This is a somewhat misleading image. Qi permeates all parts of our bodies – there is no part where qi is not – and it is probably more helpful to consider the acupuncture meridians as areas of high qi concentration. To use the analogy of a river: in the centre there will be a high volume of water and the flow will be deep and strong; towards the bank the volume reduces, the flow becomes more shallow and less vigorous. At the bank of the river there will still be water contained in the soil but it will have little active motion. Thus it is with the qi flow of the body. The meridian represents the area of the highest concentration of qi flow and although for illustrative purposes the discrete lines are useful, it should be remembered that the distribution system is much more complex than that. Along the meridians there are many key 'access' points. These are known as acupuncture points and are where the needles are inserted.

History

There are many stories about how acupuncture developed, some apocryphal and some with elements of truth in them. It was observed in ancient China that the stimulation of areas of the body, initially by pressure and later by inserting very fine fragments of sharpened bone or bamboo, brought relief to various physical problems. The practice of acupuncture has developed in an empirical manner over the centuries. It was observed that needling certain points produced consistent and identifiable effects and gradually the whole system evolved with reference to the philosophical and theoretical structures of Chinese medicine into what it has become today. Acupuncture as a practice continues to evolve and develop with new points and new point combinations being regularly reported.

Other practices such as acupressure and moxibustion also involve the stimulation of the body's energy system at acupuncture points, either with massage and pressure or with the application of heat through the burning of the herb *artesima vulgaris*, commonly called moxa.

Acupuncture in the West

There is some evidence of the knowledge and practice of acupuncture being brought back from China by European traders and adventurers, but the serious development of acupuncture in the West can only be realistically traced back to the years after World War II. Initially, the practice was developed in France, but throughout the 1960s and 70s many Westerners began to introduce Chinese medical practices into Britain and the United States. In addition there has been a consistent flow of Chinese practitioners coming West, many fleeing repression in communist China and others coming as a result of conflicts such as the Vietnam War. One or two pioneer Western practitioners have also studied in China and the Far East and brought back systems which they have developed in the West. Most notable in this regard has been the development of the five element school and the 'stems and branches' approach. The different emphasis of Japanese acupuncture has also greatly influenced practices. In addition, there have been uniquely Western developments in acupuncture, such as the trigger point theories and myofascial approaches of Mark Seem in the United States.

Different Approaches

Traditional Chinese Medicine

The TCM approach is basically the kind of acupuncture that is practised and taught in China today. The patient's disharmonies are diagnosed in terms of excesses or deficiencies of yin and yang energy and the organ systems (*zangfu*) which are most intimately related to the disharmony are identified. Once the diagnosis has taken place an acupuncture point prescription is selected. The points are needled, usually quite deeply, depending on the local anatomy and the needles themselves are often stimulated by twirling, lifting or thrusting amongst other methods. Needles are usually retained for at least 20 minutes, although in some instances this may be longer.

Traditional Chinese Medicine

Five Element Acupuncture

In the five element school, the diagnosis is based on the subtle interactions and relationships between what are described in Chinese philosophy as the five basic elements of the universe – fire, water, metal, wood and earth. The emphasis in this school tends to be at a more subtle energetic level. Needles are inserted at a more superficial level and the selection of points is different from that found in TCM. The Japanese tradition in acupuncture also emphasises the five element approach in addition to palpation of the *hara* for diagnostic assessment. The hara is considered to be the area around the abdomen from the pubic bone up to the rib cage. The area is seen as reflecting the various systems of the body and hara diagnosis involves the palpation of this area in order to ascertain where possible disharmonies may be occurring. These determine the plan of the acupuncture intervention.

Shiatsu

Stems and Branches

This particular approach develops the theory of needling and point selection through theories of Chinese astrology in addition to the more mainstream ideas of yin/yang disharmonies and the five elements.

Trigger Point / Myofascial Acupuncture

The work of the American acupuncturist Mark Seem has developed into what he describes as a 'new American school' of acupuncture. Seem has developed an approach to using acupuncture which works on the myofascial layers of tissue in certain energetic zones of the body. Seem argues that by releasing areas of myofascial congestion using acupuncture it is then possible to achieve an energetic 'domino' effect which will create a balance at a much more systemic level in the body. Seem's approach may use a large number of needles at points which have been strategically palpated and he will encourage shallow needling to achieve the energetic release that is binding the fascial tissue and consequently causing deeper levels of disharmony in the patient.

Auricular Acupuncture

A development of the TCM approach sees the whole human body as 'mirrored' in the ear. Numerous key points are identified in the ear which relate to different organ systems in the body. These points are needled or ear needles or 'seeds' are left in the ear to provide ongoing stimulation of the appropriate point. In my experience, ear acupuncture can be a useful adjunct to full body acupuncture. TCM uses it as an adjunct to other therapeutic modalities. Paul Nogier, a French doctor, brought it to Europe and developed a system exclusively using points in the ear.

Electroacupuncture

A more recent further development in acupuncture therapy is the stimulation of acupuncture needles by passing a small, pulsed DC electric current between pairs of needles. This can provide a tonifying or reducing stimulation to the needle, depending on the frequency and the strength of the electric stimulation. This low-voltage stimulation of the needle can be particularly beneficial in certain disharmonies, most especially meridian problems where the intention is to move blocked qi to relieve pain.

The Practice of Acupuncture

Diagnosis

When a practitioner of traditional Chinese medicine is undertaking a diagnosis to plan an acupuncture treatment, it is vital that a comprehensive picture of the patient's patterns of harmonies and disharmonies is acquired. The protocols adopted in acupuncture are the same as for any branch of Chinese medicine and involve: looking, hearing, smelling, questioning and touching.

The acupuncturist will glean information initially from the way the patient looks – demeanour, body shape, general behavioural patterns, etc. In addition, observing the tongue can give vital pointers to the pattern of disharmonies in the patient. Listening to the patient's voice, the sound of their breathing and other audible characteristics all add details important in identifying any disharmony. While smelling the patient may be a problem culturally in some instances, any characteristic odours can be of great importance in terms of understanding what is going on in the patient's life. The mainstay of the diagnostic process is asking the patient questions that will elicit information which enables the practitioner to identify signs of excess/deficiency; heat/cold; interior/exterior and yin/yang. Finally, the practitioner can gather much useful information by palpating the body for tender spots and, very importantly in Chinese medicine, feeling for the varying qualities of the pulse.

This information is seen against the generic backdrop of the patient's lifestyle and other relevant contextual clues which can give an important frame of reference to help make the more abstract diagnostic information more meaningful.

By adopting this comprehensive and holistic approach to understanding the patient, the acupuncturist is in a good position to identify patterns of disharmonies that will be the focus of the treatment.

Treatment

The selection of points is a matter of clinical judgement and while there are common 'point prescriptions' for particular disharmonies, individual practitioners may well alter and adjust these prescriptions according to their own experience and preferences, as well as in light of the specifics of the patient's disharmony. Point location is an interesting 'art' in acupuncture. Clearly, it is not simply a matter of describing a point as being 3 inches below the knee, for example. Human bodies are such that a simplistic method of measurement is wholly inadequate. In Chinese medicine the body is considered in proportional distances called *cun*. Individual patients' *cun* will vary depending on the local geography of their bodies. Thus, for example, the distance between the knee joint and the external ankle bone is 16 cun and leg points are located with reference to this relative distance. The practitioner will also use bodily landmarks as a means of navigation. For example, in locating the back shu points of the bladder meridian, it is useful to count down the spinous processes of the vertebrae. In addition, as a double check, other points are located by aligning them with anatomical features such as the iliac crest of the pelvis or the lower border of the scapula. Point location is unique to the individual and the general rules of location are applied in a relative manner with respect to the individual anatomy.

Modern concern in the West regarding issues such as HIV and cross infection has resulted in the vast majority of practitioners using only disposable needles, which are used once and once only, before being destroyed by incineration. The size and gauge of needle used will depend on local anatomical considerations and the clinical preferences of the practitioner.

When the needle is inserted into the body, the most common sensations are a dull ache or a tingling. The practitioner will at times move the needle in and out until the 'qi is found'. The Chinese call this practice *da qi*. Once the qi is found, the practitioner may manipulate the needle briefly – depending on what therapeutic effect is being sought, or the needle may simply be left alone. Retention times vary. Some practitioners will remove the needle as soon as da qi is achieved, while the more common practice, consistent with the system taught and used in China, is to retain the needles for up to 20 to 30 minutes. Consideration is also given to the nature of the disharmony being treated and to the 'energetic strength' and age of the patient.

Other practices such as the burning of moxa on the needle head or the electrical stimulation of the needles may also be used depending on the nature of the disharmony being treated. During the treatment the patient should remain at peace and relaxed, as someone who is very mentally agitated during acupuncture treatment may gain less benefit.

The number and frequency of treatments varies depending on the nature of the problem. A typical regime might involve weekly treatment sessions over a period of 10 to 15 weeks, but some patients will gain considerable benefit after two or three sessions, while others will require treatment that lasts for months.

Chinese medicine is a comprehensive system of health care and acupuncture, as one of its main treatments, can offer real and lasting help for a whole range of physical and emotional conditions. One of the problems which is gradually being overcome in the West is the view of acupuncture simply as symptomatic relief of conditions such as pain.

Acupuncture can be used alongside many other therapies and the potential here for genuinely complementary work is infinite.

Research

There is a considerable and growing body of evidence to support the effectiveness of acupuncture in clinical settings. In addition to a vast amount of research literature emanating from China, there is a growing body of literature based on rigorous Western research methodologies.

In particular, there has been considerable work done in the use of acupuncture with problems of pain relief, the sequelae of stroke, asthma and related conditions and also with the management of drug and alcohol dependence.[1]

Applying research protocols to acupuncture practice is far from easy, but addressing these issues is vital in the cause of bringing acupuncture into mainstream respectability and much work is being undertaken in this regard.

Research in Holistic Medicine

In the UK there is the Acupuncture Research Resource Centre in York, which actively supports research and disseminates information regarding research to interested professionals and other bodies.

Training

Acupuncture derives from a very long and respected tradition of philosophical and theoretical thought and a thorough and unique empirical approach to treatment. The models and systems of thought which underpin acupuncture and, indeed, the whole of Chinese medicine require not just to be learned, but to be absorbed into the psyche.

Training therefore should respect this tradition and requires to be theoretically thorough and rigorous in practice. It is vital that when the public consult an acupuncturist they can be confident that the practitioner is appropriately and professionally trained to standards that reflect the subject. In the United Kingdom, the Council for Acupuncture and the British Acupuncture Council set professional, ethical and training standards which withstand the closest scrutiny. All practitioners should be well versed in Chinese medicine and should demonstrate their diagnostic and treatment competencies before being allowed to treat the public. There are various colleges in the UK which offer accredited training, usually lasting up to three years for diploma status and four years for degree status. The fact that several acupuncture training courses are now accredited to degree level by universities is testament to the nature and the validity of the training offered.

Prospective patients should always be satisfied that the practitioner of their choice is appropriately registered and carries full professional indemnity insurance. In addition, there are a number of medical doctors and allied professionals, such as nurses and physiotherapists, who will have undertaken training in symptomatic acupuncture, often targeted at pain relief. While this can be useful and of benefit to patients in the short term, it must be remembered that there is usually no background knowledge of Chinese medicine and that application in this form is limited in scope.

Case Study

Sarah was a 32-year-old woman, who had been married to John for six years. For the last two years they had been trying for a baby, but within two months of their starting to try for pregnancy, Sarah's periods had ceased and had not recommenced. In addition to this she had complained of sharp and debilitating pain in her lower abdomen, especially on the left side. She had been diagnosed as having an ovarian cyst, but because of her wish to become pregnant she had wanted to avoid surgery which might have involved the removal of the ovary. She had been on ongoing drug therapy, which had eased the discomfort, but she still was not having any periods, despite the fact she felt premenstrual on a fairly regular 28-day cycle.

When she came for the initial diagnostic interview, she was very tense and upset. John, who had come along as well, and Sarah were constantly bickering and arguing about minor points of detail throughout the interview. Sarah also complained of palpitations; her sleep pattern was poor and she had a feeling of what she called 'hot tightness' in her head. She had a tendency to constipation. Her tongue was red around the sides with a red tip and it was quite dry. Her pulse was wiry. The overall impression was of someone who was very rigid and demanding in all aspects of her life.

The initial observation of Sarah showed her to be very tense and constrained. She sat continually tensing and releasing her hands and she was always at the very edge of her seat. Her eye contact was poor and her general demeanour was of someone with a very tight and rigid 'shell' around her. Her voice was terse and she was very clipped with her replies. She was easily angered when conversing with John. Detailed questioning brought out evidence of internal heat and excess patterns. The sharp debilitating pain on her side was reported to be worse for pressure and gentle palpation reinforced this, identifying a tender area just to the left and below her umbilicus.

The diagnosis from the perspective of Chinese medicine was stagnation of liver qi which was leading to stagnation in the lower jiao (part of the abdominal area below the midriff). The stagnant qi was causing internal heat which was rising up and disturbing the heart, causing palpitations and the poor sleep patterns. The head symptoms were also indicative of unregulated qi rising to the head. The quick temper and the rigidity of personality are both indicative of a 'livery' personality in Chinese medicine.

The principle of acupuncture treatment was initially to move the stagnant liver qi and to clear the stagnation in the lower jiao. Sarah came twice weekly for three weeks and then weekly thereafter. After six treatments she was feeling much calmer in herself and the palpitations and the head symptoms had markedly reduced. After 20 treatments these symptoms had vanished altogether and she had begun to show evidence of having a menstrual period. After three further months she was passing thick and clotted dark red blood accompanied by a lot of pain. After a further three months the period had settled down into a regular 28-day cycle and was less physically demanding. The symptoms from the ovarian cyst had diminished by now, although it still gave her some problems. Approximately 14 months after starting treatment Sarah fell pregnant. She went on to have a healthy baby girl and at last contact was doing well. She and John are now considering trying for another baby.

Biography

Tom Williams took his initial professional training in psychology and he has worked as an educational psychologist since 1979. He is currently the Director of Psychological services in East Ayrshire. A long term interest in taiji led him to train in acupuncture at the Northern College of Acupuncture in York. He has subsequently followed this with clinical training in Beijing and a training in Chinese herbal medicine. He is a member of the British Acupuncture Council, a member of the register of Chinese Herbal Medicine and a fellow of the British Psychological Society. He has published books on Chinese medicine and runs a part time practice in Glasgow.

References

1   I. Pain Relief

   a. T Tavola, C Gala, G Conte, G Invernizzi, *Traditional Chinese acupuncture in tension-type headaches: a controlled study,* Pain, 1992; 48 (3): 325-9.

   b. G Ter Reit, J. Kleijnen, P Knipschild, *Acupuncture and chronic pain: a criteria based meta analysis,* Journal of Clinical Epidemiology, 1990; 43(11): 1191-9.

   c. J Filshie, *The non-drug treatment of neuralgic and neuropathic pain of malignancy,* Cancer Survey 1988; 7(1): 161-93.

   d. C A Vincent, *A controlled trial of the treatment of migraine by acupuncture,* Clinical Journal of Pain 1989; 5(4): 305-12.

e. J Hesse, B Mogelvang, H Simonsen, *Acupuncture versus metoprolol in migraine prophylaxis: a randomised trial of trigger point inactivation,* Journal of Internal Medicine, 1994; 235(5):451-6.

f. W Takeda, W Wessel, *Acupuncture for the treatment of pain of osteoarthritic knees,* Arthritis Care Research, 1994; 7(3):118-22.

g. C Deluze, L Bosia, A Zirbs, A Chantraine, T L Vischer, *Electroacupuncture in fibromyalgia: results of a controlled trial,* BMJ, 1992; 305(6864):1249-52.

h. P H Richardson, C A Vincent, *Acupuncture for the treatment of pain: a review of evaluative research,* Pain, 1986; 24(1):15-40.

i. C A Vincent, *A controlled trial of the treatment of migraine by acupuncture,* Clinical Journal of Pain, 1989; 5(4):305-12.

II. Stroke

a. S Sallstrom, A Kjendhal, P E Osten, J K Stanghelle, C F Borchgrevink, *Acupuncture therapy in stroke during the subacute phase: a randomised controlled trial,* Tidsskr Nør Laegeforen, 1995; 115(23): 2884-7

b. K Johansson, I Lindgren, H Widner, I Wiklund, B B Johansson, *Can sensory stimulation improve the functional outcome in stroke patients?,* Neurology, 1993; 43(11):2189-92.

c. B B Johansson, *Has sensory stimulation a role in stroke rehabilitation?,* Scandinavian Journal of Rehabilitative Medicine (Supplement), 1993; 29: 87-96.

d. H H Hu, C Chung, T J Liu, R C Chen, C H Chen, P Chou, W S Huang, J C Lin, J J Tsuei, *A randomised controlled trial on the treatment for acute partial ischemic stroke with acupuncture,* Neuroepidemiology, 1993;12(2): 106-13.

e. M A Naeser, M P Alexander, D Staissny-Eder, L N Lannin, D Bachman, *Acupuncture in the treatment of hand paresis in chronic and acute stroke patients - improvement observed in all cases,* Clinical Rehabilitation, 1994; 8(2): 127-41.

III. Asthma & Related Conditions

a. J Kleijnen, G Ter Reit, P Knipschild, *Acupuncture & astma: a review of controlled trials,* Thorax, 1991; 46(11): 799-802.

b. K Jobst, J H Chen, K McPherson, J Arrowsnmith, V Brown, J Efthimiou, H J Flethcher, G Maciocia, P Mole, K Shiffrin, *Controlled trial of acupuncture for disabling breathlessness,* Lancet, 1986; 2(8521-22): 1416-9.

c. K A Jobst, A critical analysis of acupuncture in pulmonary disease: efficacy and safety of the acupuncture needle, JACM, 1995; 1(1): 55-85.

d. anonymous, *Acupuncture, astma & breathlessness,* Lancet, 1986;2(8521-2): 1427-8.

e. M K Tandon, P F Soh, *Comparison of real and placebo acupuncture in histamine-induced asthma: a double blind crossover study,* Chest, 1989; 96(1):102-5.

f. K P Fung, O K Chow, S Y So, *Attenuation of exercise induced asthma by acupuncture,* Lancet, 19867; 2(8521-2): 1419-21.

g. D Aldridge, P C Pietroni, *Clinical assessment of acupuncture in asthma therapy,* J R Med Soc, 1987; 80(4): 222-4.

IV. Drug & Alcohol Rehabilitation

a. M L Bullock, P D Culliton, R T Olander, *Controlled trial of acupuncture for severe recidivist alcoholism,* Lancet, 1989; 1(8652): 1435-9.

b. G Ter Reit, J Kleijnen, P Knipschild, *A meta analysis of studies into the effect of acupuncture on addiction,* B J of General Practice, 1990; 40(338): 379-82.

c. V Brewington, M Smith, D Lipton, *Acupuncture as a detoxification treatment: ananalysis of controlled research,* Journal of Substance Abuse & Treatment, 1994; 11(4): 289-307.

d. A M Washburn, R E Fullilove, M T Fullilove, P A Keenan, B McGee, K A Morris, J L Sorensen, W W Clark, *Acupuncture heroin detoxification: a single blind clinical trial,* Journal of Substance Abuse & Treatment, 1993; 10(4): 345-51.

e. D S Lipton, V Brewington, M Smith, *Acupuncture for crack cocaine detoxification: experimental evaluation of efficacy,* Journal of Substance Abuse & Treatment, 1994; 11(3): 205-15.

V. General

a. J W Dundee, C McMillan, *Positive evidence for Pericardium 6 acupuncture antiemisis,* Postgrad Med J, 1991; 67(787): 417-22.

b. J W Dundee, R G Ghaly, K T Fitzpatrick, W P Abram, G A Lynch, *Acupuncture prophylaxis of cancer chemotherapy induced sickness,* JR Soc Med, 1989; 82(5): 268-71.

c. C A Vincent, P H Richardson, *Acupuncture for some common disorders: a review of the literature,* JRCGP, 1987; 37(295): 77-81.

Further Reading

Chinese Medicine - General

Kaptchuk, Ted, *Chinese Medicine, The Web That Has No Weaver,* Rider, 1983.

Maciocia, Giovanni, *The Foundations of Chinese Medicine*, Churchill Livingstone, 1989.

Maciocia, Giovanni, *The Practice of Chinese Medicine*, Churchill Livingstone, 1994.

Williams, Tom, *Chinese Medicine*, Element, 1995.

Williams, Tom, *The Illustrated Guide to Chinese Medicine*, Element, 1996.

Beinfield, H & Korngold, E., *Between Heaven and Earth*, Ballantine, 1991.

Wiseman, Ellis & Zmiewski, *The Fundamentals of Chinese Medicine*, Paradigm, 1985.

Acupuncture

Connelly, Dianne, *Traditional Acupuncture, The Law of Five Elements*, Centre for Traditional Acupuncture, 1979.

Mole, Peter, *Acupuncture*, Element Books, 1991.

Seem, Mark, *A New American Acupuncture*, Blue Poppy Press, 1993.

Worsley, J R, *Acupuncture: Is It for You?*, Harper & Row, 1973.

Jirui, Chen; Wang, Nissi (eds), *Acupuncture Case Histories*, Eastland Press, 1988.

Matsumoto, K & Birch S., *Extraordinary Vessels*, Paradigm, 1986.

O'Connor, J & Bensky, D., *Acupuncture, A Comprehensive Text*, Eastland, 1981.

Shudo, D. & Brown S., *Japanese Classical Acupuncture*, Eastland,1990.

Resources

The British Acupuncture Accreditation Board
Park House
London W10 6RE
Tel. 0181- 968 3469

The British Acupuncture Council
Park House,
206 - 208 Latimer Road
London W10 6RE
Tel. 0181-964 0222
Fax. 0181-964 0333

British Medical Acupuncture Society
Newton House
Newton Lane
Whitley
Warrington
Cheshire WA4 4JA
Tel. 01925-730 727
Fax. 01925-730 492

The Register of Chinese Herbal Medicine
P O Box 400
Wembley
Middlesex HA9 9NZ
Tel. 0181-904 1357

Feng Shui Network
P O Box 2133
London W1A 1RL
Tel. 0171-935 8935
Fax. 0171-935 9295

Acupuncture Research & Resource Centre
122A Acomb Road
York YO2 4EY
Tel. 01904-781630
Fax. 01904-782991

United States of America:

Traditional Acupuncture Institute
America City Building
Suite 100
Columbia
Maryland 21044
Tel. 301 596 6006

Affirmations

by David Lawson

Theoretical Background

The power of words, thoughts and beliefs in shaping human life has been recognised in numerous spiritual and healing traditions. Some traditions have focused on the effects that the sound vibration and the meaning of words can have on general well-being by including sacred chants or invocations in rituals of healing. Branches of both Hindu and Islamic traditions have chanted, sung, written or even carved the many names of God as a focus to support devotees on their path to enlightenment and transcendence. Buddhist chants include sounds and phrases for stilling the mind, invoking healing energy (medicine buddha) and cleansing the environment to bring all elemental forces into balance.

Sound Therapy

Eastern and Western traditions alike are filled with prayers, declarations or invocations with meanings as diverse and as colourful as the many cultures that have spawned them, whilst dealing with universal sociological, psychological and spiritual needs. The power of declaration in itself seems to underpin many practices, indicating a widespread understanding that what we ask for we attract; our words, prayers, spells and talismans invite certain experiences or solutions whilst helping us to make sense of the challenges that we face.

Today many people are recognising and using the potency of words, thoughts and beliefs in their own process of self-healing. Knowledge of the power of positive thought is not new, but the ability to stimulate self and others to think in ways that are healthy and transformational has recently become recognised by many complementary practitioners and increasing numbers of medical professionals as a significant healing art in its own right.

One of the techniques for stimulating positive thought and consequently activating the healing process is the use of affirmations. An affirmation is a simple statement or phrase that creates change through repetition. Specific affirmations are chosen for their ability to disrupt, dissolve and replace deeply held thought patterns and beliefs. The intention is to bring healing to the attitudes that have co-created or are contributing to an imbalance within the energetic, physiological or spiritual system.

The idea behind affirmations is essentially simple: we are what we think. The thoughts and beliefs that we hold make us available or magnetic to some experiences and not to others and therefore can increase or decrease our susceptibility to environmental factors, stress, infection and degeneration. They also have their own subtle energetic or vibrational field that can activate the body's ability to heal itself, or alternatively, suppress it. Thus the way that we think can help our bodies to maintain themselves in balance or it can contribute to a state of imbalance that helps to sow the seeds of disharmony and disease.

It could be said that every thought that we think is an affirmation. Every time we have a fearful thought such as, 'I am terrified of making a mistake' or 'I am not going to be able to cope', we are reinforcing underlying negative or fearful beliefs that we have learnt from our parents and the other people in our lives who have had a formative influence upon us. In these examples the underlying beliefs may be that life is unsafe, that it is not all right for us to make a mistake and that we do not trust ourselves to be able to handle the changes and challenges of our lives.

Negative belief patterns like these invite experiences that are disturbing or stressful and that reinforce fears even more. In addition, the energy of these beliefs is dulling for the entire energetic system and in time could co-create disease. The effects of negative thought patterns are emphasised if there are other areas of lifestyle that are also causing an imbalance such as poor diet, lack of exercise, excessive consumption of alcohol or other recreational drugs, an inability to acknowledge and express emotions in an appropriate manner, airborne pollutants and irregular sleep patterns.

Hypnotherapy

Famous exponents of affirmations as tools for healing include the French pharmacist Emile Coué who was born in 1857 and who, in 1920, introduced a method of psychotherapy at his clinic in Nancy that included an affirmational approach. His universal affirmation of health and well-being, 'Every day, and in every way, I am becoming better and better' has outlived him and is still in use today. Coué studied hypnotic techniques and claimed to have effected organic changes through autosuggestion. Like many who work with affirmations today, his emphasis was on teaching other people to heal themselves rather than making assertions about his own healing or therapeutic abilities.

More recently the American author Louise Hay has become famous by providing affirmational techniques through her books and audio tapes.[1] Her ability to popularise the use of affirmations and her willingness to suggest direct connections between health and self-esteem has made these ideas and practices available for many people to use without necessitating the involvement of a therapist or health care professional.

The Practice of Affirmations

One realisation that many health care professionals have made is that current practice within conventional medicine and, to a lesser extent, within complementary therapies can be disempowering for the clients and the practitioners alike. The clients have often been educated to expect to be 'fixed' by their practitioners and frequently surrender their bodies and all responsibility for their health to the doctor, healer or therapist concerned. Many believe that this tendency increases the frustrations for both parties and could actively inhibit the process of healing.

*Self-Responsibility
of the Patient*

In contrast, an approach that encourages clients to take an active role in their healing process and retain some control over their treatments could increase the effectiveness of many therapies, speed up recuperation time and help to prevent complications or a recurrence of their condition. An affirmational approach is ideal for this, providing clients with simple but powerful techniques that they can take charge of for themselves and in liaison with sympathetic healers, doctors and therapists.

*Visualisation
Transformational
Self-Healing*

For the practitioner, the use of affirmations is simple to teach, gives the client a constructive focus for healing between consultations and allows for the creation of a healing partnership where both parties are actively working towards similar goals. In addition, affirmations can be tailored to support specific treatments, help resolve the underlying causes of illness and calm individual fears or anxieties that clients may have.

The key to working effectively with affirmations lies in accurately detecting negative messages that are being reinforced and in creating suitable positive affirmations to supplant them. Examples of positive affirmations to counteract fear would focus on safety and self-trust and may include an expectation of a positive outcome or a positive response from others:

◆ I am always safe.

◆ My life is safe and supportive.

◆ I trust myself.

◆ It is easy for me to succeed.

◆ Other people are helpful and supportive to me.

◆ My life is filled with rewards.

When dealing specifically with a physical problem, such as a headache, a sprained ankle or a tumour, a wider approach needs to be taken that directly addresses the physical symptom as well as helping to transform the overall vocabulary of negative thoughts and beliefs. For example, it may be useful to affirm:

◆ I am always stable and balanced.

◆ I deserve to be happy.

◆ My ankle quickly heals and regenerates itself.

In addition, general affirmations of health and well-being are always helpful in reinforcing a belief that health is attainable and in creating a personal receptivity or availability to healing solutions. Here are some examples:

◆ I see myself in perfect health.

◆ I am always healthy and balanced.

◆ I trust my body to heal itself.

◆ My life is full of healing solutions.

Creating and Using Affirmations

When creating affirmations for specific requirements, it helps to follow some general guidelines for their construction and use. Affirmations need to be phrased in the present tense: for example, 'I now create...' (present simple tense) or 'I am always...' (present continuous tense). If we affirm something as if it is already true, then our minds can more readily make the changes that will alter our experience of life. Whereas, if we affirm that something is going to happen in the future, that is where it will stay, constantly out of reach.

In most cases affirmations need to be positively focused on the desired outcome rather than on the situations or conditions that are wanting release. For example 'I am healthy and relaxed' is a more effective affirmation than 'I am never sick or tense'. The latter will keep attention unduly focused on the negative outcome, continuing to make it a reality.

Affirmations often work best when they are short and easy to remember.

The negative or limiting thoughts are the raw material for creating positive affirmations. Each negative thought contains the foundation for positive change and growth. 'I will never be free of back pain' can become 'My back is free, healthy and comfortable'.

The effectiveness of affirmations is most dependent on the frequency of repetition. An affirmation that is used once will create a small shift of consciousness, whereas an affirmation that is repeated regularly will facilitate a change of underlying beliefs and expectations that can stimulate a process of healing or significantly alter destructive patterns of behaviour and life experience. There are many ways to use affirmations; here are some suggestions.

Affirmations can be written, typed, spoken aloud, sung, chanted and said in front of a mirror as well as being repeated over and over in the mind. Many people find that they benefit from filling their homes with affirmational thoughts, perhaps writing or painting them out in bright colours and pasting them on the bathroom mirror, the refrigerator, on the doors or anywhere else where they will be constantly visible.

Affirmations are wonderful when they are used in conjunction with meditation or physical exercise. Choosing one or two affirmations that are easy to remember and repeating them silently with the rhythm of the breath or in time to the repetition of a familiar exercise can help them to become second nature. Affirmations may be repeated when walking, pacing them out with every step taken.

Affirmations can be easily recorded to be listened to while meditating, relaxing, having a bath, pottering around at home, travelling or at any other time.

Some Useful Affirmations for Common Needs

Relief from frequent headaches – suggested affirmations:

◆ My head is relaxed and comfortable.

◆ I value myself.

◆ My thoughts are always peaceful.

Relief from depression – suggested affirmations:

◆ I am safe with all my feelings.

◆ It is safe for me to express my needs fully.

◆ I have the power to change my life for the better.

Cancer prevention – suggested affirmations:

◆ The cells of my body are always healthy.

◆ My body re-creates itself in health and balance.

◆ My life-force is vibrant and powerful.

Prevention of AIDS related infections – suggested affirmations:

◆ My immune system is strong and healthy.

◆ I am always safe and protected.

◆ It is safe for me to be alive.

Re-awakening the body's ability to heal itself – suggested affirmations:

◆ My body knows perfectly how to heal itself.

◆ I trust my body to heal and recharge itself.

◆ I now activate my innate self-healing power.

Research

The effect of affirmations is subjective and will vary from person to person based upon each individual's unique vocabulary of thoughts and beliefs. For this reason it is difficult to devise scientific trials or tests which accurately prove or disprove the effectiveness of affirmational techniques. However, many practitioners have personal experience of clients who have healed themselves using affirmational techniques alone or in conjunction with appropriate medical or complementary therapies.

Visualisation
Spiritual Healing
Past Life Therapy
Counselling

In my own work I have combined the practice and teaching of affirmations with guided meditation, visualisation, hands-on healing, regression therapy, counselling and role-play amongst other techniques. I have also taught my clients to use affirmations to enhance the effectiveness and help to neutralise the damage of numerous medical procedures from chemotherapy and radiotherapy to surgery or the use of antidepressants. In this way I am able to support clients with the treatments that they themselves are choosing to use.

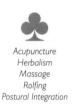

Acupuncture
Herbalism
Massage
Rolfing
Postural Integration

In my opinion, affirmations are at their most effective when used as part of a programme of preventative health care or when used in the treatment of a given condition alongside other appropriate complementary therapies such as acupuncture, body-work, herbal remedies and many others. Using positive affirmations on a regular basis can help us to support all of health care with brightness and love. What is more, the rhythms and discipline of positivity can help us to deal with and transcend the challenges of life while extending the bliss and pleasures of the good times. Affirmations are simple to use and will work for anybody who is willing to persist with them and who is open to experimenting with new, lighter expectations and patterns of thought.

Biography

David Lawson is a healer and a teacher of personal development courses who has worked chiefly in the UK, Ireland, Spain and the USA. He is an authorised facilitator of Louise Hay's 'You Can Heal Your Life' study course programme and a therapist offering hands-on healing, counselling, meditational techniques and regression. David is the author of nine books.

References

1   Louise Hay, *You Can Heal Your Life*, Eden Grove Editions, 1987.

Further Reading

Borysenko, J., *Minding the Body, Mending the Mind*, Addison Wesley Publishing Co. Inc., 1987.

Gawain, Shakti, *Creative Visualisation*, Bantam Books, 1978.

Hay, Louise, *Heal Your Body*, Hay House, Airlift Book Company, 1995.

———, *Life – Reflections on your Journey*, Hay House, 1994.

Lawson, David, *I See Myself in Perfect Health*, Thorsons/Harper Collins, 1995.

———, *Principles of Self Healing*, Thorsons/HarperCollins, 1996.

Ray, Sondra, *I Deserve Love*, Celestial Arts, 1984.

———, *The Only Diet There Is*, Celestial Arts, 1981.

———, *Loving Relationships*, Celestial Arts, 1980.

Troward, Thomas, *The Creative Process in the Individual*, DeVorss & Co., 1991.

Alexander Technique
by Duncan Coppock

The concepts and procedures of the Alexander Technique are derived from the practical methods for change developed by F. M. Alexander. Born in Tasmania in 1869, he began his investigations into how the body functions in order to solve his own vocal problems which seriously interfered with his desire to be an actor. He had developed hoarseness in performance which he realised was caused by something he did. As doctors and voice specialists were unable to help he decided to find out for himself what was amiss and so began many years of self-exploration. His journey not only solved his vocal problems but also resulted in a general improvement in health.

The underlying premise of the Alexander Technique is that the way we use our bodies affects not only our appearance and performance but also our general health. Excess tension, postural distortion and inefficient movement habits can contribute significantly to back, neck and joint pain, migraines, digestion and breathing disorders, and other medical problems. Good use means co-operating with our body's natural design and functioning, allowing its subtle 'automatic' reflexes to give us the proper support in sitting, standing and moving. The best examples, readily available for observation, are two and three-year-olds who have a general grace, freedom and energised way of moving and being. Over the years many of us learn unconscious habits which interfere with this natural co-ordination and the aim of the Alexander Technique is to recognise and release this interference in order to restore natural poise.

People learning the technique may wish to rid themselves of back and neck tension or other medical problems, to reduce stress, to improve posture and appearance, to enhance performance in sport and the performing arts, or simply to live with more awareness in a body-friendly way. What all pupils have in common is a willingness to take responsibility for the way in which they use themselves and the effect this has on their daily lives. While there is a therapeutic effect from the lessons, the real benefits come when pupils learn to apply the principles for themselves.

Background

A full account of Alexander's process of discovery is given in his book *The Use of the Self*. Many of the popular books on the technique devote whole chapters to his story as it gives perspective on what happens in a course of lessons. Here is a brief account of some of the main principles involved.

Working with mirrors, Alexander observed himself and came to realise the importance of a correct head, neck and back relationship. He referred to this as 'the primary control', meaning that the conditions in this area tend to influence the rest of the body. He was also initially surprised to see that what he felt was happening in his body was not always matched by what he observed. He described this as 'faulty sensory awareness' and realised that he could not depend on his feelings to be accurate in relation to his body. There are two aspects to this. Firstly our sense of where our bodies are in space and the relationship of one part to another is experienced in terms of what has become 'normal' for us. For instance if someone is used to to having their head over to the left, when it is brought to the centre it will initially feel to them as if it was now pulled over to the right. Secondly whatever we have become used to 'feels right' and any correction will accordingly 'feel wrong' until we get used to it. When 'trying harder' to change we invariably rely on what 'feels right' to us and it is here that the support of a teacher is invaluable. This is why learning the technique on one's own is very challenging.

As Alexander progressed with his experiments he refined his concept of the primary control and learned consciously to project thoughts or 'directions' which helped bring about the conditions which he wanted. For example: 'Let the neck be free, to let the head release forward and up, to let the back lengthen and widen.' These directions are commonly used in lessons with pupils. When properly understood they are simply reminders to let go of interference and allow the body to do what it wants to do when working naturally.

This work was sufficient to improve Alexander's condition in some situations but when attempting to recite, he found that he would go back to his old habits with consequent detrimental effects on his voice. He saw that he must take into account 'the force of habit' which was linked to the habit of 'end-gaining'. By this he meant the habit of being taken over by our desire to accomplish something, so that we not only forget but are actually unable to pay attention to the 'means-whereby' we reach our goal.

In modern society this has become such a way of life that we may not even question it and yet we are all subject to its tyranny and can feel cheated if our bodies do not live up to our expectations. In applying the technique to daily life we not only improve our physical awareness but, at the same time, examine our attitudes to living so that in a very practical way we experience the interrelationship of body and mind.

As a way of freeing himself from the domination of harmful automatic reactions, Alexander came to focus more and more on the inhibition of old patterns of interference, realising that once they were less dominant it was relatively simple to bring about new healthier conditions. Rather than 'doing the right thing' he learned to stop doing the wrong thing, so that the right thing could happen by itself.

Compared to what Alexander went through, very little is asked of a pupil taking a course of lessons with the help of a teacher. Yet many pupils find that it does take time and commitment and that his journey, and to some extent his challenges, are echoed in their own learning process. It is not a matter of a quick fix. Progress is dependent on the willingness to explore and apply what is learnt.

Learning the Technique

Naturally all teachers vary somewhat in their approach. Some will explain the process in detail and discuss with pupils their experiences between lessons. Others will work more in silence, expecting pupils to integrate the lessons in their own way. My personal preference is to emphasise conscious understanding and participation with teacher and pupil working as a team. We will consider the common factors involved in a course of lessons and then look at some particular applications.

As the technique is concerned with general co-ordination and quality of movement it can be of benefit to anyone wishing to learn and people may be motivated by a variety of reasons. These include health problems, injury prevention, posture and appearance, performance in sport and the arts, or self-awareness and personal growth.

If one is receiving treatment from a doctor or other health professional, it is advisable to talk with them before taking on a new discipline, but the technique is educational rather than a treatment, and is seldom, if ever, contraindicated on medical grounds. The real contraindications have to do with wrong motivation. If someone is expecting a quick 'cure' or having lessons because somebody else, a parent or spouse, thinks they ought to, then it is unlikely to be of much benefit. Ideally the technique becomes an ongoing personal discipline freely chosen and approached in the spirit of play and self-exploration. The right motivation comes from the realisation that choices can be made that improve our quality of life.

People of all ages have benefited, including George Bernard Shaw, who started taking lessons in his eighties. Children can also benefit provided they enjoy it and want to do it, though their short span of attention can be a difficulty. They are probably best influenced by being around adults who use it for themselves.

The technique is taught as a series of one-to-one lessons, usually on a weekly basis although it may help to come more frequently in the early stages and this can be discussed with the teacher. Introductory group courses are given by some teachers and these give an overview of the principles involved and provide prospective pupils with a sample of what is in store.

A First Lesson

A first lesson does not put the pupil under any obligation and permits a meeting with the teacher, allows an experiential sense of what is involved and gives time to ask questions. In turn, the teacher may ask about the reasons for investigating the technique and a case history will be taken. These details are not required for diagnosis but rather to understand the demands of the pupil's particular life situation, in order that the lessons may be adjusted to suit the specific needs.

The location and movement potential of major joints in the body will be pointed out and, with a combination of verbal explanation and gentle touch, pupils will be helped to be aware of and release unnecessary tension. At the same time they will be guided to experience different, simpler patterns of co-ordination and movement, and will be introduced to the Alexander directions. They will also be shown the 'Alexander rest position' which they will be encouraged to use for themselves on a daily basis. Pupils remain fully clothed during the lesson.

In the rest position, the body is supine, with knees up and head supported, while the Alexander directions are applied mentally to bring about release and opening. The effects are cumulative, with the practice done at home reinforcing the experience with the teacher. The purpose is twofold: firstly one learns to release tension and secondly it is a reference experience from which one learns to maintain the same qualities of freedom, openness and alignment in sitting, standing and movement. In a lesson teachers use their hands gently to encourage the release of interference and to establish better co-ordination. They will also teach the use of thought projection or directions, which can be used to bring about better conditions in daily living. Over a period of time most people find the rest position a very enjoyable and rewarding daily routine, which they are encouraged to continue on a preventative basis.

The touch of an Alexander teacher is very gentle and it is unlikely that anyone will be asked to do anything that causes or increases pain. There is no pressure to 'push through' resistance and pupils are encouraged to form a partnership in the learning process and to make their own decisions about what movements or activities they feel ready to do.

Ongoing Lessons

Whilst most people experience some benefits from just a few lessons, a basic course consists of 20 or more lessons. As with learning a language or a musical instrument, progress depends on individual aptitude and commitment and, as with any learning situation, there will be times of insight, times of consolidation and times when it feels as if nothing much is happening. It is important to remember that it is not a quick fix or a few treatments but rather a process of re-education involved with changing the habits of a lifetime.

Part of each lesson will be spent in sitting, standing, walking and other activities, and part will be spent in the lying down position. Often considerable attention will be given to 'chair-work' where the pupil is guided from sitting to standing and vice versa. There are a number of different things involved here which may not always be pointed out explicitly and the pupils can think they are learning 'the correct' movement for getting in and out of a chair rather than 'a way' of moving that leaves the body free and well co-ordinated. Well-balanced sitting and standing are important as is the required co-ordination of hip, knee and ankle joints to move from one position to the other while leaving the spine free and open – the same basic co-ordination as is required for squatting and lifting. What becomes obvious as lessons progress is the way that we tense habitually in response to any stimulus to action and a major part of what is then learned is to be aware of and release our unnecessary and harmful reactions. This can then be applied in other life situations whether they be participating in particular activities or interacting with other people.

In applying the principles and awareness to other activities they may be worked on directly in the lessons (for example playing a musical instrument) or else discussed with the teacher (as in the case of housework or applications to sport). In the final analysis individuals make the technique their own and integrate it into their lives in whatever way serves them. This takes time and patience and, in the beginning, pupils are often shocked to find that despite their good intentions whole days can go by with little or any awareness of body use. This is a reminder of just how strong habits can be, and what is then required is a combination of gentle persistence and realistic acceptance of ourselves. It is good to do the lying down for 20 minutes or so on a daily basis and it can also be helpful to spend a little quiet time each day 'giving oneself a lesson'. If a job involves lifting or other potentially harmful actions, then clearly attention needs to be given to body use in carrying them out. Throughout the day, attention can be given to particular activities, such as brushing teeth or making a cup of tea to increase personal awareness of movement. Bit by bit the ability to pay attention and improve use, expands, whatever is being done. In the process one can become aware of how basic attitudes to life and to ourselves can help or hinder us and in particular one may need to consider to what extent end-gaining dominates one's life.

Osteopathy Chiropractic

The Alexander Technique is educative rather than a treatment and is often suggested by doctors and other health professionals to complement their work. In particular osteopaths, chiropractors or physiotherapists, having alleviated some severe symptoms of misuse, may then recommend the technique to prevent further problems occurring.

Benefits

Ideally the technique is learned as a preventative discipline before problems occur but people frequently come to it with a history of discomfort and after conventional treatment has failed. Many complaints such as back and neck problems are strongly influenced by poor posture and excess tension and unless these causes are addressed removal of symptoms by drugs or manipulation may be short-lived.[1] Releasing tension, using the proper bending joints and allowing the natural balancing reflexes to support us takes strain off vulnerable parts of the spine. Sometimes a symptom such as a 'trapped nerve' can respond almost immediately to the Alexander approach but it is more likely that relief comes over a period of time as the pupil learns to release chronic patterns of misuse. Even when the technique on its own does not relieve pain, the release of tension and improved use will always be helpful and tend to support other approaches.

Although headaches and migraines can be caused by a number of factors they are frequently contributed to by excessive neck tension at the base of the skull. Learning to monitor and release this tension before it builds up can be a significant tool for preventing severe attacks. Similarly, general stress contributes to many other problems, both physical and emotional, and the Alexander Technique helps individuals take some responsibility for recognising and releasing tension before major traumas develop.

Poor use over a period of time produces many physical complaints and can also lead to injuries at home and work. Many back problems are caused by poor use in lifting and handling and lessons in the technique can be a very effective preventative measure. Office workers can suffer from repetitive strain injury (RSI) and other problems contributed to by chronic misuse, and whilst good ergonomic layout of desks, chairs and keyboards is important, it needs to be complemented by good posture and co-ordination. Sports injuries can also be reduced by developing a more 'body-friendly' approach to performance.

Pregnancy, birth and adapting to a new baby can place great strain on the mother's body and if misuse is already present then this can lead to backache and other problems. Lessons in the technique can be one of the greatest supports throughout.[2]

Many people take lessons because of a history of poor posture about which they want to do something effective. Conventional advice such as to 'pull your shoulders back and hold your tummy in' does nothing to remedy the causes and produces strain that can in turn lead to chronic pain. Concern with how we carry and present ourselves can be a very valid reason for taking lessons and should not be confused with vanity. Allowing ourselves to be physically open and expanded not only improves appearance, health and confidence but can also give a sense of being more fully one's self.

The major music and drama schools in Britain and America have had Alexander teachers on their staff for many years since they realise that any unnecessary tension interferes with performance and expression. The calming and grounding effects also help in mental preparation and in dealing with stage fright. Dancers find that unconscious movement habits cause them to work against themselves and that by recognising and releasing unnecessary effort they gain both greater freedom and more power.

The same principles apply in sport where learning to move with greater freedom and co-ordination results in improved performance and less injury, and many top athletes demonstrate a sense of effortlessness which is one of the aims of the technique. Horse-riders in particular have adopted many principles from the technique and some Alexander teachers specialise in working with riders.

For the majority of pupils change takes place to the extent that they are ready for it, without any emotional upheaval or therapeutic process, and the motivations to reduce pain, improve appearance or enhance performance are valid in themselves. At the same time for those wishing to work more deeply on themselves in the areas of self-awareness and personal growth, whether from a therapeutic or spiritual perspective, the Alexander Technique has an enormous amount to offer and can be explored and developed over a lifetime. Our bodies are the most tangible expression of ourselves and can be a mirror to how much we are true to ourselves. Denial, whether it be of our physicality, emotions or higher impulses results in holding and contraction, and releasing and opening up physically can inform and support us in the change process. It is helpful to think that the patterns we have developed have had some purpose, even if they are now redundant and limiting, and the technique gives new possibilities at the same time as releasing old tension and does not force change before it is ready.[3]

Biography

Duncan Coppock teaches the Alexander Technique in Inverness, Forres and Fochabers, Scotland. Before this he maintained a private teaching practice in taught Alexander studies to performance arts students at the Middlesex University, and taught Alexander courses and workshops for a variety of organisations. He has also collaborated on workshops relating the technique to voice and movement and co-led a week-long programme, for the Findhorn Foundation, in which physical awareness and the principles of the technique were related to personal and spiritual growth. He has also helped to train Alexander teachers at the North London Teacher Training School for the Alexander Technique. He has been involved with the field of personal development for over 20 years, has a background as a teacher, has been a performer, and has led business seminars in communication skills.

References

1   Deborah Caplan, *Back Trouble – A New Approach to Prevention and Recovery based on the Alexander Technique*, Triad Publ. Co., 1987.

2   Ilana Machover, Angela and Jonathan Drake, *Pregnancy and Birth the Alexander Way*, Robinson Publ., 1993.

3   Glen Park, *The Art of Changing – A New Approach to the Alexander Technique*, Ashgrove, 1989.

Further Reading

Alexander, F. Matthias, *The Use of the Self*, Gollancz, 1985 (first published 1932).

Barlow, Dr Wilfred, *The Alexander Principle*, (first published 1973), Gollancz, 1990.

Caplan, Deborah; *Back Trouble – A New Approach to Prevention and Recovery based on the Alexander Technique*, Triad Publ., Co., 1987.

Drake, Jonathan, *The Alexander Technique in Everyday Life*, Thorsons, 1996.

Drake, Jonathan, *Body Know-How – A Practical Guide to the Use of the Alexander Technique in Everyday Life*, Thorsons, 1991.

———, *Introductory Guide to the Alexander Technique*, Thorsons, 1993.

Gelb, Michael, *Body Learning*, (first published 1981), Aurum Press, 1994.

McCallion, Michael, *The Voice Book*, Faber & Faber, 1988.

Park, Glen, *The Art of Changing – A New Approach to the Alexander Technique*, Ashgrove, 1989.

Stevens, Chris, *Experimental Studies in the Alexander Technique*, Centerline Press, 1996.

Forsstrom, Brita and Mel Hampson, *The Alexander Technique for Pregnancy and Childbirth*, Gollancz, 1995.

Machover, Ilana, Angela and Jonathan Drake, *Pregnancy and Birth the Alexander Way*, Robinson Publ., 1993.

Resources

The Society of Teachers of the Alexander Technique – STAT – was established in 1958 and is the internationally recognised representative body. The Society has over 1200 members worldwide and around 500 teaching members in the UK. They are professionally qualified and adhere to a published code of ethics. Monitoring and developing standards of training are important aspects of the Society's work and all its members have completed a three-year, full-time training course and have reached a standard approved by the Society. A list of qualified teachers can be obtained by sending a stamped addressed envelope to:

STAT
20 London House
266 Fulham Road
London SW10 9EL
Tel. 0171-351 0828

Professional Association of Alexander Teachers
14 Metchley Court
Harborne
Birmingham B17 0JP
Tel. 0121-426 2108

Anthroposophical Medicine

compiled by Lori Forsyth

Historical Background

Rudolf Steiner (1861-1925), the Austrian scientist and philosopher, was the founder of a new kind of science in which both the human being and the natural world are described, not only physically but also in terms of soul and spirit. He called this science 'anthroposophy'.

During the last seven years of his life, Steiner was asked increasingly to speak on subjects which had immediate relevance for practical work, for example medicine, education and agriculture. These lectures were generally given to people who were professionally active in these fields and wished to apply the knowledge gained from anthroposophy in their work. Of the 30 or so doctors who attended his first course of medical lectures in 1921, it was with the Dutch physician Ita Wegman (1876-1943) that a very close collaboration developed. She was the founder of the first anthroposophical clinic in Arlesheim, Switzerland and was co-author with Steiner of the book *Fundamentals of Therapy*.[1]

Steiner stressed that anthroposophical medicine was no simple alternative to conventional medicine, whose achievements in its own sphere he fully acknowledged. Anthroposophical doctors will make full use of conventional medical technology when this offers benefit to the patient. He pointed out, however, that these conventional methods were the outcome of a reductionist science and that when this was applied in the areas of biology and medicine it often led to misleading conclusions. He had developed his own scientific methodology which he employed to explore how the human soul and spiritual nature influence the life and function of the physical body.

Basic Concepts

Physiology

The main aim of anthroposophical medicine is to stimulate the natural healing forces within the human being. Steiner called these 'etheric' forces. They sustain life in all its forms, including the processes of growth, reproduction and repair. The conscious life of emotions, which the human being shares with animals, is an expression of what Steiner called the 'astral body'. He also described an 'ego organisation' which is each human being's individual core. These three aspects plus the physical body are the four principles of the human being. In pointing to the corresponding affinities between these four bodies and the four traditional elements (earth, water, fire and air), Steiner was able to outline how a bridge is built between the mineral substances of the human body and the spiritual core of the human being.

From this basis Steiner proceeded to describe how the four bodies co-operate with each other within three distinct but functionally interpenetrating systems: the nerve–sense system, the rhythmic system and the metabolic system. The nerve–sense system is the basis of conscious waking life, which continually erodes the life and vitality of the physical body. This is replenished during sleep when physical and etheric forces assert themselves in the metabolism. From the tension between these two opposing dynamics, illness in the human being arises. Health is a sign that a temporary equilibrium has been established between these two systems.

While conventional medicine generally attributes all aspects of conscious awareness in human beings to the brain, Steiner suggested that all three systems (nerve–sense, rhythmic and metabolic) are of equal importance, both psychologically and physiologically. He acknowledged the brain to be an instrument of thinking, but suggested that the organs of metabolism and the limbs were to be seen as the bodily foundations for the life of the will. Feeling arises through interplay of the conscious thinking processes and the unconscious life of will and expresses itself directly in circulatory and respiratory functions. The strongly psychosomatic orientation within anthroposophical medicine is based on this fundamental picture.

Pathology

In pathology two opposite kinds of illness are distinguished. When physical and etheric forces gain the upper hand in the metabolism, inflammatory or feverish conditions occur. Illnesses of this kind are characteristic of childhood – for example measles and chickenpox – and are regarded as having an important influence in protecting the body from the hardening effects of the nerve-sense system, as well as strengthening the immune system. In contrast, degenerative or sclerotic conditions are the characteristic of the second part of life. These are seen to occur when the waking activity of the nerve-sense system has been the dominant one over a long period of time. These illnesses, which are often accompanied by sleeplessness, anxiety and a subnormal temperature, belong especially to North America and Western Europe, and are considered to be connected to the general intellectual culture of the present age, especially when this has been introduced too soon into a child's education.

Treatment

Anthroposophical medicine has developed many new forms of treatment. The most intensive area of work and research has been cancer, for which a number of medicinal preparations have been developed from the plant mistletoe (*Viscum album*).[2] Of these, Iscador® is the most well known and widely used in this country and has been prescribed by both anthroposophical and homoeopathic physicians. It has been shown to have an immunostimulant effect and research, involving increasing numbers of doctors and surgeons throughout Europe, suggests that in certain types of cancer this medicine may reduce the rate of tumour growth and the likelihood of metastatic spread. Anthroposophical medicines are prepared from substances taken from the mineral, plant or animal kingdom in which forces counterbalancing those of the particular illness may be found. In order to strengthen these forces in the direction of one of the body's main functional systems, many anthroposophically developed pharmaceutical processes are used, in addition to those which are used in homoeopathy and herbal medicine.

Homoeopathy
Herbalism

The seven metals (lead, tin, iron, gold, copper, mercury and silver) have a central importance in anthroposophical therapy through their relationship to different organs of the body. New methods have been developed of 'potentising' these metals through the use of particular plants. Steiner also drew special attention to the therapeutic activity of the essential oils of plants (for example rosemary, lavender, thyme, etc.) which are used in anthroposophical medicine to stimulate the peripheral circulation. They are especially of value in the treatment of degenerative illnesses, including cancer, multiple sclerosis, diabetes and arteriosclerosis and may either be applied directly to the skin by massage or compresses, or be finely dispersed in water and administered by way of medicinal baths.

Aromatherapy
Massage

Within anthroposophical medicine a number of schools of artistic therapy have developed, including sculpture, painting and speech, as well as a form of movement therapy called eurythmy, which Steiner was himself instrumental in creating. While most forms of artistic therapy emphasise the need to bring unconscious feelings to outward expression, the anthroposophically trained artistic therapists will also guide and direct patients into specific exercises based upon a deep understanding of the physiological effects of colour, form and movement. Artistic therapies also help patients to participate actively in the process of restoring their own health.

Art Therapy

A special form of rhythmic massage was developed by Dr Ita Wegman based on an understanding of the relationship between the nerve-sense and metabolic systems. It has a harmonising and integrating effect on many bodily functions, including breathing, circulation, digestion and muscle tone.

The Availability of Anthroposophical Medicine

In Europe there are more than a thousand doctors working with anthroposophical medicine in general practice and numerous smaller clinics, sanatoria and therapeutic centres. There are also ten larger clinics with hospital status working within the specialities of general medicine and psychiatry. Two of these are able to provide the complete range of specialist treatment expected of any general hospital, one of which (Herdecke Hospital) has been granted the status of a teaching hospital within the medical department of the University of Witten, Germany. In the UK, anthroposophical doctors work both within the NHS and privately. Residential treatment is available at two centres, one in Worcestershire and one in Kent.

Case Study: Cancer of the Breast

In 1994, Mary, age 42, was diagnosed with cancer of the breast. The following is her own account of her treatment at Park Attwood, a residential clinic in the Midlands of England.

I went to see my GP as soon as I spotted a lump in my breast. Within the week I was in the hospital for tests and within two weeks I had had my operation. The problem with this was the shock of it all. Within the space of three weeks I had a mastectomy and was facing a course of powerful drug treatment (radiotherapy, chemotherapy) to prevent any further recurrence. I remember feeling dazed, with no time and no confidence to make my own choices or even realise there may be alternatives.

Although the team in hospital was very supportive, once I left the safe and clinical environment I was very much left to cope on my own. Someone suggested I go to Park Attwood as they might be able to help me gather myself together and get swiftly on the road to recovery.

My initial experience at the clinic was really just one of peace and quiet. I was given a room looking out over the hills. I received some very valuable counselling from the medical staff, which gave me a chance to look back over my life history – my biography – and make sense of my current situation without the anger or bitterness that so many cancer patients react with initially. I began a programme that included massage, eurythmy (movement therapy) and painting therapy, all of which I found very helpful. In the painting sessions, we started with some simple exercises, applying watercolour to wet or dry paper to get different effects. I hadn't done any painting since I was a teenager. I worked with a particular style called 'veil painting' which involves building an image out of thin washes or layers of paint, brushed onto paper in broad, slow strokes. I painted with pale, subtle colours. I found the therapy very calming and drew a lot of strength from it. I tend naturally to be impatient and want to get on with things and this exercise helped me to slow down and to take stock, to be more methodical. My programme was aimed at this, learning to be less frantic.

In the eurythmy sessions, we developed movements by first visualising the gesture and then following it through physically. The mind enables the body to perform the movement more fully, so that it is more than just a mechanical action. We made various patterns, walking in a slow, methodical way, thinking about each step. There is a five-pointed star image to visualise when doing this stepping exercise. At each point of the star there is a moment of pause, both for relaxation and as preparation for the next step, so one takes stock before moving forwards, which was symbolically useful for me. I think it helped me accept the experience of my illness and the results of my operation and from there to move onwards.

My medical treatment was mainly Iscador which is a plant remedy made from mistletoe. It is based on homoeopathic principles and is used to stimulate the natural healing processes in the body and the immune system. The type and strength of Iscador may vary for each individual and also the frequency with which it is given. Although it is a course of injections, it can be administered by the patients themselves

I have never been a good sleeper, as I am not good at relaxing in any form, and I was prescribed other remedies to help me get a good night's sleep – to assist the healing process. I also received other supportive anthroposophic medicines and external applications such as warm compresses applied to the liver area, which is a very restful treatment.

I left Park Attwood after three weeks, much improved, feeling ready to get on with life. The understanding of my situation and my needs is the best thing my stay there has given me. It has helped me to come to terms with what the future may hold. Generally speaking, my health is good, I am less tired and back at work full-time. I return to Park Attwood as an outpatient every couple of months, for a consultation, for more Iscador, for massage therapy and I hope to do more painting too. This ongoing support is what makes Park Attwood special; it is counselling underwritten by solid medical understanding.

References

1   Rudolf Steiner; Ita Wegman, *Fundamentals of Therapy*, Rudolf Steiner Press, 1983.

2   Kovacs, Eva; Hajto, Tibor; Hostanska, Katerina, *Improvement of DNA repair in lymphocytes of breast cancer patients treated with Viscum album extract* (Iscador®), Eur J Cancer, 1991; 27: 12, 1672-6.

    Salzer, Georg, *70 years of mistletoe therapy and no proof of efficacy?*, JAM, 1994; 11: 2, 20-6 (originally published in Dtsch Zschr Onkologie, 1993; 25: 4, 93-7).

Further Reading

Bentheim T V., et al, *Caring for the Sick at Home*, Floris Books, 1987.

Easton, S., *Man and the World in the Light of Anthroposophy*, Rudolf Steiner Press, 1970.

Evans, M.; Rodger, I., *Anthroposophical Medicine – Treating Body, Soul and Spirit*, Thorsons, 1992.

Glockler, M.; Goebel, W., *A Guide to Child Health*, Floris Books, 1990.

Lissau, R., *Rudolf Steiner: Life, Work, Inner Path and Social Initiatives*, Hawthorn Press, 1987.

Steiner, Rudolf, *Knowledge of the Higher Worlds. How is it Achieved?*, Rudolf Steiner Press, 1985.

———, *The Philosophy of Freedom, the Basis for a Modern World Conception*, Rudolf Steiner Press, 1970.

Resources

All of the above books are available from:

Rudolf Steiner Bookshop
35 Park Road
London NW1 6XT

or:

Mail Order, Biblios
Glenside Industrial Estate
Star Road
Partridge Green
West Sussex
RH13 8LD
Tel. 01403 710971

Training Centres and courses:
Park Attwood Clinic
Trimpley
Bewdley
Worcestershire DY12 1RE
Tel. 01299-861 444
Fax. 012997-861 375

Courses for nurses:
Joan Smith
Thornbury Camphill Community
The Sheiling School
Thornbury Park
Bristol BS12 1HP

Rhythmic massage training:
Adrian Large
Park Attwood Clinic
Trimpley
Bewdley
Worcestershire DY12 1RE
Tel. 01299-861 444
Fax. 012997-861 375

Hibernia School of Artistic Therapy
Hawkwood College
Painswick Old Road
Stroud
Gloucestershire GL6 7QW

Training in biographical counselling
Centre for Social Development
Old Plaw Hatch House
Sharpthorne
West Sussex RH19 4JL

Training course for doctors and medical students:
Dr Frank Mulder
Park Attwood Clinic
Trimpley
Bewdley
Worcestershire DY12 1RE
Tel. 01299-861 444
Fax. 012997-861 375

Medical section seminar on Mental Health
Cherry Orchards Camphill Community
Canford Lane
Westbury on Trym
Bristol BS9 3PF

Training in curative eurythmy:
Linda Nunhofer
Peredur Centre for the Arts
Dunnings Road
East Grinstead
West Sussex RH19 4NF

Anthroposophical Medical Trust
Orlingbury House
Lewes Road
Forest Row
Sussex RH18 5HA

The Natural Medicines Society
Market Chambers
13a Market Place
Heanor
Derbyshire DE75 7AA

Aromatherapy

by Sue Jenkins

History

Aromatherapy in its present form began in 1928, when the Frenchman R. M. Gattéfossé coined this term for the alleviation of health problems with essential oils. Since then the therapy has blossomed, brought by a Frenchwoman, Marguerite Maury, to Britain, where it is now one of the most popular complementary therapies.[1]

The roots of the therapy go back at least 4000 years and have their origin in the use of plants as food, cosmetics, medicine, mood alterers, and in ritual. Initially plants were used in their entirety or made into macerated oils, infusions, decoctions and unguents. These were used all over the world, but most of the ancient wisdom concerning plant medicine comes from the Far East, China, India, the Middle East and the native cultures of South America. Only more recently has worldwide scientific research been carried out into the actions of essential oils.[2]

It was thought that the first distilled oil was produced in Persia in the eleventh century by an Arab doctor, Avicenna. However an ancient terracotta still, dated to 4000 years ago, has been found in the Far East.[3] Distilled oils may therefore have been used by the Egyptians, Greeks and Romans. Culinary and medicinal plants – and possibly essential oils – were brought to Britain by the Romans and then later by the returning Crusaders. Oils and the plants from which they come are mentioned several times in the literature of the Middle Ages and Elizabethan period, notably in Shakespeare's plays. In the Middle Ages apothecaries dispensed essential oils, which were used in healing in nunneries and monasteries, in large houses (where the mistress of the house would have her own still room), and in villages, where the wise woman was generally healer, counsellor and midwife.

Use decreased with the rise of medical science, and later with the chemist's ability to isolate the active ingredient in a plant and produce synthetic drugs. The synthetically produced or 'nature identical' product can never be exactly like the real thing, as the chemists cannot quite replicate the natural chemistry of, say, rose or jasmine oil, which contains up to 300 different chemical components. Although use in Britain fell off in the seventeenth century, essential oils continued to be used in the perfume

industry in France and it was from there that modern aromatherapy
now spread worldwide. It is said that Gattéfossé, a chemist in his fɑ
business, stumbled upon the healing properties of lavender oil when he bur
arm in a Bunsen burner flame and plunged it into a bowl of lavender oil. B
scientist he was intrigued by the rapid and complete healing of the burn and began
to do research into the effects and properties of essential oils. He was followed by
an army surgeon called Jean Valnet and then by other French doctors who developed
the use of essential oils in the treatment of illness.

The most common application of aromatherapy is massage with essential oils.
However, massage is not always an appropriate form of treatment and there are
many other ways of using essential oils. The French tradition uses essential oils
internally in a variety of ways; however, in order to practise in that way in France
one must first be a trained medical doctor.

Massage

Extraction of Oils

Essential oils are complex mixtures of chemical compounds, produced in different
processes: steam or water distillation, pressure extraction, solvent extraction, CO_2
extraction and enfleurage. They are obtained from many parts of plants – flowers,
leaves, twigs, roots, fruit, seeds, bark and heartwood. In steam or water distillation,
steam or boiling water is passed through the plant material which gives up its oil.
The resultant mixture of steam or water and oil is passed through a cooling chamber
and the water and oil collected. The oil is drawn off, while the water is either
recycled or sold as floral water. Plants most suitable for pressure extraction are
orange, bergamot and lemon. Oils obtained by solvent extraction are called absolutes
and some aromatherapists prefer not to use them, considering that they may have
been tainted by any residue of solvent. CO_2 extraction gives a fine oil, but is expensive
to carry out. Traditionally, delicate flower oils, such as rose and jasmine, have been
extracted by the lengthy and costly process called enfleurage, in which petals are
placed on layers of fat and left as long as three weeks for the fat to absorb the oils.
The resultant pomade is then washed in alcohol to separate the essential oil from the
fat. This process is rarely used today.[4]

How Essential Oils Work on the Client

Essential oils enter the body by inhalation and transference to the blood stream, via
the nose, lungs and skin by means of massage, baths, perfumes, etc. Essential oils,
when inhaled, affect the brain directly by means of neuro-chemical messages which
are picked up by the olfactory nerve endings in the nose and passed to the limbic
area, the oldest part of our complex brain. From there they rapidly affect our moods
and emotions. They give rise to complex chemical changes in the body, such as
increased lactation, increased or decreased libido, and the release of encephalins
and endorphins, which act as the body's natural painkillers and produce sensations

of well-being and calm. During respiration the molecules of oil pass into the lungs and thence by diffusion into the bloodstream with oxygen. This is facilitated by the small molecular size of essential oils and the single-cell thickness of the alveoli and blood capillaries of the lungs. Oils pass by diffusion into the skin during massage, crossing the stratum corneum, the outer layer of the skin, entering the epidermis and the dermis and thence into the capillary circulation. Essential oils can act very quickly, as well as over a period of time, being released into the blood stream and distributed around the body. They are then excreted in respiration, sweat, urine or faeces.[5]

Individual chemicals within essential oils are known to have certain properties and this may account for the physiological effects of a particular oil. The skill in combining certain oils for a specific treatment relies on a synergy arising from the combining of chemicals. Within any given oil, some chemicals will be beneficial in themselves, whilst others may inhibit possible unpleasant reactions, such as skin irritation. This is known as 'quenching'.[6]

It is not known exactly how essential oils do work, but their effects on high blood pressure, anxiety states, bleeding and skin problems, to name but a few conditions, are becoming more well known as more research is being carried out into the properties of the individual chemicals, the oils themselves and their effects on human beings.

The Practice of Aromatherapy

Essential oils may be used in many different ways:

♦ Massage, when usually no more than 3 drops of essential oils are diluted in 5 ml of a base oil, such as sweet almond or sunflower oil, and applied to the body. For the elderly, children and those with sensitive skins use 1 drop in 5 ml. The base oils themselves have healing properties and are chosen accordingly to complement the effects of the essential oils.

♦ Baths, when usually a maximum of 8 drops is used in a drawn bath and the person is allowed to soak for 15-20 minutes. For babies, children and the elderly 1-3 drops are used and are generally diluted first in vodka or full fat milk to ensure their dispersion in the bath.

♦ Compresses, when about 20 drops of essential oil are added to 1-2 pints of water (cool or hot depending on the condition) and the area to be treated is covered with a cloth impregnated with the oil and water.

♦ Inhalations, when 2-6 drops of essential oil are added to 1-2 pints of very hot water and inhaled, usually to clear some respiratory problem.

♦ Vaporisation, when 5-10 drops of essential oil are dropped onto water in a receptacle above a candle which is then lit. The oil and water evaporate with the heat and the fragrance fills the room.

◆ Douches, used for urinogenital infections, when about 5 drops of essential oil is added to 1 litre of boiled, cooled water and used in a sitz bath, bidet or as an external, local wash. Suppositories and pessaries may also be used.

◆ Toiletries and cosmetics, when creams, lotions, aftershaves, hair products and gels containing essential oils may be used to alleviate skin and hair problems.

◆ Internal use, at the present time, is a rare form of treatment in the UK, only provided by practitioners with extensive further training and special insurance cover by the Aromatherapy Association.

At a first treatment the aromatherapist will take a detailed medical history and also question the client about lifestyle in order to build up as complete a picture of the individual as possible. This is to enable the therapist to provide a specific and holistic blend of oils and treatment.

Massage is likely to form part of the treatment and the client may be given oils in some form to use at home. A patch test may be used to ascertain the client's skin sensitivity to particular oils.

Duration of treatment is from 30 minutes for a consultation to at least 90 minutes for consultation and full body massage.

Frequency of treatment varies with the individual, the severity and duration of the condition and the individual's response to treatment. In some cases weekly treatment may be necessary, and usually treatment can gradually be spaced out more and more. Aromatherapy is also a preventative or maintenance therapy and most people would benefit in some way from treatment, especially massage, approximately every four weeks to alleviate stress and promote well-being. It is advisable to vary oils used on a continual basis in order to prevent adverse reactions or intolerance.

Treatment is for the whole person – mind, body and spirit – as essential oils work on all levels and affect the whole being. It can also be used for the alleviation of specific physical symptoms.[7]

Applications

Aromatherapy is most definitely a complementary therapy in that it can be used alongside allopathic medicine and most other therapies. One exception may be homoeopathy as there is a risk of the essential oils nullifying the effect of the homoeopathic remedy. Research is currently being carried out in this area.[8] Aromatherapy works particularly well alongside Bach flower remedies and in conjunction with colour[9] and crystal healing, and with herbal and traditional Chinese medicine.[10]

Homoeopathy
Flower Essences
Colour Therapy
Crystal Healing
Herbalism
Traditional Chinese
Medicine

Aromatherapy may be useful for all manner of problems, particularly stress-related conditions. It can be used to alleviate many kinds of discomfort – from skin problems such as acne or eczema to painful or irregular menstruation. Muscular aches, rheumatism and insomnia all respond well to treatment with essential oils. Essential oils are especially good for boosting the immune system, for example, lavender, titree, manuka and thyme oils. Dr Daniel Pénoël once classed aromatherapy as the 'immune system of mankind'.[11] It is interesting that essential oils seem to affect the mind-body interface and influence cells and cell structure at the level of neurotransmitters, thus affecting cell memory and effecting physical, mental and emotional changes.[12]

Aromatherapy is a kind of energy medicine, where the vibrational energy of plants may be used to improve the energy of humans (as well as animals and other plants) in terms of mind, body and spirit. On a subtle level it is thought that essential oils influence the aura and chakra energies. For instance, rose and bergamot seem particularly good for the heart chakra and frankincense for the base chakra, for 'grounding'. Some oils seem to work on several chakras, for example rose and jasmine seem to work on both heart and sacral chakras. It is thought that illness is detectable in and affects the auric levels before it manifests in the physical, so if essential oils act in this area, they truly are a preventative medicine.[13]

Cautions

It would seem that essential oils may be used externally at any time, although it may be prudent for women to avoid certain oils during early pregnancy, if they are prone to miscarriage, are breastfeeding or are on certain drugs (see tables 4 and 5). Some of the so-called 'banned' oils are now thought to be safe in the small external doses used in aromatherapy, but owing to lack of proved safety it is best to err on the side of caution.

Bitter almond	Cinnamon bark	Dalmatian sage
Armoise	Costus	Sassafras
Basil (high estragole)	Elecampane	Snakeroot
Sweet Birch	Fig leaf	Tansy
Boldo	Horseradish	Tarragon
Buchu	Lanyana	Thuja
Cade	Melaleucabracteata	Verbena
Calamus	Mustard	Wintergreen
Camphor	Pennyroyal	Wormseed
Cassia	Ravensara anisata	Wormwood

Table 1: Oils to be avoided

Tisserand, a world leader in aromatherapy, recommends that certain oils should be avoided altogether (see table 1).[14] Some of these oils may be available to the general public and it would be prudent to avoid them. It is interesting to note that the herb may be safe, but the oil may not be, due to greater concentration of certain chemicals or the presence of different ones in the oil.

It is suggested also by Tisserand that the oils in table 2 should be used with caution in the following conditions and then only by trained and qualified professional practitioners.[15]

Cardiac fibrillation	Cornmint, Peppermint
Uncertain toxicity	Cangerana, Elemi, Khella, Lavender Cotton, Oakmoss, Savin, Treemoss
Epilepsy	Balsamit, Ho leaf, Hyssop, Lavender cotton
Kidney disease	Indian dill, Parsley leaf and seed
Prostatic hyperplasia	Lemongrass, May chang, Melissa

Table 2: Oils to be used with caution in listed conditions

To avoid the risk of inducing cancer one should only use the oils in table 3 below a given maximum.[16]

Basil (low estragole)	2. 0%
Fennel	1. 5%
Ho leaf	2. 0%
Nutmeg (East Indian)	2. 0%

Table 3: Oils to be used only below maximum dose

Training

Aromatherapy uses potent substances and therefore proper training is essential. The therapist should be a member of a national professional body and have full insurance cover. I encourage clients to ask about length of training (usually at least one year), which course was studied, and what postgraduate training the therapist has undergone since qualifying. Members of the International Society of Professional Aromatherapists (ISPA) are required to complete at least two days update per year. Clients may contact the professional bodies, which hold lists of all qualified members.[17]

The therapist should blend oils on the spot for each client and not use premixed blends. They should refer to a doctor or other therapist as necessary.

Therapists practise in a variety of situations – from home, in complementary and GP health centres and within hospitals and nursing homes. Some are nurses or physiotherapists who have also completed a training in aromatherapy. However, in my experience as an aromatherapy teacher, the best complementary therapists do not necessarily come from a health care background. I have often found that those with no previous experience in professional health care make more holistic therapists: they are more easily able to look beyond symptoms and treat the whole person.

Aromatherapy is being used increasingly in hospitals. It is demonstrating some success, not only in terms of patient response, but in terms of the reduction of drug bills, particularly in some departments, such as intensive care, oncology units,[18] labour wards and in the palliative care of the long-term sick and geriatric.[19] While this is excellent, it must be remembered that hospital patients are often very sick and their responses may be very different from those we would expect from a normally healthy person. Also we must be aware that in a ward of 20 or more people, all (including the staff) will inhale some oil in some degree, if it is used on any one individual. So it would make sense to be very careful when introducing oils onto hospital wards.

Much research continues to be done into the efficacy of essential oils and aromatherapy, some in the framework of clinical trials and others with a more qualitative 'feel good' basis. The results of research are available in the aromatherapy journals,[20] from professional organisations and from other medical journals, as well as from the UK database.[21] Conferences and symposia are held all over the world and reports on research findings are presented at these. Conference proceedings are usually available from the organising body and make exciting and thought provoking reading.

Home Use of Essential Oils

Here are some oils which may prove useful for home use, although the lay person should not attempt to treat any serious complaint. I have included the Latin name of each oil as different varieties may have the same common name and be very different in action. One should ensure one is buying pure essential oils, not diluted. Oils should be in dark glass bottles to prevent the continued action of light on the oils and sold with droppers to prevent overdose. They should be clearly labelled as to content, carry the warnings 'Keep away from children' and 'Not for internal use' and there should be explanatory information about possible hazards or contraindications.

◆ Lavender (*Lavendula vera*) is an invaluable standby in my first aid box for cuts and burns, for headaches, insomnia and panic attacks. It is one of the few oils which may be used neat in small amounts (1-2 drops).

◆ Roman chamomile (*Anthemis nobilis*) may be used in conjunction with lavender for insomnia (ratio 2:1) in baths or massage, or even directly onto the pillow. It is also good in creams for dry skin and eczema. German chamomile (*Chamomilla recutita*), with its high content of azulene, is excellent for inflammation and may be used in the bath or in compresses.

◆ Rosemary (*Rosmarinus officinalis*) is a good cephalic – it aids concentration. But it can also be used in baths and massage to energise and to ease muscle pain. It is useful when vaporised during the day to ward off flu viruses. In similar vein, titree (*Melaleuca alternifolia*), ravensara (*Ravensara aromatica*), eucalyptus (*Eucalyptus globulus*) and manuka (*Leptospermum scoparium*) are all good for colds, flu and infections – in inhalations, baths and vaporisers. Titree is a powerful antifungal agent and will help to relieve athlete's foot and veruccae.

◆ Geranium (*Pelargonium roseum*) is a useful hormone and sebum regulator, so is good to help balance an oily or dry skin and to help with irregular menstruation and premenstrual tension. Sweet marjoram (*Origanum majorana*) may help relieve headaches and muscle pain. It can also be combined with lavender to promote a good night's sleep.

◆ Finally bergamot (*Citrus bergamia*) is widely used as an antidepressant,[22] mostly in vaporisers, as it can cause skin sensitisation in the presence of sunlight. It is thought that it may be useful in cases of SAD (seasonally affective disorder), its pleasant fruity aroma mimicking the effects of sunlight on the spirit.

Aromatherapy in Pregnancy and Childbirth

Aromatherapy can be very useful for the expectant mother during pregnancy and in labour, as well as for both mother and baby after the birth. The majority of oils are safe to use in pregnancy. Tisserand, however, cites certain oils which should be avoided or used with caution in pregnancy (see Tables 4 & 5).[23] The reasons for avoiding these oils is that they are generally rich in chemicals thought to be neurotoxic – safrole and thujone – and might injure both foetus and mother.

Camphor
Hyssop
Indian dill
Parsley leaf
Parsley seed
Spanish sage
Savin

Cangerana
Lavandula stoechas
Lavender cotton
Oakmoss
Rue
Treemoss

Table 4: Oils to be avoided during pregnancy

Table 5: Oils to be used with caution during pregnancy

Oils may be used to alleviate many of the minor discomforts of pregnancy, such as backache, oedema and vulvar varicosity and to help prevent stretch marks. They may be used in perineal massage to encourage the elasticity of the perineum, facilitating stretching during the birth and reducing the risk of tearing or episiotomy, and should either of these occur, to speed the healing process.

A combination of lavender and rosemary in the bath or in massage may be used to ease backache caused by the pressure of the uterus on the ligaments. Spearmint (1 drop) may be inhaled to lessen the feelings of nausea. For stretch marks 2 drops of neroli or mandarin diluted in 5 ml sweet almond oil may be massaged daily into the abdomen. Alternative oils might be rose and lavender and good base oils, borage, carrot or wheatgerm. Oedema can be treated again using lavender and rosemary

(2 drops in 5 ml) or ginger, cypress and lavender (3:2:2 in 30 ml). For varicose veins, haemorrhoids and vulvar varicosity – use lemon (2 drops in 5 ml), geranium or cypress (3:1 in 10 ml base oil). Sandalwood or rose (2 drops) may be used in the bath for heartburn. For flatulence, 15 drops of fennel or spearmint diluted in 30 ml base oil may be massaged into the abdomen. Coriander or cardamom may be used in the same way for indigestion. Constipation may be alleviated by rubbing one of the following blends clockwise into the abdomen, either marjoram and rose (4:1 in 10 ml base oil) or patchouli (5 drops in 10 ml). A footbath with geranium, lavender and cypress (5:10:2 in hot water) will help alleviate leg cramps. For exhaustion a bath with lavender, grapefruit and coriander (2 drops each) will revive. Perineal massage with 1 drop rose in 5 ml almond oil will soften and tone the perineum.

Labour

The partner might help by using lavender or bergamot – 6 drops in 1 pint warm water – for sponging down the woman in labour, or just to have in the room to calm and soothe her. Massage oil with clary sage, rose, ylang ylang (7:2:3 in 25 ml vegetable oil) or with lavender and jasmine (6:1 in 25 ml vegetable oil) may be massaged gently into her abdomen or lower back as requested. When labour starts bathe her with lavender and jasmine (1 drop each) or massage lavender into her temples or use in a compress. Pain relief may be given with a hand hot clary sage compress applied to her lower abdomen.

Postnatal Care

For infection or healing use lavender and German chamomile (3 drops each in bath) or lavender and cypress (4:1 in bath). Cracked nipples may be massaged gently with 1 drop of rose in 20 ml sweet almond or sweet almond, wheatgerm, calendula (8:1:1). To increase milk flow massage fennel, geranium, clary sage (3:3:2 in 10 ml vegetable oil) gently into breasts. For mastitis try geranium, lavender, rose (1:1:2 in 1.5 pints cold water) for a compress. For postnatal depression either of the following blends are lovely in the bath (6 drops of the mix) or in a vaporiser.

◆ Nutmeg, rosewood, frankincense, lemon, rose (7:6:2:9:6)

◆ Grapefruit, geranium, mandarin (10:10:5)

They can also be mixed with vegetable oil to make a massage or perfume blend.[24]

Babyhood and Childhood

During babyhood and early childhood the most useful oils I have found are chamomile (Roman) and lavender. A mixture of them (2 chamomile: 1 lavender) will aid sleep if used in the bath. Chamomile will ease teething, toothache, earache and digestive upsets and lavender may be used as a first aid measure for all kinds of cuts and burns, etc. For babies up to two years one drop should be diluted in a teaspoon of full fat milk or vodka and dispersed in the bath. Both oils may also be used in massage – 1 drop in 5 ml sweet almond oil – with very gentle finger pressure. Yarrow is yet another oil useful for teething problems – 1 drop to a tablespoon almond oil – massaged into the cheek. It is of the same family as chamomile and it is not therefore surprising that it contains the anti-inflammatory chamazulene, also present in German blue chamomile. The same oils are useful for nappy rash – 1 drop to 1 pint of water for bathing or 1 drop in a dessertspoon of cream base and almond oil.

Additional oils useful in childhood are frankincense, bergamot, eucalyptus, thyme, linalol, titree, rosemary, niaouli and ravensara – whenever there are coughs, colds, or infections. These may be used in vaporisers or electric diffusers and the more gentle ones in massage and baths. I have found a blend of equal parts of lavender, frankincense and niaouli good in a vaporiser for childhood coughs, eucalyptus or rosemary for blocked noses and lavender, thyme and ravensara together reduce the discomforts of flu, the first in a steamer or over a bowl of hot water and the second in a vaporiser.

I have used a blend of frankincense and Roman chamomile in equal parts in a cream for eczema and on a tissue after an asthma attack to aid breathing and calm the child. For eczema I have used a blend of rose otto and German chamomile, again in a cream. Rose oil in almond can be effective too for cradle cap, as can equal parts of eucalyptus, citriodora and geranium (1 drop essential oil blend to 2 tablespoons almond oil). For colic 1 drop of dill in 15 ml almond oil may be rubbed clockwise around the tummy.

Essential oils may be used throughout childhood – one blend which seemed to work rather well was lavender, chamomile and titree in equal parts in a dabbing lotion for chicken pox. The mother of two of my young patients used the lotion on her daughter, but not on her son and found that the blisters were less itchy and healed much more quickly on the girl than on the boy.[25]

Biography

Sue Jenkins has a BA and postgraduate certificate in education. After several years in teaching, she trained as an aromatherapist with the London School of Aromatherapy in 1988 and in 1989 went into practice in Fife, Scotland where she also studied for the school's advanced diploma. She moved to Aberdeenshire with her family in 1993 and now practices from home and at the Findhorn Foundation.

She has taught aromatherapy for the LSA since 1990 and is principal of the Edinburgh School of Holistic Aromatherapy. A member of the IFA, ISPA, RQA and ICM, she works for the unification of the therapy and towards consistently high standards in training and research, and is involved with building links with the medical profession. She gives talks, workshops and lectures on aromatherapy and related subjects.

In practice her main interests lie in immune system functioning, pregnancy and childbirth, and the psychospiritual aspects of aromatherapy. At home she enjoys walking, dancing, music, swimming and gardening as well as trying to develop a more environmentally friendly and holistic lifestyle.

References

1   Robert Tisserand, *Opening Address, Aroma '93*, Brighton, 1993. Proceedings from Tisserand Institute, P O Box 746, Hove, Sussex.

2   Julia Lawless, *The Encyclopaedia of Essential Oils*, Element, 1992.

    ——, *Aromatherapy & the Mind*, Thorsons, 1994.

3   Roger Jallois, *Bref Survol geo-historique*, in Roger Jallois Ed. 'L'Aromatherapie Exactement' Limoges.

4   Op.cit. in 2.

5   Robert Tisserand, *The Art of Aromatherapy*, C W Daniel & Co., 1989.

6   Robert Tisserand, *Essential Oil Safety*, Churchill Livingstone, 1995.

7   Julia Lawless, *The Encyclopaedia of Essential Oils*, Element, 1992.

    Shirley Price, *Practical Aromatherapy*, Thorsons, 1987.

    Robert Tisserand, *The Art of Aromatherapy*, C W Daniel & Co., 1989.

8   Sue Young, *No conflict*, International Journal of Aromatherapy, 1994; 6: 4, 6-7.

    Liz Madelin, *Energies in conflict*, International Journal of Aromatherapy, 1994; 6: 2.

9   Shirley Price, *Aromacolour*, Aromatherapy World, Autumn 1993, p 7-9.

10 Gabriel Mojay, *The Chinese Energetic Model*, International Journal of Aromatherapy, 1993; 5 : 3.

11 Op.cit. 8.

    Dr Daniel Pénoël Aroma 93 conference Op.cit.1, also in International Journal of Aromatherapy, 994; 6 : 1.

12 Robert Tisserand, *The Art of Aromatherapy*, & Tony Balancs, *The Psychopharmacology of Essential Oils*, Papers at Aroma 95, Proceedings from International Journal of Aromatherapy.

13 Patricia Davis, *Subtle Aromatherapy*, C W Daniel & Co., 1991.

    Julia Lawless, *Aromatherapy & the Mind*, Thorsons, 1992.

    Christine Page, *The Frontiers of Health*, C W Daniel & Co., 1992.

14 Robert Tisserand, *Essential Oil Safety*, Churchill Livingstone, 1995.

15 ibid.

16 ibid.

17 There are three main professional organisations:

    The International Federation of Aromatherapists, Stamford House, 2-4 Chiswick High Rd., London W4 1TH.

    The International Society of Professional Aromatherapists, Hinckley & District Hospital & Health Centre, The Annex, Mount Rd., Hinckley, Leics. LE10 1AG.

    The Register of Qualified Aromatherapists, P O Box 6941, London N8 9HF.

    These come under the umbrella organisation called The Aromatherapy Organisations Council.

    There are other smaller organisations and aromatherapists may also register with the Institute for Complementary Medicine.

18 *An evaluation of the use of massage and massage with the addition of essential oils on the well-being of cancer patients* from The Centre for Cancer and Palliative Care Studies, the Royal Marsden NHS Trust.

    Barbara Evans,*The Effects of aromatherapy massage and the cancer patient in palliative and terminal care*, Complementary Therapies in Medicine, 1995;3:239-41.

    Peter Gravett, *Aromatherapy rescue from chemotherapy*, Aroma 95 conference proceedings, International Journal of Aromatherapy. 1995.

19 R. Hudson, R.N, *The value of lavender for rest and activity in the elderly patient*, Complementary Therapies in Medicine,1996;4:52-7.

20 The International Journal of Aromatherapy; Aromatherapy world; Aromatherapy Quarterly; The IFA Times.

21 Natural Therapies Database UK., (Tel. 081-391 0150); as well as various nursing and medical journals.

22 Gabriel Mojay, *Aromatherapy for Healing the Spirit*, Gaia, 1996.

23 Robert Tisserand, *Essential Oil Safety*, Churchill Livingstone, 1995.

24 Valerie Ann Worwood, *The Fragrant Pharmacy*, Bantam, 1995.

    Jane Dye, *Aromatherapy for Women & Children*, C W Daniel & Co., 1992 .

    Maggie Tisserand, *Aromatherapy for Women*, Thorsons, 1995.

25 Sue Jenkins, *Redressing the Balance - Aromatherapy* & Men, London School of Aromatherapy Advanced Dissertation, 1995. Available from the author.

Further Reading

Davis, P., *Aromatherapy: an A-Z,* C W Daniel & Co., 1988.

Lawless, J., *The Encyclopedia of Essential Oils,* Element Books, 1992.

Price, Shirley & Len, *Aromatherapy for Health Care Professionals,* Churchill Livingstone, 1995.

Tisserand, R., *Aromatherapy for Everyone,* Arkana, 1990.

Tisserand, R.; Balacs, T., *Essential Oil Safety,* Churchill Livingstone, 1995.

Valnet, J., *The Practice of Aromatherapy,* C W Daniel & Co., 1992.

Resources

The International Federation of Aromatherapists
Stamford House
2-4 Chiswick High Road
London W4 1TH

The International Society of Professional Aromatherapists
Hinckley & District Hospital & Health Centre
The Annex
Mount Road
Hinckley
Leics. LE10 1AG

The Register of Qualified Aromatherapists
P O Box 6941
London N8 9HF
Tel. 0181-341 2958

The above mentioned come under the umbrella organisation called:

The Aromatherapy Organisations Council
3 Latymer Close
Braybrooke
Market Harborough
Leicester LE16 8LN

*There are other smaller organisations and aromatherapists may
also register with the Institute for Complementary Medicine.*

Addresses of Journals:

The International Journal of Aromatherapy
P O Box 746
Hove
E. Sussex BN3 3XA

Aromatherapy Times
The IFA
Stamford House
2-4 Chiswick High Street
London W4 1TH

Aromatherapy World
c/o ISPA
ISPA House
82, Ashby Road
Hinckley
Leics LE10 1SN

Art Therapy
by Karin Werner

*Psychological
Therapies
Anthroposophical
Medicine*

Over the past 50 years two main streams of art therapy have developed. One stream has come out of depth psychology, mainly through the work of C.G. Jung, and the other stream (called artistic therapy to emphasise the artistry itself) comes from the philosophy of Rudolf Steiner and anthroposophy. It is Steiner's approach which this article will focus on.

Art Therapy

When art therapy is used as part of psychotherapy, the ability to bring inner images from the unconscious to the surface is encouraged, and the free expression of these archetypal images and colours is a healing process in itself. The therapist's role is to help reveal and interpret the symbolic meaning of the clients' pictures of themselves and their problems, and to support them in their growth. Through painting, the psyche will find ways to adjust to change, so that the client can become more inclusive and flexible. C.G. Jung called this the process of individuation.

Artistic Therapy

Colour Therapy

Working with colour, paint brush, paper, pencil, stone, clay, etc. can be a method of inner striving to be harmoniously connected to a greater whole. All disharmony, on whatever level, can be related to three aspects: thinking (nerve-sense system), feeling (rhythmic system) and will (metabolic system and limb system). Artistic therapy practised in this context helps people to use colour, form and imagination to create living relationships with all these aspects and to bring them into balance.

In a hospital or rehabilitation centre, artistic therapy follows from the diagnosis of a specially trained medical doctor who co-operates with a team of different therapists. Often, artistic therapists, eurythmists (movement and sound therapists) and massage therapists are employed. In holistic diagnosis and treatment, the organs of the body are looked at in their physical functions as well as their non-physical processes. Organs are connected to the rhythms in nature, like day and night, the seasons, the elements, growing and fading, expansion and contraction, and planetary cycles. Ideally, the doctor will have an insight into the nature of each individual patient and where the imbalances occur. Homoeopathic or allopathic remedies will be prescribed accordingly. The art therapist supports the treatment by focusing on appropriate artistic exercises. These can evolve from free paintings or drawings to precise transformative sequences. The exercises, and the choice of art materials, very much depend on the individual who comes for therapy.

Homoeopathy

The Practice of Artistic Therapy

As a general outline, an art therapy session takes about 45 minutes. The therapist prepares the studio in advance and encourages the client to get familiar with the medium. This can take one or more sessions. It is important, as in all therapeutic relationships, that a trusting, peaceful climate is established. Artistic therapy is not a verbal therapy and the client needs space and time to explore the nature of these possibly unfamiliar tools. It is a very different mode of expression to release form out of a stone as in sculpture, or to put watery colour onto a brush and paint with it, although both the brush and the hammer are felt as extensions of oneself. The therapist is there for the client, to assist skilfully and in non-intrusive ways. Towards the end of a session, the therapist and client share observations regarding the work done. One painting or sculpture can evolve over several sessions.

The great benefits of artistic therapy have been documented in cases of chronic illnesses, such as cancer, MS, ME, AIDS, and also of the so-called psychosomatic illnesses, such as allergies, asthma, eczema, colitis and anorexia.[1] A patient with a serious illness might be too weak at times to do much artwork. In such a case, the therapist might paint for the patient or show the patient a piece of art which has the qualities needed for healing.

It is an unfolding process with no prefixed boundaries. If the patient is in a hospital where art therapy is part of the treatment, they will typically have one session per day and stay about a month. Afterwards they can continue to work with an independent art therapist once or twice a week to complete the treatment. Chronic conditions often respond well initially to the new influence coming in through art and the creative process, but then need a longer time of continual art exercises. As an example, a sclerotic process which surfaces in one of the organs, the bones or the brain, might not be reversible on a physical level, but through the activity and practice of art, through the use of subtle colour combinations and through precise and clear picture observation, something can shift within the patient which leads to greater flexibility on emotional and mental levels. In other words, by engaging in this form of artistic therapy, specific creative activities can stimulate a different process of suppleness and therefore create a balance within the wholeness of the person.

The human being cannot be treated by formula, and the patients in their wholeness must be at the centre of any treatment. One person might need something completely different from another person with the same condition.

While there are no fixed recipes, there are general principles. For example, a patient in a state of mental confusion with overwhelming inner pictures or agitation may require pencil form drawings or clay work rather than free imaginative painting. Alternatively, the detailed copying of an old masterpiece in pastel drawing may be the most appropriate form of therapy, to give the mind a sense of beauty, order, composition, a balance of light and dark. Similarly, a patient who has a breathing problem and a 'wet' chest infection should not be given fluid watercolours on damp paper because it may aggravate the condition. Instead, a 'colour-breathing' exercise using sequences of appropriate colour combinations would be applied on dry paper, with wax crayons or colour pencils. Colour-breathing involves applying the inhalation/exhalation, expansion/contraction principle to the subtle levels through working with the colours of the rainbow. In a sequence of paintings, the patient would be guided to move certain colour arrangements up and down the rainbow scale with a brush, arriving at finer tonalities and blending each time. Shapes and motif may or may not result. In contrast, if a motif is drawn on paper and then filled in with premixed colours, it is a thought process, not a breathing process.

Although a finished product is not the main goal in artistic therapy, it is important that the client has a sense of accomplishment and individual creativity. There should be a sense of completed transformation from one state of being to the next, as the paper is transformed from a pure white sheet to a picture of a tree in its lively seasonal colours, complete with foliage and dimensions. Artistic activity in this way can strengthen the *I* or *ego* (not to be taken as egotism, which is a different matter). It is the client's ego and the art therapist (who supports the client) who together are able to overcome imbalance or one-sidedness, which is one of the roots of illness. The exploration of the tension of extremes, of polarities – hard and soft, light and dark, curved and straight line and many more – is one of the functions of art therapy.

In artistic therapy we examine how nature deals with extreme states and restores its balance. By painting nature's moods – the seasons, the elements (fire, air, water, earth), growing and fading, expansion and contraction – patients experience nature and get closer to their own natural rhythms and changes, which leads to balance. The elements in their diverse forms of expression restimulate a sense of acceptance of who we are – each of us, a living piece of art.

On a feeling level, art can be used to connect to the *soul moods*: joy, anger, laughter, crying, love, hate, devotion, etc. Patients paint their life situations using colours to express different states of feeling and responses to these situations. Through the process of painting, patients transform the energy and expression of their feelings, liberating stuck energy which then becomes available for healing. Colour is food for the soul. It stimulates creative solutions in a complex world.

Soul moods can be described as the essence, or pure quality, of feeling. It is essential for the health of a human being to be able to experience the whole scale of human feelings. Depth of feeling leads to imagination and a creative life. Soul moods can be worked with and transformed through working with colour. It is not important to arrive at a 'good' mood, for example to go from anger to love, but to explore the richness of feeling and where it serves life in its wholeness. Fairy tales are a fine example of the expression of soul moods and have been a rich source of wisdom and healing for the human condition. Fairy tales are frequently used in painting therapy. In the fairy tale the beautiful princess and the wicked queen each have their place and transformation happens in the dynamic interaction between the two.

Case Histories

The following case histories of two patients, both diagnosed with depression, may illustrate how art therapy can take different routes with the same illness, depending on the patient's personality, outlook on life, habits and preferences. In the beginning, both patients were given the choice of what they would like to paint.

In her first painting session, the first patient chooses to paint with watercolours. She uses a dense and dark Prussian blue, almost neat from the tube. In the finished painting there is no movement, hardly any lighter areas. When we talk about her experience, she feels that she is unable to use more water with her brush or to use any other colours. Through a gradual process of more blue paintings, she arrives at a point where the blue is divided into a lighter tone at the top and a darker one at the bottom. My suggestion is to have a conversation with another colour at this point. Then a pale red is 'allowed' to make a few horizontal stripes in between the blue but not to touch or mix. There is a turning point for her when I offer to take care of the blue while she experiments with a second colour. By then our contact is deep enough for her to trust me, and she feels greatly relieved. She fills a big central space with red, pulling and pushing the blue into more of a supporting role in her picture. She gradually transforms the burdensome darkness into a moving, dramatic scene.

The second patient shows little initiative and direction in her first paintings. She keeps asking whether she is doing all right and what to do next. One day she paints in washed out watercolours, hardly visible. The next day she puts thick blobs of yellow and red on paper but does not know what to do with them. She communicates her feelings of despair and agitation. At night she is restless and cannot sleep. Together we discover her love of landscapes, trees, flowers and fruit, but she is unable to come anywhere near these images in her paintings. I suggest a cycle of connected paintings in different moods of day and night, beginning with an evening mood. This is very difficult for her. It takes several sessions to arrive at different shades of blue and then only through the image of a blue mountain scene with a cave. There is still a lot of light in the back of the cave. But from now on she takes it into her own hands to develop a story – how she stands in the blue cave and then emerges from it to go for walks in the mountains. Finally she paints her night-blue house on top of a hill. The sun is just about to rise. Her house changes from different shades of blue to light orange. In the end, a dark green leafy tree protects the house with its shade. In her case it was important to befriend the darkness in order to come to her own sense of self, peace and balance.

Application of Artistic Therapy in a Social and Cultural Context

One of the basic tenets of artistic therapy is that illness and artistic therapy together awaken individuals to a path where they can find their way back to the creative source. This same process can prevent illnesses of society. Rudolf Steiner described the artistic healing process as arising from a purely physiological state into a life enhancing activity. It is not that the unconscious physiological function itself should rise into our awareness; for instance, we do not need to experience every detail of the liver's immense alchemy. However, when the liver ceases to function correctly, we are poisoned from within and we get depressed in all senses of the word. The role of artistic therapy in this context would be to work through and transform the liver processes.

Steiner's vision was to transform the culture as well as the individual. In our post-industrial electronic information era there is imbalance which creates unhealthy states in organisations and work. Many companies nowadays employ counsellors to help people cope with the stresses of rapid change. The problem for many is that the cultural change happens in a non-physical reality, a microchip reality, where there is seemingly nothing to connect with once the routines of the day are accomplished, unless one practises perceiving the greater context of this reality. Artistic therapy can guide people towards a perception, integration and expanded imagination of realities, once there is an acceptance that the therapeutic process assists in cultural change and healing as well as in the understanding of individual illness.

If artistic therapy were applied in groups and organisations, in particular those in the business of promoting health and healthy social and educational structures, then the creative impulse could work through the individual into the larger whole. M. Altmaier proposes a seven-step model as an artistic and cultural process:

1 collecting the material, putting some paint on paper;

2 connecting the colours into a balanced combination;

3 allowing chaos to emerge through polarities, contrasts, randomness, conflict, separation (this is often the stage where modern art sees its completion or human relating gets stuck);

4 making a decision about what direction to take, what motif to follow;

5 allowing higher principles to create order, for example through light and dark areas, balanced colour perspective, overall composition and rhythm;

6 completion of the picture;

7   from the entire experience of the first six steps a whole new picture is created, either as a metamorphosis of the old motif or as a completely new impulse.[2]

The process can be entered and left at any step. Between steps 3 and 4 a shift from physiological functioning to conscious cultural processes occurs. Step 5 is a transformation of step 2.

To summarise, it is possible to apply art as an agent for health-giving change through a variety of exercises, according to the need of the organisational culture. Artistic therapy is an evolving discipline which supports creative humanness and consciousness in illness and in health.

Training

In the UK the training requires a background in the visual arts as well as inspiration and dedication to use them for working with people and their needs. Ideally, one would have professional experience in both the visual arts and in social or therapeutic environments. Usually, the training takes three to four years full-time. A large part of the training develops one's own artistic skills, particularly in the first two years, and a recognition of how these are interconnected with inner development and understanding of the whole human being. Practical placements during the third and fourth years help to build a bridge between one's own experience of the artistic process and assisting others in their exploration. A diploma in artistic therapy will be given after thorough assessments by teachers and supervising art therapists.

Different streams of working with artistic therapy can be followed afterwards. As described earlier, therapists may work in a hospital or clinical setting in the areas of physical and mental illness or disabilities and learning difficulties. Another area is the school where artistic therapy is applied with individual children. Although the therapist can work from their own studio, their clients will mostly come through referrals from teachers or doctors.

Apart from working directly with organisational structures and cultures, there is also an application in environments such as prisons, homes or deprived inner city areas to help rebuild a sense of soul life and community. The direction chosen depends very much on the art therapist's initiative, inclinations and abilities.

Biography

Karin Werner has been involved in the healing arts and in personal and group development since her early teens. She qualified and worked as a nurse and as a social worker and educator in social skills where she applied a range of complementary therapeutic skills. Her personal life and work led her to the visual arts and a qualification in artistic therapy.

References

1   Der Merkurstab, *Gesellschaft Anthroposphischen Art in Deutschland*, Stuttgart.
2   Marianne Altmaier, *Der Kunsttherapeutische Process*, Urach Haus Verlag, 1995.

Further Reading

On artistic therapy:

Hauschka, Dr M., *Fundamentals of Artistic Therapy*, Rudolf Steiner Press, 1985.

D'Herbois, L Collot, *Light, Darkness and Colour in Painting Therapy*, The Goetheanum Press, 1993.

Steiner, Rudolf, *Colour*, Rudolf Steiner Press, 1992.

On art therapy in general:

Dalley, Tessa (ed.), *Art as Therapy*, Routledge, 1990.

Jung, Carl G., *Man and his Symbols*, Penguin, 1990.

Liebmann, Marion, *Art Therapy in Practice*, Jessica Kingsley Publ., 1994.

McNiff Shaun, *Art as Medicine*, Piatkus Books, 1994.

Waller, D.; Gilroy A. (eds.), *Art Therapy: A Handbook*, Open University Press, 1992.

Resources

For artistic therapy:

Association of Artistic Therapists
Park Attwood Clinic
Trimpley
Bewdley
Worcestershire DY12 1RE
Tel. 01229-861 444

Tobias School of Art
Coombe Hill Road
East Grinstead
West Sussex RH19 4LZ
Tel. 01342-313 655
Fax. 01342-323 401

Hibernia School for Artistic Therapy
Hawkwood College
Painswick Old Road
Stroud
Gloustershire GL6 7QW

For art therapy:

British Association of Art Therapists
11a Richmond Road
Brighton
Sussex
Tel. 01734-265 407

Edinburgh University Settlement
School of Art Therapy
Wilkie House
37 Guthrie Street
Edinburgh EH1 1JG
Tel. 0131-650 6311

Goldsmiths College
University of London
New Cross
London N1 8QL
Tel. 0171-919 7171

Sheffield University Centre for Psychotherapeutic Studies
16 Claremont Crescent
Sheffield
Yorks S10 2TA
Tel. 0114-276 8555

University of Hertfordshire
School of Art and Design
Manor Road
Hatfields
Herts AL10 9TL
Tel. 01707-285 300

Autogenic Training
by Rita Benor

While Western medicine has conditioned us to rely on the outer physician, Autogenic Training enables us to find and develop an intimate relationship with our own inner physician and healer.

Autogenic Training (AT) is a simple, powerful and effective technique which brings about a profound level of relaxation and relief from the negative effects of stress. AT has been described as a Western rediscovery of the basic principles of Eastern meditation.[1]

Relaxation Therapy
Transcendental
Meditation

Autogenic Training is based on a series of simple exercises. The process is cumulative and can eventually lead to a sense of balance, reflected in improved stamina, concentration, intellectual performance, physical co-ordination, emotional stability and ability to cope with physical illness, and in diminished arousal and reduced symptoms in most diseases.[2]

Autogenic Training was introduced in the 1920s by a German psychiatrist and neurologist named Johann Schultz. He noted the physiological changes in patients who were hypnotised. They reported feeling very relaxed and warm, with increased feelings of well-being. Schultz wondered whether these positive changes could be achieved without the patient being hypnotised or practising self-hypnosis. He developed a series of self-instructed mental exercises which became the basis of what was later known as Autogenic Training. The key to them was to be detached and simply observe the process, which differed from hypnosis and its concerns with outcomes.

Hypnotherapy

This passive state of mind is achieved by changing the level of consciousness from the usual 'active' state to a gentler 'passive' state. Passive concentration is the ability to have a relaxed attitude to the exercises, to become the 'passive observer', simply noting everything that happens in an accepting way, without judgement, preference or criticism.[3] Passive concentration greatly reduces and eases the censorship role of the ego. This in turn encourages a shift between the active and passive levels of consciousness. The mind is then in a position to alter physiological functions.[4]

Stress Management

Patients benefited from these profoundly effective exercises. A German physician, Wolfgang Luthe, joined Schultz in refining the training. Luthe was interested in helping patients to understand the importance of responding to and releasing their natural feelings and emotions, thereby preventing the unnecessary holding in of emotions which can lead to increased stress levels, and, in the long term, to disease or illness. AT proved to be an invaluable aid in the management of stress and illness.

A British doctor, Malcolm Carruthers, assisted by his wife and a committed team of colleagues, pioneered the introduction of AT into the United Kingdom in the early 1970s. Standardised training for clients and therapists was established through and by the British Association for Autogenic Training and Therapy.

All AT therapists are themselves experienced in using the technique before embarking on their therapist training. Therapists come from health care backgrounds, particularly medicine, nursing, psychology, psychotherapy and medical social work.

Stress Responses and Effects of Autogenic Training

The term 'autogenic' means generated from within and refers to two aspects of the one process. The first is the basic shift from the over-aroused flight and fight stress response. The second is to bring about specific restorative, healing, readjustment responses mediated by the brain, central nervous system, endocrine system, immune system and muscular systems.

The flight and fight response includes basic biological, chemical and emotional reactions which are set off when a person perceives a threat. Threat can appear in many forms, for example the startling experience of crossing a road and realising that the oncoming car is not making an effort to reduce speed, causing the person to sprint to safety. The heart is pounding. There is shallow, rapid breathing, and maybe a feeling of nausea, accompanied by emotions of anger.[5]

Threat comes also in more subtle forms. It can occur in circumstances when choice is reduced, such as: when one is stuck in a demanding and unsatisfying job, with too much pressure to actually enjoy the process of one's work; when facing a difficult ongoing relationship with a partner or family; when considering redundancy; or having to cope with chronic, disabling conditions or illness and treatments. Whatever the threat to the body, the nervous and chemical systems react to protect the individual. These reactions are primitive. The long-term effects of these reactions, if they are not reduced, can lead to serious imbalances. These set up a situation where the person may become ill as a result of the body's automatic response to various threats.

When stress is brief, the inbuilt mechanisms reverse the reactions of flight and fight to rest, or homoeostasis. However when the stress is prolonged these mechanisms are unable to cope. For instance blood pressure remains high, creating the conditions of hypertension, or tense muscles go into spasm, creating backaches or headaches. The first shift with AT is to reverse the over-aroused state which keeps the chronic flight or fight response going.

AT affects both consciousness and behaviour as both are directed by the brain. The left side of the brain is associated with rational logical thinking, linear measurements and language, and frequently has the ability to dominate individuals and their behaviours. The right side of the brain is associated with the creative, artistic, spatial, patterning aspects of awareness. Under the dominant influence of the left side, people can often find themselves enslaved by logical, rigid routines and can be over-aroused and stressed, the right side only being allowed to function partially. Research has shown that brain waves can be positively affected by AT, helping the individual to switch into a restful, recuperative state.[6]

> *Once it is possible to reduce excessive tension a sense of wholeness and well-being is brought about by better communication between the two hemispheres of the brain which takes place during the exercises.*[7]

Psychoneuroimmunology and Autogenic Training

Autogenic Training is an effective form of self-care and self-healing and is increasingly relevant in the light of the newly emerging science of psychoneuroimmunology (PNI).[8] PNI teaches us through an impressive body of research that there is communication and co-operation between the mind and the body and that there is a relationship between health, dis-ease and the potential for healing.[9] PNI is being practically demonstrated in the increasing use of complementary therapies with people with cancer.[10]

Research has shown that there are proteins called neuropeptides which carry messages between one part of the nervous system and the other. The very same neuropeptides are found in the immune system. This strongly suggests that the brain and the immune system communicate with each other.[11]

When a person feels compromised in some way, by illness or stress, the mental reaction produces changes in the immune system and in emotional biochemical systems. Just as the stress biochemical and PNI mechanisms can be triggered to set up imbalances, they can also be set up to redress the balances. In many instances the proteins are identical even though the systems are different, for example the nervous system and the immune system. Pert states that emotions bridge the gap between mind and matter, and asks which comes first, the peptide or the emotion?[12] Dossey, writing about holism, suggests a hypothesis about the power of reversal, transforming what might appear to be negative activities into positive.

We know that disease states themselves generate changes in our mental lives, that in turn affect the disease states, producing a spiral of events that defies an ultimate distinction between mind, body and spirit, If our minds can produce illness, can our minds also be used to prevent illness, diminish complications and promote healing.[13]

The proof of science and PNI can only be experienced in the real world through proven human success. Amongst the most respected clinicians and authors, Lawrence LeShan and Ian Gawler describe remarkable results in reversing illness and dis-ease by changing attitudes and states of mind, through regular use of relaxation and meditation.[14]

PNI gives the knowledge that empowers individuals to be actively involved in the harmonisation of their mind, their body systems and their psyche, promoting health, well-being and greater possibility of wholeness. Similarly, Autogenic Training can make a major contribution to such harmonisations, particularly in instances where chronic, disabling and life threatening illness exists. AT can help people to manage and survive stressful life events.[15] In many instances AT is used preventatively to maintain a healthy lifestyle.

AT is gaining recognition and acknowledgment for contributing to the body of PNI research on mind-body connection and in the treatment and prevention of psychosomatic disorders. Derived from a psychological model, AT is maturing into a highly researched and validated model affecting the whole person.

Responses to Autogenic Training

Autogenic Training may not be suitable for everyone. It is unsuited to children under the age of five years, individuals with severe mental handicap, personality disorders or acute psychoses and to those with no motivation.[16] Clients who have unstable physical conditions, for example diabetes or hypertension would not be excluded but close co-operation between AT therapist and treating physician would be essential. Anyone who wishes to undertake a course will be invited to meet with an AT therapist first. If they are found to have no contradictory conditions, the therapist will undertake a full assessment of their health and history of illness and lifestyle. Every AT client is encouraged to inform their GP of their AT course, and for those with illness or chronic conditions the AT therapist will seek to liaise with the family doctor. Autogenic Training is never used as a substitute for conventional treatment of illness or disease. It is always used in conjunction with or as a complementary approach to allopathic treatments.

AT has already been described as helping to overcome stress responses. It has also been proved to bring about improvements in such conditions as high blood pressure, insomnia, migraine headaches, asthma, anxiety[17] and irritable bowel syndrome.[18]

Clients are encouraged and supported in acquiring their competence over an eight to ten week period. Emphasis is placed on regular practice and in the event of a client experiencing an adverse effect, the therapist is able to assess and offer suggestions on modifying or postponing an exercise according to the individual's tolerance or circumstances. It is possible for clients to experience adverse effects and important to recognise the powerful effects AT can bring about. It is recommended that clients should always be taught by a qualified AT therapist who has been trained in the use and management of the technique. There are self-help manuals, but these cannot provide the richness or proficiency for maximum safety that the experienced therapist brings. This is the reason for not including instructions with this chapter.

The Autogenic Training Programme

A standard course of AT lasts approximately eight to ten weeks. It is available on an individual or small group basis. Both options have their advantages – availability and cost are often the determining factors. Would-be clients will need to be able to commit time and energy to practise regularly, to understand the instructions, to be able to concentrate, to apply the exercises three times a day for a few minutes and to keep a daily diary of their practice and its effects.

The clients are taught to transfer their level of concentration from active to passive. Passive concentration is the simplest and yet most important concept in AT. This process is not achieved overnight. Throughout the training the person becomes more competent at simply letting go of striving for results. The brain's inherent, self-regulatory mechanism changes and the left and right sides of the brain harmonise.[19]

The setting for AT is important. The therapist will endeavour to create a comfortable environment which is warm and peaceful, and where the client is given time and attention to enjoy the session and to practise the process. No special equipment or clothing is required. AT is practised in a series of postural positions, for example sitting on a hardback chair, sitting in an armchair, lying horizontally and sitting on the floor resting one's back against the wall. These positions have been selected to avoid creating tension by poor posture which becomes an unnecessary distraction.

Clients will talk with the therapist about the events which have been important in relation to their situation and their AT practice and its effects. It is important that clients have fully understood the instructions and explanations. With each new formula the manner and means of explanation is the same, with exact wording, to avoid mistakes and poor technical use of the exercise. After each session clients are given written notes, a step-by-step description of the exercise to be practised. It is important to set realistic expectations of the programme and what the clients can hope for; motivation is crucial for success.

This programme will, of course, vary according to the individual client and therapist and will be influenced by the client's progress, and can last between one and two hours weekly. When the standard training is completed clients will practise AT independently for several weeks, attending one or more follow-up sessions until they are confident and proficient in the uses of AT.

Exercise Format

The core of Autogenic Training is the six standard exercises. These are built up weekly to involve all four limbs, improving circulation and releasing tension from the muscular system, aiming to promote the sensations of warmth, relaxation and calmness. It is important to note that not all individuals using AT experience these sensations; however they frequently report the overall effects of relaxation, for example reduced heart rate, loosening of muscular tension, slower breathing rate, reduced gastro-intestinal activity, improved concentration and improved sleep.

The exercise series progresses from relaxation of the peripheral extremities to include regulation of the heart and circulatory system and regulation of breathing and the respiratory system. Further development includes: the visceral organs, for example the solar plexus area in the abdomen, and in contrast to the warmth and vasodilation of the muscular exercises, the forehead, where coolness and clear-headedness rounds off the process, moving into the final phase of peace. At the end of the sequence the client will stay quiet, resting in the autogenic state, cancelling the passive consciousness, in order to return to the daily activities.

The Autogenic State

The state is one of restful alertness. The two hemispheres of the brain are harmonising and the brain waves are inducing a state of peace and tranquillity. Clients have described this state as feeling very calm, meditative and detached, feeling well and balanced, and being able to let go of striving.

The Intentional Exercises

Intentional exercises help clients to recognise the importance of feelings and emotions and to respond to them. Often beliefs, values and childhood conditioning lead to feelings and reactions being held back or suppressed. This may lead to blocks and tensions which can contribute to stress and dis-ease. By giving full attention to one's feelings, a more natural pattern can emerge with better coping abilities when facing conflict or distressing or hurtful experiences. These exercises are simple to apply and take only a few minutes; they are not intended to be practised every day, as are the six standard exercises, but are to be applied when needed.

Motivational and Personal Formulae

Affirmations are not uncommonly talked about today. It is suggested that positive attitudes to life are enriching and life enhancing. These formulae are introduced at the end of the standard training when the client has experienced the quietening of the mind and body and is gaining confidence in life-affirming behaviours and attitudes.

Affirmations

They are practised within a state of passive concentration. The client can select from three kinds of formulae: 'neutralising', which are intended to take the sting out of a situation or condition; 'reinforcing' which help the client to support an action or intention; 'abstinence' which are used when the client has a habit or is in a rut and needs help to change the pattern, or their attitude to it.

Autogenic Training is woven around self-awareness. It addresses the physiological, psychological, emotional and spiritual aspects of people's lives. It helps them address maladaptive beliefs, habits and circumstances of their lives. It is a holistic approach.

Biography

Rita Benor is a psychotherapist and Autogenic Training therapist and lecturer in complementary therapies, practising in South Devon.

References

1   M Carruthers, *The psychodynamic approach*, British Journal Holistic Medicine, 1984; 1: 1, 42-5.

2   Brian O'Donovan, *Autogenic Training in Organic Illness: a handbook for therapists*, Brian O'Donovan, Chichester, 1989).

    M Carruthers, *Health promotion by mental and physical training*, British Journal Holistic Medicine, 1984; 1: 2, 142-7.

    Kai Kermani, *Stress, Emotions, Autogenic Training and AIDS: a holistic approach to the management of HIV-infected individuals*, British Journal Holistic Medicine, 1987; 2: 203-15.

3   A Green, *A guide to running an eight week course*, (trainers notes) published by author, 1994.

4   L Seward, *Autogenic Training in Managing Stress*, Jones and Bartlett, 1994.

5   L Seward, *The Physiology of Stress in Managing Stress*, Jones and Bartlett, 1994.

6   G Jacobs, J Lubar, *Spectral analysis of the central nervous system effects of the relaxation response elicited by Autogenic Training*, Behavioural Medicine, Fall 1989, 125-32 .

7   M Carruthers, op cit.

8   *Psychneuroimmunology* (editorial), Lancet, July 1985.

9   K Pelletier, D Herzing, *Psychoneuroimmunology: towards a mindbody model*, Advances, 1989; 5: 1, 27-56.

    B Dorian, P Garfinkel, *Stress, immunity and illness – a review*, Psychololical Medicine, 1987; 17: 393-407.

    R Booth, K Ashbridge, *Is the mind part of the immune system?*, Advances, 1993; 9: 2, 4-23.

    S Baur, *Psychoneuroimmunology and cancer: an integrated review Journal of Advanced Nursing*, 1994; 19: 1114-20.

10 O C Simonton et al, *Getting Well Again*, Bantam Books, 1978.

    J Archterberg, B Dossey, L Kolkmeir, *Rituals of Healing – Using Imagery for Health and Wellness*, Bantam Books, 1994).

11 C Pert, *The wisdom of the receptors: neuropeptides, the emotions and bodymind*, Advances, 1986; 3: 3, 8-16.

12 C Pert, *Psychoneuroimmunology – presentation at the Bristol Cancer Help Centre conference HOPE*, October 1995 .

13 B Dossey et al., *Holistic Nursing: A Handbook for Practice*, Aspen, 1988.

14 L LeShan, *Cancer As A Turning Point*, Dutton, 1989.

    Ian Gawler, *Peace of Mind*, Presim Press, 1991.

15 W Linden, *Autogenic Training: A narrative and quantative review of clinical outcome*, Biofeedback and Self Regulation, 1994; 19: 3, 227-64.

G Rose, J Carlson, *The behavioural treatment of Raynaud's Disease: a review*, Biofeedback and Self Regulation, 1987; 12: 4, 257-72.

E Blanchard et al., *The USA-USSR collaborative cross-cultural comparison of Autogenic Training and the thermal biofeedback in the treatment of mild hypertension*, Health Psychology, 1988; 7 (suppl): 175-92.

16   Brian O'Donovan, op cit.

17   W Linden, op cit.

18   R Benor, *Autogenic Training: Towards a Whole Person Approach*, in press (1997).

19   J Coleman, *Luthe's Cathartic Autogenic Training: A Therapists Handbook*, published by author, 1988.

Further Reading

Archterberg, J, Dossey B, and Kolkmeier L., *Ritual of Healing – Using Imagery for Health and Wellness*, Bantam Books, 1994.

Davis, M., Eshelman, E., McKay, M., *The Relaxation and Stress Reduction Workbook*, New Hargbinger, 1988.

Kermani, K., *Autogenic Training: the Effective Holistic Way to Better Health*, Souvenir Press, 1996.

Linden, W., *Autogenic Training*, The Guildford Press, 1994.

Macbeth, J., *Moon Over Water*, Gateway Books, 1994.

Seaward L., *Managing Stress*, Jones and Bartlett, 1994.

Sutcliffe, J., *The Complete Book of Relaxation Techniques*, People Medical Society, 1991.

Zahourek R (ed), *Relaxation and Imagery: Tools for Therapeutic Communication and Intervention*, W B Saunders Co, 1988.

Resources

The Secretary
British Association for Autogenic Training and Therapy
Heath Cottage
Pitch Hill
Ewhurst
Nr Cranleigh
Surrey
GU6 7NP

Centre for Autogenic Training
Positive Health Centre
101 Harley Street
London W1
Tel. 0171-935 1811

Wirral Autogenic Training Centre
Wirral Holistic Health Care Services
St. Catherine's Hospital
Church Road
Birkenhead
Merseyside
Tel. 0151-678 5111

Bioenergetic Analysis
by Ulla Sebastian

Historical Background

Bioenergetic analysis was officially founded in 1956 in New York by Alexander Lowen, John Pierrakos and William Walling. It has its roots in the theories of Sigmund Freud and Wilhelm Reich.

Psychological Therapies

Reich, a student of Freud, a passionate, warm-hearted but also belligerent and 'difficult' man, became one of the most controversial and creative figures within the psychoanalytic movement. He realised in his work with patients that certain themes and words were connected with certain body postures and expressions. He started to investigate those connections and realised that they form specific patterns which he called characters. These characters are the result of blockages in the free flow of energy, life or bio-energy, and are a survival response to social conditions. Being a man of extraordinary perception and compassion, Reich got involved with the healthy upbringing of children, as well as focusing his attention on investigating the make-up and dynamics of life energy itself. He investigated ways to unblock, condense and strengthen that energy. He discovered that all life forms follow a natural pulsating rhythm that he called the 'orgasm-reflex'. He turned to natural science and got involved with cancer research, developing an 'orgone accumulator' to help the body to restore its cellular functions. He was prosecuted by the US federal authorities, being falsely accused of peddling his accumulators as a fake cancer cure. He died in prison of a heart attack shortly before he was due for release.

Lowen, a student of Reich, adopted Reich's notion of humans as unified body/mind entities, refined Reich's character analytic concept, introduced the notion of 'grounding' and applied it to the treatment of emotional problems. He called his approach 'bioenergetic analysis'.

Theoretical Model

Humans are unified body/mind entities. This can be symbolised in the figure of the centaur. In healthy people, the expressions of the physical, emotional, mental and spiritual levels work in harmony with each other. They act in an integrated way, guided by an impulse of love and harmony, while considering the rational demands of the situation. Such people will have emotionally appropriate responses, will feel well and balanced within themselves. They are connected to the universe and grounded in their bodies, their sexuality and their relationship to the earth. Such individuals find meaning in their lives and fulfil their life purposes.

All four levels (body, emotion, mind and soul) are fuelled by the same energy, called bio-energy or orgone energy in the West. It is the same life energy that is referred to as prana, chi or kundalini in the East.

Social conditions in the upbringing of children usually prevent us from developing this harmonious way of being. Conflicts within the realms of thought, feeling or behaviour interrupt the free flow of energy. We may be told to stop crying because it upsets mother; to be nice little girls or boys who do not get angry; or to focus all our attention on doing and achieving instead of feeling and being.

Children depend on their parents. They love and want to please them. Therefore they may adopt breathing and muscular holding patterns that suppress the feelings that are not welcome. If sadness or anger arise, it is choked down to prevent the emotional expression. The chin tightens and tucks in as part of the effort to restrict flow in the throat. The arms and shoulders may tense against the impulse to hit, contracting the neck even further. Mucus forms and the throat may ache, but the child keeps a grip on itself. In an environment which continually asks for suppression of those emotions, the grip gets programmed into the body. What started as a protective device to keep the parent's love for the child becomes a prison, preventing the adult from experiencing love, joy and fulfilment, as unfortunately not only the 'bad' emotions get repressed through this mechanism, but the 'good' ones as well.

In addition situations may arise that are so overwhelming for the infant organism that the only way to survive is to leave the body and make the mind their home. This, for example, happens in cases of sexual abuse. Abuse is an attack on emotional and physical integrity, an abandonment or even an assassination of the soul. If the attack is continual or traumatic, the soul withdraws, freezes or splits. The body/mind entity – the centaur – gets split in two: the rider (mind) and the horse (body). The body becomes the object of shame, especially if it experienced pleasure during the abusive situation. The mind takes over as a base of identity, often riding the body into the ground out of shame, guilt and punishment. The mind may not recognise this self-destructive behaviour, especially if it is supported by culturally accepted patterns, such as smoking, alcohol or medical drug abuse and workaholism. All these are an attempt to avoid feeling pain and loneliness. This gets compounded and perpetuated as the body remembers the attacks – even if the mind doesn't – and shies away from human contact. As a result, life may become a desert.

The body may also respond to the split between body and mind and the repression of emotions by developing chronic pains, such as back or headaches; eating disorders, such as bulimia or anorexia; psychosomatic diseases, such as stomach ulcers, asthma, high blood pressure, heart attacks; or chronic diseases, such as cancer or ME.

The goal of the therapeutic intervention in bioenergetic analysis is to bring back the natural pulsation of life, the free flow of energy. To do so, it is necessary to re-establish the natural breathing pattern, called by Reich the 'orgasm-reflex', to loosen up muscular blocks, to reactivate frozen energy and to repattern movement, so that the body can regain vitality, motility (the inner flow of energy) and co-ordination. This process involves confronting those childhood experiences that produced the specific holding patterns, muscular tensions and splits within the body/mind unit. It requires re-experiencing, embracing and integrating the associated basic fears and emotions into everyday life, bringing to maturation infantile parts and adjusting the perception of life to adult reality. The process involves surrendering to self, moving through pain instead of running away from it or fighting it, and shifting perspective from growing through pain into growing through joy and grace.

There are basically two types of problems that need to be dealt with within the therapeutic process: a need for restructuring and a need for expression or letting go.

In cases of traumatic events, the infant development gets arrested at the stage where the trauma occurred. Resulting deficiencies can affect the general energy level, the body functions or the psychological structure. An important part of the work is to rebuild that which did not develop properly. This re-education or post-maturation process requires daily practice to increase the general energy level and to strengthen the body. It is necessary to learn self-assertion and boundaries in social interactions and to rebuild and reframe thought-forms and perceptions about reality. The aim is to empower people to take charge of their lives and to create a satisfactory reality for themselves.

If emotions have been suppressed, often a restricted breathing pattern and chronic muscular tensions result which prevent certain movements and expressions in the body. This is known as 'body armour'. Alongside this, there frequently operates a rigid 'I' that is terrified of letting go and excludes from its awareness everything that could threaten its self-image. In this case, the therapist supports the person to loosen up the body armour and revitalise the blocked energy and encourages the self-expression and a re-examination of the self-image. The aim is to expand the person's capacity to embrace all of their feelings and to surrender to the flow of life.

Procedures and Techniques

The therapeutic process usually starts with the therapist doing a 'body reading'. The therapist will look at the general energy level, posture, muscular holding and breathing patterns, facial and eye expression, contact ability and co-ordination. All these elements get related to the person's life story, their actual situation and their awareness of the different levels of their being (body, emotions, mind and spirit). The therapist helps the clients to become aware of their tensions and deficiencies, to activate their muscle functions, to express the emotions that are held within the muscular structure and to integrate memories that are associated with those holding patterns. The therapist also serves as a model for a healthy, warm contact, providing clear boundaries and strategies of how to deal with reality.

On a technical level, the therapist has four ways to mobilise blocked energy.

- ◆ By talking to the client and giving feedback on what is seen and perceived, which can elicit emotions that release tension from parts of the body.

- ◆ By working with the client to establish the orgasm-reflex, which increases the motility and helps the body to shake off chronic tensions. (The basic in-breath/out-breath movement of the orgasm-reflex is common to all humanity. In the Chinese system it is called 'spinal cord breathing'[1], and it is the primary movement in African tribal dancing.)

- ◆ By making direct interventions into the muscular structure (massage, acupressure, etc.) to help release deep-seated tensions.

- ◆ By placing the client in stress positions, such as standing as if sitting on a chair, which forces the muscles to surrender and to shake off tensions.

All these techniques help to build up or mobilise arrested energy. What the therapist chooses in any given situation depends on the actual problem, the character structure of individual clients and their response to the technique. More important than the technique is the understanding and empathy of the therapist for the situation and the client's psychological process.

The predominant setting for long-term therapeutic work in bioenergetic analysis is the one-to-one situation between the therapist and the client. However, a lot of the techniques for grounding, building up energy levels and expressing emotions can be taught within exercise classes and practised at home. Workshops are a valuable tool to increase awareness of the four 'bodies' (physical, emotional, mental and spiritual) and to come out of isolation and silence through the realisation that many others share similar problems. A group context can help to sustain a daily practice, to share insights and awareness and to find comfort and encouragement in difficult times.

Case History

The work I describe here reaches beyond the traditional forms of bioenergetic analysis but is a good illustration of the fundamental shifts which can be made through applying the techniques in combination with other skills.

Barbara, 39 years old, came to me for a two-week intensive therapy programme. She was full of anger and hate towards her father, who had sexually abused her during her puberty, and towards her depressive mother, who had not protected her against the father. She had undergone a client-centred therapy for five years aiming to increase her ability to engage in close relationships. The incest was not treated in that therapy. In a letter she wrote me:

> *At the moment I am feeling miserable. I desperately search for my identity. And I want to come home into my body. Every day I have to watch how the old Barbara disintegrates into many pieces. There is so much pain in me that I just get numb. Who am I?*

I met a very slim woman who, though normally proportioned, looked like an 18-year-old adolescent. She had been anorexic during her puberty, which can be seen as an unconscious attempt to prevent the development of a female body. In the first interview it became apparent that her mind, her body and her soul had developed separate identities. For instance, she told me that they (her mind, body and soul) had decided to trust me, as the mind had failed to run Barbara's life in any satisfactory way so far. I started to negotiate with all three aspects in an attempt to create a new inner balance between these three parts and help them to integrate. I told the mind, which had morally sentenced the body, that the body functions according to the principles of pleasure and displeasure and cannot be made responsible for the sexual abuse. We negotiated that the soul and heart would take over the mind's role and lead the 'team'. The mind would support the soul through its sharp perception in creating safe situations with others, especially men. We also agreed that both the mind and the soul would nurture the body and support its development. The soul agreed to return into the body and to fill it with life again.

This procedure is a core element in healing the separation between the body, mind and soul. It requires the therapist's empathy and understanding for all the parts, and patience and stamina to support the parts in their struggle of being heard and acknowledged.

I told Barbara that she had reached a point in her life where she could choose to keep attached to her parents through anger and hate, or use the energy that was bound in these feelings to strengthen her own inner core and build up her boundaries. I helped her to see clearly the damage that had happened to her life through these events, but also to see that her inner goodness, beauty and light and not her 'badness' had drawn these events to her. She understood that she had the choice to stay miserable or to turn those weaknesses and deficiencies into inner strength, using her experience to help others to cope with similar situations. She chose the latter, decided to make peace with her life story and to use her intense feelings to build up her own life. In an inner image she saw herself as a round, full woman, and after some struggle she was able to let that image fill her body. I introduced her to some techniques of the Chinese Healing Tao, as taught

Chi Nei Tsang

by Mantak Chia, that help to get in loving touch with the inner organs and systems, rebuild and strengthen the inner core, and balance the energy in the body. I showed her how to re-establish the basic pulsation of life in her body, and how to build up her body functions. When she left after two weeks, she felt that the abuse was healed, but she was also aware that it would take many more months to rebuild the structure on all levels. She agreed to do the work, and has worked steadily since then.

The challenge on the body level was to bring life back into a body that had gone numb. She had had several abdominal operations removing cysts and separating adhesions from the womb and intestines. At 35, she had had an ectopic pregnancy. The belly was a wounded area, and it took time and effort, working intuitively with various techniques and methods, to bring some vibration and sensation back into this part. The other problem was that she didn't feel that her feet and lower legs were part of her body. It took a few more months to re-establish the connection. She now feels alive, is exploring a new relationship and is making new friends. But the work isn't over yet. In a letter that I received a few months after our work together she wrote:

> *Every day I do my exercises... I usually succeed... at least for a few minutes, to feel my feet and lower legs and to experience a grounded flow of energy through my whole body... On the other side, I experience a lot of resistance to getting in touch with my body. I understand now that I can only take in small doses, perceiving how numb my body is... Soul and mind stand there full of action, the body wants to join in, all three get going, and then the body gets numb and speechless. It feels like a dry sponge. Its neediness shocks mind and soul, and it costs them a lot of effort to stay with the body. Sometimes horror just paralyses them; sometimes they just run off...*

Biography

Ulla Sebastian, Dr rer. soc. (social science) trained in psychoanalysis, bioenergetic analysis, group dynamics and group therapy. She is a writer, educator, psychotherapist and trainer for bioenergetic analysis at the German Institute for Bioenergetic Analysis. From 1979-1986 she held a professorship in clinical psychology in Germany, training social workers in psychopathology and supervising their work in crisis intervention, work with addicts and psychosis. She is also trained in African dance by an African medicine man from Ghana and practises the healing tao as taught by Mantak Chia. She has written many books and articles about 'pathways to life', the relationship between the genders and spiritual awakening. In her therapeutic work she helps people to shift basic patterns in their lives so that love, joy and fulfilment become part of their daily activities.

References

1   Mantak Chia, *Iron Shirt Chi Kung I*, Healing Tao Books, 1986.

Further Reading

Alexander Lowen:

> *The Language of the Body*, Collier-Macmillan, 1971.
>
> *The Betrayal of the Body*, Macmillan, 1967.
>
> *Pleasure*, Coward, Mc-Cann, 1970.
>
> *Bioenergetics*, Penguin, 1994.
>
> *Fear of Life*, Macmillan, 1980.
>
> *Narcissism. Denial of the True Self*, Macmillan, 1983.

Wilhelm Reich: All books are published by Farrar, Straus, & Giroux. The first date given refers to the Farrar publication, the second to the earliest publication.

Genitality, 1981, 1927.

Character Analysis, 1972, 1933.

The Sexual Revolution, 1974, 1936.

The Cancer Biopathy, 1973, 1948.

Listen, little Man! 1975, 1948.

The Murder of Christ, 1979, 1953.

Books about Reich:

Baker, Elsworth F., *Man in the Trap*, Avon Books, 1967.

Boadella, David, *Wilhelm Reich: the Evolution of His Work*, Contemporary Books, Inc., 1973.

Sharaf, Myron, *Fury on Earth. A Biography of Wilhelm Reich,* St. Martin's Press, 1983.

Resources

British Association of Analytical Body Psychotherapy
47 Dean Court Road
Rottingdean
Brighton BN2 7DL

The Bioenergetic Partnership
c/o Dr John Andrew Miller
22 Fitzjohn's Avenue
London NW3 5NB
Tel. 0171-435 1079

The Open Centre
188 Old Street
London EC1V 9FR
Tel. 0181-549 9583

International Training in Bioenergetic Analysis
Dr David Campbell
Davidson Clinic
Charing Cross Mansions
12 St George Street
Glasgow G3 6UJ
Tel. 0141-332 6371

Bio-Energetic Regulatory Medicine
by Julian Kenyon

New Methods of Diagnosis – The Concept of Energetic Pathology

The hypothesis of energetic pathology may be as difficult to grasp today as was the concept of radio waves before the advent of radio or television. Energetic pathology postulates that the first thing to go wrong in the body is an electrical change. Only when this electrical (energetic) change has been present for a considerable period of time does actual physical organic change in the body begin to occur.

Conventional investigations used in modern medicine, such as X-ray examination or more recently 'magnetic resonance imaging' (MRI), all look at structure in the body. Despite the fact that this can be in extraordinary detail, the investigation remains, in the conceptual sense, structural. The energetic (electrical) properties of a tissue or organ are not considered to be important.

Traditional Chinese Medicine Homoeopathy

The view of those practising alternative medicine, be that Chinese medicine or homoeopathy, is that energetic parameters are of primary importance. If pathological change can be detected at an energetic stage, then diagnosis can be made much earlier. This means that detected disturbances are potentially more easily reversible, and by implication curable. The findings of Bio-Energetic Regulatory medicine (BER) indicate that electrical (energetic) pathology often predates actual structural damage by many years. Therefore as the ideas and technologies used in BER medicine are developed, further researched and refined, the possibility of early diagnosis will open dramatic improvements for health care.

There are various methods available at the present time for energetic or electrical diagnosis. BER uses specific electrical measurements made over acupuncture points in order to determine diagnosis. The diagnosis is prinicipally cause-oriented, tracking the root cause of a presenting illness. Especially in chronic illness this may mean uncovering layers of causes (like the layers of an onion), providing insight into which treatment will address the relevant cause in an attempt to cure the symptoms rather than just suppress them.

BER medicine provides the beginnings of a viable causally oriented medicine, but is in its early stages of development. A lot more research is required into this approach, which promises to revolutionise health care.

BER Techniques

The Segmental Electrogram (SEG)

This is one of the most objective BER techniques, and of all these methods the easiest to relate to conventional diagnosis. The SEG records skin impedance (which equals a combination of the resistive effect of the skin and the capacitative resistance of the internal body structures) over eight body quadrants. The recording electrodes are placed on specific body areas.

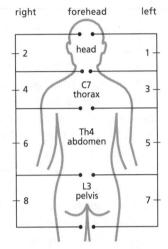

Fig. 1: Electrode placement for SEG

A 13 cycles per second (hertz) exploratory voltage (too small to be felt by the patient, as it is only 2 volts) is applied via circular silver electrodes over each quadrant in sequence. The response in terms of change of impedance with time over each quadrant is recorded on a moving paper recorder. As the diameter of the electrodes is relatively large (6 cm), it can be assumed that the skin resistance beneath the area of the electrodes is more or less equal over the whole electrode area. This means that the change of the exploratory voltage, which is subsequently recorded as a SEG recording, is largely brought about by the impedance of the major internal organs situated in each quadrant. It therefore serves as a useful pointer to organ dysfunction.

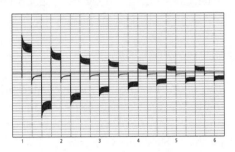

Fig. 1: Typical SEG readout

From many years of experience the following organs are the most likely to be involved if the relevant SEG quadrant recording is abnormal:

◆ Head quadrants – sinuses, tonsils (in young adults), teeth (in older people)

◆ Chest quadrants – diaphragm, lung, heart (if left quadrant)

◆ Abdominal quadrants – left: pancreas; right: liver

◆ Pelvic quadrants – colon (particularly in left quadrant), right: appendix

All the other organs located in the quadrants can, of course, also affect the reading. Therefore the SEG provides limited information in terms of which organs are involved. It does, however, enable many chronic illnesses to be worked out in a causal chain.

The next piece of equipment provides the extra detail not shown by the SEG in order to reach a complete causal diagnosis.

Diagnostic Device for Functional Medicine (DFM)

In DFM, measurements are also taken over quadrants. After establishing a baseline measurement, electrical stimulation and the observation of the changes in the measurements are an essential element of assessing the functional state of the main organs. The electrical stimulation involves passing a 13 cycles per second voltage first in a negative and then in a positive polarity from the head to the toes (that is, right down through the head and trunk) at tingling intensity for one minute in each polarity. On doing this the electrical abnormality due to underlying organic pathology becomes clearer. The change in the DFM following electrical stimulation is of major importance as it gives indication of the functional capacity of the main organs. It is a negative indication if the DFM parameters decrease following stimulation. In these cases a more dramatic approach may be necessary from a therapeutic angle. In practice this means often a surgical rather than a conservative approach, which is often based on complex homoeopathy (a combination of herbal medicine and homoeopathy). If the amplitudes of the DFM recording increase following stimulation, it indicates that the body has a good energy reserve and the patient is likely to respond to a homoeopathic approach. This is termed positive regulatory capacity.

The Vegatest Method

Complex Homoeopathy

The Vegatest method relies on changes in the resistance to the flow of electricity over acupuncture points on the ends of fingers or toes brought about by bringing particular substances, in glass phials, into series in the circuit. Electrically this is a Wheatstone bridge circuit, which is a standard electrical circuit for comparing resistances. In practice a tiny DC voltage of 0.87 volts is applied via a ball-shaped silver electrode on to an acupuncture point. The patient holds a silverplated cylinder to complete the circuit. The electricity flows from the end of the finger or toe through various complicated pathways through the body and out by the hand-held electrode.

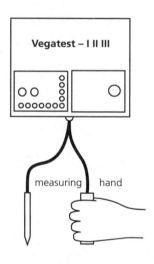

Fig. 3: The Vegatest method

The Vegatest method evolved from techniques for measuring acupuncture points developed by the German doctor Reinholdt Voll in the early 1950s. He decided to

Acupuncture

test whether electrical measurement of acupuncture points on specific meridians bore any relation to the organs to which the measured point belonged. He postulated that the measurements over certain points reflected the function of the related area of an organ. The acupuncture point is electrically negative with respect to the surrounding skin. The positive side of the measurement circuit is placed on the point via a point probe. As opposite charges cancel each other out, in order for the reading on the point to remain steady the electro-motive force (measured in volts) of the acupuncture point must exactly balance that of the measurement voltage. In order to do this the electro-motive force of the point (which behaves rather like a battery) must be constantly replenished. It is assumed that this replenishing of charge to the battery-like acupuncture point is produced by a flow of bio-electric energy moving along the appropriate meridian connected to the acupuncture point under examination. If this replenishment does not occur, an 'indicator drop' is measured. Voll then discovered that if he put medications which could help the patient's problems into series in the circuit the recorded indicator drop would disappear. This was the birth of medicine testing, which is a cornerstone of bio-energetic regulatory medicine. For the first time the effects of homoeopathic remedies, allopathic drugs and allergens, foods or chemicals to which the patient might be sensitive, could be measured.

Dr Helmut Schimmel evolved the methods further. Instead of taking the acupuncture point itself as being the main diagnostic indicator, he used homoeopathic extracts of normal mammalian organs to act as the main indicator, and tested for all organs using acupuncture points on the end of fingers or toes. The Vegatest is now commonly in use for testing of causes, allergens, organ function and medication. Of all the BER techniques the Vegatest may be seen as the method of choice. It is certainly the most accessible of the techniques as the equipment requirements are less extensive than other systems. However, there is the disadvantage that the method is prone to operator error. In many ways it is similar to using a stethoscope, in that the most important part is the bit between the ears.

Computerised Testing Systems

At the present time there are two main computerised testing systems, the *Eclosion* and the *Listen* systems. The Eclosion system is highly sophisticated containing a number of matrices which are basically plastic blocks under which tiny metal tubes are sealed at one end. In each tube there are substances such as bacteria, viruses, parasites, remedies, minerals, vitamins, and a whole range of medicinally relevant substances. The patient is connected up to the equipment via electrodes on the forehead, wrists and middle finger and a very small voltage (DC) is passed through the patient and each substance in turn. The change in amperage, voltage and resistance (that is, not just resistance as in the Vegatest) is measured. The EEG is also measured at the same time and a Fourier transformer (for frequency analysis) of the EEG is carried out every five seconds.

All of this information is assessed by the computer and a score for each substance from one to ten is made. Substances giving a score of ten are the ones taken note of by the therapist. The first run through which gives this objective analysis is known as the xerroid screen. This gives a guide as to what is going on in the patient. The key to this analysis, however, is dependent on a clear in-depth knowledge of a whole range of complementary therapies, as well as conventional medicine. As this system is so sophisticated, the essence is in the analysis.

The other main computerised system available today is the Listen system. This is a very interesting system as it simply contains in the software a computer code which is indicative of each particular remedy in the system. In the Listen system there are a vast number of remedies available (about 12,000). The computer code relevant to each substance has been derived electromagnetically by passing an electromagnetic field through the actual remedy. Based on this, an algorithm is derived from each substance and from this algorithm it is a relatively short step to devise a computer code which corresponds to that substance. The code is essentially a sequence of zeros and ones on the computer. The treatment under this system is either given by potentising a bottle of water with the appropriate remedies that come out of the system or the practitioner can actually order these remedies from the vast range of supplies of substances that are on the Listen system database. Clinically this approach seems to work, but from a scientific point of view it is extremely difficult to understand the mechanism.

Other Systems

This chapter would be incomplete without mentioning the AMI apparatus developed over 20 years ago by Hiroshi Motoyama from Tokyo. To give it its full title it is the 'Apparatus for the Measurement of the functions of the Internal organs'. Motoyama measured amperage over terminal acupuncture points using very fast circuits. He measured current over terminal acupuncture points every ten thousand billionths of a second. These readings were then plotted against time and a graph was obtained. He found that after ten microseconds polarisation of the tissues had occurred, which applies by the process of polarisation an equal and opposite voltage to the measurement voltage applied, thereby lowering the initial current recorded before polarisation had occurred. Initial current measurements can be as high as 300 milliamps and after ten microseconds this decreases to 20 or 30 milliamps.

All currently existing measurement apparatus used over acupuncture points measures after polarisation has occurred. Motoyama claimed, and indeed has shown through a number of clinical studies, that the pre-polarisation value represents electrical activity in the meridians, although he says that there are other processes as yet little understood going on in the meridians. The AMI must therefore represent a very important step forward in this field of the measurement of subtle energies.

Research

The accuracy of measuring conductivity over acupuncture points and relating the results to organ function have been subjected to experimental testing. The most recent study was at the UCLA School of Medicine which looked at the evoked electrical conductivity of the distal lung acupuncture point in 30 patients, 4 of whom had confirmed lung cancer on X-ray examination. The testing was carried out in a single-blind manner, the tester only having the patient's hand to test and seeing no other part of the patient. The results showed 4 true positives – in other words all the patients with lung cancer were identified on the basis of measurement of the distal lung acupuncture points – and 22 true negatives and 4 false positives were found.[1]

The study showed the significant level of agreement between the electro-acupuncture point measurement and the chest X-ray findings. It is interesting to note that one of the false positives showed an inconsistent shadow on the chest X-ray. This was shown not to be a malignancy; however, it is interesting to note that the electro–acupuncture measurement pointed to the presence of some lung disorder.

A number of other studies have demonstrated that electrical changes over acupuncture points seem to have some diagnostic value. For example Rosenblatt showed that acute physiological changes in heart rate may be reflected in changes in conductivity at heart acupuncture points, although no change in conductivity at another acupuncture point nearby and at a non acupuncture point was noted.[2] Matsumoto and Hayes have shown that vagotomy selectively changes the skin resistance in rabbits at the relevant acupuncture points.[3] Serisawa studied 50 patients with pulmonary tuberculosis and found an accumulation of low electrical resistance points, relative to healthy controls, on the radial side of the upper arm, in other words on the lung meridian.[4]

At the Centre for the Study of Complementary Medicine the doctors submitted themselves to accuracy tests: the objective was to find in a blind fashion substances poisonous to a test subject when using the Vegatest method. Ten bottles were filled by a third party with water or with Paraquat (a weed killer toxic to any living system), this being based on the toss of a coin, and numbered one to ten. The third party had the code for which bottles contained Paraquat and which contained water. Three testers measured these ten bottles on test subjects. Any bottle which gave a lower reading indicated that, based on testing, this bottle contained Paraquat. All testers obtained the same degree of accuracy of 70%. Therefore the hit rate was higher than chance. In the clinical situation testers are not working in a double–blind fashion, as each substance that is put into the honeycomb in the Vegatest contains a known substance. In a further test this fact increased the hit rates as they were drawing on their previous medical knowledge, experience and intuitive abilities.

In the Vegatest the operator is of major importance: the method has a subjective element which can be considered the observer effect. An insight into this mechanism has been obtained recently through the very painstaking work by Roland van Wyjk at the University of Utrecht. He showed that experienced testers could pick out appropriate remedies as opposed to placebos at a statistically significant rate in double-blind studies. He also found that changes in conductivity were brought about by subtle changes in the muscle tone of the tester, that is, the pressure of the electrode on the point. Roland van Wyjk points out that there is an unconscious change in the tester's muscle tone in response to the appropriate remedies, which then changes the conductivity of the acupuncture points by means of slightly more or less pressure on the point when retesting.

Recent work being carried out by the Dove Healing Trust, a research charity, is showing promising developments, which may possibly lead to an explanation of this phenomenon. The hypothesis is that these so-called *scalar fields* essentially are information which is carried in phased differences in the electrons rather like a voltage pattern on a capacitor. This is basically a quantum phenomenon and because of this there can be no direct electromagnetic observation of it.

Much of the work being done in the Dove Healing Trust at the present time is in some way connected with detecting scalar fields. This is highly innovative work and is a long way from any form of publication in journals. Current developments look promising, however. As a result of current scalar theory we have been successful in discovering an objective way of measuring over acupuncture points using an electrode placed over the point. This seems to be an objective method which avoids the difficulties of the difference in pressure intuitively applied by the tester in the Vegatest.

Conclusion

BER medicine is the result of many innovative discoveries. Advances have been made and understanding of the nature of subtle energies is increasing. More research is needed to understand the mechanisms further and to create more technologies for the practical applications. At the present time we stand at an important watershed, on the brink of being able to carry out objective studies. The next ten years should be very interesting indeed as far as these developments are concerned.

Biography

Dr Julian Jessel Kenyon is the co-director of the Centre for the Study of Complementary Medicine and director of the Dove Healing Trust UK and Dove Health Alliance, California, USA. He is involved in eclectic complementary medicine, and is a surgeon by training, with research interests in the scientific nature of subtle energies and the bringing together of science and spirit. The Dove Healing Trust and the Dove Health Alliance are co-ordinating approximately eighty research groups, both basic science and clinical, world wide, principally in Russia, America and Europe, to look at the scientific nature of subtle energies, and also research into complementary medicine. The ultimate aim of this research work is to have a cultural effect and be part of the process that brings science and spirit closer together.

References

1 S G Sullivan, *Evoked electrical conductivity on lung acupuncture points in healthy individuals and confirmed lung cancer patients*. Am J Acu, Vol 3,3, September 1985; 261-6.

2 S Roseblatt, *The electrodermal characteristics of acupuncture points*. Am J Acu, 1981; 10:131-7.

3 T Matsumoto, F H Hayes, *Acupuncture, electric phenomenon of the skin and post-vagotomy gastro-intestinal atony*. Am J Surg, 1973; 125: 176-80.

4 K Serisawa, *An approach on meridians and acupuncture points in modern medicine*. J Comprehensive Rehab, 1978,;11:789.

5 Roland van Wyik, *Homoeopathic medicines in enclosed phials tested by changes in conductivity of the skin: a critical evaluation*, V S M Geneesmiddelen, B V Alkmaar, The Netherlands, 1992.

6 Julian N Kenyon, *Preliminary studies revealing structure in water connected with homoeopathic remedies*. Presented to the third annual conference of the ISSSR-WEM Monterey, California, June 1993 (paper 35-34 in conference proceedings).

Further Reading

Dumitrescu, I., *Electrographic imaging in Medicine and Biology*, CW Daniel & Co., 1983.

Kenyon, Julian, *21st Century Medicine: A Layman's Guide to the Medicine of the Future*, Thorsons, 1986.

——, *Modern Techniques of Acupuncture – a scientific guide to bio-electronic regulatory techniques and complex homoeopathy*, Vol 3, Thorsons, 1985.

——*Modern Techniques of Acupuncture, A Practical Guide to Holistic Healthcare*, Heinemann Butterworth, to be published in 1998.

Lerner, E J., *Biological effects of electro-magnetic fields, a review paper*, IEEE Spectrum 1984, 57-69.

Resources

The Centre for the Study of Complementary Medicine
51 Bedford Place
Southampton
Hants SO15 2DT
Tel. 01703-334 752
Fax. 01703-231 835

Chi Nei Tsang
by Gordon Faulkner

Taoism (or Daoism) is one of the major indigenous religio-philosophical traditions that have shaped Chinese life for more than 2000 years. The term *tao* meaning 'way' or 'doctrine' was employed by all Chinese schools of thought. The universe has its tao; there is a tao of the sovereign – his royal mode of being; while the tao of humanity comprises continuity through procreation. Each of the philosophical schools had its own tao. One of the most important concepts of Taoism is the interconnectedness of nature and humanity.

The 'Healing Tao' is the name Master Mantak Chia gave to the system of mental and physical health care he devised using Taoist *chi kung* (also spelled 'qigong') and meditation practices. The Healing Tao, while independent of any religion, offers the potential for spiritual development in addition to improving health.

Historical Background

Since childhood, Master Chia has been studying the Taoist approach to life. His mastery of this ancient knowledge, enhanced by his study of other disciplines, resulted in the development of the Healing Tao system. This is now being taught worldwide.

Master Chia was born in Thailand to Chinese parents in 1944. When he was six years old, Buddhist monks taught him how to sit and 'still the mind'. While at school, he first learned traditional Thai boxing. He then was taught yoga and the martial arts of tai chi chuan and aikido. As a student in Hong Kong he was introduced to his first Taoist teacher, who eventually authorised him to teach and to heal. Later, Master Chia studied a variety of Buddhist practices (kundalini, Taoist yoga, and the Buddhist palm) and was soon able to clear blockages in the flow of energy within his own body. He also learned to pass life-force energy through his hands to heal patients. He went on to study Chi Nei Tsang (internal organ energy) massage which is the main physical therapy of the Healing Tao system. This is an extremely powerful technique which can produce very rapid results.

Theoretical Background of Chi Nei Tsang

The ancient Taoists saw the importance of working on three levels of being – the physical body, the energy body, and the spirit. Through a series of meditative and internal energy exercises, Healing Tao practitioners learn to increase physical energy, release tension, improve health, practise self-defence and gain the ability to heal.

Practitioners first learn to heal themselves, and then to heal others. Self-healing is achieved through the practice of chi kung routines, such as the 'chi self massage' for encouraging energy flow, the 'six healing sounds' for cooling the internal organs and balancing the emotions, 'spinal cord breathing' for opening joints, and the meditation techniques of the 'inner smile' and 'microcosmic orbit' for relaxation and the gathering and moving of internal energy. Once these have been mastered the practitioner can then begin to develop the skill of moving healing energy through others. The Taoists believe that unhealthy therapists can themselves be affected by the patient's 'sick energy' or they can actually drain the 'healthy energy' from their patients, leaving the patient in a worse condition.

Traditional Chinese Medicine

Chi nei tsang (CNT) is an entire system of Chinese deep healing massage that makes use of the energy flow of the five major systems in the body: vascular, lymphatic, nervous, tendon/muscle, and acupuncture meridian. CNT directly massages the internal organs and digestive tract through the abdomen. It is a comprehensive approach to energising, strengthening and detoxifying the internal systems. *Chi* (or 'qi'), which is also known as 'prana', moves through the body's internal channels, nervous system, blood vessels and lymphatic system. These systems concentrate and cross paths in the abdomen. Tensions, worries and stresses of the day, month or year accumulate there and are seldom dispersed. These disturbances can cause physical constrictions in the nerves, blood vessels and lymph nodes. The result is the gradual obstruction of energy circulation, resulting in areas of congestion in the navel area, best described as 'knots and tangles'.

When knots and tangles occur, internal organs store unhealthy energies. The ancient Taoists realised that negative emotions cause serious damage to health, impairing both physical and spiritual functions. They also identified a specific cycle of relationships between the emotions and the organs. For example, the experience of a 'knot' in one's stomach indicated the presence of worry, the negative emotion that accumulates in the stomach and spleen. They also discovered that most maladies could be healed once the underlying toxins and negative forces were released from the body.

The Practice of CNT

Only doctors practising CNT are allowed to give diagnosis. However, to determine the course of the treatment, CNT uses the four basic diagnostic tools – looking, listening, asking and touching – of traditional Chinese medicine, but emphasises touching, and in this context diagnosis and treatment become one.

A treatment begins with taking note of the shape of the navel. This gives an indication of the areas of underlying tension. The first procedure in CNT massage is known as 'opening the wind gates'. This involves applying pressure at appropriate points, so that the wind can be released and passed from the body. Wind is air or gas. The process of breathing, of moving air in and out of the body, involves wind. Each organ has an intrinsic wind. The wind becomes sick only when it is inappropriate to the part of the body in which it is found, or when it has been trapped and becomes stagnant. For example, if the intrinsic wind of an organ is 'warm' and that wind is then found in an organ that should be 'cool', then it is in the wrong location and therefore is now a 'sick wind'. Also, if intestinal gas is lodged in a tight corner of the colon it is called a 'sick wind'. The trapped energy, as blockages or knots, needs to be released, so that the life-force wind can flow freely throughout the body.

In order to clear toxins deep in the abdomen the surface must be dealt with first. This is achieved by detoxifying the skin and superficial lymph nodes with gentle and shallow massage. Work then begins on the large intestine followed by the other organs in the abdominal cavity – spleen, pancreas, stomach, small intestine, bladder, liver, gall bladder and the kidneys.

Alongside work with the organs, knots and tangles in nerve, blood vessel, and lymphatic system are also searched for and released. The filtering action of the lymphatic system is very thorough, but if it is overwhelmed with toxicity, it becomes congested with mucus and this impairs the immune system. Lymph nodes are everywhere in the body, but the largest concentration is in the abdomen. Therefore massaging the abdomen stimulates the lymph nodes and causes them to drain. Massaging specific nodes directly stimulates the detoxifying process.

Length of treatment can vary, with some chronic cases, such as ME, responding slowly, although results are often noticeable after just one or two sessions. Acute cases respond quickly; sciatic pain caused by pressure on the nerve in the abdominal region is one such example. In general, the more toxified a person is, the more treatments are required – although part of the treatment is also teaching individuals how and where to detoxify themselves. Like some other massage systems, CNT makes people feel good and so some people have regular sessions as an enjoyable preventative measure.

Traditional Chinese medicine is holistic in nature and as CNT is a branch of this it works well in conjunction with all other Chinese therapies and Western holistic treatments.

Like other Chinese therapies CNT is used to treat a wide range of problems. It can help process and integrate negative thoughts and emotions; it can be used for centring and balancing the pulses, which is done by working on the abdomen; for harmonising energy; and for using the blood flow to flush out debris and toxins. It drains the lymphatic system and is particularly effective in relieving conditions such as internal blockages, cramps, scar tissue, headaches, menstrual cramps, poor blood circulation, lower back pain, sciatica, infertility, impotence, stress, chronic fatigue and many other problems.

Training

Healing Tao centres exist in many countries, where training is provided by teachers who are certified by the International Healing Tao Association. Depending on the extent of the training, people acquire varying levels of competence. Some may simply master basic self-help techniques while others go on to obtain full professional status. Training takes place throughout the world and courses may be ongoing, part-time or full-time. Requirements for professional status include knowledge of traditional Chinese medicine, anatomy and physiology, daily practice of chi kung and meditation. Supervised practice and clinical experience is required, followed by the presentation of a series of case histories and a thorough testing of the student's knowledge at all levels, by a committee. Recently opened in Thailand is the new headquarters and training centre of the Healing Tao. It is there that full-time training can be obtained.

Case Studies

A 33-year-old athletic male was suffering from severe cramps in the left inner thigh. He was experiencing several attacks each day and this had been steadily worsening in the previous six months. CNT examination of the abdomen revealed a large knot of tension on the left side of the navel which was trapping the femoral nerve. Pressure on this spot brought immediate cramping of the left thigh. He came for six sessions, each one of which brought relief and longer intervals between cramps. This slowly built up until he was able to return to physical training with no further discomfort.

A 40-year-old male presented with irritable bowel syndrome and ulcerative colitis. CNT examination revealed a very tight abdomen, which was painful to a light touch. The first session consisted of light skin and intestinal detoxification massage. The second session revealed that although there had been some discomfort after the previous session, his general condition was now much improved and he felt better and happier. His abdomen was not so tight and therefore work could go deeper and include lymph and liver detoxification. After this session the client considered that his symptoms were manageable and he did not return for more treatment.

Biography

Gordon Faulkner, ex RAF, started training in martial arts in the late 1960s, coming across the Taoist schools in the early 1970s. He has made many trips to China and has studied with Master Chia in New York. He is a fellow of the Royal Asiatic Society and a member of the Society for Anglo-Chinese Understanding. He now works full-time as a Taoist arts teacher.

Further Reading

Chia, Mantak, *Iron Shirt Chi Kung I*, Healing Tao Books, 1986.

————, *Taoist Ways to Transform Stress into Vitality*, Healing Tao Books, 1985.

————, *Chi Self-Massage: The Taoist Way of Rejuvenation*, Healing Tao Books, 1986.

————; Maneewan, *Chi Nei Tsang: Internal Organs Chi Massage*, Healing Tao Books, 1991.

Matsumo, Kiiko; Birch, Stephen, *Hara Diagnosis: Reflections on the Sea*, Paradigm Publications, 1988.

Resources

Master Mantak Chia
Healing Tao
274 Moo 7
Luang Nua, Doi Saket
Chiang Mai 50220
Thailand

Giles Marin
Chi Nei Tsang Institute
2315 Prince Street
Berkley, CA 94705
USA

Gordon Faulkner
Healing Tao Foundation Scotland
Inver House
Bogton Place
Forres
Moray
IV36 0EP

Chiropractic
by Karin Robertson

The word chiropractic comes from two Greek words, *cheiro* meaning 'hand' and *prakos* meaning 'done by'. The literal translation is done by hand or manipulation. The art of manipulation was practised and its effects appreciated long ago. The Greeks, ancient Egyptians, Assyrians, Babylonians, Chinese and Hindus used manipulation as a form of therapy more than 3000 years ago. Indeed, Hippocrates himself, often referred to as the 'father of healing' stated, 'Look well to the spine for the cause of disease.' He understood the importance of maintaining good health by keeping the spinal column functioning correctly.

Chiropractic is a manipulative art based on an understanding of the spinal column and the nervous system and its role in maintaining normal health, without the use of drugs or surgery. Chiropractors believe that much dis-ease or abnormal function is caused by interference with nerve transmission due to pressure, strain or tension on the spinal cord or spinal nerves as a result of vertebral segment malposition.

Historical Development

The accidental rediscovery of chiropractic was made in 1895 by Daniel David Palmer in Davenport, Iowa. Palmer, a Canadian born in Ontario in 1845, practised magnetic healing, as taught by Franz von Mesmer, using the body's energy field as healing modality.[1] Palmer possessed a deep interest in the different ways of healing the sick. One day Harvey Lilliard, a janitor in the building where Palmer practised, complained of deafness. Palmer examined Lilliard's spine and on finding a displacement in the man's neck he manipulated the offending vertebra and the man's hearing was restored. From this one incident the entire principle and science of modern-day chiropractic was born.

Restoration of Harvey Lilliard's hearing by adjusting a displaced neck vertebra made Palmer deduce that correction of other spinal misalignments should restore health to the organs and other parts of the body supplied by that particular vertebral nerve. To summarise Palmer's theory: correction of any malfunctioning vertebral segment through manipulation relieves the pressure on the spinal nerve root and restores normal nervous supply to the affected areas.

In 1896 the first school of chiropractic was set up in Davenport, Iowa. Student numbers in the Palmer College of Chiropractic soon flourished, growing from 24 students in 1906 to 3100 students in 1923. Palmer's son, Bartlett J. Palmer, also became a chiropractor and then president of the college and under his influence the development of the chiropractic profession grew. In Britain, the Anglo-European College of Chiropractic was established in Bournemouth in 1965, although there already had been a British Chiropractic Association in existence since 1925.

Modern Chiropractic

Today chiropractors prefer the word 'adjustment' to 'manipulation' as this term signifies something more precise and controlled. Chiropractors refer to any spinal dysfunction as a 'subluxation'. They see themselves as specialising in the diagnosis and treatment of mechanical disorders of the spinal joints and muscles. Drugs and surgery are not used. Evaluating patients consists of putting them through a series of orthopaedic, neurological and radiological examination procedures in order to assess any neuro-muscular involvement which may be caused by limitation of joint mobility.

Lack of flexibility in the spinal facet joints which lie posterior to the disc in the spine places considerable shearing stress on the associated intervertebral discs and this may in turn lead to discal tears, prolapse or chronic disc degeneration. By restoring flexibility to the fixed joints, the stress is removed from the disc thus facilitating healing and preventing any long-term degenerative changes.

Spinal manipulation is an assisted passive motion applied to the spinal facet joints. During this manual procedure the motion segment is suddenly carried beyond its normal physiological range of motion without exceeding the boundaries of anatomical integrity. The amount of force used is a carefully applied high velocity short amplitude thrust given usually at the end of the normal passive range of movement. A cracking sound often results.

This phenomenon was examined in 1947 by two British anatomists.[2] They studied the effect of adding graduated longitudinal traction to the third metacarpo-phalangeal joint (the cracking knuckles phenomenon) using serial radiographs. Further studies were completed in 1971.[3] It was found that when two joint surfaces are being forced apart past the initial resistance barrier, the intra-articular pressure drops to a point where it reaches the partial pressure of carbon dioxide. Carbon dioxide and other gases are suddenly released from the synovial fluid within the joint and form a bubble of gas within the centre of the joint space. The audible 'crack' is a result of the fluid flowing into this low pressure region and collapsing the gas bubble. 'Cavitation' is the name physicists give to this process.

Different Forms of Manipulative Therapies

These days there are many practitioners who practise manipulation – chiropractors, osteopaths, manipulative physiotherapists and even some medical doctors. The two main manipulative professions are chiropractic and osteopathy. A commonly asked question is what is the difference between a chiropractor and an osteopath?

Osteopathy

One clear difference between the two professions is the use of X-ray. Chiropractors usually have X-ray equipment in their clinics or at least have direct access to X-ray facilities (via local hospitals). Chiropractors use X-rays to help diagnose the condition and thus decide on appropriate treatment. Chiropractors also believe adjustments help to restore proper nervous supply to the affected areas whereas osteopaths believe the vascular supply is rebalanced whenever manipulation is applied. But on the whole there are more similarities between the two professions than differences. Chiropractors and osteopaths both undergo a long specialised training – at least four years full-time – and this is usually followed by a postgraduate year in an established practice. In recent times many osteopaths have given lectures to chiropractors about different spinal techniques and vice versa. Undoubtedly technical skills in both professions overlap and it is likely that in future chiropractors and osteopaths will continue to learn from each other.

The manipulative physiotherapists, as I understand it, mainly study mobilisation techniques using the Maitland concept. In this method of treatment the physiotherapist uses a thumb contact over the vertebra and gradually increases pressure while using rhythmic oscillatory movements until reaching grade 5. Each stage of increased pressure is graded 1, 2, 3 and 4, with 5 consisting of an actual manipulation. Use of the McKenzie method of self-help exercises is also taught to physiotherapists. Robin McKenzie, a physiotherapist from New Zealand, innovated this form of treatment. Based on the assumption that people are hypolordotic (flat lumbar spine curve), passive mobilisation through exercises and lumbar roll supports is thought to increase and maintain the lumbar curve and thus alleviate back pain. Physiotherapists are usually involved with the physical rehabilitation of hospital patients after surgery and accidents. In general, physiotherapists are not trained to diagnose musculo-skeletal disorders.

Some medical doctors who have undertaken postgraduate courses in manipulation also treat the occasional spinal problem manually, although from my experience they tend not to practise on a regular basis. Many GPs are increasingly willing to refer patients to chiropractors or osteopaths.

The Practice of Chiropractic

The most common conditions treated successfully by chiropractic are low back pain, disc problems, sciatica, neck pain, whiplash injuries, headaches, migraine, and arm and leg pains.

Diagnosis

On the patient's first visit, the chiropractor will take a thorough case history and carry out a full neurological and orthopaedic examination. Reflexes and nerve stretch tests are routine neurological testing procedures and cranial nerves are also tested when necessary.

During the orthopaedic tests the spine is taken into its different ranges of motion to see if any position reproduces the pain. The chiropractor is trained to palpate the joint movements and to recognise any abnormal motion. Hip joints are also routinely tested with any low back problem.

Blood pressure is usually taken, especially in patients presenting with symptoms such as headaches, nausea, vertigo or those with familial histories of increased blood pressure, thrombosis, heart problems or strokes.

The two main reasons for taking X-rays are to exclude any pathology, which is of particular importance in the older patient, and to exclude any fractures, particularly it there is a history of any recent accident. X-rays are also taken when it is thought necessary to assess the condition of the patient's spine prior to manipulation.

Chiropractors differ from hospitals in X-ray positioning of the spine. Hospitals usually take spinal X-rays with the patient lying down. Chiropractors take spinal X-rays with the patient in weight-bearing positions, i.e. standing or sitting. This enables the patient's 'normal' posture to be assessed.

Treatment

Massage

There are many different ways of adjusting or manipulating the spine. The type of manipulation varies from patient to patient depending on the area of the spine requiring treatment. Chiropractors also work on the muscles of the body using deep therapeutic massage techniques. I personally have found 'muscle work' to be of great value and of particular importance in treating chronic cases.

Most neck problems are treated with the patient in the supine position. Sitting, prone and side posture positions can also be used. The chiropractor usually contacts the vertebra's posterior joints with either index or middle finger of one hand while supporting and slightly tractioning the opposite side of the neck with the other hand. The whole neck is flexed slightly forward, then laterally flexed and lightly rotated until a 'locking' of the joint has been felt, before a quick thrust is given. The force is directed through the joint articulation.

The thoracic spine is usually treated in the prone position but treatment can also be given with the patient in a sitting or supine position. Manipulation in this area consists of contacting the affected segment bilaterally on the posterior facets via pisiform (a small bone in the wrist) or edge of hand contact from the chiropractor. The patient is usually asked to inhale and exhale deeply. On reaching the end of exhalation the chiropractor quickly makes a thrust, usually in a downwards and slightly headwards direction.

The classical way of treating the lumbar spine is with the patient in the side posture position. This is referred to as 'the lumbar roll'. Contact is made on the mamillary process of the offending lumbar vertebra, again with the chiropractor's pisiform. The patient's top shoulder is rotated backwards and pelvis forwards. Manipulation is again usually assisted by the patient breathing in and out. This position is also used for pelvic treatments.

An important feature for treating patients correctly is the use of the 'Hi-Lo' – the chiropractic table. This table is specifically designed for patient and chiropractor comfort. The height of the table is adjusted hydraulically to suit the chiropractor when giving treatment. Modern tables usually have 'drop mechanisms' for each spinal level, i.e. cervical, thoracic and lumbar/pelvic areas. 'Toggle drop' is a commonly used technique which involves 'cocking up' the different segments of the table, i.e. cervical, thoracic or lumbar so that it just holds the patient's weight and no more. When the adjustment is given the table segment 'drops', thus assisting to 'open up' the two articular surfaces.

The number of treatments required for each patient varies considerably. Many different factors determine this – type of condition, the amount of time the problem has been present, age and lifestyle of the patient seem to be the main influencing factors. Patients who are thought to have a condition which usually responds well to chiropractic treatment will probably find relief within six to eight treatments. This is only a generalisation and some patients will require a lot more treatments and others perhaps less.

Conditions Treated

Many patients complaining of low back pain will ask if their disc has slipped out. There is no such thing as a 'slipped' disc; however, there are 'floppy' discs. The disc comprises an outer tough layer of fibrous tissue called the annulus and a soft watery type centre called the nucleus. The disc acts as a cushion between adjacent vertebrae.

Basically there are two types of disc herniations – contained and uncontained. In an uncontained herniation the soft nucleus penetrates the torn annulus and seeps out pressing on the nerve roots. In a contained herniation the disc bulges causing nerve root pressure but the nucleus is still intact. The chiropractor views the spinal joint segment as a whole and thus sees the protrusion of disc material as a complication of spinal joint dysfunction.

An argument put forward against lumbar manipulation when the patient has a suspected disc herniation is the fear of increasing the protrusion. However, apart from any indication of progressive neurological involvement or bladder and bowel problems, chiropractors have found that careful manipulative management of discal problems improves the condition. From my own clinical experience in dealing with discal problems, any patient suffering from severe leg pain which increases when the patient takes up the premanipulation position would not be manipulated. Very often in serious prolapses the patient is too uncomfortable to be 'handled' and manipulation can only be performed when the acute phase is well under control.

There are certain conditions where manipulation is clearly contraindicated. The obvious ones are recent fractures of the spine or spinal pathologies and these patients are usually referred for medical care. Other clear contraindications are cauda equina syndrome, urinary deficit and a history of progressive neurological deficit.

One concern to the chiropractor when using cervical manipulation is the risk of vertebral artery injury. The risk rate is about two cases per million.[4] This must be compared with the risk rate of paralysis from neurosurgery for neck pain which is 15,000 per million.[5] However, the chiropractor is trained to use specific testing procedures prior to cervical manipulation and from that result a decision is made whether or not manipulation will be beneficial to the patient.

Acupuncture
Homoeopathy

In 15 years of practice I have seen a wide-ranging variety of spine-related conditions. Generally speaking, most problems of a biomechanical nature are treated successfully. However, as in all professions, we sometimes come up against certain conditions which may respond more quickly with the help of another form of treatment. Often patients' symptoms may be too acute to manipulate immediately and in these cases referral to a qualified acupuncturist can help the acute situation and enable the chiropractor to continue with treatment. Homoeopathy can also be of value when treating acute patients.

Training

In Britain, the Anglo-European College of Chiropractic in Bournemouth offers students a five-year full-time course leading to a BSc degree in chiropractic and a postgraduate diploma. Training is consolidated with a year's postgraduate course at an established clinic. Once qualified, most chiropractors become members of the British Chiropractic Association. There is also the Scottish Chiropractic Association. There are two part-time courses in chiropractic offered by the Oxford College of Chiropractic and the McTimoney College of Chiropractic, both situated in Oxford. The McTimoney college was set up in 1972 by John McTimoney, who trained for three years with Dr Mary Walker, DC, a Palmer College graduate. He received treatment after injuring his neck in a fall and decided to train as a chiropractor. The four-year part-time course also includes the treatment of animals.

Chiropractors are at times referred to as doctors. This term is usually qualified as in 'doctor of chiropractic' (DC). This is purely a courtesy title and has been used since chiropractic began.

Young people entering the Anglo European College of Chiropractic must have at least three science A levels or the equivalent. Mature students must also show some knowledge of science subjects. Chiropractic is the third largest health care profession in the Western world following medicine and dentistry. There are approximately 1000 fully qualified chiropractors in Great Britain today.

Research

In Britain, most research is carried out by academic staff at the Anglo-European College of Chiropractic. As it is a relatively young profession, the research department has some very innovative and sophisticated ongoing programmes, particularly in the fields of biomechanics, neurophysiology and field research.

One of the most detailed and comprehensive independent studies ever undertaken into the efficiency of chiropractic was carried out by the New Zealand Commission in 1978-79. The commission comprised government representatives, educational representatives, one MD and one chiropractor. The end result was the publication of a 377 page report called *Chiropractic in New Zealand*.[6]

Some of the main findings

◆ Chiropractors are the only health practitioners who are equipped by their education and training to carry out spinal manual therapy.

◆ Spinal manual therapy can be effective in relieving musculo-skeletal symptoms such as back pain, as well as other symptoms, for instance migraine.

◆ Although the precise nature of the biochemical dysfunction that chiropractors claim to treat has not yet been demonstrated scientifically, and although the precise reasons why spinal manual therapy provides relief have not been scientifically explained, chiropractors have reasonable grounds, based on clinical evidence, for their belief that symptoms of the kind described above can respond beneficially to spinal manual therapy.

Since the New Zealand report in 1979 there have been major developments in chiropractic research, particularly into the effects of manipulation and the cost-effectiveness of treatment.

In 1990 the British Medical Research Council funded the first feasibility study, which compared the effectiveness of chiropractic treatment to hospital outpatient management for low back pain.[7] The full results were published in the *British Medical*

Journal in August 1995.[8] The evidence showed a 29% greater improvement in patients treated by chiropractic than in those patients treated by the hospitals. The results of these independent trials were so convincing that the medical profession itself, to its great credit, is now advocating inclusion of chiropractic services in the British National Health System.

The Management of Low Back Pain

Each year 46 million working days are lost in the UK because of back pain. The majority of these patients present with low back pain classically referred to as 'lumbago'.

Surveys of chiropractic practice in a number of countries confirm that approximately 90% of chiropractic patients have headaches and neck and back pain as the main presenting complaints: 50-60% have acute or chronic low back pain.

Gordon Waddell, a well-known and respected orthopaedic surgeon from Glasgow's West Infirmary, is now considered one of the foremost international spinal researchers. He concludes:

1   The main theme of management must change from rest to rehabilitation and restoration of function.

2   There is no evidence that rest has any beneficial effect on the natural history of low back pain. On the contrary, there is strongly suggestive evidence that rest, particularly prolonged bed-rest, may be the most harmful treatment ever devised and a potent cause of iatrogenic disability. There is clear evidence that activity is not harmful and active rehabilitation not only restores function but also reduces pain.[9]

Medical[10] and chiropractic[11] research reports a greater than 90% success rate with skilled specific spinal manipulation for treatment of acute low back pain.

Kirkaldy-Willis, an orthopaedic surgeon, and Cassidy, a doctor of chiropractic, who have been researching chiropractic treatment of chronic low back and leg pain for many years, considered a group of 171 patients who were examined by chiropractors in a hospital setting and found to have 'facet syndrome' or 'sacro-iliac joint syndrome'.[12] These were patients who had been totally disabled by chronic lowback pain for an average of 7.6 years. Over that period they had proved unresponsive to a wide variety of medical treatments. Following a two to three week regime of daily chiropractic manipulation, 87% returned to full function with no restrictions for work or other activities. More importantly at twelve months follow-up that success rate was maintained and no patient was made worse.[13]

In 1982 Nwuga compared the relative efficacy of conventional conservative medical care and manipulation in the management of patients with disc herniation and back and leg pain.[14] The 51 patients on trial had confirmed disc protrusion by myelography and electrodiagnosis. All were experiencing back pain and pain/numbness in the leg arising from apparent nerve root compression. Altered leg reflexes were also evident. 25 patients received rotational lumbar manipulation and back education three times weekly for a month. The comparison group of 26 received conventional physical therapy – heat and exercises – at the same time frequency over the same time period. It was found that all measurements of lumbar flexion, extension, side bending and rotation and straight leg rise tests prior to both treatments showed no significant changes. However after the four weeks' trial the patients who received the rotational lumbar manipulation from chiropractic showed significant changes in all measurements.

Research has demonstrated that more than 50% of patients with sciatica will be greatly improved with conservative care[15] and that even where there are good early surgical results, over the long-term patients do not do significantly better than when treated conservatively with bed-rest and exercise.[16]

Through my 15 years' experience as a chiropractor, I have had to refer a number of patients to neurosurgeons for surgery. This, of course, is a last resort as spinal surgery is irreversible. In practice I have found that one of the main criteria when considering referral for spinal surgery is the pain factor. Potential spinal surgery patients suffer intractable and persistent pain which usually involves nerve roots, most commonly the sciatic nerve. The intensity of the pain is unbearable and very little relief is given by taking analgesics or anti-inflammatories. Although the majority of patients may have a neurological involvement, such as reduced reflexes and parasthesia, this would not necessarily be so in all cases.

Surgery has a rightful place. However, before contemplating spinal surgery, I would recommend that patients first consider an adequate trial of manipulative therapy or, at the very least, a thorough examination should be performed by a qualified chiropractor.

Biography

From an early age, Karin Robertson was interested in health matters. The peace, freedom and tranquillity of a Highland upbringing helped to nurture the feelings she had of keeping healthy through natural methods. When she was 17, she was introduced to a chiropractor, Dr Ken Correll DC, which inspired her to begin training. Five years later she qualified as a chiropractor at the Anglo-European College of Chiropractic. After graduation she spent three years as an assistant to a chiropractor in Plymouth, then returned to her native Scotland to start two practices, one in Huntly and the other in Elgin.

References

1   *Alternative Medicine: a report to the National Institutes of Health on alternative medical systems and practices in the United States*, US Government Printing Office, 1994.

2   J B Roston; R Wheeler-Haines, *Cracking in the metacarpo-phalangeal joint*, J Anat., 1947; 81: 165-73.

3   A Unsworth, et al., *Cracking joints*, Ann Rheum. Dis., 1971; 30: 348-58.

4   D J Henderson, *Vertebral artery syndrome*, Chapter 6 in *Chiropractic Standards of Practice and Quality of Care*, Aspen Publishers, 1992; 115-143.

A G J Terrett, *Vascular accidents from cervical spine manipulation: report of 107 cases*, J Aust Chiro Assoc., 1987; 17: 15-24.

J Dvorak; F Orelli, *How dangerous is manipulation to the cervical spine?*, Manual Medicine, 1985; 2: 1-4.

WG Carlini et al., *Incidence of stroke following chiropractic manipulation*, Abstract, American Heart Association's 19th International Joint Conference on Stroke and Cerebral Circulation, San Diego, 1994 and AHA news release.

5   Harris v Roch, *A Canadian case expert testimony of Dr Lawrence Clein, neurosurgeon*, 1987; 39 CCCT 279-83.

6   P D Hasselberg, *Chiropractic in New Zealand*, Government Printer, Wellington N. Z., 1979.

7   T W Meade et al., *Low back pain of mechanical origin: randomised comparison of chiropractic and hospital outpatient treatment*, BMJ, 1990; 300: 1431-7.

8   T W Meade et al., *Randomised comparison of chiropractic and hospital outpatient management for low back pain: results from extended follow up*, BMJ, 1995; 311: 349-51.

9   G Waddell, *A new clinical model for treatment of low back pain*, Spine, 1987; 12(7): 662-44.

10   R Bosshard, *The treatment of acute lumbago and sciatica*, Annals Swiss Chiro Assoc., 1961; 2: 50-61.

J Potter, *A study of 744 cases of neck and back pain treated with spinal manipulation*, J Can Chiro Assoc., 1977; 21(4): 154-6.

11   J W Fisk, *Manipulation in general practice*, NZ Med J, 1971; 74: 172-5.

G G Rasmussen, *Manipulation of treatment of low back pain*, Manuelle Medizin 1979; 17(1): 8-10.

12   W H Kirkaldy-Willis; J D. Cassidy, *Spinal manipulation in the treatment of low back pain*, Can. Fam. Phys 1985; 31: 535-540.

13   W H Kirkaldy-Willis (ed.) *Managing Low Back Pain*, Churchill Livingston, (2nd Edition), 1988.

W H Kirkaldy-Willis; J D Cassidy; M McGregor, *Spinal manipulation for the treatment of chronic low back pain and leg pain*, an observational study. Chapter 9 in Empirical Approaches to the Validation of Spinal Manipulation, Bürger AA et al (eds), 1985.

Team effort between MD and DC produces results at Canadian university, an interview, ACAJ. Chiro, 1984; 21(7): 36-48.

14   V B C Nwuga, *Relative therapeutic efficacy of vertebral manipulation and conventional treatment in back pain management*, Ann J Phys Med, 1982; 61: 273-8.

15   A Nachemson, *A critical look at the treatment for low back pain*, Scand J Rehab Med, 1979; 11 (suppl): 143-7.

16   H Weber, *Lumbar disc herniation: a controlled prospective study with ten years of observation*, Spine, 1983; 8: 131-40.

Further Reading

Coplan-Griffith, Michael, *Dynamic Chiropractic Today: The Complete and Authoritative Guide to This Major Therapy*, Thorsons, 1991.

Howitt Wilson, M B., *Chiropractic*, Thorsons, 1991.

Leach, R A., *The Chiropractic Theories – A Synopsis of Scientific Research*, Williams and Wilkins, 1986.

Moore, S., *A Guide to Chiropractic*, Macdonald Optima, 1988.

Palmer, Daniel D., *The Chiropractor's Adjuster*, Palmer College Press, 1992.

———, *The Science, Art and Philosophy of Chiropractic*, Portland Printing House, 1910.

Palmer, D D and B J., *The Science of Chiropractic: Its Principles and Adjustments*, Davenport, Iowa, Palmer School of Chiropractic, 1906.

Koes B W et al., *Randomised clinical trial of manipulative therapy and physiotherapy for persistent back and neck complaints: results of one year follow up*, BMJ, 1992; 304: 601-5.

Little P et al., *General practitioners management of acute back pain: a survey of reported practice compared with clinical guidelines*, BMJ, 1996; 312: 485-8.

Shekelle P G et al., *Spinal manipulation for low back pain*, A Int Med, 1992; 117: 59-68.

Resources

The British Chiropractic Association
Equity House
29 Whitley Street
Reading
Berks RG2 0EG
Tel. 01734-757557 or 0800-212 618

The Scottish Chiropractic Association
30 Roseburn Place
Edinburgh EH12 5NX
Tel. 0131-346 7500

McTimoney Chiropractic Association
21 High Street
Eynsham
Oxon OX8 1HE
Tel. 01865-880 974
Fax. 01865-880 975

Anglo-European College of Chiropractic
13-15 Parkwood Road
Boscombe
Bournemouth
Dorset BH5 2DF
Tel. 01202-431021
Fax. 01202-436 312

McTimoney Chiropractic College
14b Park End Lane
Oxford OX1 1HH
Tel. 01865-246786

The Oxford College of Chiropractic
The Old Post Office
Cherry Street
Stratton Audley
Near Bicester
Oxon OX6 9BA
Tel. 01869-277 111

Co-Counselling

by Hazel and James Jarvie

Background

Psychological Therapies Counselling Psychotherapy

Like many other humanistic psychology growth movements, co-counselling started in the USA. Around 1950, Harvey Jackins, who ran a personal counselling agency in Seattle, Washington, began to develop a process of psychological healing based on emotional discharge (catharsis). By 1970 he had established what was known as 're-evaluation counselling' based on the principles of reciprocal peer counselling between non-professionals. However, the organisational structure appeared to some of his appointed teachers to be too centralised and hierarchical and in contradiction to the principles underlying the teaching. So in 1975 a breakaway group established Co-Counselling International (CCI) as a peer network. One of the founders was John Heron, the director of the Human Potential Research Project at the University of Surrey, who initiated the teaching of co-counselling there and in the British Postgraduate Medical Federation. He has also been influential in spreading some of the basic concepts of co-counselling in other counselling and management situations. Co-counselling ideas and methods are taught in further education and in various kinds of group work including within the caring professions.

Theoretical Base

The theoretical base of co-counselling is that human beings have an innate need and potential for love, understanding and co-operative self-direction. These qualities can become blocked early in life by adults who have themselves accumulated distress experiences from the blocking of their own needs. Nature's way of releasing the fear, anger and grief which result from such experiences is the cathartic discharge. Society suppresses this and our behaviour becomes distorted as we react to situations in rigid, stereotyped ways. Any situation that reminds us of past distressing experiences can throw us into the defence mode which we have adopted for such situations, instead of meeting it with fresh confidence and active, flexible intelligence. When, as adults, our own distress is restimulated by, for example children's anger and other expression of emotion, we may react by forbidding or ridiculing them with such phrases as: 'Control yourself', 'Don't be a cry-baby', 'Scared? don't be so silly.' This creates a cycle of distressed and distorted behaviour.

When our needs are blocked we are no longer able to use fully our potential for love, understanding and co-operative self-direction. Co-counselling believes (and shows in practice) that by exploring past distress experiences we can release the suppressed feelings which lie at the root of our inappropriate behaviour patterns, and so gain access to more of our potential.

Training

As the 'co-' in the name implies, co-counselling is about counselling together. Two people come together in order to have a reciprocal counselling session. Each will act as 'counsellor' and each as 'client', in turn. This co-counselling sets it apart from other forms of counselling where there is a strict delineation of roles. In co-counselling both participants have received the same training and are abiding by the same protocol whereby the 'client' counsels him or herself while the 'counsellor' sits in. The concept is that the 'client' knows more about their own case than anyone, and so is in the best position to direct the session. In this way the 'client' is in charge. However, the 'counsellor's' role is essential, as in any therapeutic situation the presence of an accepting, attentive, supporting listener is vital to the process. The pair allocate equal time where one works as 'client' on their own issue, supported by the other as 'counsellor', then swap roles. This can be replicated in a group situation.

The basic training is a 40 hour course covering the theory and practice of co-counselling. It sets up the safe, supportive environment which is the prerequisite of all co-counselling work, and uses confidence-building and 'loosening-up' exercises to ease beginners into the challenge of accepting full responsibility for their own lives. Groups are small, which helps participation. Students are encouraged to 'own' (speak in the first person) what they say and feel. They are encouraged to listen to others without comment or judgement. The techniques are learned experientially. By the end of the course participants are ready to go out with their skills and can work with any other co-counsellor.

Individuals make their own counselling arrangements, and CCI consists of a loose network of regional or local groups, who organise themselves by mutual agreement and arrange practising groups, peer workshops and workshops on specific themes. There are also regional, national and international workshops. It speaks well for the peer model taught by co-counselling that these take place very efficiently, in spite of the fact that there is no overall organisation as such. The principles of co-counselling are distinctive enough to ensure a large measure of acceptance and practice, and CCI members worldwide work easily together.

The Practice of Co-Counselling

This is self-help counselling. It requires that people have the capacity to give good attention to others. It is not meant for deeply disturbed individuals, but it can deal with very deep-seated problems, as well as ongoing daily stresses and immediate upsets. A five-minute session can result in laughter and lightness instead of building up for future trouble. People use telephone sessions in the same way. Co-counselling methods are very direct, powerful and rapid.

The cultural setting in which a co-counselling session takes place is important. Since safety is an essential condition for successful therapy, complete confidentiality is an absolute requirement. No verbal or physical violence against persons or property is permitted and there is to be no sexual exploitation of the counselling situation. Because self-empowerment is the goal of this therapy, there is complete acceptance of the client. This is not just client-centred counselling, but client-led. The counsellor generally gives no advice or interpretation, and offers no judgement or opinion, allowing the client space to find their own way, make their own decisions and generate their own interpretations. Working in reciprocal pairs not only makes these conditions essential, it also ensures them, since only then can people feel safe enough to reveal their private thoughts and feelings to each other and begin to find their own power. Each partner experiences the other in the role of client, with both distresses and the ability to deal with them, and in counsellor role as a supportive, accepting human being. This engenders empathy and trust.

As well as the conditions already mentioned, there are other explicit rules governing any co-counselling session. The length of time is agreed and shared equally in both roles.

There are three types of contract: free attention, normal and intensive; the client decides the type (and can change it at any time during the session) which the counsellor must adhere to.

Free attention means the counsellor offers the client maximum caring attention and acceptance without interventions, being always available for eye contact or supportive touch if required. As a 'counsellor' giving free attention, one learns how simple support can powerfully enable the client to direct their own healing process without the need for advice or helpful interpretations. The counsellor learns from observation to trust their own ability and power when they change to the role of client. The client learns from the experience to be a more effective counsellor by being non-intrusive and non-directive.

This style of counselling underlies the *normal* contract also. As its name implies this is the usual counselling asked for. It calls for interventions where the client is so influenced by the distress being worked on that they are unable to remember, or are failing to notice, the clues that call for the techniques learned in training. Then the counsellor suggests an intervention reminding the client of the appropriate procedure, but there is no insistence, no direction; the client, who can accept or reject the suggestion, is still in charge.

An *intensive* contract is required in the special situation where the client becomes so swamped by distress that all ability to be self-directing is lost. The counsellor will then apply simple techniques to bring the client safely back into present time. Experience shows this to be very exceptional.

Interventions Used

In addition to the foregoing theory and principles underlying co-counselling, there are various interventions and techniques taught in the training. These can be placed in various categories.

◆ **Celebration**
Working from strengths is crucial to success in dealing with distress, so clients are encouraged to celebrate their positive qualities, skills and achievements, either at the beginning of a session, or towards the end by appreciating their work and finishing in a positive state of mind. This is an attitude which co-counsellors carry out into the world, applying both to themselves and to others.

◆ **Discharge**
The major strategy in co-counselling is catharsis, or discharge of emotions suppressed during past distressing experiences. This group of interventions is the most varied, but a prerequisite for discharge in co-counselling is called a 'balance of attention'. This simply means that, along with awareness of the distress experience, the client must be aware that here-and-now it is safe to discharge. This entails directing some attention outward, to the counsellor, to present reality, or possibly to raising physical energy. As long as this prerequisite is met, discharge is encouraged by techniques that increase arousal. They focus on reliving the experience vividly enough for discharge to happen. This may require contradicting avoidance patterns that can be part of the client's defence armour. An important result of discharge is that the client achieves insights, enabling re-evaluation of the past distress experience and relating it to subsequent and present behaviour.

Many people fear that if they let out emotions they will lose control. The experience of co-counselling is reassuring. Understanding the theories and following the techniques of co-counselling, especially with regard to maintaining a 'balance of attention', makes it almost impossible to lose control, even though the cathartic experience can be powerful and complete.

◆ **Attention Switching**

These are simple techniques to switch mentally or physically from negative feelings to positive ones. They can restore a 'balance of attention' and are used also to finish the session in a positive frame of mind. This leads to celebration which is not only beneficial to the client's self-esteem, but is essential for the client who is now to fulfil the role of counsellor, able to give proper free attention.

◆ **Target Practice**

The final group of techniques is directed to dealing with inappropriate behaviour patterns as they arise in everyday life. Using the insights and clear thinking which come spontaneously after discharge, a client may use a session to plan strategies for this purpose. Role-play of such situations can enable discharge of distress feelings around them, and give opportunity to try out new thoughts or actions which could be applied in meeting these events. This can make it possible to separate with more awareness the past causal distress from present time events, and so improve response to restimulating situations when they occur.

Case Study

The following is one of the authors' case study in his own words.

Before I came to co-counselling I was deeply introverted, very level and controlled; never angry; never scared – except of authority figures, and groups of people; never sad – until one event that threw me into a long and deep depression. Until this happened, I imagined myself to be fine. This was very difficult for Hazel, my wife, who never knew what I was feeling but desperately wanted to know. I didn't know either. It was late in life when I came in contact with co-counselling. It brought up long-forgotten memories highly charged with suppressed emotions. A traumatic incident of early childhood of which I knew only in factual terms emerged in all its original pain.

When I was three my wonderful, loving, 15-year-old sister died without warning. My mother, also deeply loving, suddenly became inaccessible because of her own overwhelming grief and I was left without support of any kind when I most needed it. My only remedy was to switch off all feelings of my own, and take on myself the responsibility of protecting my mother's feelings. The effect of this was a lifetime of looking after other people's emotions while being totally unaware of my own. I lacked any sense of my own importance and in a group of people would retreat into a corner.

In co-counselling I became aware of and was able to re-experience that devastating event. I discharged, in progressively reducing intensity, the terrible grief and anger, over two or three years. Insights flooded in; adult intelligent reactions took over from the ingrained childhood pattern. I came out completely changed, in touch with my emotions, alive. To my wife's delight, and mine, I am able now to feel angry or sad without having to bottle it up through fear. I have discovered a new sense of my own value and power, have completely lost my fear of people, and have rediscovered my long-lost energy and joy in living.

Of course, not everyone has such a single causative problem to deal with. If there have been repeated distress experiences leading to a long build-up of chronic patterns of inappropriate response, there may be many layers to come off. In such cases, co-counselling helps to deal with these on a daily basis, in addition to effecting long-term change.

We ourselves regularly use sessions in our daily life together, and with others in pair or group meetings. We can resolve difficult decisions by letting go of any distress reactions that prevent us from thinking clearly. We discharge the negativity of the upsets that arise in daily life and regain our light and positive outlook. We delve deeper when we find persistent behaviour patterns repeatedly marring our capacity for spontaneous and flexible response to the challenges of living.

The basic training alone regularly produces a noticeably more positive outlook and a greater understanding of self and others. The more co-counselling is used, the more benefits accrue, and the more its value is appreciated. This explains why this voluntary self-help non-organisation has stood the test of time and continues to spread its influence into different spheres.'

Biographies

Hazel Jarvie, B. Ed., started her career as a pharmacist, has a degree in education and considerable experience of teaching and adult group tutoring. She has taken a course of training for teachers of co-counselling under John Heron at Surrey University, and a two year course on "Human Relations and Counselling" run by the Scottish Institute of Human Relations in association with the University of Edinburgh's Department of Extramural Studies. She is an active and experienced co-counsellor of 13 years' standing, and has been active in running co-counselling training courses for the last seven years.

James Jarvie, with art and teaching qualifications and experience, has been active in co-counselling for only six years, but that has so released his potential that he is now able and delighted to co-operate with Hazel as assistant, support and consultant in her teaching projects.

Further Reading

Dryden, E.; Rowan, J., *Innovative Therapies in Britain*, Open University Press, 1988.

Ernst, S.; Goddison, L., *In Our Own Hands,* The Women's Press Ltd., 1981.

Evison, R.; Horobin, R., *How to Change Yourself & Your World*, Co-Counselling Phoenix, 1985.

Heron, John, *Co-Counselling*, Human Potential Research Project, University of Surrey, 1979.

———, *Catharsis in Human Development*, Human Potential Research Project, University of Surrey, 1977.

———, *Co-Counselling Teacher's Manual*, Human Potential Research Project, University of Surrey, & Postgraduate Medical Federation, University of London, 1978.

Jackins, Harvey, *The Human Side of Human Beings*, Rational Island Publishers, 1977.

Postle, Denis, *The Mind Gymnasium*, Macmillan Publishers Ltd. & Papermac, 1989.

Resources

UK contact:

CO-COUNSELLING INTERNATIONAL
John Talbot
The Laurels
Berry Hill Lane
Donnington-le-Heath
Coalville
Leicester
Tel. 01530 836 780

London area:

Peter Birtwell
79b Ferme Park Road
Crouch End
London N8 9SA
Tel. 0181-348 8516

Courses in the Fundamentals of Co-counselling in Scotland:

CCIS
6 Comely Bank Place
Edinburgh
EH4 1DU
Tel. 0131-332 8661

CCIS
146 Park Road
Glasgow G20
Tel. 0141-357 5210

CCIS
8 Bonhard Road
Scone
Perth PH2 6QL
Tel. 01738-551696

CCIS
Lunga Mill
Ardfern
Argyll PA31 8QR
Tel. 01852-500 526

RE-EVALUATION COUNSELLING
For a list of UK contacts please write to:

International Reference Person
Harvey Jackins
719 Second Avenue
North Seattle, Wa 98109
USA
Tel. 206-284 0311

Colonic Irrigation (Hydrotherapy)
by Roger Groos

History

Colonic irrigation, or hydrotherapy, may be laughed at by some, but for sufferers of constipation or irritable bowel syndrome, it offers great relief. Nowadays it is justly finding recognition as a useful treatment and management tool for a range of bowel disorders and associated conditions.

Colonic irrigations and enemas are amongst the oldest recorded medical treatments; implements for giving enemas and descriptions of their use are recorded in Egyptian artefacts over 4000 years old[1] and Aramaic texts over 2000 years old emphasise the importance of internal cleansing using a trailing gourd as a means of giving a retention enema.[2]

Since these early times enemas were used extensively as part of the treatments given by lay-healers until the mid-1800s, when the rise of scientifically based medicine and practice occurred. Enemas and colonics continued to be used in the home and hospitals, usually administered by nurses or midwives, to ensure daily bowel movements – a recognition of the importance of maintaining regular elimination to allow the body to heal. With increasing pressures on time and money in the health services, the administration of enemas and colonics has, for some time, been curtailed in favour of pills. Powerful laxatives prior to operations, or fibre supplements for constipation are much cheaper than employing trained staff to administer colonics.[3]

Theoretical Background

The primary reason for cleansing the colon is to avoid internal toxicity or autotoxicity; and in 1918 a meeting of the Royal Society of Medicine concluded that 'death begins in the colon', documenting connections between autotoxicity and heart disease, nervous disorders, eye problems, skin conditions and rheumatic disease, to name a few.[4] Popularised by Dr Kellog[5] early this century, and further promoted by Dr Gray[6] and Dr Jensen[7] in the USA, enemas and colonics are very much a part of cleansing programmes to restore health. The effect can indeed be instant. I have personally seen lethargic people, who arrived with black bags under their eyes, walk out after treatment feeling lighter, more energetic and with no shadow under the eyes. After a series of treatments, the colour of the iris of the eye becomes significantly brighter, and the white (sclera) becomes whiter.

The theory behind using water to improve elimination is simple: constipation, or bowel stasis, leads to higher levels of toxic substances within the body (present in the bloodstream, lymph and liver particularly) which in turn affect the other organs of elimination within the body: the lungs (bad breath), the skin (spots, dryness, eczema, etc.) and the kidneys (highly coloured urine). In cases where there has been a long history of constipation, these toxins may affect the muscles, the eyes, the stomach and digestion, giving rise to secondary illnesses such as diverticulitis and colon cancer.

In practice, enemas simply introduce water or dilute solutions into the lower bowel for retention, softening the stools which are then passed out. Colonic irrigation differs by having an inlet for water and an outlet for the water and waste, which enables water to be fed around the whole bowel, and offers the ability to alter the peristalsis, or muscular rhythm, of the bowel muscle itself.

The Practice of Colonic Irrigation

Colonic irrigation treatment can perhaps be described as undignified, but not uncomfortable. No special preparation is necessary, although it is not recommended to eat a large meal beforehand. After a case history is taken, the therapist will describe the process and hand the client an open-backed gown into which to change. The client lies on their left side on a couch while the therapist, using sterilised or disposable equipment, gently inserts a speculum about 3.5 cm into the rectum. Filtered water at low pressure is introduced through an inlet tube connected to the speculum and fed progressively in waves around the colon, whilst the water, waste; and gas is piped away through the outlet tube. The feeling one has during treatment is of wanting to pass a motion, which can be a little disconcerting but is seldom painful.

The outlet tubing is see-through, so the therapist can make observations of the nature of the waste passed during treatment and judge the bowel muscle action by the rhythm and speed of the elimination.

The water temperature may be adjusted during the process to influence the bowel muscle action. Warmer water relaxes and slows peristalsis while cooler water stimulates bowel action. Antispasmodic herbs or soothing salt solutions may be given during treatment. Gentle massage over the abdomen helps to stimulate peristalsis and promote the evacuation of waste. In all, about 30 minutes are spent on the couch. A small amount of water is sometimes retained, and patients are given time afterwards to pass this in the toilet.

One important quality of the bowel is the environment it provides for friendly bacteria. The principal ones present in the bowel are anaerobic (survive without oxygen), and their numbers are vast – indeed they exceed the number of cells which make up our entire body, and around 50% of our stool's weight is bacterial waste, and not food waste at all. The presence of a normal, balanced population of these bacteria is very important for proper bowel health and general immune function, and it can easily be upset by antibiotic therapy, food poisoning, poor diet and yeast overgrowth. When the bowel is more or less empty after a colonic, the ideal opportunity exists to repopulate the bowel, using a nucleus of high-count human-origin bacteria[8], and this is routinely done by therapists at the end of the treatment.

The number of treatments required is dependent upon many factors, including how long the condition has existed and how bad it is, how relaxed the client is during treatment, their individual constitution and what efforts they are able to make regarding diet, exercise and fluid intake to support the treatment. I have successfully treated people with spastic colon in only one treatment, but others take more; chronic constipation always takes a number of successive treatments to restore some natural bowel activity, with follow-ups at about three-monthly intervals for a year or so.

Compatibility with Other Therapies

A colon hydrotherapist is required to have been comprehensively trained in and practising a body-based therapy previously; therefore often this treatment is an adjunct to others. Diet is of great importance, herbs are useful, as are massage, acupuncture, manipulative therapies, homoeopathy and psycho/hypnotherapy. In my practice, I treat many people referred to me by other practitioners to reinforce their efforts and to speed up the healing process. Information gathered during treatment is reported back to the therapist so that their treatment may be modified if necessary.

Nutritional Therapy
Herbalism
Massage
Acupuncture
Chiropractic
Osteopathy
Homoeopathy
Counselling
Psychotherapy
Hypnotherapy

Conditions Treated

Any condition which is accompanied by or exacerbated by poor bowel elimination is helped by colonic hydrotherapy. Obviously, primary bowel conditions like classic constipation, diarrhoea, irritable bowel syndrome, candida, diverticulosis or remission colitis are prime candidates. Secondary conditions are not so obvious, but again problems involving the other eliminative organs (skin, kidneys, bladder, lungs) are helped. Inflammatory diseases such as arthritis may be improved, and any toxic condition involving the liver, cardiovascular system or nervous system often responds.

Contraindications

Treatment is not indicated during the first three months of pregnancy, and if there is a history of unstable pregnancies (for example miscarriages), not during pregnancy at all. High blood pressure (systolic above 180, diastolic above 110) must be reduced before treatment can commence, although improving bowel function does lead to a lowering of blood pressure itself. Treatment is not carried out during the active phase of any bowel inflammation or any acute infectious disease process. In such situations medical treatment is indicated.

Training and Availability

Naturopathy
Aromatherapy
Iridology

Colon hydrotherapists practise all over the UK, and usually work according to naturopathic principles, incorporating dietary and lifestyle recommendations with treatment. Practitioners include dietary therapists, chiropractors and osteopaths, massage and aromatherapists and iridologists. Training is carried out in four colleges whose syllabus has been approved and recognised by the Colonic International Association, an independent grouping of therapists who seek to maintain high standards of practice and safeguard the public. The training naturally covers all the theory, including autotoxicity, fasting regimes and cleansing programmes, but most importantly includes a minimum of six practice sessions during which treatment is both given and received. At least ten supervised treatments are mandatory before taking the written examination, which must be submitted for final assessment. A period of one year's probationary membership of the Colonic International Association follows college success, during which time advice and information is freely available from experienced members. Professional contact is encouraged between members and this includes annual study weekends.

Colonic Irrigation and Irritable Bowel Syndrome (IBS)

The supportive role of colonic irrigation, together with diet and herbs is well illustrated in the treatment and management of the irritable bowel. About 70% of my patients suffer from IBS, and an improvement in their symptoms is always achieved. More importantly, they always leave with the knowledge and tools to manage their condition.

IBS is not a life-threatening condition, but to sufferers it is either permanently or periodically uppermost in their minds. The symptoms include abdominal pain which is relieved by defecation, together with altered stool frequency, altered stool form (lumpy, hard, narrow, or loose watery stool) and/or altered stool passage (straining, urgency or feeling of incomplete evacuation). This may be accompanied by the passage of mucus and/or bloating or abdominal pain.[9]

The patient can experience variable pain, discomfort, abdominal bloating and irregular bowel habits, with either constipation or diarrhoea. Pellets, like sheep's droppings, or ribbon stool (narrow, flattened) are symptomatic of a region of spasm often associated with IBS. They have often had conventional diagnostic investigations carried out: a barium enema with X-rays and possibly a sigmoidoscopy, although there is now a move away from expensive hospital-based tests to symptomatic diagnosis.[10] They are likely to have tried medications with varying success, none of which have shown convincing benefit in clinical trials[11] and their GP's dietary advice is usually restricted to adding more fibre, which is far from a proven treatment.[12] It is a very common complaint, with an estimated 50 million people within the EC suffering from the above symptoms at some time.[13]

IBS is regarded as a functional disease because at present the cause is unknown. There are many theories, but the most likely is a disturbance in the nerve control of the intestinal muscles which are part of the autonomic nervous system over which we have no conscious control.

The parasympathetic branch of the autonomic nervous system is the main controlling influence on the bowel. This branch co-ordinates peristalsis by exciting muscle movement, promoting alternate contraction and relaxation of circular and longitudinal muscles, forming wave actions which travel along the bowel. There are many drugs, herbs and foods which affect the parasympathetic nerve branch, and studies have been made of conditions attributable to an overstimulated parasympathetic nervous system.[14] The picture is further complicated by the presence of two more neurological pathways: the mesenteric nervous system, which covers the whole of the intestines and is thought to have a co-ordinating role, and the central nervous system, which controls voluntary action. An imbalance in any one or all of these can lead to disordered or inappropriate peristalsis.

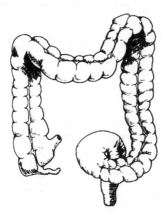
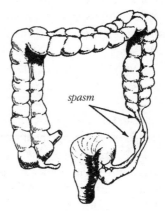

Fig. 1: Normal colon   *Fig. 2: Colon in spasm*

One important aspect of treatment of IBS is explaining to the patient what it is. Patients often believe that the pain and discomfort is something serious, and having a better understanding of their body and its functions helps them to cope with its management.

Colonic irrigation has two major treatment benefits for IBS: it is a simple and painless way to relieve the acute effects of a full bowel, voiding gas and the contents, and more importantly, it allows for local treatment of the bowel muscle itself with warm water to relax spasms, slow peristalsis and begin restoration of normal bowel muscle function. In addition, it allows antispasmodic herb solutions to be infused into the colon. During treatment, the outlet tubing of the colonic apparatus reveals the nature of the peristalsis, whether the bowel is in spasm, and whether it is overactive, so that treatment may be varied accordingly. Most spasms occur on the left side of the bowel just above the rectum. Here the hard pellets are found, and it is these which are usually felt at the start of a bowel movement, sometimes followed by most of the rest of the bowel contents in a liquid state – hence the common description given by patients of explosive bowel movements. The spasm causes bloating across the waist and down the right side, since sufferers find gas generated in the bowel very difficult to pass.

Treatment supporting colonics can relieve the acute effects: this may include dietary advice tailored to the individual (which, against current trends, often involves reducing fibre intake to reduce wind and irritation of the intestinal mucosa), herbal infusions and an oral herbal regime for everyday management.

Herbalism

The herbal element of treatment typically includes Dr Christopher's bowel tonic formula containing a balance of eight herbs which is taken at night to ensure a bowel movement the following morning. Another herbal compound containing cramp bark, wild yam and valerian, is taken at breakfast and lunch to ensure a relaxed bowel during the day. In cases where magnesium deficiency is evident, I suggest taking small amounts ($^1/_4$ teaspoon) Epsom salts (magnesium sulphate) in warm water daily, since magnesium is an excellent smooth muscle relaxant. The avoidance of stimulant drinks helps, and teas such as fennel, peppermint and raspberry leaf further help to relax the muscle. If nervousness is part of the picture, some calming herbs may be included and also chamomile or verbena tisanes.

Psychotherapy
Hypnotherapy
Autogenic Training
Counselling
Stress Management

It must be stated that IBS is a variable condition, and linked to outside stresses, so that the aim is often management rather than cure. Colonic irrigation aids flare-ups and relieves spasm, herbs enable everyday management and dietary advice usually makes an improvement. Other therapies that have been found to help include psychotherapy, hypnotherapy, Autogenic Training, biofeedback and stress counselling – all of which aim to alter the effects of the subconscious on the bowel.[15] Other alternative treatments for IBS exist but all can be complemented by colonic irrigation which can speed up progress and break the vicious circle of discomfort and distress.

Biography

Roger Groos graduated in botany, zoology and biochemistry at degree level and spent 15 years working in agriculture before further studying and obtaining a diploma in holistic medicine. He combines the practices of reflexology, colon hydrotherapy, manual lymph drainage and nutritional therapy into a natural treatment approach to health problems. He is a member of the Association of Reflexologists, past chairman and present committee member of the Colonic International Association and a council member and trustee of the Natural Medicines Society. He lives in Woolacombe, North Devon, and runs private practices there and in Truro, Cornwall. He lectures regularly and teaches at the European School, Eastbourne.

References

1   J Glen Knox, *Enemas and colonics*, Health Freedom News, Jan 1990: 38-44.

2   Edmond Bordeaux Szekely, (trans.), *The Essene Gospel of Peace, Book One*, International Biogenic Society 1981, pp 15-16.

3   J Glen Knox, op cit.

4   A Immerman, *Evidence for intestinal toxaemia*, ACA Journal of Chiropractic 1979; 13: 21-36.

5   John Kellog, *Autointoxication or intestinal toxaemia*, Modern Medical Publishing Co. 1922.

6   Gray, Robert, *The Colon Health Handbook*, Emerald Publishing, 1990.

7   Jensen, Bernard, *Tissue Cleansing Through Bowel Management*, Bernard Jensen, 1981.

8   Nigel Plummer, *The Lactic Acid Bacteria, Their Role in Human Health*, Biomed Publications, 1992.

9   W G Thompson et al., *Functional bowel disorders and functional abdominal pain*, Gastroenterology Int., 1992; 5: 75-91.

10   Sorting out Symptoms, *Gastroenterology in Perspective*, March 1989; 1: 4, 1.

11   K B Klein, *Controlled treatment trials in the irritable bowel syndrome: a critique*, Gastroenterology 1988; 95: 232-241

12   I J Cook, E J Irvine, D Campbell et al., *Effect of dietary fiber on symptoms and recto-sigmoid motility in patients with irritable bowel syndrome*, Gastroenterology 1990, 98: 66-72.

13   J F Erckenbrecht, *IBS – a motility disorder of the colon?*, Motility, Sept 1993; 23: 13-14.

14   Tom and Carole Valentine, *Medicine's Missing Link*, Thorsons, 1987.

15   Geoff Watts, *The Irritable Bowel Syndrome*, Cedar Press, 1991.

Further Reading

Baker, Mark, *Colon Irrigation: A Forgotten Key to Health*, Mark Baker, 1989.

Collings, Jillie, *Principles of Colonic Irrigation*, Thorsons, 1996.

Janowitz, Henry D., *Your Gut Feelings*, Oxford University Press, 1989.

Jensen, Bernard, *Tissue Cleansing Through Bowel Management*, Bernard Jensen, 1981.

Trickett, Shirley, *Irritable Bowel Syndrome and Diverticulosis*, Thorsons, 1990.

Walker, Norman, *Colon Health: Key to Vibrant Life*, Norwalk Press, 1979.

Resources

For further details and membership list
(please send a SAE)

The Colonic International Association
6, England's Lane
London NW3 4TG
Tel. 0171 483 1595
(24 hour answerphone)

Training Schools
National College of Holistic Medicine
32A, Wessex Road
Lower Parkstone
Poole
Dorset BH14 8BQ
Tel. 01202 717727
Fax. 01202 717787

UK College of Colonic Hydrotherapy
515 Hagley Road
Birmingham B66 4AX
Tel. 0121 429 9191
Body Management
16 England's Lane
London NW3 4TG
Tel. 0171 722 9270

The European School of Colon Hydrotherapy
Harding House, 57
Upperton Gardens
Eastbourne
Sussex BN21 2AF
Tel. 01323 412855 or 01271 870436
Fax 01323 412855

Colour Therapy
by Elinor Kolbeck

Light is the original substance of the physical cosmos. All matter is light energy in a denser form. The contemplation of light and colour has inspired many poetic and metaphoric observations. 2500 years ago, Pythagoras said, 'A stone is frozen music.' More recently the physicist David Bohm wrote, 'A rock is frozen light.' Both music and light are pulsing energy fields, vibrating frequencies of energy. When the human eye sees the colour yellow, the cone cells of the eye vibrate at 500 trillion cycles per second. When the eye vibrates at 1000 times faster than that, it perceives the colour blue.

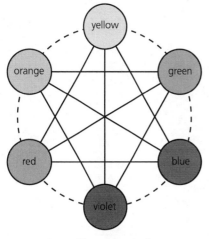

Fig. 1: The colour wheel

Diversity in terms of light and shade, colour and form, images and objects is created by light splitting into rays. Colour is the primary expression of light when it is split up and differentiated. When hitting matter, light rays are reflected back and the reflected radiation appears to the human eye as a specific colour, according to its wavelength or frequency. The beam of light diffused by prisms creates colours in the order of the rainbow; this is called the spectrum or spectral colours. Each beam of colour has a specific wavelength, that is to say frequency. The frequency of red is the longest and slowest; purple is the shortest and fastest.

The primary pigment colours are red, blue and yellow, unique identities which cannot be split further. All the other colours arise from them. When two primary colours are mixed in equal amounts, the secondary colours – orange, green and purple – are created. Red and blue create purple. Red and yellow create orange. Yellow and blue create green. The secondary colour is complementary to the primary one opposite it on the colour wheel, which is not contained in it.

The poet Johann Wolfgang von Goethe (1749-1832) bequeathed us the most comprehensive study on colours there is, the *Farbenlehre* (The Theory of Colour),[1] published in 1810, which he himself valued more than his poetical works. Goethe proposed that light symbolises the divine in the physical world. He observed the laws of harmony of colours in nature and the influence of colours on the human psyche. His approach was contrary to the way in which Newtonian science, with its abstract mathematical laws, perceived the world. For Goethe, the quality and significance of colours derived from experience and observation of the pure and simple original expressions of nature.

Many ancient civilisations knew about the specific energies of colours and their healing qualities. Egyptian, Chinese, Greek, Arab and other Oriental physicians made use of the healing powers of colours to restore health and vitality in their patients.

Following are some characteristics of the specific energies of colours:

◆ **Blue**
Of all the colours this is the most healing. It is cooling, soothing, anti-inflammatory and pain relieving. It creates an atmosphere of peace, openness and unlimitedness. It releases stress, encouraging exhalation and sighing and reduces blood pressure. It is useful in cases of headaches, migraine and also asthma. Related organs: bladder and kidney.

◆ **Red**
The most powerful of the colours, red should be used advisedly. It is vitalising, warming, activating and can be stimulating and aggressive. It prepares the body for action, therefore promoting inhalation and raising blood pressure. Related organs: heart, small intestine, circulation and triple warmer (glandular system).

◆ **Violet**
In this colour the relaxing energy of blue and the stimulating energy of red meet. It is the colour of balance and stability. It is purifying, furthering transcendence, mysticism, spirituality and inspiration.

◆ **Orange**
This is the colour of joy, acting as an antidepressant. It is stimulating, life-embracing, positive, warm and sensual, inspiring enthusiasm. It is beneficial to most of the metabolic system, promoting good digestion. Rejuvenating and revitalising, it can also raise blood pressure.

◆ **Yellow**
Radiant, gay, cheerful, alert, optimistic, lucid and light, this colour promotes a sense of detachment and stimulates the nervous system. It can help with the treatment of arthritis by removing dense deposits in the body. Related organs: spleen and stomach.

◆ **Green**
Soft, friendly and refreshing, this colour is also calming, peaceful and balancing. As it is the complementary colour to red, green must also be used carefully. In

some cases, it may trigger heart palpitations by stimulating the cardiac plexus. Related organs: liver and gall bladder.

◆ **Turquoise**

Refreshing and cooling, this colour is restful on the nervous system. It helps reduce inflammations and is useful in cases of eczema.

◆ **Magenta**

This colour draws one into spiritual awareness. It should be used rarely and carefully.

◆ **Brown**

This colour implies commitment, sacrifice and martyrdom.

◆ **Grey**

The opposite of brown, grey promotes non-commitment, evasion and denial, non-involvement and escape from responsibility.

◆ **Black**

It is the colour of self-denial; it swallows light altogether, it absorbs the entire light energy.

◆ **White**

It insulates against all intrusion and represents purity. Related organs: lungs and large intestine.

The Practice of Colour Therapy

Through colour therapy it is possible to achieve harmony within our physical and psychological being. Colour stimulates an increase of the body's defences and it can bring about cure or at least an improvement in physical and psychological illnesses.

Acupuncture
Homoeopathy
Flower Essences

There are a variety of ways to apply colour treatment. I mainly use a colour-puncture pencil with a source of light which enables me to combine 14 different colours in order to attain a totally individual tone. Using a rock crystal attached to its tip (which can be exchanged according to the required size), I shine this coloured light on certain acupuncture points, reflex zones, organs, chakras or areas influenced by these. In addition I can place a small glass bottle with a homoeopathic remedy or flower essence into the colour device and, by doing so, use the frequency of the healing substance alongside the chosen colour for the treatment. In addition the whole body can be bathed in colour via a lamp with different coloured screens.

Massage
Psychotherapy

The number of sessions required differs, depending on whether the illness is acute or chronic. Often it is helpful to combine colour therapy with other therapies, for example with homoeopathy, flower essences, massage or psychotherapy.

There is an art in choosing the right colour according to the illness presented and observing the exact duration of the radiation, which is generally between 30 seconds and 2 minutes, on acupuncture points. For example, a patient with reduced kidney function, water retention and exhaustion may be treated with red on acupuncture point K1, on the sole of the foot. Someone suffering from hyperactivity, anxiety and restlessness might be treated with blue and green on a point two fingers above the navel and at the edge of the ribcage in a line below the nipples. Often I will also needle these points and radiate the needles where they are inserted. For sinusitis, in acute cases the colour chosen would be blue or green, in chronic cases, orange or red, applied for 30 seconds each to five points around the eyes and nose and to the acupuncture point LI4 on the hand.

I also use colours in my psychotherapeutic work by asking patients to visualise healing colours, by working with colour charts and by having patients do paintings. Sometimes I ask them to close their eyes while I encourage them to get in touch with certain emotional states such as fear, panic, disappointment, rage, hatred, a feeling of being deserted, etc. This is then expressed by the clients with colours on paper and I support them in recognising their feelings and in expressing them verbally and with sounds. This is a very successful approach especially with children.

Visualisation

Colour tests have been used in psychology and as therapeutic aids for decades, for example the Lüscher colour test in which the client is asked to select eight colours in order of preference. The order they select is interpreted and can provide significant insight into their current psychological state. In other contexts, colour is mentioned in medical literature as being used successfully in psychiatry for treating neuroses and psychoses.[2] In a residential home for emotionally disturbed teenagers, they have painted the dormitories green, on the advice of a colour therapist, with the intention of creating a soothing environment.

Colour therapy is being increasingly researched for its effectiveness and potential in the treatment of various illnesses. Through this, the method is becoming more well known.

Self-Help with Colours

It goes without saying that everyone can apply colour healing on themselves.

Visualisation

Colours can be visualised. The visualisation can be combined with breathing exercises, imagining the colour being taken into the body on the in-breath. One can imagine the colours of the chakras which follow the sequence of the rainbow – violet, indigo, blue, green, yellow, orange, red – starting at the crown chakra. One might imagine the colour assigned to a specific chakra as a flower and breathe and let it sink into that spot. For relaxation, visualising a colour that is attuned to and 'lying down in it' is extremely effective, especially if accentuated with quiet music and a pleasant fragrance, such as essential oil of lavender.

Bathing

Aromatherapy

Human beings have a natural affinity with water as the body consists largely of water. Therefore, water is an ideal medium for carrying the healing vibrations of colour. It is possible to bathe with colours by suffusing the bathwater with coloured light from a lamp, or covering the normal light source in the bathroom with a coloured screen. Colour vibration can be added to the water by adding a few drops of essential oils which carry the same frequency as the colour, for example lavender oil for blue, to promote relaxation and help with cold symptoms; rosemary or orange oil for a revitalising and refreshing orange bath; pine essence in place of green to help with arthritis and rheumatism. With fresh flowers floating on the water, the lighting of a coloured candle, and a coloured beverage which harmonises with the colour of the water, add, perhaps, some beautiful music and a truly sensuous healing experience is created.

Food and Drink

A therapeutic effect can be gained by being aware of the colours of the food and drink one takes in. If, for example, orange is required, carrots, pumpkin and orange juice should be on the menu. Alternatively food can be suffused with a specific colour vibration by leaving it under a coloured light for a few minutes before eating it. Food can be decorated with herbs, flower petals and the like; this aids digestion.

Cosmetics and Clothes

Colours have, of course, been used cosmetically for centuries. Women have always been intrigued by the effects of different shades on their skin and hair. New colours in one's wardrobe will create noticeable changes in mood and reactions. In recent times colour analysts will test for skin tone and advise on colour usage appropriate to the personal type. While doing wonders for the self-esteem, this may not provide the colours required for healing, and the opposite may be true. For example, it has become fashionable to have tinted contact lenses, usually blue or green. People wearing these are unwittingly overstimulating specific internal organs (blue: kidney and bladder; green: liver and gall bladder) thereby creating potentially grave problems for themselves. Equally, when a specific colour is 'in fashion', as black was for young people a few years ago, this may have serious consequences on their outlook on life. On a positive note, cosmetic creams, oils and face packs can be irradiated with the colour necessary for healing and the vibration can be absorbed in that way.

Living Areas

The use of colour in living areas is part of daily life, but people seldom realise the effect this can have on their health and well-being. I once heard of a woman who was chair-bound and who spent most of her time in the sitting room. Her favourite colour was red and the wallpaper, chairs and carpets in this room were all red. In Chinese theory, red is the colour of the fire element which governs the small intestine, the circulation, the triple warmer (glandular system) and the heart. This lady died of a heart attack. While not suggesting that the decor was the primary cause of the heart problem, it might well have been a contributory factor. Another woman with spleen problems had been treated by an acupuncturist over a long period of time. The acupuncturist was mystified as to why so little improvement was taking place. A visit to the client's home solved the mystery. The predominant colour in the house was yellow, the colour which stimulates the spleen, which in this case was recreating imbalance after each acupuncture treatment.

To experiment with colours, one can hang big coloured pieces of cloth on the wall or look at colour charts for a few minutes. To sense the different colour vibrations with eyes shut is enjoyable and increases one's perceptive sensitivity. This can allow an educated choice of colour schemes which may have a positive effect on the living environment of an individual.

Colour and Plants

Research has been done with plants to establish their reaction to colour radiation.[3] The results of one experiment, growing cress,[4] were as follows:

Red	Growth:	Even but stunted and small foliage, almost no offshoots from stems of plants 2.5" high.
	Colour:	Light green to white stems.
	Taste:	Very bitter, unpleasant to eat.
Green	Growth:	Only 14 very weak plants were left, 2" high, no offshoots.
	Colour:	Almost white.
	Taste:	Sharp, no defined taste.
Clear	Growth:	Well-developed with offshoots from stems of plants 3.5" high.
	Colour:	Strong, even green.
	Taste:	Sweet, sharp (normal).
Blue	Growth:	Very well-developed, up to 4 offshoots of each plant, very regular development, 5.5" high.
	Colour:	A clear, strong green.
	Taste:	Sweet, sharp, enhanced flavour.

Table 1: The effect of different coloured light on the growth of cress seedlings

Conclusion

Following in the footsteps of Goethe, my experience has borne out that the energy of colours enables us to bring about positive, healing changes on a physical as well as on a psychological level. This experience is typified in the almost universally positive response to looking at a rainbow – a glimpse of the divine in the physical world.

Biography

Elinor Kolbeck, 49, works as a homoeopath, psychotherapist and colour therapist in Munich, Germany. She has been in practice for 10 years.

References

1   Johann Wolfgang von Goethe, *The Theory of Colours*, Mit Press, 1970.

2   L Eberhard, *Heilkräfte der Farben*, Drei-Eichen-Verlag, 1974.

3   Peter Tompkins and Christopher Bird, *The Secret Life of Plants*, Harper and Row, 1973.
     E F Schumacher, *Small is Beautiful*, Vintage, 1993.

4   Theo Gimbel, *Healing Through Colour*, CW Daniel, 1980, p164.

Further Reading

Amber, Reuben, *Color Therapy*, Aurora Press, 1983.

Billmeyer, F W.; Saltzman, M., *Principles of Colour Technology*, Wiley, Interscience, 1981.

Bragg, Sir W., *The Universe of Light*, Bell, Peter Smith Pub., 1959.

Dalichow, Irene; Booth, Mike, *Auro-Soma – Healing Through Colour*, Plant and Crystal Energy, Nataraj Publ., 1996.

Dinshaw Darius, *Let There Be Light*, Dinshaw Health Society, 1985.

Gimbel, Theo, *Healing Through Colour*, CW Daniel, 1991.

————, *The Book of Colour Healing*, Gaia Books, 1994.

Goethe, J W von, *Theory of Colour*, Mit Press, 1970.

Heel, A C S van, *What is Light?*, World University Library, 1968.

Liberman, Jacob, *Light: Medicine of the Future*, Bear and Co., 1993.

Lüscher, Max, *The Lüscher Colour Test*, Pan Books, 1971.

Ott, John, *Health&Light*, The Devin-Adair Co., 1988.

Steiner, R., *Spiritual Science and Medicine*, Rudolf Steiner Press, 1975.

Wall, Vicky, *The Miracle of Healing*, Aquarian, 1993.

Warson, L., *The Romeo Error*, Hodder and Stoughton, 1974.

Resources

International Association for Colour Therapy
P O Box 3688
London SW13 0XA

Centre of New Directions
White Lodge
Stockland Green Road
Speldhurst
Nr Tunbridge Wells
Kent TN1 2DY
Tel. 01892-863 166
Fax. 01892-861 330

Auro-Soma
Dev Aura
Tetford
Lincolnshire LN9 6QL
Tel. 01507-533 581
Fax. 01507-533 412

The Hygeia College of Colour Therapy
Brook House
Avening
Tetbury
Glostershire GL8 8NS
Tel. 01453-832 150

College of Chromotherapy
Jan Davidson
228 Hendon Way
London NW4 3NE
Tel. 0181-202 7545

Complex Homoeopathy
by Julian Kenyon

Complex homoeopathy is the use of combinations of generally low potency homoeopathics together with herbs and in some cases other preparations and extracts.

The Argument for Complex Homoeopathy

Homoeopathy

Although using homoeopathics in this way began towards the end of the life of Samuel Hahnemann, founder of homoeopathy, it has never been accepted by the establishment of classical homoeopathy. Classical homoeopathy can have astonishingly good results if the remedy is correct. However, to put forward the argument for complex homoeopathy, there are a number of situations in which classical homoeopathy does not work and in my experience these clinical situations include:

◆ where there is an excess of toxins in the body or, indeed, outside the body if the patient is working in a polluted environment;

◆ where long-term conventional drugs such as steroids or antidepressants have been used;

◆ where the patient is immuno-depressed, which means that the immune system is working at less than optimal level. The most common group of patients who are like this are those who suffer from chronic fatigue syndrome, of which ME is one example.

The numbers of patients suffering from these conditions has grown vastly since Hahnemann's death, and therefore classical homoeopathy is, it could be argued, becoming less applicable. One way to resolve this situation is to use homoeopathic complexes.

Herbalism

It has been found that low potency homoeopathics potentiate the action of herbal medicines and vice versa. Therefore the use of these complex preparations produces very effective medications. Essentially, complex homoeopathics bring out the best from both worlds, that of herbal medicine and that of homoeopathic medicine combined in one medication.

History of Development

Complexes originated in Europe, and 30 years ago a number of homoeopathic manufacturing pharmacies were producing well over a thousand complexes for a whole range of practitioners. When legislation came in, requiring the pharmacies to register these preparations, they decided to select only the most popular ones to keep costs down. By implication this means that the preparations that worked best were retained. Therefore most pharmacies ended up producing between 100 and 200 well-tried complexes for a range of clinical situations. The most recent addition to the range of complexes has come from America and seems to be of very high quality.

Organ preparations derived from animal sources are often added to these mixtures. These have the effect of targeting the medication at a particular organ, depending on which organ preparations are added. In clinical practice this is very effective, and the American complex homoeopathics develop this potential to its fullest. The majority of complex homoeopathics, however, do not have organ preparations in them and so are suitable for vegetarians.

Treatment with Complex Homoeopathy

A very efficient way of using complexes is to treat the patient using an organ-based approach as in traditional Chinese medicine, which sees the patient's illness as being due to the malfunction of one or a number of organs. The cause of the organ dysfunction is often toxic, but can be emotional or spiritual in some cases, and in others a combination of all three.

Traditional Chinese Medicine

Isolating the organs can be achieved by making electrical measurements over acupuncture points as in bio-energetic regulatory medicine (such as Vegatesting). Appropriate complexes are then chosen to treat these organs. As a rule, complexes which are directed at digestive organs, such as the liver, pancreas, stomach and colon, are taken just before a meal, and complex remedies which are directed at the non-digestive organs, such as the lungs, heart, kidneys, etc., are taken after a meal. The patient is advised to drink plenty of water while taking the remedies to detoxify the body.

Bio-Energetic Regulatory Medicir

Detoxification is a major part of complex homoeopathy and the use of nosodes is integral to this. Nosodes are homoeopathic dilutions of toxins. These toxins may come from the outside in the form of pesticides, hydrocarbons, conventional drugs, heavy metals, etc. or can be generated inside the body, by bacteria, viruses and a whole range of internal pollutants.

Various complex nosodes contain a whole range of potencies of the same toxin; this is known as a potency accord. The argument is that if the body is presented with a whole range of potencies it picks out those which it actually requires at the time.

This seems to work very well from a clinical point of view. Nosodes have the effect of releasing the toxins from an intracellular position and causing them to be excreted into extracellular fluid, as shown in several studies.[1] Once the toxin is in an extracellular position it needs to be excreted. Complex remedies assist this, particularly the class of remedies called drainage remedies, which improve excretion from the body via the kidneys, the colon and the skin (through sweating). Drinking plenty of water and having a low-stress, non-toxic (organic) diet are essential to encourage detoxification.

Homotoxicosis

This process has been encapsulated in the theory known as homotoxicosis proposed by Dr Hans Reckeweg, a German doctor who did most of his work during the 1930s. It has generated the whole clinical approach as described here involving complex homoeopathics.

The theory of homotoxicosis assumes that illness is the end result of a battle between homotoxins (poisons) and the body's natural defences. The most important part of the body's defences lies in the immune system, which has two main methods of dealing with invasion by foreign material. Immunoglobulins, which are large protein molecules (known as antibodies), are manufactured by special white cells against specific foreign bodies (known as antigens). In cell-mediated immunity, specialised white cells engulf the foreign material (known as phagocytosis) and digest it. A great deal is known about the immunoglobulin system but relatively little about cell-mediated immunity. Complex homoeopathy makes use of combinations of herbal and homoeopathic remedies which stimulate both immune system responses in order to facilitate the body's immune competence. The autonomic nervous system (the part of the nervous system controlling unconscious internal bodily functions such as heart rate, muscle contractions, etc.) has a major part to play in balancing the body's natural defences between activity (stimulated by the sympathetic division of the autonomic nervous system) and quiescence (encouraged by the parasympathetic division of the autonomic nervous system). Many of the natural therapies work through the autonomic nervous system and therefore can be expected to improve the body's natural defences.

Naturopathy

The second line of the body's defences lies in its methods of getting rid of toxins via three main routes of excretion: the colon, the kidneys and the skin. Methods of encouraging elimination via these routes using bowel stimulants, diuretics and diaphoretics (substances that increase sweating) are the cornerstone of naturopathic and herbal practice. The fundamental feature of complex homoeopathic therapy embodies these principles by including herbal components to encourage elimination.

The third line of our natural defences is the lymphatic system. The consists of a vast network of tiny capillaries which permeate all the connective tissues of the body.

The lymphatics drain tissue fluid away together with toxins into large aggregations of lymphatic tissue known as lymph nodes. The toxins carried by the lymph are largely excreted into the intestinal lumen via the so-called Peyer's patches, aggregates of lymphatic tissues situated just below the internal lining of the small intestine. The lymph system acts like an internal connective tissue cleansing system. Anything which impedes its flow or overwhelms it with toxins will soon give rise to a local accumulation of toxins. Also a slight rise in pressure inside the small intestine may prejudice the fine balance which allows the lymphatics to discharge into the intestine via the Peyer's patches. Many complex homoeopathic medications contain effective lymphatic stimulants; this is one of the important mechanisms contributing to the effectiveness of this form of therapy. Habitual constipation can be a major problem as it predisposes to toxins remaining in the lymphatic system. We have a lot to learn from the Victorian obsession with bowels and unfortunately much modern medicine has lost sight of these simple facts.

The Natural History of Disease Due to Toxins

The body is constantly striving towards homoeostasis or balance. The different processes which we consider as disease, are in effect ways for the organism to defend itself against toxins which are damaging to the human body (called homotoxins). Homotoxicology describes six distinct phases of disease grouped together as the humoral (Phases 1-3), when the toxins are present in the extracellular fluid, and the cellular (Phases 4-6), when the toxins are deposited in the cells and cause increasing degeneration.

Phase 1   Excretion phase – the physiological elimination of toxins via the gastro-intestinal tract, kidneys, lungs and skin, etc.

Phase 2   Reaction phase – pathologically augmented elimination, associated with symptoms such as fever, pain or inflammation.

Phase 3   Deposition phase – deposits such as gout, obesity, edema, benign tumours, etc. are seen to help the body deal with the toxin load through storing them.

Phase 4   Impregnation phase – toxins penetrate into the cells. Cell enzymes and structures are damaged, cell membrane functions are disturbed. This phase may remain latent and can later develop into a weak spot in the organism. Illnesses such as migraine, asthma, ulcers or toxic liver damage are manifestations of this phase.

Phase 5   Degeneration phase – destruction of intracellular structures through toxins, leading to an accumulation of degeneration products. This can manifest illnesses such as tuberculosis, osteoarthrosis, liver cirrhosis, nephrosis, etc.

Phase 6   Neoplasm phase – the degeneration has led to uncontrolled growth of one particular cell cluster at the expense of all other cells and the organism, and cancer develops.

After Phase 3, attempts by the body to excrete toxins have no effect as the most damaging toxins are locked away inside the cells. Complex homoeopathy treatment attempts to reverse these six phases by using nosodes to make the toxins accessible again for the elimination process. Through the effects of the nosodes, toxins move from the intracellular fluid to the extracellular fluid. The organs of excretion are stimulated with complex remedies and can now perform the task of ridding the body of the toxins which threaten its integrity.

Lay Use of Complex Homoeopathy

Lay people can choose a complex remedy according to their particular condition, such as a sore throat or chest infection. In addition there are books on traditional Chinese medicine which give simple explanations of the function of each organ, and by studying these, lay people can decide which organs are mainly involved in their case. The appropriate complexes to stimulate these organs can then be chosen. The most common organs involved are the liver, kidneys, large intestine and lungs, more or less in that order. More complicated problems such as irritable bowel syndrome or asthma require a trained practitioner to decide what remedy the patient should take.

Cautions

Whereas in Germany and France complex remedies are licensed, in the UK they are available over the counter. They are usually sold as food supplements without any medical claims made in their advertisements or packaging. Therefore the market in complex homoeopathics is largely unregulated, as it is in classical homoeopathy. This has to be taken seriously because complexes from India, Asia and South America may contain heavy metals, such as mercury or lead, which are toxic and tend to accumulate in the liver. Also there have been two deaths from liver failure due to the ingestion of complex mixtures although this is a very rare occurrence.[2] This must be set against the number of deaths from the use of allopathic medicines, such as non-steroidal anti-inflammatory drugs in the treatment of arthritis which runs into the thousands every year in the United Kingdom alone.[3]

Complex homoeopathy has a potential for aggravating the condition, as do many complementary therapies. However, proving of a homoeopathic complex, which can happen in classical homoeopathy if a single remedy is continued longer than it is required, is very uncommon.

Research

Several clinical trials have been done with complex homoeopathic preparations showing them to be effective.[4] A randomised, placebo-controlled, double-blind trial demonstrated significant benefit in the prophylaxis of flu or the common cold. The onset of the symptoms was delayed in the test group and the severity of symptoms was reduced.[5]

Biography

Dr Julian Jessel Kenyon is the co-director of the Centre for the Study of Complementary Medicine and director of the Dove Healing Trust UK and Dove Health Alliance, California, USA. He is involved in eclectic complementary medicine and is a surgeon by training, with research interests in the scientific nature of subtle energies and the bringing together of science and spirit. The Dove Healing Trust and the Dove Health Alliance are co-ordinating approximately eighty research groups, both basic science and clinical, world wide, principally in Russia, America and Europe, to look at the scientific nature of subtle energies, and also research into complementary medicine. The ultimate aim of this research work is to have a cultural effect and be part of the process that brings science and spirit closer together.

References

1   J C Cazin; N Gaborit; J L Chaoui; J Boiron; P Belon; P Cherruault; C Papapanayotou, *A study of the effect of decimal and centecimal dilutions of arsenic on the retention of mobilisation of arsenic in the rat.,* Human Toxicology 1987; 6: 315-20

    P Fisher et al., *The influence of the homeopathic remedy plumben metallicum on the excretion kinetics of lead in rats,* Human Toxicology, 1987; 6: 321-4.

2   Veterinary Human Toxicology, 1995; 37: 6, 562-6.

3   Vernon Coleman, *The Betrayal of Trust,* Europ. Med J, 1994: 4.

4   M Weiser; P P E Clausen, *Controlled double blind study of a homeopathic sinusitis medication,* Biological Therapy. 1995; XIII: 1, 4-11.

5   A Heilmann, *A combination injection preparation as a prophylactic for flu and common colds,* Biological Therapy 1994; XII: 4, 249-253.

Further Reading

Clausen, C F., *Homotoxicology - The Core of a Probiotic and Holistic Approach to Medicine,* Aurelia Verlag, 1988.

Kenyon, J N., *Modern Techniques of Acupuncture - a scientific guide to bio-electronic regulatory techniques and complex homoeopathy,* Vol 3, Thorsons, 1985.

Schimmel, H., *Guidelines for the treatment of chronic disease using complex homœopathy,* Vol I, Pascoe Pharmaceutical Preparations, Gießen (Germany), 1984.

Schmid, F., *Biological Medicine - Scientific Position, Medication and Therapeutic Techniques,* Aurelia Verlag, 1991.

Reckeweg, H H., *Homotoxicology - Illness and healing through Anti-homotoxic Therapy,* Menaco Publishing Co., 1980.

Journal

Biological Therapy - Journal of Natural Medicine, Menaco Publishing Co., USA.

Counselling

by Jim Murray

The increasing awareness of and demand for counselling is reflected in the fact that there are 43 different approaches to counselling offered in the UK at present.[1] A survey carried out by the British Association for Counselling (BAC) in 1993 showed that their membership included practitioners of 22 different types of counselling.

The BAC's own definition of counselling, however, is uncomplicated:

Co-Counselling

> *People become engaged in counselling when a person occupying regularly or temporarily the role of counsellor offers or agrees explicitly to offer time, attention and respect to another person or persons temporarily in the role of client.*

In other words, everyone can use counselling skills and anyone can be counselled, because counselling is a form of therapeutic listening based on the exercise of ordinary human communication skills and everyone's need for human relationship.

The BAC makes a careful distinction between people, such as doctors, teachers, nurses or social workers, who often use counselling skills in the course of their work (but rarely receive any formal training in counselling) and people who are trained and accredited to work as professional counsellors. An important distinction between the two is that the counsellor 'offers or agrees explicitly' to counsel whereas doctors, for example, find that counselling is implicit in their role as doctor. Another distinction is that those who use counselling skills in the context of another profession usually do so in a consultative way, which means they are using their expertise to advise or prescribe. The professional counsellor is a specialist rather than an expert and does not usually offer advice, but facilitates clients finding out for themselves the right course of action.

The second part of the BAC definition explains that:

Health and Wellness
as the Focus of
Health Care

> *The task of counselling is to give clients an opportunity to explore, discover and clarify ways of living more resourcefully and towards greater well-being.*

The aim of counselling is to enable clients to exercise the right to take responsibility for living their own lives. So, a final distinction between the person who uses counselling skills and the professional counsellor is that the person who uses counselling skills is usually primarily responsible to the organisation for which they work. The professional counsellor, on the other hand, is primarily responsible to the client. For these reasons, the BAC publishes separate codes of ethics and practice for those who use counselling skills in their work, and for those who practise as professional counsellors.

The Background to Counselling

The methods used by counsellors have developed in a number of different settings. The first important source is the psychoanalytic tradition based on the medical research of Dr Sigmund Freud and his associates into the causes of mental illness. A second is the behavioural tradition based on experiments carried out into animal behaviour by Ivan Pavlov in Russia and by J. B. Watson and his associates in America. A final important source is the humanistic tradition which emphasises the importance of putting man in touch with his own nature. The most influential figure in this movement has been the American Carl Rogers whose 'non-directive' style of counselling both questions overemphasis on technique and focuses on the importance for the counsellor of simply being human.

Psychological Therapies

Freud's Contribution

It was as a result of listening to his patients that Freud came to the conclusion that what he had observed to be emotional disturbance, irrational behaviour and breakdown in relationships in adult life could often be explained by examining the conflicts in relationships with parents which his patients had experienced in childhood. According to Freud, the reason why such behaviour was difficult to understand was because his patients were unconscious of the original conflicts which continued to 'contaminate' their adult behaviour and experience. The aim of Freud's method, which he called 'psychoanalysis', was to give his patients insight into the reasons for their difficulties by encouraging them to talk: hence the 'talking cure'.

Freud's ideas have had a major influence in shaping our contemporary, more compassionate attitude towards kinds of behaviour and experience which in previous ages had been condemned as either mad or bad. He emphasised the importance of an open approach towards sex and sexuality, of the free expression of emotions and of self-awareness. Freud considered all of these things to be necessary for the full development of human personality and for the maintenance of the mental health of the individual. Central to Freud's approach were the values of openness, respect for feelings, honesty and self-awareness. It was such values which the counselling movement represented by such figures as Rogers inherited.

The ordinary person's image of how counselling and therapy take place is often based on the ritual which Freud used with his patients. He asked his patients to lie on a couch while he sat behind them making notes as they told him about their dreams and childhood memories. Unfortunately, Freud's methods required a lengthy and expensive medical training for the therapist and a lengthy and expensive treatment for patients (four or five times a week for several years). As a result it is popularly believed that counselling and therapy are only for the rich.

While there are traditional psychoanalysts who continue to work in this way, a shorter and more inexpensive form of therapy called 'psychodynamic' counselling has developed from Freud's methods. This kind of counselling is provided by lay therapists for people who have not been diagnosed as suffering from mental illness. It takes place less formally, face to face. What has not changed is the counsellor's approach of encouraging clients to talk about the past in order that the counsellor can help to provide an explanation of how past experience continues to determine the client's present behaviour.

Behavioural Change

Psychoanalysis developed from Freud's attempt to show that even apparently irrational behaviour can be understood and that understanding can lead to effective behaviour change. In one sense, all counselling is about helping people change their behaviour, and this is the view of another approach to counselling called 'behaviour therapy'. This approach was developed not in the doctor's consulting room, but in the scientist's laboratory. It is based on the pioneering research of the Russian Ivan Pavlov and the Americans J. B. Watson and B. F. Skinner into how animals learn and adapt to their environment.

Behaviour therapy is based on the age-old, common sense observation that even wild animals can be trained to change their behaviour by the application of reward and punishment. This is the mechanism by which all animals (including human beings) can learn to adapt to their environment in order to survive. There are a large number of techniques which can be described as behaviour therapy (for example assertiveness training, aversion therapy, desensitisation), but all have one feature in common: they are based on learning and adaptation. The behaviourist sees the client as a product of conditioning, so the counsellor's task is to design a programme to modify problem behaviours. The programme is then applied methodically.

A further development of behaviour therapy is known as the cognitive-behavioural approach. Cognitive therapies are based on the idea that we can change our behaviour by changing the way we think. For the cognitive therapist, it is false beliefs which cause behaviour problems. For example, I may have learned to think that I am ugly or unlovable, so I avoid people. Since problem behaviours (in this case, avoidance) often result from the feelings of anxiety caused by the false belief system, cognitive approaches to counselling frequently use relaxation techniques such as hypnosis as part of the learning programme. They also encourage clients to rehearse mentally the change in behaviour they want to achieve, in a similar way to athletes preparing for a race.

The Humanistic Approach

What psychoanalysis and cognitive and behaviour therapies all have in common is that they make the assumption that it is the therapist's expertise which causes change in the client. The aim of these styles of counselling is to correct some kind of abnormality.

Such assumptions are challenged by the 'person-centred approach' to counselling, developed by the American psychologist Carl Rogers. Rogers suggested that counselling is an ordinary and natural activity. All of us potentially possess the ability to counsel and to benefit from being counselled by others. He also suggested that humans are self-regulating organisms. The counsellor's function is therefore a holistic one: to help clients to access their own resources. The person is at the centre of the counselling process and the aim of the process for ordinary people is personal growth.

Hypnotherapy
Relaxation Therapy
Affirmations
Visualisation

Research into the Effectiveness of Counselling

Rogers was one of the first to carry out research into the effectiveness of counselling. He believed that there were certain 'core' conditions which had to exist in the relationship between counsellor and client for counselling to be effective. The counsellor needed to be able to communicate total acceptance of his clients, accurate understanding of their feelings, and complete honesty. Rogers came to the conclusion that these were the 'necessary and sufficient' conditions for all effective counselling.

Recent research has shown that most practising counsellors would agree that the core conditions which Rogers identified are necessary for effective counselling and that the relationship between counsellor and client is of primary importance.[2] A review of 500 evaluative studies[3] has shown that modest claims can be made that counselling is effective and this is confirmed by other researchers.[4] A conservative estimate seems to be improvement in about 10% of the cases.

One famous study into reduction in absence from work due to counselling after an average of three sessions, among post office workers in the UK, showed an improvement of 50%.[5] An equally famous study by Eysenck (1952) dismissed counselling and psychotherapy as 'an unidentifiable technique applied to unspecified problems with unpredictable outcomes'.[6] However, McNeilly and Howard (1991) found an improvement of 50% after about 15 sessions compared with 2% in people not counselled, when they re-examined the same data that Eysenck used to demonstrate the ineffectiveness of counselling.[7] Such research does not show the degree to which counselling may speed the rate of improvement or change, or affect its duration, and this is the subject of current research, particularly in medical settings.

Counselling and Psychotherapy

Psychotherapy

Rogers suggested that there is no fundamental difference between counselling and psychological therapy. As a result, the terms 'counsellor' and 'therapist' are considered to be equivalent in the United States. This is not so in the UK and can cause confusion. 'Psychological therapy' in the UK still means the same as clinical psychology and is only practised in hospitals by clinical psychologists who are chartered and registered with the BPS (British Psychological Society). There are also a number of people who describe themselves as 'psychotherapists' who practise privately in non-medical settings, and have been trained in different schools. Those who have trained for a minimum of four years can be registered with the UKCP (United Kingdom Council for Psychotherapy).

The BAC publishes a register of accredited counsellors practising in the UK and sets training standards (at least one year full-time training, or part-time equivalent, and an additional period of supervised practice and further professional development, which often includes personal experience of being counselled). In Scotland, an equivalent body, COSCA (The Confederation of Scottish Counselling Agencies) has been set up to standardise the training and practice of counselling in Scotland. The BAC and COSCA recognise one another as equivalent and they meet together twice a year. An important development in 1996 has been the creation of a United Kingdom Register of Counsellors which will eventually contain a list of every accredited counsellor practising in the UK.

The Practice of Counselling

The style of counselling used by a counsellor (psychoanalytical/psychodynamic, cognitive/behavioural/person-centred/humanistic, etc.) may depend on the organisation for which they work, and how they trained. Counsellors who work in medical settings, for example, often use cognitive/behavioural methods. Those who specialise in family or marital problems frequently use psychoanalytic/psychodynamic methods. Those who work in educational settings, or in the voluntary sector, tend to use a person-centred approach. It is difficult to generalise. Currently there is a movement towards what is being described as 'eclectic', 'multimodal' and 'integrative' approaches which use a mixture of methods. A good counsellor will always explain how they work to the client during the introductory session.

The number of sessions required varies. This is a result of the recognition that most people may only need to see a counsellor for one or two sessions, and of the pressure on counsellors who work for statutory bodies to shorten waiting lists. The 'two plus one' system is used increasingly, particularly by those working in health care settings. This means that clients are offered two sessions in order to explore their problems, then reassess with the counsellor the need for further counselling. Counsellors in independent practice usually offer an introductory session which leads on to 'brief' counselling lasting from three to six sessions. Sessions usually last an hour, but some counsellors use the 'fifty-minute hour' to leave ten minutes between sessions. Brief counselling is not suitable for people with chronic (i.e. long-term) disturbances such as drug or alcohol addiction, personality disorder or mental health problems.

It would be unrealistic to expect counsellors to be specialists in helping people deal with every kind of problem. Individual counsellors and organisations specialise in counselling people who are experiencing a particular type of problem: for example CRUSE specialises in bereavement counselling and RELATE (known as Marriage Guidance in Scotland) focuses on marital and relationship counselling. However, organisational policy varies: CRUSE counsellors are not allowed to counsel people who are not bereaved, whereas RELATE now offers general counselling as part of their services. All professional counsellors work in accordance with a code of ethics and practice which forbids them to work outwith their training and competence. If a counsellor recognises that someone is suffering from a clinical condition they will work towards helping clients to acknowledge this. Then, with the client's permission, they will be referred to a doctor or to a clinical psychologist to receive appropriate help.

As a general rule, most voluntary bodies do not yet charge fees for counselling, although there is increasing pressure on them to do so in order to survive, because of lack of funding. Counsellors in private practice do charge, but fees vary (they tend to be higher in urban areas) and most counsellors operate a sliding fee scale to match each client's means. However, the fee is not the major investment required for counselling. The personal investment of time and attention by both client and counsellor in the counselling process is illustrated in the following case study, which also demonstrates both the effectiveness and the limitations of counselling. Counselling cannot cure all ills, but it does offer an opportunity for clients to work towards living in a different, more resourceful and satisfying way, and taking control of their own life.

Case Study: Bereavement Counselling

Alice came for counselling because she found it difficult to cope with the fact that her father was dying and her marriage was breaking up. She was becoming depressed, was not sleeping or eating and was having frequent nightmares. She chose her counsellor on the recommendation of a friend and because she knew he was an experienced counsellor who was accredited by the BAC.

After her father died, Alice found herself in a state of inner turmoil and confusion. She felt intense anger and frustration and was disturbed by nightmares of violent death. She was particularly disturbed by the fact that she felt no sadness and was unable to cry. She thought this made her unnatural.

The counsellor encouraged Alice to keep a diary of her sessions. Alice found this not only helped her to provide a structure for her often confused thoughts and experiences, but also provided an overview of the process and of her own progress.

The death of her father had also reawakened memories of her mother's death. Her mother had died when Alice was 13, but her father had not allowed her or her sister to grieve. Alice still found herself unable to shed tears for her mother and attributed this to her father's influence as she grew up. She felt that, if she were able to grieve properly for her mother, her distressing feelings and nightmares would disappear. She was particularly concerned about experiencing increasingly frequent and pronounced involuntary muscle spasms, but refused to see a doctor.

Alice blamed her husband, who was much older than her, for getting her pregnant when she was only 17 and entrapping her in marriage. Her mood was unstable, alternating between anger and depression. Her feelings of intense anger towards her husband and her father became confused to the point that her counsellor often found it difficult to distinguish to whom she was referring. In mid-life (at the age of 42) Alice felt outrage at the realisation that both men had abused her gender and her inexperience to meet their needs, as housekeeper and wife, while robbing her of the opportunity of living a full and satisfying life.

Because Alice felt that a key element in her difficulties was her unresolved grief for her mother, the counsellor asked her to bring a photograph of her mother. When asked what she would like to say to her mother when looking at the photograph, she burst into tears, but was unable to articulate anything. She visited her mother's grave in the middle of the night on more than one occasion and had fantasies about digging her up in order to speak to her face to face.

During this time Alice suffered a further bereavement, that of a friend and ex-employer who had treated her as a daughter. To her surprise, she found that she grieved his loss 'naturally' and openly, which contrasted sharply with the confused and conflicting emotions she experienced when grieving for both her parents.

Alice continued to keep her diary and began to make sense of the recurring dream images and daytime flashback images she had been having, particularly since she had wept for her mother. Alice found it difficult to acknowledge what these were, and the counsellor offered no interpretation, asking her to describe as accurately as possible what she saw. She finally recognised that she did not 'allow' herself to remember having been raped by a neighbour when she was a child. This incident was witnessed and reported to the police. Her mother had punished her (she was four) and no action was taken. She was raped by the same neighbour on several occasions between the ages of four and thirteen. This stopped when she moved away after her mother died. Alice was meticulous in checking out her memories with other family members and even found the woman who had witnessed the first assault.

Alice could now understand her lack of tears for both of her parents and was able to reassess her relationship with them. The involuntary spasms ceased. She was able to resolve her grief over the deaths of her father and mother. She also ended her relationship with her husband and, in buying her own home, she established her own safe space and began to establish her own identity by changing her name to that of her grandmother, the one person in her childhood who had really cared for her, thus dissociating herself from both her father and her husband.

Alice received counselling for more than a year. Since she had originally come for bereavement counselling, her counsellor discussed with her whether she needed a different kind of help, since she could now recognise she had been damaged by years of sexual abuse and the apparent indifference of her parents. Alice decided to go to her doctor and was referred to a psychiatrist and then to a clinical psychologist to help her deal with the traumatic effects of her early experience.

In Alice's case bereavement counselling was successful and led to the resolution of her grief at the loss of her father and of her mother. The further outcome of counselling was Alice's re-evaluation of her relationship with both her parents and her husband and her decision to seek clinical help as the most appropriate next step in her journey towards wholeness.

Conclusion

The counselling movement is often seen as a response to the effects of the increased rate of technological and social change now being experienced by ordinary people in their everyday lives. The current soaring rates of unemployment and divorce are examples of how people's lives have become increasingly vulnerable to upheaval. However, the wider context within which such changes have taken place is war and destruction on a scale unparalleled in any other age, and the threat of nuclear annihilation. In such a context it may not be too fanciful to see the counselling movement as part of twentieth century humanity's attempt to understand itself and to meet its need to find adequate ways of explaining and changing human behaviour, not only to improve the quality of life, but to ensure the continuation of the species.

Biography

Jim Murray trained as a person-centred counsellor and for twelve years was a student counsellor in a college of further education. He was accredited as a counsellor with the Association for Student Counselling Division of the British Association for Counselling in 1992. He now works as staff counselling psychologist in the Department of Clinical Psychology at the West Cumberland Hospital.

References

1   The 1993 edition of *The Counselling and Psychotherapy Resources Directory* published by the BAC.

2   Fiedler, F E., *A Comparison of Therapeutic Relationships in Psychoanalytic, Non-Directive and Adlerian Therapy*, Journal of Consulting Psychology, 1950; 27(4): 310-8.

Raskin, N., *Studies on Therapeutic Orientation: Ideology in Practice*, American Academy of Psychotherapists Psychotherapy Research Monographs, Orlando, Florida: American Academy of Psychotherapists, 1974.

3   Smith, M.; Glass, G; and Miller, T., *The Benefits of Psychotherapy*, John Hopkins Press, 1980.

4   Stiles, W B.; Shapiro, D A.; and Elliot, R., *Are All Psychotherapists Equivalent?*, American Psychologist, 1986; 41: 165-80.

Barkham, M., *Research in Individual Therapy*, in *Individual Therapy. A Handbook* (ed. Dryden, W.), Sage, 1990.

————, *Research and Practice*, in *Questions and Answers on Counselling in Action* (ed. Dryden, W.), Sage, 1993.

5   Allinson, T.; Cooper, C L.; and Reynolds, P., *Stress Counselling in the Workplace, The Post Office Experience*, The Psychologist, 1989; 12(9), 384-88.

6   Eysenck, H J., *The Effects of Psychotherapy: An Evaluation*, Journal of Consulting Psychology, 1952; 16: 319-24.

7   McNeilly, C.; Howard, K., *The Effects of Psychotherapy: A Re-Evaluation Based on Dosage*, Psychotherapy Research, 1991; 1: 78-9.

Further Reading

Burningham, S., *Not on Your Own, The MIND Guide to Mental Health*, Penguin, 1989.

Einzig, H., *Counselling and Psychotherapy: Is it for me?*, BAC, 1993.

Jenkins, Peter, *Counselling, Psychotherapy and the Law*, Sage Publications, 1996.

Kovel, J., *A Complete Guide to Therapy*, Pelican, 1978.

Knight, L., *Talking to a Stranger: A Consumer's Guide to Therapy*, Fontana, 1986.

Dryden, W.; Feltham, C., *Counselling and Psychotherapy: A Consumer's Guide*, Sheldon Press, 1995.

Palmer, Stephen (ed), *Counselling, The BAC Counselling Reader*, Sage Publications, 1996.

Quilliam, S.; Grove-Stephenson, I., *The Best Counselling Guide*, Thorsons, 1990.

Resources

The following directories of practitioners are published every year:

Counselling and Psychotherapy Resources Directory published by:

The British Association for Counselling
1 Regents Place
Rugby
Warwickshire CV21 2PJ
Tel. 01788 578 328
Fax. 01788 562 189

Directory of Chartered Psychologists published by:

The British Psychological Society
St Andrew's House
48 Princess Road East
Leicester
LE1 7DR
Tel. 0116 549 568

The National Register of Psychotherapists
published by:

The United Kingdom Council for Psychotherapy
Regent's College
Regent's Park
London
NW1 4NS
Tel. 0171 487 7554

Cranio-Sacral Therapy
by Donald Howitt

Cranio-sacral therapy is widely regarded as a new therapy, but its inspiration lies in the field of cranial osteopathy which was developed in America in the early part of this century by an osteopath – William G. Sutherland. It began with an idea which occurred to him while studying a human skull. Sutherland was struck by the possibility that the many interlocking bones which make up the skull might be designed to permit a slight degree of movement. This notion turned out to be the starting point for the development of a new form of treatment, and was the first of many radical challenges to orthodox teachings in anatomy and physiology. If these bones were designed to move, he reasoned, perhaps trauma to the skull might wedge them and restrict their natural excursion. If this were the case, what might be the effect on the health of the patient? Sutherland began to test his hypothesis by self-experimentation. He fashioned a number of devices to reproduce the possible effects of trauma to the skull and noted the results on himself. He catalogued various possibilities and then developed a technique to deal with them.

Osteopathy

This alone was a revolutionary step in structural manipulation. In the course of his experimentation, however, Sutherland discovered something of even greater significance – that the bones seemed to be moving in a gentle rhythmic way as if the whole head were expanding and contracting in a motion that resembled breathing. Sutherland had in fact stumbled upon a new physiological system – which has now been named the cranio-sacral system.

Theoretical Background

The cavity of the skull and the spinal canal contain and protect the most delicate system in the body – the central nervous system – comprising the brain and the spinal cord. This organ is wrapped in a triple layer of membrane known as the meninges. The spaces between these layers of tissue are filled with cerebro-spinal fluid – a clear fluid that has the double function of providing some buoyancy and support for the central nervous system, as well as fulfilling a nutritive function. This membrane lines the inside of the skull and connects it to the sacrum. Collectively these structures form a core mechanism which we call the cranio-sacral mechanism. The rhythmic motion (which Sutherland called primary respiration) seems to originate here, expanding outwards through the connective tissues to the rest of the body. A comprehensive understanding of the cranio-sacral system is still a long way off, but it is thought that primary respiration is a fundamental expression of the life energy of the human being.

Chiropractic Osteopathy

Primary respiration provides a tool for diagnosis. By placing a hand on the skull and other parts of the body, different structures can be palpated and their inherent motion determined. Restriction in body structure caused by muscular spasm, fascial adhesions, locked spinal joints, as well as restrictions in the motion of the skull bones can be determined – in fact, structural disturbance of the sort that osteopaths and chiropractors deal with are detectable. The body directly reports variations in the range, pattern and quality of rhythm to the listening hand of the therapist. A free, easy quality to the pattern implies energetic and structural health.

Through influencing this energy system, the healing potential to resolve many of these problems can be utilised. With very subtle techniques the fluid drive of the system can be directed. It has the power to gently unwind and release restrictions, restore fluidity to body structure and revitalise our life energy.

For many years cranial osteopathy remained something of a well-kept secret. This was due in part to the considerable scepticism of scientists and doctors; indeed, many osteopaths found such a revolutionary idea a threat to their credibility, and cranial osteopathy was considered an obscure specialist treatment.

Around 1980 another osteopath, John Upledger, decided that this attitude was inhibiting the development of a system of healing that he knew to be deeply effective and yet so gentle that it could be used on a newborn child. He decided that it should be developed as a separate discipline outwith the osteopathic profession and having established his own form of cranial work, he began teaching it to interested therapists from different backgrounds. He called it cranio-sacral therapy. Many of the techniques and concepts were those already developed by Sutherland. However, Upledger made it his task to apply the gentle techniques of cranial work to the whole body.

A further development was the recognition that releasing the restrictions and contractions of the physical body brings to the surface deeply held tensions of emotional origin and cranial work can be an effective method of approaching and resolving them. Cranio-sacral therapy is thus a powerful and gentle therapy for mind, body and emotions.

The Practice of Cranio-Sacral Therapy

In treatment the patient, usually fully clothed, lies on their back, while the therapist gently places their hands on the body, starting perhaps on the head or under the sacrum. Leaving the hands there for minutes at a time allows the therapist to sense the complex tidal rhythms of the body and the resistance to them within and around different structures. It is possible, quite literally, to feel the contours of the energy system of the patient. Moving around the body, the practitioner builds up a dynamic picture of the body's energy pattern and the structural landscape underlying it. A range of techniques, involving subtle adjustments in hand pressure, amplify and direct the healing potency of this primary energy system towards old patterns of tension and contraction. The expansive motion separates and releases contracted tissues – muscles, ligaments, joints, bones, even organs. At the same time the hands gently support the inertia of these tissues as they respond to the tidal influence of the fluids. Reaction to treatment can vary; often the patient will feel nothing more than a sense of relaxation, but over a number of sessions old injuries – physical and emotional – are dissipated and the body restored to a higher level of function.

Applications

The practitioner is working with fundamental energetic processes in the body and the cumulative effect can radically alter disease patterns. It is thus effective in many different disease conditions and not simply musculo-skeletal aches and pains. It is particularly of use where there is damage to the cranio-sacral system itself through injury, for example trauma to the head, dental work (particularly extractions), etc. Problems arising during the birth process can leave their imprint upon the baby causing a range of symptoms from irritability and colic to serious neurological disorders. The gentleness of the technique means that such problems can be addressed within minutes of birth. Left untreated these problems continue to exert a profound effect throughout life. In these circumstances the condition may still yield to skilled cranial treatment, though it is obvious that the earlier it is addressed the more complete is the resolution.

Holistic Dentistry

A difficult birth can be a trauma also for the mother. Postnatal depression often has a physiological basis that can be detected and treated by these methods. In adulthood such diverse conditions as high blood pressure, migraines, tinnitus, problems of balance (especially after trauma), digestive problems, hormonal imbalance, have been known to respond. Stress-related conditions usually respond very readily. The gentleness of the technique and its reliance on the internal energies of the body to do the work, rather than outside force, attracts many grateful patients of all ages who have been traumatised by overenthusiastic manipulation.

Often patients use cranio-sacral therapy when dealing with transitions in their lives and when working towards personal growth. Cranial work has an ability to put clients in touch with their body and its emotional patterning, educating them into an experience of both their inner vitality and their resistance to it.

Treatment is uniquely tailored for each individual and depends on the condition of the patient and the therapeutic goals which are negotiated. Weekly treatments are common in the beginning as this helps to build a therapeutic momentum. Treatment is cumulative and while some conditions have been known to respond to one or two sessions, the depth of this kind of work means that this is the exception rather than the rule.

Problems are dynamically structured into the body and treatment needs to go at a pace which takes into account the patients' vitality, their structural condition, their mental preparedness, and the present circumstances in their lives. Tackling some fundamental issues may require considerable preparation.

Training

The structure and duration of training in cranio-sacral therapy is as yet unstandardised. It is practised in some cases as an auxiliary technique by practitioners qualified in other therapies and in other cases by practitioners for whom cranio-sacral therapy is the primary discipline.

Co-operation with Other Disciplines

Homoeopathy
Acupuncture
Counselling
Psychotherapy

Cranio-sacral therapy may work in tandem with other therapies, though there can be problems. A considerable amount of analysis of the structural and energetic patterns is involved, and account must be taken of the response of the patient to the treatment. This becomes part of the ongoing refinement of diagnosis and treatment. Other treatments can confuse the picture. Conversely, powerful treatments such as cranial work can confuse practitioners of other disciplines. For example classical homoeopathy relies heavily on the report of the client from session to session, and the effects of cranial work can cloud the process. Treatments such as acupuncture which have an independent marker of change from week to week (the pulses) are more compatible. Counselling and psychotherapy can be useful adjuncts and many cranial workers combine these skills.

Contraindications

There are few cases where treatment is contraindicated. Acute illnesses require skilful management as there is a risk of depleting the patient's resources at a time when the body is already committed to a particular healing strategy. It has been suggested that certain techniques be avoided when there is a history of cerebro-vascular accidents (strokes) or a risk thereof; though in such cases there is still much that can be done to improve a patient's general resistance to disease – whatever its manifestation.

Case History: Glue Ear

Patrick was 4 years old when his mother brought him to see me. He was a serious though good-natured child, but it was immediately evident that his hearing was very poor. It had been deteriorating for one year due to 'glue ear', an after-effect of recurrent middle ear infections which were unable to drain adequately. In such conditions we pay particular attention to the temporal bones forming part of the floor and sides of the skull. Problems here can interfere with drainage from the ear. As is usual with such a young patient, finding out about his mother Susan's pregnancy and the circumstances of the birth itself were important. Patrick was her first child and the pregnancy had been remarkably trouble-free. However, for no particular reason the labour was long (about 23 hours) and arduous. Susan had an epidural and forceps were used.

In the ensuing months no problem was evident and the baby fed well. When he was a year old, however, he began having recurrent ear infections. By the time he came to see me his hearing was poor in both ears, particularly the right.

Before each treatment I used to play a little game with him, clicking my fingers, moving them closer and asking him to say when he could hear anything. It amused him and gave me a crude measure of his deafness. He was keen to co-operate.

As is so often the case with birth trauma, the occipital bone, one of the key bones forming the base of the skull and extending up the back of the head, was compressed on to the top vertebrae of the spine. This often introduces a distortion into the structure of the occipital bone itself. This can in turn introduce a torsion or twist into the spinal membranes and is commonly the primary problem underlying certain types of spinal curvature. In addition, in Patrick's case, I could literally feel the squeezing effect of the forceps on his temporal bones. The very act of resting my hands there, adjusting the pressure to the tidal rhythms, was enough to allow his whole body to begin the process of unwinding – a gentle sense of ease and release gradually passing down his back.

The following week Susan felt that his hearing was better. I wondered if this was wishful thinking. However, three more treatments followed at fortnightly intervals and by the end of this period he was evidently much improved. The effects were visible not only as regards his hearing, but as a general improvement in his health and vitality. Parents often notice that the child is happier or more active at a particular stage in the series of treatments, and this indicates a major turning point. When he returned a month later, Susan reported that Patrick's doctor had pronounced his hearing normal. Several more treatments were required to stabilise the profound changes that this kind of treatment can set in motion and he has since had no relapse. For adults such a quick resolution of a deep-seated pattern is unusual, but young children often respond speedily.

Biography

Donald Howitt was born in Dumfries and studied philosophy at Edinburgh University and then trained in adult education. In 1977 he enrolled at the European School of Osteopathy where he studied under a number of leading osteopaths including John Upledger. He practised for a number of years in Wales and then moved to Edinburgh and now practises at The Whole Works Therapy Centre. He has taught cranial work in Britain and Europe and presently runs a 2-year training course in cranio-sacral therapy in Germany (Lübeck). He is also on the teaching staff of the Edinburgh College of Classical Homoeopathy.

Further Reading

Sutherland, William G., *Teachings in the science of osteopathy,* edited by Anne Wales, Sutherland Cranial Teaching Foundation, 1990.

Upledger, John, *Your Inner Physician and You: CranioSacral Therapy and SomatoEmotional Release*, North Atlantic Books, 1992.

Manheim, Carol; Lavett, Diane, *Craniosacral Therapy and SomatoEmotional Release: The Self Healing Body*, SLACK Inc., 1989.

Upledger, John E.; Vredevoogd, Jon D. *Cranio-sacral Therapy*, Eastland Press, 1983 (A practitioners manual).

Resources

Carnio-Sacral Therapy Association
8 Warren Road
Colliers Wood
London SW19 2HX

The College of Cranio-Sacral Therapy
160 Upper Fant Road
Maidstone
Kent ME16 8DJ
Tel. 01622-729 231

The Craniosacral Therapy Education Trust
67 Tritton Gardens
Dymchurch
Kent TN29 0NA
Tel. 01303-873 641

The Upledger Institute UK
52 Main Street
Bridgend
Perth PH2 7HB
Tel/Fax. 01738-444 404

Karuna Institute
Natsworthy Manor
Widecombe in the Moor
Devon TQ13 7TR

Cranio-Sacral Practitioner Training, Scotland
The Whole Works
Jacksons Close
209 Royal Mile
Edinburgh EH1 1PB
Tel. 0131-225 8092

Crystal Healing
by Jacqui Cullen and Robin Robinson

Crystals are everywhere, in snow, sand, steel, sugar, salt, aspirin, plaster, pottery, even in the human body. Apatite crystals (a calcium phosphate) are in bones and make up tooth enamel, while some people develop much larger crystals of tetrahedral silicate, more commonly known as kidney stones. There are two million species of animals, 300,000 species of plants, but only 3000 varieties of minerals on the planet.

Geological Background

Planet earth is approximately 4,600 million years old and is composed of three types of rock – igneous (volcanic), which has crystallised from a molten state; sedimentary – formed by the accumulation of material produced by the breakdown of other rocks (in, for example, lake, ocean and river beds) and metamorphic – which are igneous or sedimentary rocks altered by heat and/or pressure. As the rocks settle and cool, they produce within their matrix cracks, fissures and spaces where oxygen has been released, and it is within these spaces that crystals and gemstones grow. Liquid minerals are contained in the boiling geothermal waters deep within the heart of the earth, and when certain conditions of temperature and pressure prevail, the geothermal waters pour through the ancient gas chambers and flood the fissures, lining them with the seeds of various crystals and gemstones. The larger the space the larger the crystals will be able to grow. Different crystals (sulphur, gypsum) are formed when the geothermal waters rise to the surface of the planet and slowly precipitate their contents, while others are formed on the surface by their reaction to the atmosphere and weather (malachite, bornite).

The Theory of Crystal Healing

Crystals can absorb, transmit and transform energy. Each crystal contains a precise internal symmetry which can influence chaotic energy. This quality is used not only in healing but in everyday life. In the common wristwatch, a piece of quartz is connected to a battery; the energy from the battery sets up a vibration within the molecules of the crystal at a specific and regular frequency. All rock crystal quartz vibrates at the same speed. The energy from the battery, however, is unpredictable and irregular. The quartz becomes a transforming energy medium and creates consistency and regularity.

Applying this analogy to the body, the body is an organism which, like the battery, fluctuates in energy from moment to moment, depending on the demands put upon it. Energy is vibration; all life is composed of vibrating molecules. Connecting the body to a crystal will establish interaction with the vibration of the crystal. The body and the crystal become part of the same circuit. As the character of quartz is harmony and regularity, the quartz will affect any disharmony including that which is the result of illness.

A child with cerebral palsy was treated with crystal therapy. He could only move his eyes, make a single sound with his voice and smile. When he became aware that the crystals were being placed around his body, he would relax and become peaceful. Children are particularly responsive to crystals and the most chaotic and uncoordinated will, when given a crystal to hold, become still and look at the object with uncharacteristic concentration.

Colour Therapy

Crystal healing works in many ways. One of them is by the absorption of the colour vibrations of the crystal into the relevant chakra. Chakras are vortices within the body's energy field through which energy can enter or leave. There are seven main chakras and seven main layers of the aura, each related to a gland within the physical body and responding to a particular colour vibration.

Crown chakra:	layer 7 of the aura divine	pituitary gland pineal gland	white/violet/gold
Third eye chakra:	layer 6 of the aura spirit	pituitary gland pineal gland	indigo
Throat chakra:	layer 5 of the aura spirit	thyroid gland	blue
Heart chakra:	layer 4 of the aura mental	thymus gland	green/pink
Solar plexus chakra:	layer 3 of the aura emotional	pancreas	yellow
Sacral chakra:	layer 2 of the aura vitality	ovaries/prostate/ testes	orange
Base chakra:	layer 1 of the aura physical	adrenal glands	red

Table 1: Corresponding layers of aura, glands and colours

The earth produces a wide range of crystals in each colour, each having a different chemical structure and form and consequently having slightly different vibrations and regularity of vibration, so the crystal therapist can make a choice based on other relevant factors. For example, if working with a stressed client whose adrenal glands are overactive, the therapist could choose to treat the client with a red jasper – a member of the quartz family, a volcanic gemstone the energy of which relates to the element of fire. If, however, the source of the client's imbalance lies in unresolved anger or resentment, then the therapist is more likely to choose a red calcite, a crystal holding the energy of the water element which would help to balance the anger.

The Practice of Crystal Therapy

Crystal therapists use their own gifts of intuition to read the client's auric field for areas of imbalance. Having scanned the energy bodies – without touching the physical body – therapists may then choose to place crystals in the client's hands and/or upon the fully clothed body. They may choose to place crystals in a configuration around the physical body, activated by a quartz crystal to produce an energy network or grid running through the client's auric field.

Light, when shone through a crystal, is transformed. Light treatment can be given by shining light through a colour filter into a clear or milky quartz crystal in a darkened room. Healing qualities are activated which are not apparent if only coloured light fills the same darkened room. Light can also be beamed with a torch through a crystal onto the client's body. While seemingly harmless, this can have powerful effects, clearing headaches or muscular pain, assisting digestive disorders, etc.

Some Qualities and Uses of Different Crystals

◆ **Rock (clear) crystal** has a penetrating, clear, focused energy which can contribute to physical change within specific places in the body. For example it can be used when there is a known problem with an organ or on affected tissue. While being a general cure-all, it is specifically indicated for heartburn and digestive problems.

◆ **Milky quartz** has a softer, quieter, slower, more feminine energy which can affect the body both physically and on an emotional level and is therefore suitable for balancing the body systems, for example the nervous or circulatory system.

◆ **Rose quartz** is the gem of self-love. It aids with the development of forgiveness and compassion. It produces soft healing energy which can be used for dispersing stored anger, guilt, fear and jealousy. It is suitable for cases of asthma, fatigue, MS and conditions involving the bones. It can be helpful in improving eyesight and in stimulating personal creativity.

◆ **Amethyst** is spiritually transforming, cleansing and balancing, evoking strength and determination in the patient. It is used in a wide range of disorders, including mental stress and sluggish metabolism. It can help curb addictions. It has anti-nightmare properties and promotes restful sleep.

◆ **Smoky quartz** absorbs negativity and brings a balance between spirit and body.

◆ **Ferruginous quartz** can help in clearing infections.

◆ **Green aventurine** stimulates physical healing by encouraging the body to release its blocked energy and begin its own curative process in the direction of energetic harmony and personal evolution.

◆ **Brown aventurine** brings an 'earthing' quality to the body.

◆ **Morion** will absorb energy.

◆ **Citrine** is good for timid people who need to increase their confidence.

Crystals and Minerals

The main role of minerals within the body is as co-factors for enzymes. Enzymes are the keys of life, because they turn one substance into another. For example, enzymes break down proteins into amino acids ready for absorption, and then rebuild proteins to make body cells. The mineral co-factor is an essential part of this process. Without a mineral co-factor there would be no enzyme function, so sufficient minerals are essential to our health and well-being. When a gemstone or crystal is in direct contact with the skin – whether held in the hand or placed upon the body – the mineral content will he absorbed (via the skin) into the bloodstream. This gentle form of absorption is ideal for those who do not like taking tablets, or whose digestion is easily upset.

Sodium	sodalite, tourmaline, lapis lazuli, tiger's eye
Potassium	biotite, muscovite, amazonite
Phosphoros	turquoise, apatite
Magnesium	biotite, tiger's eye, tourmaline, garnet
Copper	dioptase, turquoise, azurite, malachite, chalcopyrite
Iron	pyrite, carnelian, biotite, red jasper, bornite, hematite, garnet, tiger's eye, tangerine agate, tourmaline, bornite, chalcopyrite
Manganese	tourmaline, garnet, moss agate, rose quartz

Table 2: Minerals and the crystals which contain them

Contraindications and Effects

Crystal healing will complement and increase the effectiveness of most kinds of medication and treatment. The only times crystal healing should not be used are on broken bones before they have been set and just prior to surgery, as crystal energies can interfere with the anaesthetic.[1]

It has been scientifically proven that members of the quartz family of crystals if held in the hand for more than 30 minutes promote a change in brain wave pattern from beta (fully alert) to alpha (relaxed). Over a longer period of time there is an increase in theta and delta brain waves (deep relaxation).[2]

Gemstone and Crystal Cleansing

Crystals absorb negative or pain vibrations, so it is important to cleanse them regularly, especially if they have been used for healing. Cleansing can be done in a variety of ways, all equally effective.

◆ Light is a potent cleansing force. The crystal is left outside for a full 24-hour period (outside only, window glass does not allow the full light spectrum through). Direct sunlight will burn away the unnecessary energies during daylight hours, while the reflected sunlight of the moon's gentle rays will cleanse and rebalance during the hours of darkness. The gemstone or crystal is now once again ready for use.

◆ Sea water is a cleansing medium, and tap water with added sea-salt works almost as well. The crystal is placed in a container full of water and left for 24 hours. The crystal then needs to be dried, point downwards, for 8 hours.

◆ Fresh water on its own is an excellent cleansing medium for those gems which are rich in iron; red jasper, golden jasper, carnelian, hematite, bornite, etc. Crystals which are not suitable for water cleansing are those which change colour in water due to their porosity: malachite, turquoise, fluorite, moonstone and lapis lazuli.

◆ Crystals can also be buried in order to cleanse them. Again, they need to be left for a full 24-hour period before being removed and wiped or washed clean.

◆ Crystal clusters can themselves provide a potent cleansing force for other stones. The gemstone needing cleansing is placed on top of the cluster or very close to it with the crystal points facing the gemstone and left in this position for 24 hours.

Bonding with Crystals

The active hand (for right-handed people, the right hand; for left-handed people, the left hand) is the projective hand – with which positive vibrations can be beamed out, while the passive hand (the left hand in right-handed people, but the right in a left-handed person) is the receiving hand through which a sensitive person can have access to the love vibrations of the entire universe.

The crystal is placed in the projective hand and focused on, as other thoughts dissipate and the breathing becomes deep and even. With eyes closed, a thought-form of pure unconditional love is sent to the crystal. This vibration can be visualised entering the body through the top of the head (crown chakra) and travelling down through the centre of the body until it reaches the heart (heart chakra), and from there down the arm to the hand and into the crystal. Many people then feel warmth, tingling or a pulse (like a heartbeat) coming from the gemstone or crystal. It is now ready for use.

The projective hand, amplified by the electromagnetic energy released by the gemstone or crystal, can be used to send positive vibrations anywhere in the universe. Distance healing can be accomplished in this way.

To receive vibrations the crystal is placed in the receiving hand. This can assist in times of stress or vulnerability, when positive energy is required to amplify one's own flagging spirit.

Gemstones and crystals are personal things, and having bonded with them the practitioner should not to allow others to touch or handle them, as others' thought vibrations – albeit not deliberately – may enter them and lessen their effectiveness as personal amplifying tools.

Programming Crystals

The practitioner may activate or programme the crystals; this is achieved by intentional prayer or meditation. Empirically it is noted that when positive thought patterns are projected through crystals, they respond with an almost instantaneous release of electromagnetic energy. There seems to be a far lesser effect or energy interchange when crystals are simply held, without being programmed or used to amplify thought patterns.

Crystals and Houses

Crystals can be used to heal places as well as people and can affect the vibrations in a space – a room, a house or an office. This was applied to a school staffroom where the teachers were experiencing a high degree of negativity. A crystal was programmed to clear negative energies, placed in the staffroom in a decorative capacity, and within two months a noticeable change had taken place. Some of the teachers remarked that they felt happier at school than they had previously.[3]

Crystals for Dreamwork

Some people find that if they sleep with their activated gemstone or crystal in their receiving hand overnight, in the morning they feel refreshed, energised and relaxed and they can often remember their dreams with greater accuracy and for a longer period of time before they fade. It is also noticeable that the gemstone or crystal will instinctively be found without trouble, no matter where in the bed it may be.

Trying it for Yourself

Those who work with crystals and those who have had treatment will vouch for their transformative power, but words are never as powerful as a personal experience. Therefore, if you wish to explore this further, find a selection of crystals, look at them, allow yourself to be drawn to one, pick it up and close your eyes. If there is an affinity with this particular crystal, a physical and/or visual effect may be detected. This will provide proof, through personal experience, that humankind can be affected and healed by a crystal.

It is important to be aware that there are some synthetic, heat-treated and dyed specimens on the market which react in a different way from natural crystals. Crystals for healing need to be assessed and prescribed by a qualified crystal therapist.

Case Reports

A woman of 24 tried to commit suicide by taking an overdose of tablets with alcohol three days before coming for crystal therapy. She was suffering from very low self-esteem with destructive thought patterns, perceiving her life to be out of her control. Nutritionally she was very imbalanced. The crystals chosen were rose quartz to raise self-esteem; aventurine for mental clarity and to strengthen the immune system and promote balance; and smoky quartz to aid with overcoming depression and self-destructive tendencies. Soon after these treatments the woman separated from her husband, moved abroad, trained as an aromatherapist and began to use the wisdom she had gained from this experience to help others to help themselves.

Aromatherapy

A woman of 52 presented with a deep racking cough. The GP's diagnosis was chronic obstructive airways disease. She had been using a steroid inhaler daily for the last three years. In the night she had a frequent need to urinate. She feared she would be housebound within six months. Emotionally this woman was suffering from a painful separation from her first husband and had feelings of betrayal and worthlessness. She had a difficult relationship with her second husband's ex-wife, and with his son who now lived with them. The throat chakra was almost completely blocked with fear, guilt, anger and resentment towards both herself and others. The crystals chosen were blue lace agate, a form of quartz which changes the brain wave pattern while soothing the throat chakra; turquoise – a powerful auric protector – which teaches one how to accept beauty within and without while promoting balance within the throat chakra; moonstone which teaches one how to receive and promotes balance within all body fluids; and rose quartz to promote self-love. After the treatment the woman left with hope in her heart, choosing to use supportive thought patterns. The cough was gone and therefore medication could be reduced. She has since done a training in Reiki healing and is finding her own healing gifts. Follow-up treatment is being continued.

Biographies

Jacqui Cullen, TM, Crys., HM, IACHT, HPAI, is a crystal healing therapist and a spiritual healer. She works with colour therapy, relaxation techniques and Hawaiian shamanism combined with nutritional knowledge. Jacqui endured an illness herself for five years, and now shares with others some of what she learned on her journey back to health. Jacqui and her husband Paul offer therapy sessions, residential weekends at their healing centre, introductory workshops in crystal healing and a two year (part-time) qualifying course as the Scottish branch of the IACHT.

Robin Robinson is a spiritual healer and crystal healer. He is a member of the NFSH and has been practising for 12 years.

References

1   IACHT Code of Conduct.

2   Melody, *Love is in the Earth*, Earth Love Publishing House, 1991, p334.

3   R Robinson's personal experience.

Further Reading

Bonewitz, Ra, *The Cosmic Crystal Spiral*, Element Books, 1986.

Gerber, Richard, *Vibrational Medicine: New Choices for Healing Ourselves,* Bear & Co., 1988.

Melody, *Love Is In The Earth – A Kaleidoscope Of Crystals*, Earth Love Publishing House, 1991.

Palmer, Magda, *The Healing Power of Crystals*, Rider, 1988.

Resources

The Affiliation of Crystal Healing Organisations (ACHO)
46, Lower Green Road
Esher
Surrey KT10 8HD

The International Association of Crystal Healing Therapists (IACHT)
Hazel Raven
50, Birchfield Drive
Boothstown
Worsley
Manchester M28 4ND
Tel. 0161 702 8191

The International Association of Crystal Healing Therapists (Scotland)
Jacqui & Paul Cullen
P O Box 727
Glasgow G12 9QQ
Tel. 01659 58319

Dowsing

by Roy and Ann Procter

Dowsing has traditionally been used to find water. This ancient skill is now being applied to many other functions. This includes searching for mineral deposits, lost objects or missing persons. Despite its unorthodox image, the services of professional dowsers are used by businesses and public institutions who would obviously not be prepared to pay if the success rate were not high. Although Scotland Yard do not publicise the fact, once in a while they are reported by the media to have used a dowser to successfully complete a case. Dowsing is also used as a means of providing answers to questions which would be difficult or impossible to deduce by logical means.

In the field of health, dowsing is used in a variety of ways in many different therapies, for example to assist in the choice of aromatherapy oils or homoeopathic remedies or in the healing of geopathic stress – subtle earth energies which affect human health. Dowsing is not in itself a curative therapy, but is a means by which therapists can access their intuition to enhance and expand their work in a chosen modality, including, albeit in rare cases, allopathic medicine.

Aromatherapy
Homoeopathy

The mechanism of dowsing lies within the mind of the dowser, who uses intellect and logic (left brain) to ask suitably detailed and unambiguous questions, then allows the intuitive faculty (right brain) to provide a yes/no answer. Some work has been done with EEG monitors which detect the various electrical rates in the brain while the subject adopts different mental modes.[1] It has been discovered through this work that problem-solving uses beta wave frequencies, over 16 cycles per second, while meditation, dreaming (asleep or awake) and imaging use the alpha frequencies of between 8 and 16 cycles per second. It seems that the dowser needs to ask his questions logically while in the beta range, then switch into the alpha range to receive the answers.

Radionics

There is no generally accepted theoretical basis explaining the dowsing response, but most agree that an involuntary muscular action gives a signal which is augmented by the dowsing instrument to make it clearly visible. The tool is merely the indicator of the internal mechanism, as are the hands on a clock.

Kinesiology

Instruments range from the traditional forked stick used by water dowsers, of which a version made of plastic rods is now available, to simple muscle checking which requires no outside instrumentation, but involves testing for weak or strong response from the dowser's body.

When using a dowsing fork, the two legs of the fork are held between fingers and thumbs, palms upwards, with the point forward and the fork under strain.

When the dowser walks over a spot where there is water (or whatever they are looking for) underground, there is a very slight rotation of the wrist and the springiness of the fork causes it to flip up or down. Other suitable tools for finding underground features or subtle energies 'in the field' include a pair of rods each bent at right angles. One part of the rod is held upright in the dowser's hand, the other points forwards, parallel to the ground and the two rods are held shoulder-width apart. Again a small rotation in the dowser's wrists when walking over the sought substance will be magnified and the rods will cross or separate. More sophisticated manufactured tools can also be used for field work, and dowsers have been very inventive in designing customised devices to clarify their questioning and receive accurate answers.

Different tools may be used when dowsing indoors, for example over a map to locate a place, person or subtle energy system, or for choosing remedies. In these instances a bobber or a pendulum might be more suitable. A bobber is a long, flexible rod with a weight on the end, which magnifies the muscle movement by nodding horizontally for 'no' or vertically for 'yes'. A pendulum is a weight on a string which makes a rotational movement or swings in different directions for positive and negative answers. Some practitioners impose a pattern of swing, for example clockwise is 'yes', anticlockwise is 'no', but we prefer to help our students to find the motion which comes naturally to them, and then use those signals.

Dowsing for Geopathic Stress

There are many applications which benefit from the use of the dowsing skill, so most dowsers have their speciality. Ours is searching for geopathic stress – mapping the subtle earth energies which are found to be detrimental to human beings, so that we can assist in healing these energies.

As far back as 1932, a German aristocrat called Gustav von Pohl researched this phenomenon and published his results in a book called *Earth Currents: Causative Factor of Cancer and other Diseases*. An English translation was produced in 1987. Unfortunately von Pohl overstated his case, and claimed that just about every disease was due to these harmful earth currents, which discredited the general validity of his work. Since then numerous researchers have looked at the subject in many different ways, and called these currents black streams, negative earth energies, bad ley lines, and more. The terminology is not yet fixed, but it is likely that 'geopathic stress' will become the most acceptable.

Development of our Practice

The subject was brought to our attention in 1979, when attending a summer school run by Bruce MacManaway, celebrated Scottish dowser and healer. During the first session the group was troubled by one member, John, who spoke very slowly, taking a laborious time to pose his questions. MacManaway used him as the subject for an experiential healing exercise, after which John became much more lively, sped up his speech, and practically danced into dinner. At the next session MacManaway told us that he had dowsed John's home and found it crisscrossed with negative earth energy lines, which he undertook to heal.

We were also told about research on a remote Scottish island.[2] Dowsers had mapped negative energy lines and then submitted their findings to the local GP who counted the incidence of chronic illness and cancer amongst residents living along the lines. The figures seemed to support the theory that when energy lines are negative, causing geopathic stress, they drain and deplete our vital energies and therefore make it more difficult for bodies and minds to maintain balance and health and to resist infections and internal anomalies such as cancer. However, when the energies are positive, they are life-enhancing and they charge us up.

At the summer school the following year we learned to map and heal the energies in the way MacManaway had developed, and have been working with these techniques and developing them since then.

One of the earliest requests for help we received was from the family of a woman in England, who had suffered clinical depression for about five years. She had been admitted to hospital several times, but on her return home became worse again and had to go back in for more treatment. We dowsed on a sketch plan of her home and found two large negative energy lines going through her house, with the crossing point in her kitchen. We went along and did what MacManaway had taught us. This involved driving two iron stakes into the ground at exactly the right places, having dowsed for the length they should be. This changed the polarity of the energy lines from negative to positive, so that they enhanced the atmosphere in her home rather than draining her energy. At the time she was menopausal, which made her more vulnerable to subtle energies. It is apparent that some people are more sensitive to these influences than others. The woman did not need hospital treatment again, and we have heard that she has kept relatively well in the 15 years since.

One of the great pioneers in this field of work was a Herefordshire gentleman called Alfred Watkins. Having a keen eye for the subtle aspects of landscape, he was the first to moot a system of ley lines which run across the countryside apparently picking up on ancient pathways connecting earthworks or sacred sites such as Stonehenge and the Rollright Stones.[3] Some people see the negative earth currents as relating to these larger ley lines. To test this theory, we traced the larger pattern near this woman's home on an ordnance survey map. We found that one of her lines originated in a hilltop site about ten miles away. It was positively charged at that point but changed to negative about six miles from her home where a lot of deep digging had been done for a lead-in road to a new bypass. We asked the family when this work had happened. 'About six years ago,' they said, 'not long before Mother became ill.' This hypothesis, that major earth works affecting earth energy lines can be detrimental for miles downstream, has subsequently been confirmed many times.

Spiritual Healing

We have since done healing work on many hundreds of places and developed a way of healing from a distance, using our spiritual healing capabilities in a finely focused and meditative way.

Research

Research in this country is very scant, but in Austria ongoing work is being done by Dr O. Bergsmann, a Viennese medical consultant, funded by the government.[4] Bergsmann asked three dowsers to locate places in eight hospital rooms, in various parts of Austria, which were either neutral or affected by geopathic stress. Twenty-four medical tests were undertaken on 985 subjects who had simply sat in each of the different places for 15 minutes. Reduction of the neurotransmitter serotonin, which has been connected with depression, was especially noted in the stressed areas. The statistics so far are highly significant in proving that geopathic stress affects the human organism.

Colour Therapy
Sound Therapy

The Austrian research covers diagnosis and does not address treatment, which is a common situation. Dowsers sometimes get as far as diagnosis and advise people to move their chairs, beds, etc., away from the deleterious location, which can be impossible in a small home. Moving house is not a very helpful suggestion either. Wherever possible healing treatment needs to be instigated, and increasing numbers of practitioners are finding ways of doing this at various levels. Dowsers who are not spiritual healers may work with imaging, for example. Others may use artifacts, ranging from electronic gadgets to colour coding or sound vibration. The fact that there is no set way of effecting the healing work can undermine its acceptability, but pragmatism speaks for itself. Even though dowsers work with the intuitive faculty of the mind rather than with scientific mechanisms, the results are proven, and hopefully more serious research will, in time, be initiated. Dowsing is a developing skill.

Biography

Roy Proctor is an aeronautical engineer, officially retired, who does consultancy work. Ann Proctor is a BAC counsellor and psychotherapist using her qualifications in transpersonal psychology and psychological astrology. Both are registered healers with the NFSH.

References

1   for instance the 'mind mirror', a device constructed by Geoffry Blundell and described in Maxwell Cade, Nona Coxhead, *The Awakened Mind*, Delacorte Press, 1979.

2   A Bruce Macmanaway, *Healing, the Energy that can restore health*, Thorsons, 1983, p150.

3   Alfred Watkins, The Long Straight Track, 1925.

4   O Bergsmann, Risk Factor Place, *Dowsing Zone and Man, Scientific study investigating place-related influences on man*, University Publishing House Vienna, 1990 (German edition).

Further Reading

Bailey, Arthur, *Dowsing for Health*, Quantum 1990.

Bird, Christopher, *The Divining Hand*, EP Dutton, 1979.

Cowan, D.; Girdlestone, R.; *Safe as Houses?*, Gateway, Bath, 1996.

Davies, Rodney, *Dowsing*, Aquarian Press, 1991.

Graves, Tom, *The Diviners Handbook*, Aquarian Press, 1986.

Havelock Fidler, J, *Earth Energy*, Aquarian Press, 1988.

Jurriaanse, D., *The Practical Pendulum Book*, Samuel Weiser Inc., 1986.

Lethbridge, Tom, *Ghost and Divining Rod*, Routledge and Kegan Paul, 1963.

Lonegren, Sig, *Spiritual Dowsing*, Gothic Image, 1986.

Maby, J C., Bedford Franklin, T., *The Physics of the Divining Rod*, Bell, 1939.

MacManaway, Bruce, *Healing, the energy that can restore health*, Thorsons, 1983.

Ross, T.; Wright, R., *The Divining Mind*, Inner Traditions, 1991.

Scott-Elliot, James, *Dowsing – One Man's Way*, Jersey, Neville Spearman, 1977.

Thurnell-Read, Jane, *Geopathic Stress*, Element, 1995.

Wright, R and P., *The Divining Heart*, Millenium Books, 1994.

Resources

The British Society of Dowsers
Sycamore Barn
Tamley Lane
Hastingleigh
Ashford
Kent TN25 5HW

The American Society of Dowsers
Dowser's Hall
Danville
Vermont 005828 0024
USA
Tel. (802) 684 3417

Drama and Movement Therapy
by Sue Rickards

Historical Background

In 1964, in the early hours of morning, Marian Lindkvist, an actress and social activist, awoke from a dream which was to change her life and the lives of many others. She dreamt of a hospital ward in which patients were moving together, creating drama and participating in the enacting. Marian, or Billy, as she is affectionately known, had been working with groups of actors, taking drama performances into institutions, hospitals, prisons and schools. She felt that the dream clarified questions she had been asking about the content and quality of this work, reinforcing her sense that more interaction was required, rather than the people simply watching a performance.

Billy's work was funded by various charities and mental health organisations interested in establishing community support systems for the sick, disabled or marginal members of society. With their help, she established a group called KATS, which involved volunteers taking drama into residential institutions as a therapeutic activity. They used story and mime and everyone could be included in the creativity, both patients and staff.

KATS learnt and grew on its feet, metaphorically and physically. They toured Britain, including the Edinburgh Festival Fringe, taking drama and movement and promoting its therapeutic effects wherever they went. Staff were fascinated by the transformations that took place. They saw and experienced how people responded and changed (for example patients feeling more empowered and becoming more communicative) and a demand for training to use this method grew.

The first training course in drama and movement therapy took place at Guy's Hospital, London. Twenty-five occupational therapists attended and thereafter several hundred short courses were held in various parts of the UK. During the 1970s interest and acknowledgement grew rapidly and it was increasingly recognised that the depth of what KATS and other groups embodied could not be covered in short courses.

In 1975 the full-time study of drama and movement as a therapy began, recognised by the Department of Education and Science. The organisation promoting the combined use of drama and movement as therapy was called Sesame, which offers a one year full-time post-graduate diploma. Drama and movement therapy is practised worldwide by Sesame practitioners with many groups of people, including children with special needs, people living with HIV, survivors of sexual or emotional abuse, elderly people, people with learning difficulties and others.

Theoretical Background

Drama and movement therapy has its roots in Jungian theory. Jung stated that the psyche is self regulating, seeking homoeostasis in much the same way as the body does. A body, for example, recognises and signals overheating, which is then balanced by sweating until a healthy temperature is restored. Similarly, the psyche can signal an imbalance as, for instance, when neurosis or depression signals the need for issues to be addressed. This can be done through psychotherapeutic or other means, one of which might be drama and movement.

Psychological Therapies

One of Jung's discoveries was the use of 'active imagination' to stimulate creative potential. This can include dancing, drawing, moving or in some other way giving form to the inner experience. The act of creation, by marrying inner experience with outward expression, can in itself be healing, regardless of the technical quality of the final outcome. When unconscious material is brought to light and assimilated, verbally or otherwise, it no longer has power over someone's feelings and actions. As a result, the person becomes more balanced, aware and empowered.

One way drama and movement therapy uses this knowledge is through the enactment of myths. Myths express humankind's psychological experience, using metaphor and symbol. They have been used the world over throughout history to give understanding and meaning to psychological experiences. There are universal similarities in every culture which enable myths to speak to that which all humankind has in common. By enacting a myth it is possible to experience, rather than simply understand intellectually, the metaphor. Participants enacting their part in the story bring their own history, their own personality, their own psyche, and so each time it is performed with different people as actors, the experience will be entirely different.

Drama and movement therapy also uses movement. Bodies hold memories of all earlier experiences that did not get expressed or released at the time: they store unexpressed and unexplored feelings. Through movement it is possible to explore and express these feelings in non-intellectual ways. Everyone's movements are unique, like fingerprints.

Bio–Energetic Analysis

Some patterns of movement, though individually coloured, are universal. When people are sad or angry, it is usually possible to recognise this by their body language.

The core emotions seem to express themselves in ways universally recognisable to us all. The second fundamental theory embraced by drama and movement therapy is that of Rudolph Laban, whose analysis of movement makes it possible to notice which qualities are predominant and strong in an individual and which are less so.[1] Laban provided a map which clarifies the way in which people move from one set of movement qualities to another. He trained people to observe which movements come easily and which do not and in re-establishing balance suggested that the psyche is freed as the body resolves its constricted movements. More recently, Gabrielle Roth (whose Five Rhythms work will be discussed later) says the first task in healing ourselves is to free the body.[2]

The Practice of Drama and Movement Therapy

Prior to the session, a 'main event' will have been carefully planned by the facilitator. It might be in the form of enacting a myth, moving to music (made by the group or recorded) or in the form of a piece of drama, improvised or prepared. It might be in the form of movement with touch, a technique devised by Marian Lindkvist, which involves the practitioner interacting with the patients, dancing with them, using touch to assist them in responding and freeing up their own creative energy and movements.

There is always a warm-up to make the transition from 'outside' and to loosen up the group or the individual's imagination, voice and body. This may involve moving to music or to a rhythmic beat and will also include exercises to warm up the imagination, asking the participants, for example, to imagine they are a field of wild flowers in the wind, and to move accordingly. There is also always a 'grounding' at the end, to enable them to come out of their roles. An example might be the instruction to touch four objects in the room that are red. This type of activity ensures that people are ready, safe and able to leave the session.

Realising that we have many ways to resist our fearful (because unknown) unconscious material, drama and movement therapy works obliquely, often non-verbally. Rather than hammering on the door of the unconscious shouting, 'Come out, we know you're in there!', therapists trained by Sesame seek to invite and allow – hence the institute's name 'Sesame' (as in the story when 'Open Sesame' opens the door to reveal treasures within) and its logo of an ancient key.

Personal Example

I will give an example from my own training sessions of how a myth enactment might unfold, and the implications it might have for the players.

One afternoon we enacted a 'coyote' myth twice. There is no sense or fear that we might 'get it wrong' because it is understood that each time it will be different, so we all feel free to improvise spontaneously. Coyote myths have cunning, tricky coyote as their central character. In our myth, coyote is well meaning. His friend's wife has died and he tries to coax her across the river Styx, back to the land of the living, to be reunited with her husband. However, she no longer wishes to return, so all coyote's trickery and scheming come to nothing. The first enactment left coyote and his friend sad, but able to get on with the healing process of grieving. In the second, I volunteered for the coyote role as I was feeling a bit cheeky and tricky myself. Because of the way I played coyote, not only did he not manage to reunite the couple, he also incurred the wrath of the people he had tricked along the way, including his friend. Coyote ended up alienated and so the enactment ended.

In this instance, I had unconsciously evoked a huge fear of mine – I had been 'bad' as coyote, in a way I would never allow myself to be in the 'real' world, and had been rejected. This brought up much material for me, which I began to acknowledge, with support, in the feedback time before the end of the session. Since that session I have noticed a marked difference in myself. While I am not totally free of the fear of rejection, I am more able to make clear choices, even risky ones, rather than being unconsciously dominated by my fear of rejection. I can choose to do something that may alienate me from others, for instance speak my mind when I know I am not with a group of like-minded people. I am confident that my fear of standing alone will pass.

At times people can experience very deep psychological healing, as I did in this instance, and at other times they may just try on a role for size – taking the part of a hero or an incensed goddess, a mischievous animal or a saintly traveller. When enacting or moving, everything and nothing is true. It is a story and yet, by taking part, we can only describe, enact, move from that which is within us. Our own truth unfolds, beautiful and ugly, wild and contained, bold and timid.

No two movement sessions are ever the same. They are planned to allow spontaneous, organic connections – with oneself, with others, and with the therapist – to arise and be expressed and explored.

Case History

A woman of 45 had learning difficulties; speech did not come easily, and during this session she was in her wheelchair. We began with some warm-up movement and imagination exercises – stretching, pulling, throwing a soft ball to one another (laughing shyly, both of us) then moving as if we were throwing something heavy then featherlight, fast or sticky… I had brought a selection of music with me of varying qualities, tempos and textures and invited her to choose one. First she chose a very calm piece and we began sitting slightly adjacent to one another, moving our fingers and hands, sometimes mirroring or repeating each other's actions. We chose a second piece, a livelier one. This time we deliberately formed our movements together. I would be with her movements, almost copying until I got the feel for them; then I would add some of myself, lightly changing, emphasising a different quality – larger, softer, shakier... not leading on ahead but easing and stretching our repertoire, always paying attention. As she picked this up, I would surrender to her lead and later, following my intuition take it up again. As the music became more energetic, we linked hands, pushing and pulling one another. (I was no longer able to stay sitting beside her but was kneeling in front.) Our eyes would meet, stay for a few moments until the music and the organic changing of our movement led us on. At one point as we wrangled our hands and arms, she withdrew one hand and punched the air, with a loud 'Hah!' I joined her and we punched the air with our free hands, the sounds changing, growing louder, more aggressive, then softer and finally becoming a gentle 'hah, hah, hah' as we began to dissolve into laughter. We kept moving as the music ended, just paying attention as we got slower, more tender and then stopped. We waited, fingers touching for a few moments and she said gently, 'Yeah.' We both grinned.

Together we had been on a journey with energy arising from what we created between us. We had expressed ourselves in simple ways, raw and honest as our dance unfolded and what we shared changed us as we established in the outer world that which had been a private aspect of our inner, perhaps unknown, world.

We 'grounded' by rubbing each other's shoulders, our own arms and hands, stretching and shaking our muscles and flesh.

Psychotherapy

Drama and movement therapy can be used by groups or individuals, often, though not necessarily, once a week. It can be used alone or in conjunction with other therapies, especially psychotherapy, material from each being utilised to inform and balance the other. Its uses are widespread and growing: for people with learning disabilities; for people who move freely or hardly at all; for people who can understand and communicate using language; for those for whom language is difficult; and for people going about their everyday lives just wanting to learn more about themselves and others in a creative, supported way.

Some Examples of Work in Institutions

◆ A group of elderly people in a hospital might come together once a week and dance in their chairs, on their feet, in their imagination – music and movement reaching past their confusion or dementias, uniting them with one another or with the therapist.

◆ A group of people with learning difficulties might take an imaginary trip on a magic carpet to a land where anything might happen. Relying on their imaginations to take them where they need to go, they might take the chance to explore through enactment what it is like to be a robot or a bully, to walk along a quiet beach, or to be able to fly, etc.

◆ A group of children might create an imaginary home, with the seashore just outside and a football team in the sitting room who cannot go into the kitchen because... that is where the wicked hag is making football stew! Through using their imagination, hopes and fears, worries and delights can be expressed, become manageable, and be witnessed and accepted.

◆ A group of young women living together might create their own piece of music using instruments or things from the kitchen – bags that rustle, wooden spoons, saucepans, plastic tubs, cutlery. From shyness and experiments, a rhythm emerges, tentative but becoming bolder. Together they create something unique that can never again exist in exactly the same way. They can feel it as they finish and grin at one another and the therapist. For a while defences are dropped and they meet one another in a way that is alive and vibrant.

Whenever imagination is involved, psyche evoked and expressed, creation takes place and through creation, transformation. The group has changed and so has the inner and often the outer world of the participants.

Training

Drama and movement therapists are trained through the Sesame Institute. Training includes the study of practical drama; myths and legends; movement; voice work; movement with touch; music; analytical psychology; clinical studies; human development; group process. Each student must be in personal therapy and is given professional support and ongoing assessment, including clinical placements.

One may need tolerant people to live with while training as a drama and movement therapist. As we explored the stages of growth of the personality and examined what was needed at each age, I would often come home grounded, but with a strong urge to play, sing and lark about. The course is largely experiential, so in exploring what needs to be addressed at each age through movement and drama, energy gets freed up and spills over into other areas of one's life, in what may be considered a positive, if unconventional, way.

Sesame is the only organisation for combined drama and movement therapy. Both drama therapy and dance/movement therapy can be studied individually.

The Work of Gabrielle Roth

Gabrielle Roth is an American shamanic dancer who uses dance and ritual theatre as a way of encouraging people to use their bodies more freely as a primary means of communication.

Describing her work is like trying to describe good food – no matter how detailed the description, there's nothing like the taste of it. Like food, her work is nourishing, delicious, not always easy to swallow and sometimes takes a while to digest.

Gabrielle Roth calls to people's hearts and souls, encouraging and enticing people to wake up, move out of inertia and into the unique and vibrant life that is possible for each person. For over 30 years, Gabrielle Roth has learnt, by watching, sensing and creating what enables people to experience the ecstasy of a heart, mind, soul, spirit and body in unity.

Movement is her medicine. Movement is healing. The first time I moved to music by Gabrielle Roth and her group, 'The Mirrors', I began by having a wonderful, enjoyable, no steps dance. Gradually as the music seeped into me, I moved less and I realised, with surprise and a little horror, that I felt like crying. I was mortified. I didn't cry. I just moved less and less until I didn't feel the impulse any more. This was a metaphor for my life. I didn't know that I had a choice: to suppress the feeling or to move and release what was probably a stored-up, unexpressed emotion from an earlier experience and, in so doing, to move on, a little lighter, a little less defended against living life to the full.

People are all unique and yet there are places where there is connection. People all have to deal with similar psychological processes. There is hurt, laughter, longing to be authentic and longing for honest connections with others. Everyone wants to love and be loved. Gabrielle Roth's work offers a map through universal themes and processes.

Movement and breath are used as a means to heal. The work begins by encouraging people to free their bodies. This is not dependent on how much or how little a person is able to move. Young people and grandparents, people in wheelchairs, gymnasts, everyone can free their body a little bit more, learning to trust and make new discoveries.

The Five Rhythms

Roth has identified five rhythms that constitute a complete range of movement and expression. These are flow, staccato, chaos, lyrical and stillness. It is essential for health on all levels that we can access and learn to let these rhythms emerge. They are intrinsically part of everyone, five shoots of potential in each individual's personal garden. One or two may have been watered and encouraged; the others are still there, waiting.

The rhythms flow into one another and by practising them as a unit of movement, people can begin to learn to move from one to the next, getting less stuck in places that don't serve them. Moving helps to release old stored-up and unexpressed feelings, leaving people more free to be authentic in each moment. It is also a reminder not to hang on to anger, fear or sadness, but to let them serve their purpose and change. Clinging on to joy makes it brittle; flowing through the five rhythms provides a metaphor for trusting the inevitable return of joy as the cycles of life revolve.

Practising the five rhythms expands the capacity to flow, to be able to move smoothly and confidently in the world, to be able to take in and assimilate that which nourishes and to learn to trust. People may have an affinity with one particular rhythm which comes more easily than the others as they move through the sequences. The staccato rhythm involves percussive movements, creating boundaries, knowing where the body ends and someone else begins. It embodies the ability to communicate honestly and simply, from the heart. Chaos involves the ability to move lightly through the contradictions, paradoxes and surprises of life, finding them exciting challenges rather than a threat. Lyrical rhythm is of comfort to those who are willing to be moved to tears or laughter, open to possibilities. For others, stillness is their home rhythm, not stuck or inert, but vibrantly available to themselves and others, moving from trust and love.

Everyone has all of these qualities within them, and more. When working with the five rhythms, people dance or move through each rhythm, physically exploring shapes and ways to dance them, paying attention to their bodies, learning to listen to the wisdom within. This may be with or without music and for everyone their experience of the rhythms will be exquisitely, excitingly different.

People are practising these rhythms in many places: in schools, hospitals, with the elderly, with people with learning difficulties, in homes for adolescents, in the streets, in people's front rooms, in workshops; it is an exciting practice with potential to help anyone to become more alive and expressive.

Biography

Adventurer and traveller for many years, Sue Rickards eventually 'settled down' and trained and worked with small children for six years, but then felt in need of another adventure. She trained as a drama and movement therapist at the Sesame Institute and the adventuring and exploring became internal. She is a humanistic counsellor and a practitioner of tai chi. Whilst working as a therapist, she began dancing with Second Wave and, in 1994, became apprenticed to Gabrielle Roth.

References

1   Rudolph Laban, *The Mastery of Movement*, Northcote House, 1988.
2   Gabrielle Roth, *Maps to Ecstasy*, Thorsons, 1995.

Further Reading

Payne, Helen (ed), *Dance Movement Therapy: Theory and Practice*, Routledge, 1992.

Roth, Gabrielle, *Maps to Ecstasy*, Nataraj Publishing, 1990.

Stanton-Jones, K., *An Introduction to Dance Movement Therapy in Psychiatry*, Routledge, 1992.

Resources

Sesame Institute UK
Christchurch
27 Blackfriars Road
London SE1 8NY

British Association of Drama Therapists
5 Sunnydale Villas
Durlston Road
Swanage
Dorset BH19 2HY

Association of Dance Movement Therapy
c/o Arts Therapies Dept.
Springfield Hospital
Glenburnie Road
London SW17 7DJ

Teachers of Gabrielle Roth's Wave (5 rhythms) in Britain are:

Second Wave
Susanne Perks, Administrator
Nappers Crossing
Staverton
S. Devon TQ9 6PD
Tel. 01803 762655

Gabrielle Roth's book, video and cassettes are available from:

Staccato
Bridham
Kents Road
Wellswood
Torquay
Devon TQ1 2NN

Family Therapy

by David McNamara

Our families are our primary communities and yet are also sources of pain and confusion. All too often, they are something from which we seek escape rather than a cause of celebration. Yet, we cannot escape. When we are ill or hurt or emotionally overwhelmed, the hurt ripples out to affect and potentially damage those to whom we are close and with whom we share our lives. When others in our families are hurt, likewise, we are affected. Just as our parents' pain influences us deeply in our growing, our own hurt deeply shapes our children's experience. Conversely, the strength of the family unit can support and bolster us as individuals, and one family member's healing process can bring positive change to the rest of the family. Often health practitioners tend to overlook the broader context of the lives of clients; that whatever trauma, illness or block is being treated in the individual can strongly affect the whole network of their family.

Usually, we get little training or support for our roles as partners and parents. We are somehow expected to know what to do with our children, how to keep our relationships working, and how to deal with trauma in our lives.

The work of family therapy, as complementary medical practice, is to heal and support individuals in these webs of interrelationship and interdependence which are families, and to guide the resolution of problems in those patterns of relationship as they affect an individual's illness, trauma or emotional difficulty. Family therapy is a way of understanding and changing these patterns of interaction, of helping to create more fulfilment in this basic – and inescapable – area of life.

History of Family Therapy

Family therapy developed in the 1950s and 60s, as some alternative-seeking psychiatrists in the US began to realise that many emotional problems could not be easily separated from interpersonal relationships, that the web of family relationship supported, even contributed to, the problems. What they noticed was a particular quality to the communication and relationship patterns that characterised certain emotional problems. People with the illness of schizophrenia, for example, were thought to come from families in which there was a particular style of communication.

Likewise, the families of teenagers suffering from anorexia nervosa showed a specific pattern of interaction that in some way related to the symptom of refusal to eat. At that time, some 30 to 40 years ago, it was a revolutionary act to invite the entire family into the consulting room and investigate and clarify the way people dealt with one another.

The development of family therapy from these early experiments was a complex, often contradictory one. Family therapy is not, and has never been, a single, discrete and unified method of healing. Rather, it developed from the theoretical and practical explorations of several individuals, each with a particular background and theoretical orientation.

Psychological Therapies

One such method of observing and facilitating family interaction had roots in psychoanalytic theory, shifting its emphasis from the in-depth analysis of individuals to the interactions between family members. Based in psychoanalytic object-relations theory, this approach sees current situations as repeating and playing out early parent-child relationship patterns. Applied to the interactions of parents and children, as well as to couples, these theoretical formulations led to the concept of the family as a group of interlocking, intrapsychic systems, in which each individual acts out unresolved patterns from their early childhood. Such pioneer figures as Nathan Ackerman,[1] Theodore Lidz,[2] Helm Stierlin,[3] and Ivan Boszormenyi-Nagy[4] each developed his own perspective, concerns and approach to treatment.

At the same time, the insights from 'general systems theory', originally developed in application to engineering, were being seen as highly applicable to human systems. Here, the family is viewed not as a collection of individuals, but as a mutually interacting system of individual members in which each member affects all others and is, in turn, affected by the family as a whole. A change in one member of the system produces change in other members, since all react to restore equilibrium – reverting to known, if uncomfortable, old patterns of relating. In addition, family functioning is influenced by its interrelationships with the cultural or community system of which it is a part. This systemic view, while also largely implicit in psychoanalytically based family theory, became the guiding principle for several other major approaches.

Murray Bowen developed an approach which focused on such factors as the multigenerational transmission process, whereby the family pattern of dysfunction in the current generation can be understood as the result of an emotional problem that has been in the family for generations; triangulation, whereby two individuals avoid dealing with a conflict between them by involving a third person to relieve tension; and the family projection process, whereby the family uses one or more members to contain and express its emotional disturbance.[5] Bowen's contributions in these concepts were some of the most profound and far-reaching understandings of family emotional illness, and are still central in the understanding of family processes.

The concepts of communication theory also grew out of systems theory and have come to be incorporated in much of current family therapy. This approach focuses on the exchange of verbal and non-verbal messages in relationships. Symptoms are seen as being supported by problems in communication, including such issues as unclarity and conflicting messages, and therapy is designed to alter these dysfunctional patterns of interaction.

Salvatore Minuchin developed an orientation that came to be known as structural family therapy.[6] Emphasising the organised patterns in which family members interact, structural concerns include issues of power and hierarchy, relationships within and between subsystems in the family, and family boundaries. Of particular note for the structural therapist is the nature and balance of closeness and distance between family members: families become dysfunctional when individuals are either overinvolved with one another (enmeshed) or separated by rigid boundaries (disengaged). Treatment from a structural perspective involves shifting the pattern of interactions in order to rebalance the organisational structure.

Yet another outgrowth of the systemic view of family functioning, which has come to play a larger part in contemporary family therapy, are the strategic approaches. This intentionally short-term method, or group of methods, intervenes in systemic functioning by interrupting specifically targeted behaviour patterns associated with the symptom by confronting the family – or an individual within the family – with novel situations or tasks, often confusing, paradoxical or seemingly nonsensical, in order to stimulate new, more adaptive behaviours.

If these are some of the major strands in the web of theory and practice that has become the field of family therapy, it is important to note that this is by no means a complete portrayal, but merely a rough sketch. Such powerfully influential figures as Virginia Satir,[7] who developed her own humanistically-based approach, and Carl Whitaker,[8] who evolved a radical approach to exploring the family's unconsciously driven behaviour, shaped the development of the field as well.

Central Elements of Family Theory

Despite the range of theories about how families function and misfunction, there are some basic underlying assumptions that are common to all branches of family therapy. Perhaps most important is that of the family as system: the wholeness of the family is more than the sum of its individual members, and the behaviour of any one individual affects and is affected by other family members and the family as a whole. From this insight the concept of circular causality was developed. This is the understanding that symptoms are caused and sustained by a pattern of interaction processes rather than by any simple singular cause. In turn, such concepts as responsibility and blame take on quite a different meaning. Another shared assumption within family therapy is that those interactional patterns are strongly related to physical symptoms and, therefore, to medical problems within the family. Behaviour of an individual can affect the system by bringing about physical symptoms in another family member, the system expressing its stress through physical illness. Vice versa, the physical illness of any family member strongly impacts and reverberates through the whole family system.

Indications for Family Therapy

From this perspective, family therapy can be seen as a method of treatment not just for relationship problems within the family, but for seemingly individual emotional problems and physical illness. Many research studies have demonstrated the relationship between paediatric illnesses, such as headaches, gastro-intestinal problems and asthma, and family stress. One such study showed clear relationship between marital distress of parents and the level of stress hormones in five-year-old children.[9] Compliance by children with medical treatment for such chronic childhood illnesses as diabetes, cystic fibrosis, renal disease and attention deficit hyperactivity disorder is strongly related to levels of either emotional support or interactional stress within the family. Children in highly stressed families often refuse or 'forget' to take their medicine, which in turn creates more stress. At the same time, chronic or catastrophic illness such as cancer in either children or parents powerfully impacts families and can cause imbalance and dysfunction in the relationship of family members. Family therapy can be essential for helping the family cope with the terribly demanding and threatening burden of illness and potential death. Emotional problems or mental illness of a family member, from schizophrenia to depression to alcoholism or eating disorders, also have powerful effects on the system, and so family therapy can help each person deal with its meaning for themselves.

Another equally important – and often overlooked – value of family therapy is teaching and supporting the family through the negotiation of normal life cycle stresses. In this aspect, family therapy becomes more a kind of family psycho-education. It is here that the insights into family functioning gained over the past half century can serve to assist families in not simply surviving various developmental stress points, but in finding ways to bring out the fullest potential in all members, often in significantly more healthy patterns than in earlier family generations. Change is always a challenge to any system, even normal and healthy changes, from the transition of being single to being married, the birth of children, the onset of adolescence, to the leaving home of late-adolescent children. These normal developmental stages of family life can bring tremendous and unexpected upheaval to a family, even to the point of breaking it apart. Approaching such life cycle transitions consciously, finding ways to seek support and guidance in dealing with the intensity of feelings that are aroused, can be an invaluable use of family therapy.

While the effects on children of family stresses are profound, perhaps even more significant for family functioning is the couple relationship. Equally in two-parent families and in divorced families, the emotional health of the marital or ex-marital relationship powerfully impacts the emotional health of the children. Dealing with marital stress, whether it be the normal stresses of any two people living together or the more pathological conflicts that can arise within couples, is of vital importance in raising emotionally healthy kids. Single parent families also bring with them their own unique stresses and needs. The field of marital therapy, often seen as a subset of family therapy, has developed its own insights and techniques for supporting healthy couple relationships and helping work through dysfunctional and destructive patterns of relating.

Seeking Help from Family Therapy

It might be apparent that seeking family therapy is perhaps a more complex endeavour than choosing other complementary practices. While all family therapists have as their goal the helping of families, how they go about that task can vary widely.

In the course of family therapy, it would be usual to meet weekly or perhaps bi-weekly. The longer-term therapeutic approaches or tackling more difficult, pervasive problems can take more than a year of solid work, while symptom-focused approaches often seek specific behavioural changes in ten to twelve sessions. Some therapists insist on all members of the family being present, occasionally including grandparents, while others will work with a single individual. The nature of the therapeutic conversation, the focus of therapy and the methods employed all depend on the approach of the therapist and the needs of the situation.

Seeking help from a family therapist is a matter of finding out from the prospective therapist how they think about family change and the methods they use to bring this about. The training and certification of family therapists is quite variable. In the US there are specific training programmes for marital and family therapy and a certifying group which sets professional standards, the American Association of Marital and Family Therapists. AAMFT certification guarantees a high level of training and supervised experience. Licensure and standards for psychologists are regulated in the US by individual state law. In the UK, training for family therapy tends to be included in other professional preparation programmes or in training institutes, such as London's Tavistock Institute or the Institute for Family Therapy. Accreditation and certification are currently in the process of being formulated through the British Association of Counselling.

Toward Optimal Family Health

If family therapy is a relatively new addition to the field of health care, thinking about preventive care for family mental health is an area which has been still less explored. While a few popular books have been written to coach families on how to enrich their lives together, little research or professional attention has been devoted to this focus. Largely it must be the responsibility of conscious, self-aware families to seek the help they desire to make their families work more smoothly, consciously and lovingly. It goes without saying that even the most self-aware and caring families face crises, even normal and expected developmental crises, the destructive impact of which can be transformed through counselling, education and communication.

Building Health

From this perspective, holistic family health care looks at how to support the family to grow and develop optimally as well as to maintain physical health. This involves both supporting individual growth and freedom and maintaining cohesion and a sense of unity and wholeness for the family. The holistic view of families sees the inherent unity, the systemic wholeness of the family, as a particularly significant – and largely ignored – aspect of family life. This awareness of family unity demands particular care and nurturing, especially in a time of social fragmentation and stress on the family structure. So, as well as supporting the interrelationships within and between families, the holistic view supports the unity and wholeness of individual families: the essential power of family life.

Case Study

The family had been referred by their GP for counselling when the thirteen-year-old son's juvenile diabetes could not be stabilised and the stress on the family relationships, and the boy's illness, seemed to be getting out of control. In the referral, the doctor had mentioned the concern with non-compliance with the medical regimen and conflict between the parents over control of the son's treatment. She had also told the therapist that while the boy overtly seemed upset at the life-threatening nature of the insulin-level swings, he seemed somehow gratified by the upset this was causing his parents and the central role in which it placed him in the family.

It was for all of these reasons that the therapist saw the issue as concerning the whole family system and had insisted that the younger sister be present at the initial session, despite the parents' protests that she was not part of the problem and should be shielded from the stress. The insistence that the grandmother – mom's mother – who lived with the family, also attend, brought more discomfort and resistance, further suggesting to the therapist that somehow the medical issue had important psychosocial family relational significance. Exploring these relationships, how each family member understood and was affected by the boy's illness, would guide the course of the family counselling.

The family filled the therapist's consulting room: As often happens, the seating arrangement they chose spoke eloquently about the family. The grandmother and the younger sister sat together on one sofa while the mother and the boy sat on the other. The father sat alone in a chair. As each spoke in turn about their perceptions and concerns for the boy's health and the family in general, the patterns of interaction, belief, connectedness and disconnectedness gradually made themselves clear. If the process of family therapy is that of finding ways for each family member to clarify and meet their own needs as well as those of the family as a whole, the weekly sessions for this family gradually revealed a pattern of stress and disappointment and anger which kept those underlying needs from being understood and fulfilled. The son's medical condition and the family's reaction to it, while certainly having a medical reality of its own, also served to express these patterns of need and disappointment.

The picture emerged of a family system in which the mother and her own mother had never worked out their differences and existed in a state of unexpressed, but deeply felt, tension, while the father experienced that tension in his relationship with his wife. Over the years, especially with the introduction of children, the patterns of emotional stress became interactional patterns of closeness, disconnectedness, alliances, and unspoken feelings. With the parents' difficulty in maintaining their own emotional closeness, each found alternative focuses for their caring and involvement. The father began working late and spending time with his mates in the pub. The mother maintained a closeness with her first child, the now thirteen-year-old diabetic boy. When the daughter arrived a few years later, the grandmother found a focus for her own love and neediness. It was with the death of her own husband, and her moving in with her daughter's family that these not atypical patterns became more intense, difficult and pathological for the family. With the increasing tension of the physical closeness, the emotional patterns became more exaggerated and problematic. The father further withdrew, the grandmother found her ally in her young granddaughter, and the mother became more and more concerned with her son's medical problems. From one perspective, the boy's medical non-compliance provided the family system with a focus for its emotional stress: everyone could be worried about his health without having to deal with the more personal pain of long-standing unmet needs and simmering, unexpressed resentment.

Family therapy allowed the family to gradually understand and come to express those underlying feelings, to move through the pain and fear and anger, to speak what had been unspoken, and craft new ways of interaction. The mother and her mother were helped to work through old resentments, father and mother were supported to try and rebuild their relationship, and the son was encouraged to take responsibility for his own medical needs and leave his parents out of it – while also to include his father more in other aspects of his life. Both the daughter and grandmother were freed to build their own lives rather than relying solely on each other. The family was pushed, encouraged and allowed to find its true strength – a group of individuals who were each able to speak and meet their needs and support each other out of caring and freedom rather than resentment and fear.

This was not an easy or brief process. Its description might sound neat, sweet and simple whereas the truth was months of struggle and tears and resistance. Change is not easy and years of pain are not easily faced. Whether mother and father were able to rebuild their relationship remained questionable and the central remaining danger for the family. But, communication had been opened, real needs seen and spoken, and the process of healing begun.

Biography

David McNamara, Ph. D., is a licensed child, adolescent, and family psychologist currently in private practice in a multidisciplinary preventive medicine clinic in the Seattle, Washington area of the USA. David lived at the Findhorn Foundation during the late 1970s and early 1980s where he was involved in the creation and facilitation of 'The Findhorn Family Workshop', a residential workshop for families. Having met and married his wife, Alexandra, at the Foundation and having their first child, Geoffrey, they left Findhorn to explore living in the 'outer' world. After settling in the U. S., David achieved a Ph. D. in clinical psychology from the Fielding Institute in Santa Barbara, California with training in family therapy in a variety of mental health settings. Currently, David, Alexandra, Geoffrey, daughter Erin and assorted animal friends live on Bainbridge Island, Washington.

References

1   N W Ackerman, *The Psychodynamics of Family Life*, Basic Books, 1958.

2   T Lidz, *The influence of family studies in the treatment of schizophrenia, in Green*, R. & Framo, J., *Family Therapy: Major Contributions*, International Universities Press, 1981.

3   H Stierlin, *Separating Parents and Adolescents: A Persepctive on Running Away, Schizophrenia, and Waywardness*, Quadrangle, 1974.

4   I Boszormenyi-Nagy & G Spark, *Invisible Loyalities*, Harper & Row, 1973.

5   M Bowen, *Family Therapy in Clinical Practice*, Jason Aaronson, 1978.

6   S Minuchin, *Family Healing*, Free Press, 1992.

7   V Satir, *Conjoint Family Therapy: A Guide to Theory and Technique*, Science and Behavior Books, 1964.

8   C Whitaker & A Napier, *The Family Crucible*, Harper, 1978.

9   J R Springer & R H Woody (eds.), *Health Promotion in Family Therapy*, Aspen Systems Corporation, 1985.

Further Reading

Ackerman, N W., *The Psychodynamics of Family Life*, Basic Books, 1958. (One of the first discussions of applying psychoanalytic principles to families, by a pioneer of family therapy.)

Bowen, M., *Family Therapy in Clinical Practice*, Jason Aaronson, 1978. (The primary articulation of Bowen's theory of multigenerational family therapy.)

Carter, B.; McGoldrick, M. (eds.), *The Changing Family Life Cycle: A Framework for Family Therapy*, (Second edition), Gardner Press, 1988. (A collection of papers on family life and therapy from the life cycle perspective, the normative developmental phases that families go through.)

Curran, D., *Traits of a Healthy Family*, Winston Press, Minneapolis, MN, 1983. (A popular approach to what makes families healthy, written in a very readable style. Very useful for families seeking insight into how to be happier together.)

Doherty, W J.; Baird, M. A., *Family therapy & family medicine: Toward the Primary Care of Families*, Guildford Press, 1983. (The key text in the field of medical family therapy, the application of family therapy principles and practices to counselling and supporting families with medical illnesses.)

Elkind, D., *Ties that Stress*, Harvard University Press, 1994. (A discussion of the stresses facing the contemporary family and potential ways for family health in the face of overwhelming social change.)

Engel, G., *The clinical application of the biopsychosocial model*, American Journal of Psychiatry, 1980; 137: 5, 535-44. (The application of systemic conceptualisation in the orthodox psychiatric medical model of health and disease.)

Green, R J & Framo, J L (eds.), *Family therapy: Major contributions*, International Universities Press, 1981. (A collection of the early seminal scholarly papers in the development of the field.)

Gurman, A S.; Kniskern, D P (eds.), *Handbook of Family Therapy*, Brunner/Mazel, 1981. (A compilation describing the principles and practices of various 'schools' of family therapy, each chapter written in consistent format by a leading developer or practitioner of the particular approach. A good way to compare and contrast the various methodologies.)

Minuchin, S., *Family Healing*, Free Press, 1992. (A non-professional, popular-press book on families and family mental health by one of most insightful and erudite founders of the field.)

Minuchin, S.; Rosman, B L.; Baker, L., *Psychosomatic Families: Anorexia Nervosa in Context*, Harvard University Press, 1978. (One of the earliest works by the founders of structural family therapy on the application of structural therapeutic principles to medical illness.)

Napier, A.; Whitaker, C., *The Family Crucible*, Harper & Row, 1978. (A fascinating description of Carl Whitaker's idiosyncratic, but highly effective approach to family therapy, through the description of one family's struggles and successes in treatment.)

Nichols, M., *Family therapy: Concepts and Methods*, Gardner Press, 1984. (A comprehensive introduction and overview of the variety of approaches to family therapy. Readable and well-organised by a single author.)

Scott-Samuel, A., *Total Participation, Total Health: Reinventing the Peckham Health Centre for the 1990s*, Scottish Academic Press, Edinburgh, 1990. (A description of an experiment in creating a centre for community-based family health, and a discussion of the lessons of the project and the application of the principles of the Peckham Experiment to contemporary approaches to family-based health care.)

Springer, J R & Woody, R H (eds.), *Health Promotion in Family Therapy, Aspen Systems Corporation*, 1985. (An edited volume of articles on physical and emotional health as seen from a family systems perspective. One of the few books that includes a holistic perspective on family health.)

Journals

Family Process, P O Box 6889, Syracuse, NY., USA. (The pre-eminent scholarly journal in the field. Quarterly.)

Family Therapy Networker, 8525 Bradford Road, Silver Spring, MD, 20901, USA. (A popular format magazine for therapists, on both issues in family therapy and family life, written in very accessible and interesting style.)

Resources

Institute of Family Therapy
43 New Cavendish Street
London W1M 7RG
Tel. 0171-935 1651
Fax. 0171-224 3291

Feldenkrais Method

by Chantal Kickx with the help of Lawrence Goldfarb

By being aware, Feldenkrais believed, we can understand how much unnecessary tension we have, how much pleasure and grace we miss, how inefficiently and stressfully we live our lives. Through awareness we can learn to move with astonishing lightness and freedom – at any age – and thereby improve our living circumstances not only physically but also emotionally, intellectually and spiritually.

History

Moshe Feldenkrais was born in the Ukraine in May 1904 and died in Israel in 1984. Ju-jitsu was the first alternative discipline in which he became interested, and in 1936 he was the first European to become a black belt judoka. It was his experiments in applying judo concepts to the learning of movement combined with his thorough knowledge of system mechanics that was at the origin of his 'Feldenkrais exercises'. He used the basic concept taught in martial arts of never going against the mechanisms of another human's resistance but instead working with it positively in order to bring about change.

The turning point in the life of Moshe Feldenkrais came when he injured his knee in a soccer match. Having been told that he could neither stand on nor bend his leg for several months, he began developing a new way of understanding how the body functions, through practical application of system mechanics. For example, he was initially unable to reach the foot and toes of his injured leg because his hamstring was too tight; however, when he began to think about releasing his shoulders and his chest, and involving his whole body in the movement, the parts that could be flexible operated better and enabled the movement to be carried out.[1]

Psychological Therapies Alexander Technique

He coupled this exploratory information with that which he had gathered from psychology and psychoanalysis, and also expanded his study into anatomy and neurophysiology. Seeing how we move and understanding how we can move, Moshe Feldenkrais understood how dysfunction arises from our limitations – in imagination, perception and motion – and how our difficulties are embedded in the very ways we sense and move. A significant influence on this work was that of F. Matthias Alexander, whose techniques stemmed from similar questioning.

Theoretical Background

One of the principles on which the Feldenkrais Method* is based is 'the less effort you make, the more sensitive you will become'. To put it graphically, if I carry a fridge on my back, half a pound of sugar can be added and I won't feel the difference. But if I'm holding a feather between my fingers and a bee comes to sit on it, even if my eyes are closed I will feel the difference. So, the less muscular effort we make, the more our nervous system is free and available to feel and to become aware. In doing so it will be engaged in the process of learning.[2]

In traditional learning, achievement is the aim, not the process of learning itself. In the Feldenkrais Method it is the process that is the important thing and should be as general and aimless to the adult learner as it is to the baby.

The Feldenkrais Method deals with *function* rather than with posture. It is concerned with the way we function and how to do it with ease, avoiding useless effort and becoming aware of how we prevent ourselves from being in motion gracefully, physically as well as emotionally and spiritually. Its point of view is systematic rather than reductionist. Instead of finding a localised cause, it looks at how a problem or limitation *lives* in the student's movement. It situates the problem in a pattern of relationships and tries to understand how the system is organised.

Thought plays an important role in this system. In blind subjects, active imagery elicits brain activity in the visual cortex, even though they cannot see.[3] Just imagining a movement creates the necessary muscular tone to set it into action. New interneuronal pathways can be forged by thought, to allow new movement to occur. The process itself is slow and introspective. However, functional changes occur very quickly.

The Practice of the Feldenkrais Method

There are two ways of experiencing the Feldenkrais Method: in classes called 'awareness through movement' or in a one-to-one lesson known as 'functional integration'. Both these sessions provide an efficient, short and general way of learning to learn.

Those who benefit range from professional dancers, singers, actors and musicians, to those with neuromuscular disturbances (this work particularly benefits any child or adult suffering from brain damage or stroke), as well as anyone with aches and pains who would like to experience less tension and stress in their lives. It is also most appreciated by those who are interested in psychology and mind/body interconnections. There are no contraindications, as movements are always done within the student's range of ease and comfort. I have seen elderly people over 80

---

*The Feldenkrais Method is a registered trademark.

and even 90 years old greatly enjoying the benefits of this work. As this method is above all about awareness, any other method or therapy can be complementary to it.

Awareness Through Movement

In an 'awareness through movement' class, the students are guided verbally to move slowly and gently, mostly lying on the floor, sometimes sitting or standing. They are invited to focus on sensory awareness. We usually look at one particular function, for example lifting the head.

A number of students are lying on their backs on the floor. To start with, they are asked to listen to the floor's feedback about the way they are lying. Then I ask them to lift their heads. For some students this might be very hard work. I ask them to bend their knees and interlace their fingers in order to carry their heads with their hands, using the hands and arms like a sling. I ask them to lift their heads again with their hands, so that they do not have to use their neck muscles to do this movement, several times, back and forth. At the same time, I ask them to notice what they do with their eyes, whether they are looking towards the floor, the horizon, or up towards the ceiling. Even the position of the eyes affects the ease of movement. We explore all possibilities. They rest for a moment. In that quiet space, they listen to the possible changes of pressure of their bodies against the floor, compared to the beginning of the class.

Their hands stay interlaced behind their heads, and I ask them again to lift their heads from the floor, repeatedly. Everybody has their own rhythm, their own scope of movement. I ask them now to pay attention to the movement of the breastbone. Here again there are different possibilities. I guide them verbally to explore them all, in detail. Maybe, in lifting their heads, they notice that they have been unconsciously co-ordinating their breathing pattern with this movement. This too can be playfully explored in different ways.

The explorations are interrupted very regularly with moments of rest, moments of silence, moments of letting go. Students are encouraged to cultivate no intention and to allow emptiness – wherein the nervous system can integrate the new perceptions, giving time for a new type of order to emerge.

In lifting the head, we can also pay attention to other movements, for example the movement of the ribcage; the movement of the pelvis, whether the student keeps it fixed or tilted; the way the knees move in relation to each other; the change of the pressure of the feet in relation to the floor. All these relationships are looked at in various ways.

After the lesson, we go back to the movement asked for at the very start of the lesson: 'Please lift your head.' It is amazing to see how the head is now lifting not only higher, but, more importantly, with much more ease. The nervous system has done its work – the student's mental understanding of what is best is unnecessary.

Functional Integration

To illustrate a functional integration session, the following is adapted from a case history written up by Lawrence Goldfarb, the educational director of the Strasbourg International Feldenkrais Training.[4]

Toby lies on my Feldenkrais table with his head turned to the right and his right hip slightly lifted. Searching the contours of his back, I see an asymmetry. Perhaps the right side hollows out a little more than the left? The mid-spine dips forward, arching in a continuation of the proud dancerly posture – chest up and stomach in – he takes in standing. I am curious how Toby's way of holding himself effects his movement. Gently moving parts of his body and noticing how he takes up the motion, I begin to investigate his moveability, that is to say, his readiness to act. Even though the movements are tiny, I can feel how easily he moves in each direction. Placing my hands over the crests of his hip bones, I tilt his pelvis forward and back ever so slightly, noticing the very bottom of his spine hardly moves in response. As his pelvis rocks on his legs, I feel his left hip's reluctance to lift away from the table.

I gently roll Toby's pelvis side to side. Tracking the response up through his spine and ribcage and down through his hip joints and legs, I compare his movement with what I know is possible for human structure. When his right hip lifts away from the table, his lower back arches slightly and the motion diffuses easily through his spine and chest. The left hip feels heavier and there is no ripple of movement up his spine.

Toby said he was having problems getting to relevé a dance position of standing on the balls of the feet since he injured his left foot in a bicycling accident. I asked him to walk around the room a bit.

As he walked around, the way his left foot moved caught my eye. Something was missing: rather than pushing off with his toes, before he could arch his heel away from the floor he lifted his foot keeping his ankle bent. There was no clear push-off. At the end of the step cycle, the motion of each leg differed greatly. When he stepped forward onto his left foot, his right leg stretched behind and his lower back arched in response; when he stepped onto the right, his back was still and his left leg hardly moved back.

I ask myself, how would this person move if he were doing so efficiently?

In Toby's case, certain dynamic relationships nested in the complex coordination we call walking are missing. His pelvis did not move in the way it needed to for him to push off with his left leg. He lacked the necessary moveability in his lower back. His left hip joint was hindering, rather helping, the action. The same phenomenon occurred when he attempted to rise onto the ball of his left foot: without the rest of him accommodating appropriately, his weight couldn't shift easily onto the front of his foot.

Comparing what could be with what is, I made a hypothesis about how his problem is situated in his movement. Asking him to temporarily alter his way of moving, I tested which solution would be beneficial. I continue my evaluation after he lies on the table, confirming what I observed in standing.

My hands explore the boundaries of his habit by moving his legs, pelvis, ribs, and shoulders. My hands are neither instructing or commanding, rather I suggest one movement and then another. I am asking how he moves in each direction, listening to changes in the quality of motion.. I'm getting to know Toby through my fingertips.

Thinking about the way his foot meets into the floor and the way in which the floor pushes back through the skeleton, I begin to press ever so gently on the bottom of the right foot.

Since I can elicit the appropriate response on the right side, I work to improve it. Starting with movements of the foot and working my way up to Toby's head and neck, I clarify each link's role in passing force. For example, I look at the relationship of the leg to the pelvis, investigating how slightly different angles of the leg effect the transmission of motion.

After I can elicit a response from the right side that distributes the work globally, I return to pressing through the left leg. The difference is clear: something is definitely missing on this side. The parts do not work together, some coming together just cannot happen.

The invariants, the relationships that could change but do not, appear as a corset around the body, allowing some minimal give but preventing certain patterns from ever manifesting. Tracing the movement limitations in the forefoot, lower leg, hip, back, and lower ribs, I explore how these interweave to form Toby's habit. His foot seems stiff and he holds his breath whenever I touch it. I go to his pelvis and lower back. I'm searching for a transition point from where I can elicit the missing movements and not finding one.

Moving on, I become interested in his ribs. They seem glued together. I return to the movement of pushing through the right leg and investigate how the ribs fit into the picture. Returning to the left, I begin to look for some movement, however small, that could make the ribs a part of the movement rather than a part of the problem. Ever so slowly, I encourage each rib to move, reminding it of its birthright. Toby takes a deep breath, relaxing his belly and settling a bit more onto the table.

Returning to his pelvis, I find a little more willingness to move. Starting with the areas of his low back that move with ease, I begin to evoke the various movements that are possible. Lifting the hip a bit away from the table, I explore how to call forth the movement lacking in his back. At no point do I insist, knowing that if each local motion improves a little and if the pieces start to fall into place, at some point, the boundaries will melt away and a new global organization will appear, whole and vibrant. So I continue, following the line of a motion that is not yet present, preparing each place, from toe to head, for its part.

Returning to Toby's left foot, I gently push again. I can see the motion going through to his head, making it nod slightly. His foot and lower leg are freer, allowing them to make the movements necessary for pushing off. Even more importantly, his back and hips know what to do. A new pattern has come into focus.

I slowly guide Toby to sitting and, after giving him a few moments to get comfortable, bring him to standing. He walks a few steps, stops, and comes easily to relevé.

'Hey, I can do it. How did you do that?'

My Practice

Not all Feldenkrais practitioners give attention to the emotional aspect of their students' lives. Some practitioners very consciously avoid this area, either because they are not confident about their own capacity to deal with those depths, or because they choose only to work on the body, possibly advising their students to complement their lessons with psychotherapy. In my experience, however, patterns of 'holding' in the body always relate to blocked emotions, feelings and/or fears. So part of my work focuses on how body patterns relate to mind patterns and how body reveals mind. One could say that mind incarnates – from the Latin verb *incarnare*, which means 'coming into flesh'.

Psychotherapy

I am also very conscious of my attitude as a practitioner. In quantum physics one learns that the observer influences the observed. So I am constantly observing myself as a priority. Am I comfortable? Am I at ease? Do I breathe freely? How attached am I to the outcome of this session? Am I in a 'doing' mode or can I allow myself to just 'be' with the student(s)? Do I want to impose anything on the student(s)? Am I free from any wish or aim in relation to the student(s)? Can I be a subject relating to another subject, rather than seeing the student as an object? Particularly in functional integration sessions, I keep noticing that any tension in me, any doubt or wanting a specific result does influence the student. My tension creates tension in them, and their level of trust and capacity to learn is seriously affected by my attitude.

Metamorphic Technique

I have observed time and time again that my thoughts actually alter the effectiveness of the session. While I'm working consciously with the skeletal structure of the student, I have noticed that if I think that the bones are floating in fluids (the human body is composed of about 80% fluid) the bones let me feel the relationships between them much more clearly (and fluidly) than if I think of them being solid objects surrounded by matter that is solid as well.

Gestalt Therapy
Bio-Energetic Analysis

I also consider there to be importance in acknowledging emptiness and chaos as natural and integral parts of our being. This was something I learned from Dr Stephen Wolinsky, founder of 'quantum psychology', originally a gestalt and Reichian therapist, who was of particular inspiration to me and made enormous contributions both to my personal and my professional life. First he made me aware that once a belief about ourselves or about the world is rigidified, we resist merging and losing ourselves. This creates separation and prevents us from experiencing our interconnectedness with the larger whole. He made me understand, in intelligent and touching ways, how emptiness is the underlying unity of substance.

Second, he helped me become aware of my need to organise, explain and categorise everything – to create order in me and around me and feel secure. Thanks to Dr Wolinsky, I'm learning to be willing not to know. He says: 'The resistance to chaos keeps the chaos there, makes life uncomfortable, but more importantly robs us of a higher order whereby interconnection and unity are revealed.'[5] Today it seems important for me to recognise, accept and integrate emptiness and chaos as essential elements in order to be fully me, and prepared to be of service to a bigger whole. These ideas are also shared and discussed with great interest in the community of Feldenkrais practitioners.

Here is a warning for those who believe that 'awareness through movement' is another type of fitness class. It is not. After my first experience with the Feldenkrais Method, I was so enthused about it that I thought it had all the answers. I thought it was magical, intelligent, fascinating, fun and efficient. However, in moving with so little effort, I forgot that I had muscles as well. Today I choose to complement the awareness I have gained through the Feldenkrais Method with more aerobic and gym exercises in order to enjoy a fit and healthy body.

Biography

Born in Belgium, Chantal Kickx was academically trained as an educational psychologist. While working in a psychiatric hospital with severely disturbed teenagers, she felt it was important to be able to 'touch' and invite transformation not solely with the use of words. She qualified as a Feldenkrais practitioner in Paris in 1991 after having been involved and engaged in that work for the previous ten years. She was a member of the Findhorn Foundation for 4 years. She currently teaches classes internationally, and also works privately from her home, in South Devon.

References

1   Frank Wildman, *Life with Moshe*, I. F. F. Journal No. 2, May 1994.

2   Paul Bach-y-Rita, *Brain Mechanisms in Sensory Substitution*, Academic Press, 1972.

3   Moshe Feldenkrais, *Man and the World*, Somatics, Spring 1979.

4   Lawrence Wm. Goldfarb, *The Teacher Learns*, Telekinesis, 1994; 3: 2,1-3.

5   Stephen Wolinsky, *The Tao of Chaos*, Bramble Co., 1994.

Further Reading

Alon, Ruthy, *Mindful Spontaneity*, North Atlantic Books, 1996.

Feldenkrais, Moshe, *Awareness through Movement: Health Exercises for Personal Growth*, Arkana, 1990.

———, *The Elusive Obvious*, Meta Publications, 1985.

———, *Body and Mature Behavior*, International Universities Press, 1970.

———, *The Potent Self: a Guide to Spontaneity*, HarperCollins, 1992.

———, *The Master Moves*, Meta Publications, 1985.

Goldfarb, Lawrence Wm., *Back into Action*, Therapy Skill Builders, 1994.

———, *Foundations of Learning*, Feldenkrais Resources, 1993

Rywerant, Yochanan, *The Feldenkrais Method: Teaching by Handling*, Keats Publishing, Inc., 1991.

Zemach, David; Bersin, Käthe; Reese, Mark, *Relaxercise*, Collins Aus, 1990.

Resources

For more information, please contact:

In the UK:

Feldenkrais Guild UK
P O Box 370
London N10 3XA

for trainings:

The Feldenkrais Professional Training Programme
P O Box 1207
Hove BN3 2GG
Tel. 0181 549 9583

In the USA:

Feldenkrais Guild
P O Box 489
Albany, OR 97321-0143

Feldenkrais Resources
P O Box 2067
Berkeley, CA 94702

Flower Essences

by Marion Leigh

Flowers have been a source of joy and happiness throughout time and healing with flowers is among the most ancient of healing modalities. Flowers contain the highest concentration of the life-force of a plant and by the method of sun infusion the vibrational imprint of the flowers is transferred into water. This is used to create the flower essence wherein the healing life-force is then conveyed to people.

The subtle healing properties of flower essences restore equilibrium on all levels of being: physical, emotional, mental and spiritual. They can enhance personal development and are a powerful aid to transformation. They offer us the opportunity to address outworn behaviour patterns and negative states of mind which may contribute to or cause disease, emotional imbalance and spiritual disharmony. By stimulating the body's inherent ability to heal itself, flower essences restore order from a higher level and help to strengthen desirable or positive qualities such as courage, inner peace, love and acceptance.

History

In the 1500s the great mystic healer Paracelsus collected the dew from flowering plants to treat his patients' emotional imbalances. The modern development of flower essence therapy is attributed to Dr Edward Bach, a respected Harley Street doctor, homoeopathic practitioner and sensitive who experienced emotional and physical symptoms when he was near a particular plant. He discovered that by taking an essence of the plant, the symptoms were alleviated and that the same essence would heal similar emotional patterns in his patients. Bach was among the first to see the link between emotions, stress and illness.

In the mid-1970s, nearly half a century after Bach left his legacy of the Bach flower remedies, new flower essences appeared. The Flower Essence Society in California began researching new essences, and in the 1980s and 1990s others were inspired, bringing us essences from countries around the world including Australia, New Zealand, South America, India and the Himalayas. The world has changed dramatically over the past 50 years, the stresses and demands on humanity and on the environment are reaching turbulent proportions. These new essences have surely come at a time when they are most needed, for healing and for transformation.

Theoretical Base

Vibrational or etheric medicine, views the human being as multidimensional, consisting of body, mind and spirit. It defines the energy networks linking the physical body and its subtle bodies of spirit from the perspective of vibration and energy. As with homoeopathic remedies, we do not know how flower essences actually work. However, scientific evidence of the existence of subtle energy systems is growing. Many flower essence producers are researching the efficacy of remedies. Flower essences would appear to influence the subtle energy bodies and systems which feed life into the body and mind. They transform the energy flow through the subtle bodies, the chakras and the etheric streams, affecting the energetic patterns which influence life and consciousness. Ways of measuring effects are being undertaken using electro-scanning equipment, Kirlian photography and methods such as the Vegatest.

Homoeopathy

Bio-Energetic Regulatory Medicine

Research

Dr Michael Wiesglas conducted a double-blind trial in 1979 to test the Bach flower remedies and the placebo effect. His subjects suffered from depression. Results showed that those who were given the flower remedy experienced feelings of well-being, personal growth, self-acceptance and increased creativity. Those who received the placebo reported no significant change.

The Flower Essence Society has been running a research programme for many years, encouraging people to participate in documenting self-help or client use of flower essences. This is done by case study forms, sharing observations and insights, developing controlled clinical studies, studying subtle plant properties and developing research for detecting, analysing and interpreting the presence of subtle forces within flower essences.

Treatment with Flower Essences

Some flower essences free us from negative emotions. Others help us to recognise and let go of negative thoughts and feelings which generate unconscious or outworn behaviour patterns. They can help and support us by giving strength to cope with growth and change, to be more flexible and to respond positively to life's demands and stresses. Self-adjusting and safe to use for people of all ages, flower essences do not interfere with other forms of treatment and can be used alongside any healing modality.

Normally flower essences are ingested and, like homoeopathic remedies, are absorbed through the mucus membranes in the mouth. They can also be used in other ways:

topically, applied directly to the skin, or added to creams or lotions. The forehead, the neck, the wrists, the soles of the feet and palms of the hands are good places for topical application. As bath therapy, a few drops of flower essence are added to the water. They can also be dispersed into the air using a spray bottle or by evaporation in a clean aromatherapy burner.

When choosing essences for oneself, family or friends, it is important to find the key emotional issues which need addressing. This requires honesty and self-reflection, seeking understanding and awareness of problems and challenges in the present and in the past, and looking to future goals. This is the basis for successful flower essence selection. Some areas to look at might include: crisis, childhood, emotions, energy levels, fear, fulfilment, life changes, mental clarity, motivation, outside or environmental influences, physical health, relationships, self-esteem, sexuality, stress, sleep, shock or trauma and thought patterns.

Radionics
Kinesiology
Dowsing

Other methods of selection include using intuition and vibrational techniques such as radiesthesia, muscle testing or kinesiology. These techniques need to be objectively tested and evaluated for one's ability to use them effectively. To choose a remedy intuitively, the essence description is read, or the bottles held in turn, and the remedy chosen which 'feels right'. Muscle testing or dowsing with the pendulum are techniques which will work best if used in conjunction with knowledge of the essences and the issues being addressed.

Whenever there is a serious physical or psychological problem, it is crucial to seek professional help. Working with an experienced practitioner, who has knowledge of essence qualities and the counselling and interview skills to elicit awareness of underlying soul issues, is of great benefit. Such a practitioner can also give support and insight when the essences bring up painful feelings or confront us with difficult decisions.

A professional practitioner will usually take a detailed case history including medical history, presenting physical symptoms (digestive problems, circulatory problems, sleeping, breathing difficulties and blood pressure problems): personality traits; lifestyle; stress levels at home and at work; relationships; mental, emotional and spiritual issues; predominant feelings such as anger, grief, depression, sadness and fear; purpose, direction and motivation; self-esteem etc.

The Findhorn Flower Essences

When I began developing the Findhorn Flower Essences I was guided by my contact with the intelligences of the plant kingdom. This contact had developed over many years and was growing stronger. I had been working in Australia as a homoeopath and for the Australian Bush Flower Essences company for three years when I unexpectedly felt drawn to return to live in Findhorn. I did not know then that I would be making flower essences in Scotland but almost immediately on arriving it felt appropriate. I was guided by my intuition with each essence I made. During the time of discovery and the making of each essence, I observed that I would experience its nature within myself, with the associated feelings, emotions and effects on all parts of my being. It is this first-hand experience within myself – along with information received from the higher levels and translated by my mind, and the messages received from the overlighting intelligences – that gives me a picture of the qualities of a flower. There is an ongoing process of attunement, followed by research on the essences in a variety of therapeutic settings over extended periods of time, by clients, friends and other health care practitioners, to study the indications, qualities and effects.

Repertory of Findhorn Flower Essences (in brief)

APPLE (*Malus sylvestris*)
◆ Keynote: HIGHER PURPOSE, will-to-good.
Apple helps us to integrate our desires and our willpower to realise our goals and visions positively. By aligning with higher or divine purpose we channel these powerful energies into right action.

BELL HEATHER (*Erica cinerea*)
◆ Keynote: STABILITY, self-confidence.
Bell Heather helps to access inner strength and resolve to stand one's ground after stress, trauma or conflict.

BIRCH (*Betula pendula*)
◆ Keynote: PERCEPTION, vision.
Birch helps us to broaden our perceptions and transcend limitations of mind. Through expanding our consciousness and seeing our cosmic connections we gain understanding and peace of mind.

BROOM (*Cytisus scoparius*)
◆ Keynote: CLARITY, illumination.
Broom stimulates mental clarity and concentration, facilitating ease in communication and creative thought when in a state of bewilderment.

DAISY Common Daisy (*Bellis perennis*)
◆ Keynote: INNOCENCE, grace.
Daisy allows us to remain calm and centred amid turbulent surroundings or overwhelming situations, creating a safe space in which to be vulnerable.

ELDER (*Sambucus nigra*)
◆ Keynote: BEAUTY, rejuvenation.
Elder stimulates the body's natural powers of recuperation and renewal. It helps us to contact and radiate the beauty and joy of our inner eternal youth.

GORSE (*Ulex europaeus*)
◆ Keynote: JOY, passion for life.
Gorse is a light-bringer, stimulating vitality, enthusiasm and motivation at times of apathy and low immunity, bringing light-heartedness and enjoyment of life.

SCOTTISH HAREBELL (*Campanula rotundifolia*)
◆ Keynote: PROSPERITY, faith.
Harebell is for realigning to the spirit of abundance and releasing material concerns following fear of lack.

HOLY-THORN (*Cratageus sp.*)
◆ Keynote: REBIRTH, creation.
Holy-thorn essence opens our hearts to love and the acceptance of ourselves and others, allowing intimacy and the expression of our truth and creativity.

LAUREL (*Prunus lusitanica*)
◆ Keynote: RESOURCEFULNESS, manifestation.
Laurel represents the abundance of the universe. It enables those wise in heart to empower themselves to find the resources to bring their ideas and ideals into form.

LIME (*Tilia platyphyllos*)

◆ Keynote: ONENESS, universality.

Lime helps us open our hearts to the light and love of our universal being. From this awareness we experience our interrelatedness on earth and create harmonious relationships in our lives: universality.

RAGGED ROBIN (*Lychnis flos-cuculi*)

◆ Keynote: PURITY, inner purification.

Ragged Robin aids in releasing, on all levels, congestion, obstruction and toxicity and facilitates the free flow of life-force and energies.

ROWAN (*Sorbus aucuparia*)

◆ Keynote: FORGIVENESS, reconciliation.

Rowan helps us to let go of resentments and to heal old wounds. As we learn to forgive ourselves and others, we can heal the past.

SCOTS PINE (*Pinus sylvestris*)

◆ Keynote: WISDOM, truth.

Scots pine helps us in finding directions in our search for answers to our questions. In being open to listening, we can be guided from within by the all-knowing self and the inner teachers.

SCOTTISH PRIMROSE (*Primula scotica*)

◆ Keynote: PEACE, unconditional love.

Scottish Primrose brings inner peace and stillness to the heart when confronted by fear, anxiety, conflict or crisis.

SEA PINK (*Armeria maritima*)

◆ Keynote: HARMONY, unity.

Sea pink aligns and infuses our being with Spirit. Blending and melding our life-force with Divine Will, it helps to balance the energy flow between all energy centres.

SILVERWEED (*Potentilla anserina*)

◆ Keynote: SIMPLICITY, self-realisation.

Silverweed helps us to detach ourselves from material concerns and overindulgence, by promoting moderation and self-awareness.

SNOWDROP (*Galanthus nivalis*)

◆ Keynote: SURRENDER, immortality.

Snowdrop allows us to surrender to the end of past events and attachments in life. In the death of the old we find the seed of our eternal inner light and behold new vistas.

SPOTTED ORCHID (*Dactylorhiza fuchsii*)

◆ Keynote: PERFECTION, creative expression.

Spotted Orchid enables us to go beyond pessimism and self-interest to seeing the best in everyone and everything.

STONECROP (*Sedum anglicum*)

◆ Keynote: TRANSITION, transcendence.

Stonecrop helps us to maintain inner stillness whilst in the process of breaking through inertia and resistance to change in the face of imminent transformation: transcendence.

SYCAMORE (*Acer pseudoplatanus*)

◆ Keynote: SOFTNESS, revitalisation.

Sycamore recharges and uplifts body and soul when we are stressed, allowing the emergence of a soft yet powerful new energy supply.

THISTLE Spear Thistle (*Cirsium heterophyllum*)

◆ Keynote: COURAGE, self-empowerment.

Thistle helps us to find true courage in times of adversity and to respond with positive action.

VALERIAN (*Valeriana officinalis*)

◆ Keynote: HUMOUR, mirth.

Valerian lifts our spirits and helps us to rediscover delight and happiness in living. It helps us to be at peace by taking ourselves lightly.

ROSE BAY WILLOWHERB (*Chamaenerion angustifolium*)

◆ Keynote: POWER, self-mastery.

Willowherb helps to balance the personality expressing self-seeking, authoritarian or over-bearing behaviour, bringing about the responsible integration of will and power issues.

Biography

Marion Leigh joined the Findhorn Foundation in 1976 where she was active in communications and networking with other groups and communities. She returned to her native Australia to strengthen her experience in these fields, also working with the Australian Bush Flower Essences, and qualified as a homoeopath. In 1992 she returned to Findhorn and pioneered the Findhorn Flower Essence range, based on flowers indigenous to the region and a continuation of that tradition of attuning to the angelic realms informing the nature kingdom that first made the Findhorn Community famed around the world. She subsequently founded a cottage industry based on these flower essences; developing, researching and teaching flower essence therapy and communication with nature.

Further Reading

Bach, Edward, *Heal Thyself*, C. W. Daniel Co. Ltd. 1931; reprint 1990.
Barnard, Julian, *A Guide to the Bach Flower Remedies*, C. W. Daniel Co. Ltd., 1979, 1994.
Gerber MD., Richard, *Vibrational Medicine*, Bear & Co. 1988.
Harvey, Clare G.; Cochrane, Amanda, *The Encyclopaedia of Flower Remedies*, Thorsons, 1995.
Kaminski, Patricia; Katz, Richard, *Flower Essence Repertory*, The Flower Essence Society, 1994.
White, Ian, *Australian Bush Flower Essences*, Findhorn Press, 1994.

Resources

Suppliers of flower essences:

Bach Flower Remedies
The Bach Centre
Mt. Vernon, Sotwell
Oxon OX10 OPZ
England

Healing Herbs – The Flower Remedy Programme
P O Box 65
Hereford HR2 OUW
England.
Tel. (01873) 890218

International Flower Essence Repertoire
The Working Tree
Milland
Near Liphook
Hants. GU30 7JS, England
Tel. 01428 741572

Findhorn Flower Essences
The Wellspring
31 The Park
Findhorn Bay
Forres Moray Scotland IV36 OTY
Tel. 01309 690129 Fax 01309 690933

Phoenix Apothecary
Findhorn Foundation
The Park
Forres Moray Scotland IV36 OTZ
Tel. 01309 691044 Fax 01309 690933

Flower Essence Services (FES – Californian)
P O Box 1769
Nevada City, CA 95959, USA
Tel (916) 265-9163

Pegasus Products
Box 228
Boulder, CO. 80306, USA
Tel (604) 384 5560

Perelandra, Ltd.
Box 3603
Warrenton, VA 22186, USA
Tel. (703) 937 2153

Professional Courses in Flower Remedies:

Australian Bush Flower Essences
81 Oaks Avenue
Dee Why
NSW 2099
Australia
Tel. (02) 9972 1033

Findhorn Flower Essences
& Australian Bush Flower Essences
The Wellspring
31 The Park
Findhorn Bay
Forres Moray Scotland IV36 OTY
Tel 01309 690129 Fax 01309 690933

Flower Essence Society (FES-Californian)
P O Box 459
Nevada City, CA 95959, USA
Tel. (916) 265-9163

Healing Herbs – the Flower Remedy Programme
P O Box 65
Hereford HR2 OWW
England
Tel. (01873) 890218

Perelandra, Ltd.
Box 3603
Warrenton, VA 22186, USA
USA
Tel. (703) 937-2153

Gestalt Therapy

by Sue Lieberman

*Counselling
Psychological
Therapies*

'What is Gestalt?' is the question new acquaintances invariably ask when I mention my work. Even native German-speakers can look perplexed at the application of a familiar word to an unfamiliar activity. For non-Germans, the problem is different. Most adults in this country now have a grasp of what counselling is, but Gestalt therapy, and especially Gestalt groupwork or organisational work, is much less known and understood.

Theoretical Background

Psychotherapy

The human personality, human behaviour and systems, and human interactions are a never-ending source of richness and information. Gestalt, like other psychotherapies, offers tools for understanding our own complexities and integrating rejected parts of ourselves; so that, in the Gestalt frame, people can become more alive, more aware and more 'whole' human beings in the changing circumstances of their lives.

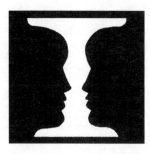

Fig.1: Figure and Field

In German, the word *Gestalt* conveys several different meanings. One of these is 'wholeness', a word that in English is linguistically related to the words 'well', 'hale' and 'healthy'. The word Gestalt therefore encompasses a belief that a psychotherapy is about helping human beings to discover their wholeness and health. The other meaning concerns the differentiation between foreground and background, or 'figure and field'. This is conventionally described by referring to the picture (Fig.1) in which can be seen either two profiles or a candlestick, but not both at the same time. If the profiles are foreground, then the candlestick is background, and vice versa. This relates to the Gestalt premise that one can only work creatively with what is in the here-and-now reality. The therapist's task is to focus the client's awareness on this reality, and then to explore its meaning in relation to the background from which it has emerged.

In terms of its theoretical understanding of the development of human personality, and the impact of early experiences on later patterns of behaviour, Gestalt does not depart significantly from its psychotherapeutic precursors. Where Gestalt differs, however, is in its approach to working with people: the how rather than the why.

Gestalt is primarily an experiential discipline. That is to say, it emphasises human experience as the vehicle through which to explore whatever needs exploring. This experience can be manifested in all the ways accessible to human perception: sensory, physical, emotional, intuitive, imaginative, intellectual and even spiritual. In this sense, Gestalt aspires to be truly an holistic method of working which accepts all aspects of a client's experience as relevant.

Gestalt is founded on several core concepts. The most important of these are:

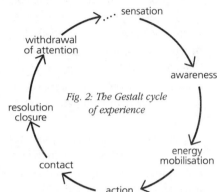

Fig. 2: The Gestalt cycle of experience

- ◆ The Gestalt Cycle of Experience

- ◆ Figure and Field

- ◆ Use of the Self

The Gestalt Cycle of Experience

Gestalt theory teaches that all living organisms are in a continual flow of energy related to needs. The diagram above shows how the cycle begins with some sensation, which grows through increasing awareness and focusing of energy until action takes place to satisfy the need (contact). Thereafter, the organism can absorb the results of the action (integration), and rest until the next need begins to claim attention.

A simple way of understanding this is to think about food and eating. I must eat every day if I am to maintain my physical health and energy system. At some point each day, I will begin to feel hungry (sensation). Initially, this may be a low-level sensation, but as my need for food increases, my awareness of being hungry pushes further into my consciousness (for example tummy rumbling, sensation of emptiness or lethargy). Eventually, I must mobilise my energy into action; that is, I have to go into the kitchen or to a restaurant to get food. Having eaten, my need is satisfied; my body can get on with the necessary process of digestion (integration), and I can rest from the quest for food and turn my attention to something else.

This is the healthy, uninterrupted cycle. It applies to all aspects of human existence; including the need for social contact; for rest; for physical affection; for exposure to stimulating work; for creative expression. Ideally, we live in a continual flow of need satisfaction, so that we are always able to respond appropriately to the current situation.

But what happens if the environment cannot deliver? For example, if there is no food in my fridge, and all the shops are closed? It is likely that, initially, my feeling of hunger will push out other claims for my attention. My need to eat remains constant, but is frustrated. If this continues, I have to start repressing my need; for a while I may experience it in other forms, such as headache, dizziness, aggression or weariness. If frustration continues for long enough, the effects take a chronic form, by which time I have probably lost touch with the original reason for my symptoms.

This frustration forms what Gestalt calls 'interruptions' to the healthy cycle. Psychotherapy, in effect, deals with the effects of early interruptions to need fulfilment; interruptions which, by adulthood, have become chronic in their effect, to the extent that people are unconscious of the original cause of the symptoms they experience. Therefore, early abandonment of an infant by its primary carer interferes with the later capacity to feel one has 'enough' love, care or attention. It probably also disrupts one's sense of power in being able to influence the world and get these needs satisfied.

In tackling this, the Gestalt practitioner's initial focus in working with a client is on raising awareness. So the client who comes with persistent but undiagnosable physical symptoms can be encouraged to explore the emotional companions to these symptoms in order to discover what hidden, unmet need lies beneath them. Identifying the unmet need is the prerequisite to being able to explore how, in present reality, that need may be satisfied.

Figure and Field

People do not like to experience life as a series of chaotic episodes. People struggle to place meaning on experience and so to create some sort of form ('figure') with which they can engage. Incomplete or 'unfinished' forms create disturbance in people, and they will automatically seek to finish them in some way. So, when looking at Fig. 3, the chances are that it will be seen as a triangle which needs closing, rather than as three separately angled and unconnected lines.

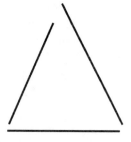

Fig. 3: 'Triangle' figure

In the process of making sense of life's experience, people attribute meanings which make sense to them at the time. The abandoned child, rather than continuing to experience the chaotic pain of loss and longing, may well draw the meaning 'I am not lovable', in order to construct some explanation for the abandonment. This becomes part of the developing adult's reality, and in some way also defines and influences subsequent experience. Clients who carry this motif deep inside are not only emotionally attuned to the abandoning aspect of subsequent experiences but continue to interact with these experiences as though the only possible explanation is that they are not lovable. This in turn affects how other people respond to them.

This explains why people will often react differently to exactly the same event – indeed, they may hear and see quite different things happening (it has long been recognised that individual eyewitness accounts of a crime will always be subject to partiality, both in the sense of being incomplete accounts and in having a particular slant). For example, in a therapy group, John may react angrily to Janet's stated intention to leave the group, seeing this as further proof that he is not worth staying for, while Louise may be sad at seeing Janet go but able to accept her reasons.

The concept of figure and field operates on several different levels. At one level, there is the immediate phenomenological experience ('I feel hungry') which, if attention is paid, becomes distinct from other sensations or emotions in that moment. At another level, there is a constant interplay between each event and the interpretation of its meaning. (For example: 'He cannot see me today because he is working. I feel abandoned, lost, lonely. He cannot love me.') At a third level, it provides an opportunity for people to explore events anew in their present environment, and redefine some old meanings in the light of present reality.

Use of the Self

Gestalt therapy departs radically from psychodynamic work in one area: that of the relationship between client and therapist. In psychodynamic work, the therapist stays as neutral as possible with the client, with the aim of bringing into sharper focus the transference which clients bring into the therapeutic relationship. Gestalt thinking emphasises that what takes place in the counselling room between client and therapist in itself provides living material relevant to the client's therapy. Gestalt practitioners therefore draw on the resources of their own individuality in order to help clients learn from their reactions to this particular person in their immediate environment.

The great value of this approach is that it offers a dynamic and creative dialogue between two people. Therapists consciously draw on themselves as a resource; for example, I may offer a personal response to what has occurred in the session in order to highlight awareness of the impact clients have had; or I may deliberately gaze out of the window in order to help my clients contact their anger at being ignored. Clients can make powerful discoveries about themselves, and even start to experiment with acting differently. This has its own risks. By bringing the therapist's own feelings and reactions actively into the room, it adds another complication into the client's field (for example, another person to please or to reject). It also means that therapists have to be highly sensitive to the appropriate management of their own boundaries – did I touch that client because I wanted to or because it was important for them?

What Might Happen in a Therapy Session

The Gestalt therapist's consulting room resembles that of other psychotherapists, with at least two chairs, a clock and a box of tissues. There may also be objects to use during the course of a session, such as cushions and drawing or painting materials.

In any session, there will be a period of 'settling in', in which normal greetings and familiarisation take place. Clients may well feel anxious at this point, either because they are bursting to tell the therapist something, or, conversely, because they apparently have nothing of immediate importance to share. Either way, this is the starting point for the session.

Typically, a Gestaltist 'follows the client'. This means that the therapist (in this example, female) follows the moment-by-moment shifts that the client (in this example, male) makes during the session. She will pause every now and again to make simple factual observations on what she has noticed. This could include a physical action which she sees the client make; or an expression on the client's face; or an emotion which the therapist herself feels. Sharing these selectively with the client allows him the opportunity to notice (a) how he is feeling; (b) how he is behaving in relation to his feeling; and (c) how he is feeling in relation to his therapist. All of these provide material to explore.

This is the kind of conversation that might take place:

C: *'I'm late. I'm sorry. The dog's unwell, and my wife wanted me to take him to the vet this morning. She insisted it had to be done immediately, though it could have waited till this evening. And it took longer than I expected, because of the traffic.'*

T: *'And now that you're here, how are you feeling about all this?'*

C: *'Well, I'm upset about the dog, I don't like him to be unwell. I'm angry with my wife for the way she controls me, and I'm angry with myself that I can't stand my ground with her.'*

The therapist observes the client for physical clues. His face is rather mild and displays no emotion, but she notices that he clenches one fist as he is talking.

T: *'I notice that you just clenched your fist. You seem to be more angry than anything else at the moment.'*

Client looks down at his fist and makes small hitting movements. He doesn't look at his therapist.

C: *'I get so frustrated, I just don't know how to deal with her when she's like that. She wants me to do everything the way she thinks it should be done. I can't talk to her at all about how I'm feeling; I've tried, but she just says, 'I thought you were over all that nonsense'.*

The therapist feels something resembling a physical blow in her chest at this last phrase. She takes a moment to decide how she wants to respond.

T: *'When your wife says that to you, she wipes you out. No wonder you're feeling angry. (Pause). Could you look at me and tell me how angry you feel?'*

Client looks at his therapist a couple of times and then looks away.

C: *'No. It's difficult to do that.'*

T: *'What do you imagine might happen if you were to look at me and tell me?'*

C: *'I'm afraid you wouldn't take me seriously either.'*

In this interchange, the client brings a wealth of feeling into the room. The therapist notes his embarrassment at being late, his distress over his dog, and his irritation at the traffic, but these are less immediate than his feelings in relation to his wife. He experiences her as controlling not only his actions, but also his feelings. He feels anger, and probably also impotence and despair. Yet he stops himself from expressing these feelings directly. He fears that his therapist will treat him in the same way as his wife treats him (and almost certainly the way a significant adult in his early life treated him).

So past and present are both in the room; along with feelings, and the repression of those feelings; and the way C. transfers feelings and experiences from his relationship with one woman (his wife) to that with another (his therapist). Part of his therapist's job is to help him feel more able to express his anger, and thus more in touch with his own power. The work is very likely to touch at some point on the client's relationship with one or both of his parents, but will always return to the present: to helping him notice the blocks that he himself imposes on his spontaneous self-expression; and to helping him discover what could happen if he tried different actions.

Becoming a Gestalt Therapist

Often people become interested in training as a Gestalt therapist through experiencing Gestalt as a client, and they may undertake the training regardless of their existing profession. However, more commonly people arrive at the training with an existing professional interest. Some people retrain in Gestalt who are already working in an equivalent field, such as in psychiatry, counselling, or another form of psychotherapy. Others come into Gestalt from a related discipline, such as social work or medicine. Generally aspiring trainees will be assessed for their suitability by the institute they approach: a suitability which will be determined as much by personal as by professional factors. Training in Gestalt requires a strong commitment, both financially and to one's own personal growth, and most psychotherapy trainings will require trainees also to be in personal therapy throughout the course of the training.

The availability of training in Gestalt is developing rapidly but unevenly throughout the UK. Most Gestalt psychotherapy trainings are now four years long on a part-time basis, although there are shorter trainings which will equip people with Gestalt skills suitable for application in other fields of work. There is, as yet (1996), no national register for Gestalt practitioners.

Conclusion

Until very recently, Gestalt had something of a reputation for aggressive confrontation. This was largely due to the considerable influence on early Gestalt practice and teaching by its co-founder Fritz Perls, and the cultural and social climate in which Gestalt initially developed. For the same reasons, Gestalt is often associated in people's experience with classic Gestalt 'techniques', such as talking to 'the empty chair'. However, as Gestalt has evolved, practice has matured and deepened. Techniques are less important than genuine contact between client and therapist; and many practitioners now work in a gentler way than hitherto. Gestalt is capable of encompassing both a vision of humanity and considerable sensitivity to individual needs. For both practitioners and clients, Gestalt offers enormous opportunity within a coherent theoretical framework for creative and fruitful exchange.

Biography

Sue Lieberman was born in London in 1949, one of the post-war generation of Jews who grew up in the shadow of the holocaust. She studied history at Bristol University, and during this period developed her interest in social justice. Her first profession was community work; over a period of several years, she became fascinated by the relationship between personal and group dynamics, and organisational health. She entered into personal therapy, subsequently trained with Gestalt Training Services (UK) as a therapist, and later with the Gestalt Institute of Cleveland in organisational applications. She escaped from London in 1974 and has lived for the past 11 years in Edinburgh where she practises as a therapist, group worker and organisational consultant and trainer. She lives with three cats.

Further Reading

Clarkson, P., *Gestalt Counselling in Action*, (in The Counselling in Action Series, ed. Windy Dryden) Sage, 1989.

Houston, G., *The Red Book of Gestalt*, The Rochester Foundation, 1982.

Latner, J., *The Gestalt Therapy Book*, The Julian Press and The Centre for Gestalt Development, 1973.

Nevis, E. (ed.), *Gestalt Therapy: Perspectives & Applications*, Gestalt Institute of Cleveland, 1992.

Passons, W., *Gestalt Approaches in Counselling*, Holt, Rinehart & Wilson, 1975.

Perls, F.; Hefferline, R F.; Goodman, P., *Gestalt Therapy*, Julian Press, 1951; reprinted by Bantam Press, 1980. The original Bible of Gestalt therapy.

Philippson, P.; Harris, J., *Gestalt Working with Groups*, Manchester Gestalt Centre, 1989.

The British Gestalt Journal appears twice annually and is invaluable as a sourcebook for current thinking in Gestalt in Britain. Contact: P O Box 2994, London N5 1UG. Publ. by GPTI Publications Ltd.

Resources

For further information about training, contact:

Metanoia
13 North Common Road
London W5 2QB

The Gestalt Centre
64 Warwick Road
St Albans
AL1 4DL

Gestalt South West
79 Effingham Road
Bristol BS6 5AY

Gestalt Education Midlands
1 Seaford Cottage
Peopleton
Worcs WR10 2LF

Sherwood Psychotherapy Training Institute
Thiskney House
2 St James Terrace
Nottingham NG1 6FW

Manchester Gestalt Centre
7 Norman Road
Rusholme
Manchester M14 5LF

The Gestalt Trust
c/o 71 Castlehill Road
Bearsden
G61 4DY

Teamwork
11 Castle Terrace
Edinburgh EH1 2DP

The Scottish Gestalt Association
c/o 31 Montague Street
Edinburgh EH8 9QS

Herbalism

by Helmut Hasso Cézanne

History

Proponents of complementary therapies often tend to claim a historically anchored 'right of existence'; many claim their therapy to be one of the oldest forms of medicine practised. In this respect, herbal medicine is no exception – since it is so closely linked to nutrition, it was inevitable that humankind would make use of it from early times. Even animals are known to choose medicinally active plants according to the specific ailment from which they may be suffering, like parasitosis; animals in the wild also generally avoid potentially hazardous plants. This no longer applies to domestic animals, which have lost some of the instincts essential for survival in the wild. Intoxications have been described in herds: with St. John's Wort in sheep, cattle and horses; with melilot in cattle; or with mistletoe in dogs and horses.[1]

Traditional Chinese Medicine

Documentary evidence shows the use of plants as medicines in ancient Egypt, by the Greeks and the Romans and during the Middle Ages. This use continues in our times, when herbal medicine still is of considerable importance: the medical treatment available to 70% of the world population, in fact, depends on it as the non-industrialised countries still rely on herbal remedies to treat their ailments. Herbs have an essential role in most cultures; some well-known examples are the Indian Ayurvedic system, traditional Chinese medicine, and the native American Indian tradition. Although different in their philosophy and diagnostic approaches, they all use the herbs from their natural environment to relieve suffering and enhance health. The appreciation of the natural world is illustrated by an Ayurvedic teaching story: the master sends his students out to find one plant which does not have healing properties. His best student travels for many months and finally returns and says: 'Master, I have failed you – I could not find the plant which you asked for.' The reply is: 'You have done very well; there is no more that I can teach you.'

In the last 50 years in the Western industrialised world, herbal medicine – also called 'phytotherapy',[2] or 'botanotherapy' – has lost its role in medicine as most of the medicinal products used nowadays are synthetic compounds supplied by the pharmaceutical industry. However, it is interesting to note that 25% of all prescription drugs are still derived from plants.[3] Indeed, there are many doctors who are unaware of the relationship between, for instance, atropine, ephedrine, pilocarpine, lobeline, digitoxin and papaverine and their herbal origin.

Some reasons for the decline of herbalism are that, by their very nature, herbs are not easily standardised and quantifiable and not all constituents of all medicinally used plants have been identified. The complex composition of herbs varies according to growing conditions (soils, weather, season), harvest procedures and storage techniques. There are pressures to regulate herbal medicines and herbalists generally use defined and pharmacologically controlled remedies. Regulation is important to ensure quality and safety, but it is essential that it does not prevent the availability of effective and unadulterated natural remedies.

There have always been a number of practitioners, more so on the European continent than in Britain, who are dedicated to the holistic approach of phytotherapy. They have preserved the traditional knowledge and have developed it further, so that it can continue to play a role in health care. It is quite likely that this role will increase as the disenchantment with synthetic drugs grows.

The Effects of Herbs

Herbs can be seen as a bridge between the inner, physiological environment and the outer, ecological environment. They help the body to sustain or regain homoeostasis, enhancing health by facilitating harmony and resonance between the inner and the outer. Therefore herbs often have gentle and long-term actions. The many different ingredients in each plant will work synergistically to balance the body. Often herbs are prescribed in a mixture, as it is known that in certain combinations herbs will enhance each other's actions.

Much research has been undertaken to establish what the active ingredients in herbs are and what action they have. This leads to a nomenclature based on the effects the remedy has on human physiology. Traditionally in herbal medicine the herb's action is more relevantly described by looking at the kind of problems it can address, for instance antihelminitic, carminative, diuretic, expectorant, laxative.

Forte and Mite Phytotherapeutica

One common misconception is that herbs are weak and slow in action, which easily gets translated into 'not very effective'. While it is true that many herbs are very gentle and can be used safely by the untrained, it is important to state that there are herbs which have powerful effects and must only be used by trained practitioners.

Herbal remedies such as belladonna (*Atropa belladonna*), ephedra (*Ephedra sinica*), jaborandi (*Pilocarpus jaborandi*), foxglove (*Digitalis purpurea*), and of course opium poppy (*Papaver somniferum*), will indeed readily convince the sceptic that herbs can have drastic effects. These 'forte' phytotherapeutics occupy one end of the range of action of medicinal plants within a given category.[4] Therapeutic categories of phytotherapeutics are essentially the same as those applied to medicines in general. So *Atropa belladonna* is a 'forte' antispasmodic remedy, whereas German chamomile (*Matricaria recutita*), fennel (*Foeniculum officinalis*) and peppermint (*Mentha piperita*) are classified as 'mite' antispasmodics.

Between these extremes of the phytomedicinal range, there are remedies with a medium strength or intensity of action, in the antispasmodic category for example rosemary (*Rosmarinus officinalis*) and cramp bark (*Viburnum opulus*). For a long-time, the remedies for the nervous system seemed to be an exception as no medium strength remedies were described. Remedies such as opium poppy (*Papaver somniferum*) are found at the one end of the spectrum, and valerian (*Valeriana officinalis*) and hops (*Humulus lupulus*) at the other end. However, individually chosen and appropriately dosed remedies such as Californian poppy (*Escholtzia californica*) and kava kava (*Piper methysticum*) are now recognised neurotropic phytotherapeutica which have their place between the more gentle (mite) and the most powerful (forte) remedies.

Synthetic Drugs – Plant Extracts – Whole Plant Remedies

When considering the benefits of herbal medicine, the usage of whole plant preparations needs to be compared with preparations that provide the reassurance of the scientific production method which can be reproduced, quantified and standardised: synthetic drugs and plant extracts containing defined quantities of the effective component.

What are the arguments for using herbal remedies rather than synthetic drugs? Quite simply, they have fewer side effects than orthodox therapy with chemical entities. It is not that there are no toxic effects but plants are natural. Humankind has co-evolved with and is adapted to them, having done particularly well with respect to the indigenous flora. The preparation of a remedy from a more toxic plant often discards (unless this is specifically required) the actual toxic component, as in mistletoe (*Viscum album)*, where the berries are not used in herbal medicine, only the leaves and young twiglets. This produces a remedy that is mainly hypotensive and used as a geriatricum.

Anthroposophical Medicine

Anthroposophic medicine uses the whole plant of mistletoe, growing on different species of trees, for an antineoplastic preparation for the treatment of different cancers;[5] whilst orthodoxy currently appears to be essentially interested in the purification and screening of the most cytotoxic components of the berries in its race for potent antitumour drugs. Another important development seems to be the spreading recognition of *Hypericum perforatum* as an antidepressant and anxiolytic remedy, on the basis of research conducted according to current orthodox standards of investigation in clinical pharmacology.[6]

Other efforts concentrate on the comparison of phytomedicines and synthetic agents in benign prostatic hyperplasia (BPH),[7] and surgical treatment of BPH, where continuous irrigation of the bladder with a herbal infusion of nettle (*Urtica dioica L.*), St. John's Wort (*Hypericum perforatum L.*), German chamomile (*Matricaria recutita L.*), plantain (*folia Plantaginis majoris*), yarrow (*Herba millefolii*), birch (*folia Betula pendula*), mugwort (*Artemisia vulgaris*) and strawberry (*folia Fragaria vesca*)) after prostatic adenomectomy appears to be beneficial.[8]

What are the arguments for taking herbal medicines containing substances which are not fully standardised and not fully investigated? This question undoubtedly applies to the more potent remedies such as *Papaver somniferum* and *Digitalis purpurea*; it is here that one wants to know how much of active constituents are contained in a certain amount of a preparation, and one wishes to have this preparation available in a stable composition. However, many herbs have been appreciated for millennia in the context of culinary use and folk medicine and have proven to be safe and effective even though not all their properties and constituents have been fully scientifically analysed. While the standardisation of whole plant remedies (for example extracts or tinctures which contain several active constituents, and often even great numbers) is possible for any remedy, for economical and practical reasons such standardised remedies are not a primary objective of pharmaceutical companies.

If we use herbal drugs at all, why should we not use well-defined, precisely dosed, purified substances rather than the plant from which these single substances are derived? In spite of a trend towards the use of single substances which has eradicated products such as *Tinctura opii* from the British National Formulary, if not from the pharmacopoeias, there is good evidence for the whole plant remedy having fewer side effects than the isolated constituents, in the treatment of diarrhoea,[9] and depressive syndrome,[10] and for its beneficial use as a methadone substitute for treating heroin addiction;[11] moreover, there is evidence of synergism of the various constituents within a complex plant remedy, or even for the interdependence and presence of various constituents to be a necessary condition of medicinal action. This appears to be recognised by more orthodox researchers for various plants to date, as for example valerian (*Valeriana officinalis*);[12] yarrow (*Achillea millefolium*)[13] and hawthorn (*Crataegus oxyacanthoides*).[14]

A more recent example of isolating the (principal) therapeutically active constituent from a plant is the substance artemether, the sesquiterpene lactone, which is at present investigated in chloroquine resistant *Plasmodium falciparum* malaria; it also seems to be efficacious in disease caused by *Schistosoma japonicum*. The compounds derived from the Chinese medicinal plant qinghao (*Artemisia annua*) appear to be the most rapidly acting of all antimalarial drugs; effective when given parenterally, orally or by suppository. No serious adverse effect has yet been reported in humans.[15] Since its discovery as an antimalarial with low toxicity, hundreds of derivatives have been synthesised. However, the whole plant appears to be more than an antimalarial remedy: aqueous extracts, ethyl-acetate, and n-butyl alcohol extracts of qinghao have antipyretic, anti-inflammatory, analgesic and bacteriostatic effects. Animal experiments have demonstrated that qinghao acid is one of the actively bacteriostatic constituents, whereas scopoletin is one of the anti-inflammatory constituents.[16] One study reports the pharmacological and clinical effects of a whole plant preparation of qinghao in a gelatine capsule compared with the extract artemisinin. The results revealed that the toxicity of the whole plant was relatively low whilst its effectiveness was 3.5 times higher than the extract.[17]

The Practice of Herbal Medicine

Preparations

The plant remedy, as used by the medical herbalist, may be administered in various forms. The basis of the remedy, however, is generally the fresh or dried whole plant or parts of it. Creams, tablets, suppositories, pessaries, tinctures, fluid extracts, herbal teas, aromatic oils, plant juices and, although less frequently, injectable preparations, are available in herbal medicine. Most commonly used are tinctures, fluid extracts and teas; the first two are water-ethanol solutions of constituents of dried or fresh plants, the latter are prepared as infusions, but steeping is a bit longer than for preparing tea, preferably 10 to 15 minutes. Macerations, using cold water, may be applied to less infusible plants or parts of plants, such as bark, which may be left in water for up to 24 hours, or even boiled for an hour or more, in order to dissolve the active components of the plant. Each plant contains a whole range of different active substances. Regularly more of them are being discovered, researched and used for new drug developments. For instance, bladderwrack, the marine alga *Fucus vesiculosus*, an old remedy well known to herbalists for its use in myxoedema combined with obesity, is currently being investigated for the isolation of anti-HIV compounds.[18]

Conditions Treated

Herbal medicine is useful in minor ailments which are amenable to self-medication: common colds and flus, headaches, mild digestive problems, menstrual problems etc. In the hands of a trained practitioner herbal medicine can treat a wide variety of diseases, especially chronic illnesses, such as gastro-intestinal disturbances, rheumatic and arthritic conditions, skin problems, hormone related symptoms, and respiratory and cardiovascular illnesses.

Case Studies

The following cases may illustrate that phytotherapy can be useful in chronic, as well as acute situations. I do not explain in detail the rationale behind each of the plants which were prescribed, but with respect to each patient's main complaint I list aspects of some of the plants which were used.[19] The prescriptions are the original ones and in no way are any of them intended as a guideline for self-medication.

First patient: *Long-standing intestinal mycosis following long-term exposure to antibiotic treatment (which was given to treat chronic prostatitis) in an otherwise healthy male adult; the current treatment consisted in the repeated application of oral antimycotic drugs and antimycotic cream to the perianal region. He spontaneously responded to the following treatment:*

I. Tinctura	Hypericum perforatum extr. fl.		10 ml
	Baptisia tinctoria	1-5	20 ml
	Calendula officinalis	1-5	20 ml
	Potentilla tormentilla	1-3	20 ml
	Gingko biloba	1-4	10 ml
	Pimpinella anisum	1-5	10 ml
	Turnera diffusa	1-5	10 ml

100 ml x 2, 5 ml tid cum aq. cal. ante cibo.

II. Infusio	Matricaria recutita	30g
	Mentha piperita	10g
	Salvia officinalis	10g
	Calendula officinalis	5g

55g, 1 cup tid ante cibo.

III. Ung. Calendulae et Hamamelidis cum Tinct. Querci 14 ml ad 60 g; bid to perianal region. 2/52

Four weeks later:

I. Tinctura	Hypericum perforatum extr. fl.		10 ml
	Baptisia tinctoria	1-5	20 ml
	Calendula officinalis	1-5	20 ml
	Potentilla tormentilla	1-3	20 ml
	Gingko biloba	1-4	10 ml
	Pimpinella anisum	1-5	10 ml
	Turnera diffusa extr. fl.		10 ml

100 ml x 3, 5 ml tid 1/52, cibo.

II. Infusio	Matricaria recutita	60g
	Mentha piperita	20g
	Salvia officinalis	20g
	Calendula officinalis	10g

110g, 1 cup bid – tid ante cibo.

POT MARIGOLD *Calendula officinalis* L.
This annual herb has been grown in gardens since the Middle Ages. Its taste is saline, slightly bitter; its odour is faint. The petals or flowerheads are used. Among the constituents are an essential oil, pigments (carotenoids), bitter compounds, saponins; the calendulosides A-D (in the root at least); lupeol, flavonoids; isorhamnetin

glycosides including narcissin, and quercetin glycosides including rutin, chlorogenic acid, mucilage and resin. It has anti-inflammatory, spasmolytic, antihaemorrhagic, choleretic, styptic, vulnerary and antiseptic properties. Internally it may be taken as an infusion for stomach disorders, gastric and duodenal ulcers and dysmenorrhoea; and externally as a lotion or ointment for cuts and bruises, nappy rash, sore nipples, burns, scalds, etc. An alcoholic extract has been shown to have in vitro antitrichomonal activity.

TORMENTIL *Potentilla erecta* L. Raeuschel
A creeping perennial, its taste is astringent and it is odourless. The medieval Latin word tormentilla stems from tormentum, pain; the herb has traditionally been used for relieving stomach pains and toothache. The rhizome is the principal medicinally active part; containing tannins (up to 20%), phlobaphene (= 'tormentil red'), the triterpene alcohol tormentol, a glycoside (tormentillin), starch, sugars, and a bitter compound (chinovic acid). Its medicinal use is as an astringent, tonic, haemostatic, anti-inflammatory, vulnerary and antiseptic remedy. It is used as an infusion in diarrhoea, dysentery, and intestinal haemorrhage. Externally it is used in compresses, ointments or as a lotion for wounds with delayed healing, sores and ulcers. It has shown a weak anti-allergenic, immunostimulating and interferon inducing activity in vitro.

Second patient: *Long-standing history of obstructive airways disease/emphysema, adult, on regular prophylactic salbutamol inhaler; had an episode of worsening, with cough, chest pain, influenza – symptoms for which he received several courses of oral antibiotic treatment, in addition to steroids.*

First treatment:

I. Sirupus	Sir. thymi glycyrr.	50 ml
	Sir. pruni serot.	50 ml
	100 ml, 5ml cum aq. cal. mane, prn nocte	
II. Infusio	Herba cham. recut.	40 g
	Herba lavand. off.	5 g
	Herba thymi vulg.	5 g
	50 g, 1 cup nocte, prn nocte	
III. Tinctura	Ephedra sinica	30 ml
	Echin. angust. extr. fl.	20 ml
	Althaea off. herba	20 ml
	Tussilago farfara	20 ml
	Foeniculum vulg.	10 ml
	100 ml x 2, 5ml tid cum aq. cal. ante cibo.	

This treatment resolved the situation within three days. It must be added that this patient has no penchant for 'alternative' medicine whatsoever.

COLTSFOOT *Tussilago farfara* L.
Tussis is the Latin word for cough. Tussilago tastes mucilaginous, slightly bitter, astringent; it is odourless. The leaves and flowers are used medicinally. Its constituents are flavonoids; rutin, hyperoside and isoquercetin; mucilage, about 8%, consisting of polysaccharides based on glucose, galactose, fructose, arabinose and xylose; and inulin; pyrrolizidine alkaloids, including senkirkine and tussilagine, in very small amounts (about 0.015%), and tannin. It is medicinally used as an expectorant, demulcent, antitussive and anticatarrhal. Coltsfoot is used for pulmonary complaints, irritating or spasmodic coughs, whooping cough, bronchitis, laryngitis and asthma. Recent research has shown that the polysaccharides are anti-inflammatory and immunostimulating as

well as demulcent, and the flavonoids also have anti-inflammatory and antispasmodic action. A total extract and antilipophilic fraction stimulate phagocytosis in mice inoculated with *E. coli*, again showing stimulation of the immune system. The pyrrolizidine alkaloids have caused hepatotoxicity in rats fed daily on high doses, but not on daily low dose regimes. They have been shown not to cause any damage to human chromosomes in vitro.

Third patient: *Hyperkinetic heart syndrome in a young adult, previously treated with propranolol, responded most satisfactorily to the following treatment:*

I. Tinctura	Valeriana off.	30 ml
	Hypericum perf.	30 ml
	Avena sat.	20 ml
	Leonurus card.	20 ml
	100 ml x 2, 5 ml tid cum aq. cal. ante cibo.	

One month later: repeat prescription.

MOTHERWORT *Leonurus cardiaca* L.
The taste is very bitter; the odour faint. The flowering stems are used medicinally; their constituents include a bitter compound (leonurin), an iridoid glycoside (leonuride), tannins, an essential oil and alkaloids. It contains flavonoids; rutin, quinqueloside, genkwanin, quercetin, quercitrin, isoquercitrin, hyperoside, and apigenin and kaempferol glucosides. Motherwort is used medicinally as a cardiac tonic, sedative, nervine, antispasmodic and emmenagogue remedy. Studies in China have shown that extracts have antiplatelet aggregation actions and decrease the levels of blood lipids; they also have an inhibitory effect on pulsating myocardial cells in vitro.

Fourth patient: *A dry eczema which developed in an adult with atopic diathesis and recurrent acne vulgaris. History of multiple orthodox dermatological treatments.*

I. Tinctura	Solanum dulcamara	20 ml
	Ephedra sinica	20 ml
	Arctium lappa	20 ml
	Rumex crispus	20 ml
	Valeriana off. extr. fl.	15 ml
	Pimpinella anisum	10 ml
	105 ml x 2, 5ml tid cum aq. cal ante cibo.	

II. Unguentum
Ung. hamamelidis cum tinct. querci 15 ml; 60 g; bid (to dry scaly eczematic lesions)
Ung. calend. cum oleo aetherol. melaleucae 30 gtt.; 30 g. Rp. prn (acne vulg.)

Three weeks later:

I. Tinctura	Solanum dulcamara	20 ml
	Ephedra sinica	20 ml
	Arctium lappa	20 ml
	Rumex crispus	20 ml
	Valeriana off. extr. fl.	15 ml
	Pimpinella anisum	10 ml
	105 ml x 3, 5ml tid cum aq. cal ante cibo.	

The response, after about one week, was most satisfactory; again in a patient who tried herbal medicine as a last resort.

YELLOW DOCK *Rumex crispus* L.

It tastes mucilaginous, bitter; it is odourless. The root is used medicinally. Its constituents are anthraquinone glycosides, about 3%–4%; tannins, rumicin and oxalates. Its medicinal use is as a laxative, cholagogue, alterative, tonic. It is used for chronic skin disease, jaundice and constipation. Large doses should be avoided due to the oxalate content.

Training

In the UK at present herbal medicine is practised by practitioners with variable backgrounds, training, experience and degrees of adherence to Eastern or Western traditions. Such a varying degree of competence amongst practitioners is certainly not helpful in establishing high quality standards of practice, and efforts are now being made to achieve regulation of practitioners, similar to the Osteopaths Act, for setting standards of education, training and practice. For Western herbal medicine this is currently being attempted by the oldest body of herbal practitioners in the Western world, the National Institute of Medical Herbalists (NIHM) which was founded in 1864. Fellows and members of this institute have undertaken the appropriate studies and carry the letters FNIMH and MNIMH respectively after their names. The NIMH is committed to promoting and maintaining high standards of education and training for its members. The institute currently accepts graduates only from training establishments which teach a certain standard of medical and phytotherapeutic skills. These courses all involve at least 500 hours of clinical practice supervised by experienced practitioners. Core subjects covered in the training include: pathology, diagnosis, pharmacology, pharmacognosy, botany, materia medica, communication skills, complementary medicine, as well as nutritional and herbal therapeutics. Critical skills and research methodology are part of the curriculum. Currently there are two institutions which run courses leading to membership of the National Institute of Medical Herbalists. The School of Phytotherapy runs a full-time BSc course and part-time correspondence course. Middlesex University runs a full-time and part-time BSc course and is developing postgraduate courses; a similar curriculum might be developed by the University of Cardiff. New members enter a three-year scheme involving postgraduate training, a mentor scheme and self-audit training.

NIMH also provides information leaflets and a regional directory of members. The information officer deals with queries from the public, professional bodies and the media.

Biography

Helmut Hasso Cézanne is a former research assistant of the Max-Planck-Institut für Biophysik, Germany. He qualified as a medical practitioner at Frankfurt University. He held a hospital practitioner post at the Centre Hospitalier de Draguignan in France, where he worked alongside Odette Fiori and Sabine Bressin, and was awarded a medal of merit. He held NHS posts in Wales and Scotland, and more recently worked as a research physician, contributing to the evaluation of the effects of new drugs. He is in independent phytotherapeutic practice in Dundee. His approach to herbal medicine is based mainly on the teachings of Rudolf Fritz Weiss and Jean Valnet.

References

1 *St. John's wort and its effect on livestock*, Agricultural Gazette of New South Wales, 1920; 31: 265-72.

N T Clare, *Photosensitisation in Diseases of Domestic Animals*, Review Series No. 3, Commonwealth Bureau of Animal Health, Commonwealth Agricultural Bureaux, Farnham Royal, UK, 1952; 11-15.

O M Radostits; G. P. Searcy; K. G. Mitchall, *Moldy sweet clover poisoning in cattle*, Canadian Veterinary Journal 1980; 21: 155-8.

J C Greatorex, *Some unusual cases of plant poisoning in animals*, Veterinary Record, 1966; 78, 725-7.

C Jean Blain, [*Mistletoe.*] Notes de Toxicologie Vétérinaire, 1977; 1: 21-2.

2 The term phytotherapy was introduced by the French physician Henri Leclerc (1870-1955), who, in his Précis de Phytotherapie, summed up his life-time experience as a medical practitioner putting herbs wholeheartedly to medicinal use.

3 NR Farnsworth et al., *Medicinal Plants in Therapy*, Bulletin of the World Health Organisiation, 1985; 63(6).

4 Rudolf Fritz Weiss, *Herbal Medicine*, translated from the Sixth German Edition of Lehrbuch der Phytotherapie by A. R. Meuss; Beaconsfield Publishers Ltd., 1991.

5 Iscador®; Weleda (UK) Ltd, Heanor Road, , Ilkeston, Derbyshire, DE7 8DR

6 B Witte; G Harrer; T Kaptan; H Podzuweit; U Schmidt, [*Treatment of depressive symptoms with a high concentration Hypericum preparation. A multicentre placebo-controlled double-blind study*]: *Behandlung depressiver Verstimmungen mit einem hochkonzentrierten Hypericumpräparat*, Arbeits- und Forschungsgemeinschaft für Arzneimittel-Sicherheit e. V., Köln. Fortschr-Med. 1995 Oct 10; 113(28): 404-8.

E Ernst, [*St. John's Wort as antidepressive therapy*]: *Johanniskraut zur antidepressiven Therapie*, Centre for Complementary Health Studies, Postgraduate Medical School, Exeter, UK. Fortschr-Med., 1995; 113(25): 354-5.

7 D Bach, [*Treatment of benign prostatic hyperplasia*]*, Behandlung der benignen Prostatahyperplasie (BPH)*, Zeitschr. f. Phytother, 1996; 17: 209-18.

8 M I Davidov; V G Goriunov; P G Kubarikov, [*Phytoperfusion of the bladder after adenomectomy*]: *Fitoperfuziia mochevogo puzyria posle adenomektomii*, Urol-Nefrol-Mosk., 1995; Sept-Oct(5): 19-20.

9 William Charles Evans, *Trease and Evans' Pharmacognosy*, 13th edition, p. 590; Bailliére Tindall, 1992.

10 J Ott; G Witzenhausen, [*Objectification of psychopathological symptoms in patients with a depressive syndrome*]: *Zur Objektivierung psychopathologischer Symptome bei Patienten mit depressivem Syndrom*, Psychiatr-Neurol-Med-Psychol-Beih., 1975; 20-21.

11 M Auriacombe; D Grabot; J P Daulouede; J P Vergnolle; C O'Brien; J Tignol, *A naturalistic follow-up study of French-speaking opiate-maintained heroin-addicted patients: effect on biopsychosocial status*, Laboratoire de Psychiatrie, Université de Bordeaux II, France. J-Subst-Abuse-Treat, 1994; Nov-Dec.

12 B Hazelhoff; T M Malingre; D K Meijer, *Antispasmodic effects of valeriana compounds: an in-vivo and in-vitro study on the guinea-pig ileum*, Arch-Int-Pharmacodyn-Ther., 1982; 257(2): 274-87.

R Della-Loggia; A Tubaro; C Redaelli, [*Evaluation of the activity on the mouse CNS of several plant extracts and a combination of them*]: *Valutazione dell'attivita sul S. N. C. del topo di alcuni estratti vegetali e di una loro associazione*, Riv-Neurol., 1981; 51(5): 297-310.

P W Thies; S Funke, [*On the active ingredients in valerian. 1. Detection and isolation of isovalerian acid esters with sedative effect from roots and rhizomes of various valerian and kentranthus species*]: *Über die Wirkstoffe des Baldrians. 1. Nachweis und Isolierung von sedativ wirksamen Isovaleriansäureestern aus Wurzeln und Rhizomen von verschiedenen Valeriana- und Kentranthus-Arten*, Tetrahedron-Lett., 1966; 11: 1155-62.

13 T Tozyo; Y Yoshimura; K Sakurai; N Uchida; Y Takeda; H Nakai; H Ishii, *Novel antitumor sesquiterpenoids in Achillea millefolium*, Shionogi Research Laboratories, Shionogi & Co., Ltd., Osaka, Japan. Chem-Pharm-Bull-Tokyo, 1994; 42(5): 1096-100.

K Zitterl-Eglseer; J Jurenitsch; S Korhammer; E Haslinger; S Sosa; R Della-Loggia; W Kubelka; C Franz, [*Sesquiterpenelactones of Achillea setacea with antiphlogistic activity*]: *Entzündungshemmende Sesquiterpenlactone von Achillea setacea*, Institut für Botanik und Lebensmittelkunde, Veterinärmedizinischen Universität Wien, Austria. Planta-Med., 1991;57(5): 444-6.

S Barel; R Segal; J Yashphe, *The antimicrobial activity of the essential oil from Achillea fragrantissima*, Department of Bacteriology, Faculty of Medicine, Hebrew University, Jerusalem, Israel. J-Ethnopharmacol, 1991; 33(1-2): 187-91.

14 G Joseph; Y Zhao; W Klaus, [*Pharmacologic action profile of crataegus extract in comparison to epinephrine, amirinone, milrinone and digoxin in the isolated perfused guinea pig heart*]: *Pharmakologisches Wirkprofil von Crataegus-Extrakt im Vergleich zu Epinephrin, Amrinon, Milrinon und Digoxin am isoliert perfundierten Meerschweinchenherzen*, Institut für Pharmakologie, Universität zu Köln. Arzneimittelforschung, 1995; 45(12): 1261-5.

M Schussler; J Holzl; U Fricke, *Myocardial effects of flavonoids from Crataegus species*, Institut für Pharmakologie, Universität zu Köln, Germany. Arzneimittelforschung, 1995g; 45(8): 842-5.

T Bahorun; V Trotin; J Pommery; M Pinkas; J Vasseur, *Antioxidant activities of Crataegus monogyna extracts*, Laboratoire de Physiologie Cellulaire et Morphogenèse Végétale, Université des Sciences et Technologies de Lille, Villeneuve d'Ascq, France. Planta-Med., 1994; 60(4): 323-8.

15 N J White, *Artemisinin, current status*, Wellcome-Mahidol University, Oxford Tropical Medicine Research Programme, Faculty of Tropical Medicine, Mahidol University, Bangkok, Thailand. Trans-R-Soc-Trop-Med-Hyg., 1994; 88 Suppl 1: 3-4.

16 K C Zhao; Z Y Song, [*Pharmacokinetics of dihydroqinghaosu in human volunteers and comparison with qinghaosu*]. Institute of Materia Medica, Chinese Academy of Medical Sciences, Beijing. Yao-Hsueh-Hsueh-Pao, 1993; 28(5): 342-6.

17 Y D Wan; Q Z Zang; J S Wang, [*Studies on the antimalarial action of gelatine capsule of Artemisia annua*]. Sichuan Institute of Chinese Materia Medica, Chongqing. Chung-Kuo-Chi-Sheng-Chung-Hsueh-Yu-Chi-Sheng-Chung-Ping-Tsa-Chih, 1992; 10(4): 290-4.

18 A Beress; O Wassermann; T Bruhn; L Beress; E N Kraiselburd; L V Gonzalez; G E de-Motta; P I Chavez, *A new procedure for the isolation of anti-HIV compounds (polysaccharides and polyphenols) from the marine alga Fucus vesiculosus*, Institute of Toxicology, Christian Albrechts-Universität, Kiel, Germany. J-Nat-Prod., 1993; 56(4): 478-88.

19 R C Wren (rewritten by E M Williamson and F J Evans, *Potter's New Cyclopaedia of Botanical Drugs and Preparations*, Potter's (Herbal Supplies) Ltd., Daniel Co., Ltd., 1989.

Further Reading

Brooke, E., *Herbal Therapy for Women*, Thorsons, 1992.

Evans, William Charles, *Trease and Evans' pharmacognosy*, 13th edition, Baillière Tindall, 1992.

Hoffmann, David, *The New Holistic Herbal*, Element, 1992.

Mills, S Y., *The Essential Book of Herbal Medicine*, Penguin, 1993.

Newall, C A.; Anderson, L A., Phillipson, J D., *Herbal Medicines*, The Pharmaceutical Press, 1996

Weiss, Rudolf Fritz, *Herbal Medicine; translated from the Sixth German Edition of Lehrbuch der Phytotherapie by A. R. Meuss*; Beaconsfield Publishers Ltd., 1991.

Wren, R C (rewritten by Williamson, E M and Evans, F J) *Potter's New Cyclopaedia of Botanical Drugs and Preparations*, Potter's (Herbal Supplies) Ltd. Daniel Co., Ltd, 1989.

Journals

Zeitschrift für Phytotherapie, bi-monthly, Hippokrates Verlag GmbH, Stuttgart.

The British Journal of Phytotherapy, bi-annually (with considerable delays), The School of Phytotherapy, East Sussex.

European Journal of Herbal Medicine, four-monthly, The National Institute of Medical Herbalists, Exeter.

Australian Journal of Medical Herbalism, quarterly; The National Herbalists' Association of Australia, Kingsgrove NSW.

Resources

National Institute of Medical Herbalists (NIMH)
56 Longbrook Street
Exeter
Devon EX4 6AH
Tel. 01392-426022
Fax. 01392-498963

General Council and Register of Consultant Herbalists
Grosvenor House
40 Sea Way
Middleton-On-Sea PO2 7SA

British Herbal Medicine Association
P O Box 304
Bournemouth
Dorset BH7 6JZ

The School of Phytotherapy
Bucksteep Manor
Bodle Street Green
near Hailsham
East Sussex BN27 4RJ
Tel. 01323-833 812/4

Middlesex University
White Hart Lane
London N17 8HR
Tel. 0181-362 5000

Holistic Dentistry

by Ian Ireland

Holistic dentistry is not taught as part of the undergraduate syllabus. It is a way of thinking and working which has developed for an increasing number of dentists, including myself, as a result of personal experience and interest, leading to a questioning of how dentistry can affect the whole person and influence the health both favourably and adversely.

One pioneer of holistic dentistry is Dr Harold Gelb of New York.[1] He has a practice which provides a multidisciplinary approach to dentistry using a variety of health care professionals. Dr Gelb has inspired many dentists in the UK to change their approach to their work and use kinesiology, osteopathy, biofeedback, reflexology, physiotherapy, etc. to augment the treatment they provide.

Kinesiology
Osteopathy
Reflexology

As more patients come to expect their treatment to be carried out with careful consideration of their overall health and well-being, more dentists will become aware of the advantages of the holistic way of thinking.

Personal Involvement

I had a lower left second molar removed in 1972 to allow a wisdom tooth to erupt. This was a standard procedure, aimed at eliminating episodes of acute infection around the impacted wisdom tooth, and is a course of action which I might responsibly carry out on my patients today. However, a side effect which was not noticed, but which I would look for in my current practice, was that the treatment produced a change in the occlusion on the left side of my mouth, otherwise known as a disturbance to the tempero mandibular joint (TMJ). This caused overclosure resulting in a myriad of other symptoms, some of which were migraines and intense pain in the neck, shoulder and lower back. These symptoms I put down to stress, not imagining that a standard dental procedure could have such devastating effects on the rest of the body.

As chance would have it, TMJ related problems were beginning to gain notice in the UK, and in the Solway area where I was working, a group of dentists formed who wished to explore this topic further. I joined them and we formed an organisation called the British Dental Migraine Study Group. Many speakers from other parts of the world gave presentations to our group, raising awareness of the fact that dental treatment can affect the whole body, causing seemingly quite unrelated symptoms unless certain precautions and checking measures are taken.

I consequently received treatment to correct my TMJ problems after which my painful symptoms cleared. I pursued my interest in these matters, learning the appropriate skills and determining to promote the ethos of holistic dentistry for the sake of professionals and patients alike, both of whom stand to gain from the broader based approach to dental problems.

The Practice of Holistic Dentistry

In contrast to the traditional approach, where the dentist is the expert and the patient a passive recipient, a visit to a holistic dentist involves a different kind of relationship. There is a partnership in which dentist and patient discuss together possible treatments. The patient's needs and desires, for example not to take antibiotics or have painkillers, are listened to and taken into account.

Investigation of any symptoms may lead to a complete health check involving a team of health care workers, medical and complementary, each using their specialised knowledge to examine the patient. The holistic dentist is one of a team of professionals whose aim is to help the patient.

Bio-Energetic Regulatory Medicine Homoeopathy

The health check may include tests to examine the sensitivity of the patient to substances such as mercury, used in dental fillings. In my practice, this involves Vegatesting, hair mineral analysis and a homoeopathic challenge with Merc. Sol. These tests have not been scientifically validated but empirically are good indicators as to whether or not it can be considered safe to use these substances.

Prior to treatment, possible side effects will be discussed openly. Nothing will be done without the full understanding and consent of the patient.

The Mercury Debate

The mercury content of dental fillings has become of increasing concern to some. Dentists worldwide have consistently stated that amalgam fillings, which contain mercury, are not poisonous and do not constitute a health hazard. However, mercury is being increasingly implicated in kidney dysfunction; neurotoxicity, contributing to multiple sclerosis; reduced immuno-competence, for example ME; increased stillbirths and birth defects.[2] Although it has been known for centuries that mercury is a poison, the dental establishment believes that when it is amalgamated with other constituents, it is rendered harmless. It is thought that in amalgam, it is irreversibly bound and prevented from leaching out. There is now evidence to suggest that this is not the case, and that mercury is released from amalgam fillings to be deposited in the body's tissues.

Alternatives to Amalgam

Composite is a completely non-metallic material, which is hardened with light and shade-matched to the tooth's colour. Its disadvantage is that it should not be used when the patient has a hard bite and, most importantly, should only be used in small to medium sized fillings. It can be strengthened by incorporating glass beads.

Inlays of various materials can be used for fillings in back teeth. Substances commonly used are porcelain, composite-type substances (isocit is one of many in use) and gold, which is arguably the best alternative. When gold is to be used, all amalgams should be removed beforehand as a mix of metals in the mouth can generate electric currents, leading to health problems, such as headaches, muscle tension, jaw clenching, etc. Inlays are suited to medium or large cavities and are costly.

Crowns and caps are made of gold or ceramic materials bonded to gold. Porcelain substitutes are available for back teeth. The procedure involved is to remove the amalgam from the previously filled tooth, and insert a composite core, held in place by titanium pins if necessary. The tooth is shaped, an impression taken and the crown fitted at the next appointment.

Removal of Amalgam

If, in the light of the prevailing evidence, the patient decides to have all their amalgam fillings removed, there is a recommended procedure to be observed. Before a decision is made, patients should be properly tested for mercury sensitivity. The level of sensitivity determines the urgency of the treatment. Amalgams need to be removed in the correct sequence, starting with the fillings which have shown through the testing to be the most negatively charged. A special instrument is available to measure charge across fillings, so that the order of removal can be established.

During amalgam removal, mercury vaporises and can be absorbed through the lining of the mouth and the lungs, into the blood stream. There are nutritional supplements which bind mercury and therefore prevent deposition in body tissue. These, which include free radical scavengers such as vitamins A, C, E and selenium, should be started prior to the procedure. Charcoal tablets should also be taken one-half hour before treatment commences. Patients should be given oxygen to breathe whilst the amalgam is being removed.

It should be stressed again: amalgam need not be removed unless the patient tests sensitive to its constituents or on the grounds of excessive negative charge due to a mix of metals in the mouth, because removal itself can further burden the body with mercury.

The Fluoride Debate

It is an indisputable, statistically proven fact that fluoride, when added to the public water supply (in areas where it is not present naturally), at one part fluoride to one million parts water, strengthens tooth enamel and inhibits dental decay.[3]

For the general population, this reduces pain and suffering because of reduced dental procedures; for the NHS it reduces the cost of treating rampant dental caries. Were these facts the end of the argument, there would be no controversy.

Problems with water fluoridation became accentuated with arrival of fluoride toothpastes in the late 1960s and early 70s. Before this, toothpaste contained no fluoride and was merely a cleaning agent. It is now argued by some that because most people use fluoride toothpaste, we do not need the substance in the water supply.

Because children ingest large quantities of toothpaste during brushing (presumably because of the good taste), they over-fluoridate themselves – even without added fluoride in the water supply. Fluoride is incorporated into developing tooth enamel and reinforces its resistance to decay, but in any concentration more than one part per million produces varying degrees of enamel deformity seen as mottling of the tooth surface. Mild mottling is grey and white in appearance; severe mottling is brown and white with variations. Enamel mottling, or fluorosis, is unsightly and disfiguring.

There is also some evidence that raises the suspicion that fluoride, in quite low concentrations, can cause a host of symptoms such as chronic fatigue, headaches, aches and pains, gastro-intestinal disturbances, etc.[4]

The antifluoride lobby is now becoming more vociferous, and its objections to water fluoridation include:

◆ No freedom of choice – an objection to mass medication.

◆ No attention paid to the needs of each individual rather than the average person.

◆ Enamel damage and subsequent psychological effect of deformed teeth, leading to the expense of cosmetic work.

◆ Possible sensitivity to fluoride with direct effects giving rise to symptoms, such as fatigue, headaches, excessive dryness of the throat, aches in muscles and bones, muscle spasms, gastro-intestinal disturbances, dizziness, skin rashes and brittle bones.

Testing can be carried out to check fluoride levels. The following steps to remove it from the everyday diet should be taken: use of bottled water or reverse osmosis water purifier (if the tap water is fluoridated); reduce intake of tea and soft drinks; reduce processed food especially frozen vegetables. The discontinuation of fluoride toothpaste is obviously crucial.[5] A holistic health check is advisable to monitor the metabolism and to provide suitable levels of vitamins and minerals to counteract excess fluoride levels (magnesium, zinc and iron).

Application of Holistic Dentistry in Head and Neck Pain

Experience indicates a definite link between headaches, neck pain, facial pain, shoulder pain and other less well-defined pains to occlusal (bite) problems. A holistic dentist will pick this up and institute treatment.

Stress, be it pleasant or unpleasant, is a primary cause of a host of symptoms because it can put the body's systems under duress, including the muscles of the jaw. This gives rise to temporo mandibular joint dysfunction syndrome (TMJ), also called cranio mandibular dysfunction syndrome (CMD).

Holistic dentists typically recognise patients with TMJ by their posture: shoulders pulled up, head pushed forward and chin set – each to a varying degree. The next step is questioning them about the nature of their pain and palpating the facial and neck muscles to determine which are the trigger points and which are the most stressed muscles. The dentist then confirms that the occlusion is a factor by examining the teeth and observing the opening and closing of the jaws.

Some patients with this problem typically have missing teeth which have not been replaced, resulting in the movement of opposing and neighbouring teeth, which causes bite disturbances. Teeth which are given space, caused by removal of neighbours, will almost always move. When this occurs, the opening and closing of the jaws alters from the genetically correct manner for the individual, causing the muscles of the head and neck to go into spasm because they are no longer functioning properly.

Other causes leading to the same end result are trauma to the cranial skeleton resulting in movement of the skull bones to which the muscles are attached. This obviously changes their mode of action with similar symptoms to those mentioned above. Restorations made without due attention to the occlusion can also precipitate the same problems. Worn dentures are a common cause of TMJ problems. Teeth which fail to achieve their proper position in the mouth as they erupt, for whatever reason, can alter the genetically correct bite and trigger pain.

Lifestyle stress can compound the problem. Stress produces adrenalin, which in turn causes increase in muscle tone. Muscles already in spasm will become more painful in the presence of increased adrenalin. It is a fact that most patients with TMJ problems are stressed individuals. In many cases, because head pain is multifactorial, its successful treatment requires a multidisciplinary approach.

The dental practitioner, having diagnosed possible TMJ problems, makes a simple bite splint to a design which ensures that the jaws are directed into their carefully worked-out proper relationship. If this position is achieved successfully, then muscle spasm will gradually cease and relief should ensue. If this occurs, permanent measures to correct the bite can be taken, or the patient may elect to continue with the splint.

If pain relief is incomplete after a period of time, other avenues have to be explored, to search for the cause and remove the symptom.

Cranio-Sacral Therapy
Osteopathy
Kinesiology
Relaxation Therapy
Nutrition

Among the most obviously indicated disciplines is firstly cranial osteopathy, to make adjustments to the skull. An osteopath can assess habits and positions leading to imbalances in the body. Applied kinesiology can strengthen muscular weaknesses which are compounding the problem. Checking hormone levels is vital as imbalance can cause muscular spasm, especially in thyroid or parathyroid hormones. Learning to relax through biofeedback is very useful. A strict review of nutrition – the cornerstone of good health – is essential.

In short, the holistic approach to head and neck pain means correcting the occlusion, reversibly at first, and then exploring all avenues possible to ensure the patient's overall health.

Biography

Ian Ireland qualified in dentistry from Edinburgh University in 1971 and was the most distinguished graduate of his year. He became interested in the holistic aspects of dentistry after he developed TMJ problems himself. He was part of the British Dental Migraine Study Group which studied the effects of and appropriate treatment methods for occlusal problems. Over time his interests in holistic dentistry expanded to include amalgam-free dentistry and the other aspects described in the chapter. He is senior partner in a progressive dental practice in Forres, Scotland and the regional dental adviser for BUPA Dentalcover at present.

References

1   H Gelb, *Killing Pain Without Prescription*, Thorsons, 1983.

        ———, *Clinical Management of Head, Neck and TMJ Pain and Dysfunction*, W B Saunders Co., 1977.

2   I D Mandel, *Amalgam hazards: an assessment of research*, J Am Dent Ass; 1991; 122; 42-65.

3   Department of Health, *Report on Health and Social Subjects*, October 1991.

4   George Walgbolt, *Fluoridation: The Great Dilemma*, Coronado Press, 1979.

5   *Good Housekeeping*, Lincolnshire, Tel. 01507-327655.

Further reading

Eley, B M.; Cox, S W., *The release, absorption and possible health effects of mercury from dental amalgam: a review of recent findings*, Br Dent J, 1993; 175: 161-8.

Gelb, H., *Killing Pain Without Prescription*, Thorsons, 1983.

        ———, *Clinical Management of Head, Neck and TMJ Pain and Dysfunction*, W B Saunders Co., 1977.

Huggins, Hal, *It's All in Your Head*, Life Science Press, 1986.

Mandel, I D., *Amalgam hazards: an assessment of research*, J Am Dent Ass; 1991; 122; 42-65.

Taylor, Joyal, *The Complete Guide to Mercury Toxicity from Dental Fillings*, Scripps Publ., 1988.

WDDTY, *The WDDTY Dental Handbook*, Wallace Press, 1993.

Yiamouyiannis, John, *Flouride, The Aging Factor*, Health Action Press, 1986.

Ziff, Sam & Michael, *Dental Mercury Detox*, Bio-Probe Inc., 1993.

———, *The Missing Link*, Bio-Probe Inc., 1992.

———, *Dentistry Without Mercury*, Bio-Probe Inc., 1993.

Resources

The British Society for Mercury Free Dentistry
Jack Levenson
Welbeck House
62 Welbeck Street
London W1M 7HB
Tel. 0171-486 3127

(This organisation provides a list of dentists *who practise mercury free dentistry*)

The British Homoeopathic Dental Association
2b Franklin Road
Watford
Herts WD1 1QD
Tel. 01923 233 336

Stockport Dental Seminars
Roy Higson
6 Union Road
New Mills
Stockport
Cheshire

Holotropic Breathwork

by Anthony Hillin

Holotropic Breathwork*, was developed by Stanislav and Christina Grof in California, USA. Holotropic Breathwork uses a combination of breathing and music to induce a non-ordinary state of consciousness (NOSC) in which physical and emotional healing, personal growth and spiritual development can occur. The word 'holotropic', from the Greek *holos* and *trepein*, means moving towards wholeness.

Historical Background

Holotropic Breathwork is a new procedure based on ancient methods of accessing NOSC found in many parts of the world, ranging from the breathing techniques of Buddhist and Hindu spiritual practices to the traditional music and rhythms in cultures as diverse as those of the indigenous peoples of Australia and the Pacific, Africa, Asia and America. Evidence in cave paintings suggests humans have been using NOSC in ritual contexts for 20,000-40,000 years. Michael Harner, an authority on shamanism, suggests that if a practice has been used for this long it is likely to have an important function.[1]

Stanislav Grof conducted pioneering research into the use of LSD in psychotherapy,[2] initially as a psychiatrist in his native Prague during the 1950s and 60s, and then as assistant professor at Johns Hopkins University and as chief of research at Maryland Psychiatric Research Center in the USA, where he conducted an extensive programme of LSD therapy sessions. He found participants had a rich encounter with their inner world which was different from external reality. The experience of a wide range of people in NOSC typically fell into three categories.

◆ The first category consists of re-experiencing biographical events, such as physical or emotional traumas.

◆ The second category includes issues of death and being reborn which emerge in forms that are closely related to biological birth. Experiences of this type often seem to involve subjects reliving their own birth.

---

*Holotropic Breathwork is a registered trademark.

◆ The third category of experiences can seem fantastical to those who have not undergone them, and include: contact with deities, mythological figures and spirit guides; events which subjects report as feeling like past lives; access to knowledge from other times and cultures of which the subject may have no conscious knowledge; and a sense of oneness or connection with other people, other species or the whole universe. These experiences are known as transpersonal; that is, they transcend the usual boundaries of personality to include what might be thought of as mystical, spiritual, religious or paranormal experiences.

Past Life Therapy

The transpersonal experiences, in particular, caused Grof to repeatedly revise his theoretical framework, which had been based in the accepted Western psychiatric view. This orthodox view only accepts the first category of experience. It does not accept that perinatal (meaning 'around birth') events have a significant effect on later mental health, believing that the infant's cortex is not sufficiently developed to allow memory of such events. Transpersonal events would be considered evidence of psychosis within the orthodox medical model. Yet a wide range of people who function perfectly well in everyday reality have these experiences in NOSC, and in addition these experiences often bring profound insights and a sense of well-being.

Stan Grof's work for more than 30 years has been about developing a map of human consciousness which includes these experiences without pathologising them. It has been a major contribution to modern psychology. Stan and Christina Grof developed Holotropic Breathwork as a non-drug based means of accessing the healing potential of NOSC.

Theoretical Basis

Holotropic Breathwork occupies territory where several fields of study merge. This includes: anthropology and the study of the healing potential of NOSC in traditional cultures, especially their use in shamanism;[3] theology and comparative religion, particularly techniques for accessing, understanding and integrating mystical experiences;[4] the new physics, as it calls into question traditional scientific notions of time and space;[5] modern consciousness research in the fields of near death, out of body and psychic experiences;[6] and mythology.[7]

The most useful theoretical framework for understanding Holotropic Breathwork is provided by transpersonal psychology, which was established by Grof, Maslow and others in the late 1960s. It builds on Jung's work in the 1930s which went far beyond the biographical model. He developed the concept of the collective unconscious to explain his findings that symbols and archetypes found in dreams, mythology and religion transcend culture and are found throughout history.[8]

Psychological Therapies

The Grofs helped develop the concept of spiritual emergency,[9] which asserts that some of the experiences labelled as functional psychosis by orthodox psychiatry, that is, those without an organic cause, can be indicative of an opening to transpersonal dimensions which, if supported and allowed to unfold, can bring the individual to a place of greater well-being. Because of lack of understanding of this dimension and limited resources, orthodox psychiatry usually uses medication to suppress such symptoms.

Rebirthing

The importance of perinatal events was acknowledged by Otto Rank and later researchers.[10] People often re-experience their birth in Holotropic Breathwork and this can bring useful insight into long-standing behaviour patterns or symptoms. Birth is a tremendous struggle for survival. Powerful physical and emotional stress builds up. The infant will rarely be able to fully express or release this. Its imprint will therefore remain and influence life. There is a sense in which the foetus dies and is reborn as an infant. This forms a prototype experience of death and rebirth which can become a template determining people's response to later experiences of major change which are beyond their control.

Grof hypothesised that by reliving the birth trauma in NOSC we can complete what is unfinished and free ourselves of associated repetitive life patterns.[11]

Perinatal Birth Matrices

The experiential nature of perinatal material corresponds with the four clinical stages of birth. This led Grof to postulate the theory of 'perinatal birth matrices' (BPM) as the organising principle for the perinatal level of the unconscious and related transpersonal dimensions.[12] This model offers new insights into the causes and nature of psychopathology and suggests innovative therapeutic options, in particular the experiential work of Holotropic Breathwork.

BPM I includes pregnancy up until labour. It may be a blissful period for the foetus. Alternatively, it may be toxic if the mother used alcohol or drugs, or if she experiences physical or emotional harm. BPM II commences with labour. The incredible pressure of uterine contractions combined with hormonal changes and no opportunity of escape mean this stage is characterised by a sense of victimisation. In BPM III the cervix dilates and passage through the birth canal is possible. This stage is characterised by struggle. Hopelessness and hope alternate in a life and death struggle. In BPM IV the foetus emerges. In the best outcome the infant is reunited with the mother. Bonding and nursing create an imprint of struggle and pain being rewarded with pleasure and success. Anaesthesia, caesarean and difficult births complicate this picture.

How Does It Work?

Bienergetic Analysis

Participants are instructed simply to increase their rate of breathing and to keep their awareness on their inner process or experiences. Stan Grof explains that this lessens psychological defences and allows unconscious material to emerge, apparently confirming Wilhelm Reich's observation that psychological defences are related to restricted breathing.[13]

In describing the effect of inducing a NOSC, Grof states, 'This tends to change the dynamic equilibrium underlying symptoms, transform them into a stream of unusual experiences, and consume them in the process.'[14]

Hyperventilation changes the physiology of the body, which brings to the surface deep-seated tensions and patterns. They are often spontaneously released through catharsis including shaking, twitching, coughing, vomiting and verbal expression, including screaming. The tensions may also surface as lasting contractions and spasms, which can consume or release vast amounts of pent up energy, accounting perhaps for the sometimes dramatic change in long-standing symptoms which can occur.

Symptoms of tetany (cramps in the hands and feet) occur in some people. However, the experience of the thousands of people who have participated in Holotropic Breathwork does not confirm the Western medical view that tetany always occurs in hyperventilation. In common with other symptoms, those who do experience tetany find that if it is allowed to build to a climactic peak, it usually releases and other experiences follow.

Music supports the process by activating and intensifying old patterns and by providing a context for the experience.[15] It helps breathers move through difficulties and blocks, allowing them to 'let go' and to enter more fully into the experience. A number of books discuss the healing effects of music. In a group context music helps mask sounds from other breathers.

Sound Therapy

What Happens During a Session?

Preparation

A Holotropic Breathwork session usually takes place in a group and lasts two to three hours, sometimes a little longer. It should always be preceded by an introductory talk which explains how the breather can get maximum benefit from the session. It also mentions the range of experiences which may arise, as these can feel very odd for someone who has not experienced them before. Participants are reminded of contraindications, which are discussed below.

People work in pairs, in turn occupying the role of breather and sitter/helper. The sitter/helper gives undivided attention to their partner, watching over them and attending to their needs, for example for tissues, blankets or to get to the toilet. Breathers lie on their back with their eyes closed and are talked through progressive muscle relaxation to help relax their bodies. They are encouraged to let go of any preconceptions about what they would like to happen in the session and to trust the ability of their psyche to bring to the surface whatever is most appropriate for them at this time. They start breathing a little deeper and faster than usual and the music commences.

The Range of Experiences

No two sessions are the same. Some people experience no turmoil. However, this is uncommon, especially in someone's first sessions. As hyperventilation affects the physiology, usually some of the symptoms mentioned previously emerge.

The spectrum of possible experiences can include: the full range of emotions; aches and pains; nausea; hypersalivation; sweating; sexual feelings; and ecstatic states. Many people experience heightened sensory awareness. Some move in apparently random ways; others in stylised or precise sequences which may emulate animals, dance or spiritual postures from a range of cultures. Others remain motionless having profound experiences.

Intensifying Symptoms

Holotropic Breathwork views symptoms which arise as indicative that unconscious or repressed material is being activated. Rather than trying to lessen a symptom the facilitator will encourage the participant to intensify it, so that they can experience it more completely. This helps bring it fully into consciousness and is likely ultimately to release it, often in a climactic fashion. Focusing attention on the symptom and breathing more rapidly are often sufficient to bring this intensification and release about.

Focused Energy Release Work

For symptoms such as pain, tension, blocked energy, numbness, or sensations of cold and heat in the body, focused energy release work can also be provided in the form of resistance or pressure to assist the breather to amplify the sensation. This is sometimes referred to as bodywork; however, it is not massage. It is only provided with the breather's consent. Nurturing touch can be provided in situations of apparent early deprivation.

Art Work

Participants are encouraged to complete a drawing or painting to represent some aspect of their experience. This is usually in the form of a mandala or circle. It can play a useful role in integrating the experience. Pictures kept from a sequence of sessions often reveal themes, particularly in relation to perinatal material. Participants are encouraged to date and keep their pictures.

Group Sharing

Ideally there is an opportunity for group sharing where participants tell of their experience. This helps with integrating and grounding the experience. Also, hearing other participants' stories can bring additional insight for the breathers into their own experience.

Concluding a Session

After the session participants are advised how further to ground themselves and integrate the experience. A Holotropic Breathwork session can be likened to major surgery for the psyche. Just as a patient would be advised to take it easy after a physical operation, participants are encouraged to allow themselves time to rest. They are urged not to attempt to drive immediately after a session.

Individual or Group Sessions

For the majority of people Holotropic Breathwork is most effective in groups. Seeing other people having experiences which may appear profound, weird or frightening, and not only survive but benefit from them, can help participants trust their process and enter more fully into their own experience. Many people find the sounds of others form a useful context for their own experience. Dimmed lights, loud music and the practice of many breathers of wearing blindfolds can minimise distractions.

A minority of individuals may find the prospect of a group too daunting or may feel too embarrassed to 'let go' in public. Often a few individual sessions will bring these individuals to a place where they are able to attend a group workshop. Workshops can take place over a day, weekend, or longer period. Many people find longer workshops, particularly residential ones, are conducive to a greater sense of trust and safety and deeper work.

Frequency of Sessions

There is no particular recommendation regarding the number or frequency of sessions. Just one session can bring benefits. Some people embark on a series of regular sessions, for example every month or two. Others have occasional sessions when they feel the need.

Usually it is possible for the breather to end a session with a sense of completion for that day. Occasionally, however, there will be an awareness that there is more of the experience close to the surface and the full emotional or physical charge has not been released. In these circumstances another session soon afterwards is likely to be beneficial.

Potential Benefits

People are drawn to Holotropic Breathwork for a variety of reasons. Some use it as a tool for physical and emotional healing, others as an adjunct to their spiritual path. I believe it also has potential for beneficial social, economic and political change.

Physical Symptoms

Twelve Steps Programme

Holotropic Breathwork cannot claim to cure physical symptoms. No research exists to prove any such claims. However, anecdotal evidence points to physical changes which include improvements in pain, menstrual cramps, asthma, obesity and joint flexibility. Some people have reported it useful in recovering from alcohol and drug addictions. Christina Grof agrees with Jung and the founders of Alcoholics Anonymous in likening addiction to a thirst for wholeness and spiritual connection.[16] Tav Sparks also describes the potential of Holotropic Breathwork in healing addiction.[17]

Mental and Emotional Health

Many participants report Holotropic Breathwork benefits their mental and emotional health, but again the research has not been done to quantify this. Breathwork seems to be particularly useful at times of major life crisis, such as bereavement or loss; changes in health or work; and in dealing with abuse, or early neglect or deprivation. Grof postulates that positive touch and nurturing provided when the subject is regressed in NOSC can help heal early deprivation.[18]

Prevention and Health Promotion

Autogenic Training Relaxation Therapy

The role of stress in a wide range of conditions is well documented and is being augmented by the new field of psychoneuroimmunology which demonstrates how attitudes and repressed emotions can suppress our immune system.[19] The profound de-stressing effect of Holotropic Breathwork suggests it can help prevent stress–related conditions.

Vascular and lymphatic constriction can change the cellular environment in ways which many complementary therapies postulate may dispose individuals to a variety of chronic conditions, cancer and immune suppression. Many people find Holotropic Breathwork helps release such constriction.

Creativity and Spirituality

Some people report renewed creativity and inspiration following a breathwork session. This is particularly attractive to writers and artists experiencing blocks, or for anyone who wants a fresh look at dilemmas or issues facing them. As already mentioned, some people are attracted to breathwork primarily as a way of deepening their spiritual experience.

Wider Implications

The increased compassion and sense of oneness with other beings, and with the whole of creation, which breathwork can bring, suggest it could play a potential role in helping humanity move to a more just and sustainable world.

Contraindications

For most people this will be a safe and beneficial practice. Because a breathwork session may trigger powerful emotions, it is not suitable for people with a history of cardiovascular problems or high blood pressure. Glaucoma is contraindicated because intraoccular pressure may increase during a session. Those who have had recent surgery, or injury, should not undergo breathwork until they are fully healed, as energetic movement may impair their healing.

Because breathwork can trigger contractions of the uterus, it is not recommended during pregnancy. Someone with epilepsy should discuss their situation with their doctor and the breathwork facilitator. It is not necessarily contraindicated.

Whilst breathwork can be beneficial for some people with a mental health history, it should be pointed out that residential or intensive outpatient support from staff with an understanding of this way of working is required. Unfortunately, this is currently rarely available. Such people should not participate in weekend workshops because this format does not provide ongoing support.

Thorough attempts are made to filter out the small number of people for whom deep experiential work may be dangerous. There have been instances of participants misrepresenting their history for fear of being refused. It is possible that a participant may be unaware of having a condition which is contraindicated, for example aneurysms. Screening for a family history of heart disease may help reduce this risk.

Standards of Facilitation and Training

Holotropic Breathwork can appear deceptively simple and this can lead people with little experience themselves to offer to facilitate others. To help maintain high standards Stan and Christina Grof have trademarked the term 'Holotropic Breathwork' and offer a training programme leading to certification. This currently involves 500 hours of experiential work, lectures, consultation and apprenticeship. Its large experiential component helps ensure that facilitators have worked through a significant amount of their own unresolved issues. The minimum completion time is two years in order to allow integration of the profound experiences which usually emerge when someone engages in breathwork over an extended period.

Usually a facilitator will need to have come to a position of deep trust in the psyche's healing ability in NOSC, grounded in their own experience, in order to maintain a posture of acceptance, non-judgement and compassion, whilst avoiding over-identification, in the face of the powerful material presented by participants.

The training related to focused energy release work instructs facilitators in how to avoid injury to themselves and the breather. An untrained facilitator will not necessarily have this information. As with any qualification, it does not guarantee the quality of the work of those who have completed the training. In addition to checking that facilitators have completed certification, participants are advised to look for indicators of good practice.[20]

Members of the Association of Holotropic Breathwork International subscribe to a code of ethics agreement.

Biography

Anthony Hillin, BSS, CQSW, has a background in social work. He was the first co-ordinator of PACE, London's gay, lesbian and HIV counselling and training organisation. For the last eight years he has been a freelance trainer and consultant working on issues of HIV, holistic approaches to well-being and empowerment, sexuality, bereavement, stress and burnout. His work is commissioned by health and local authorities, voluntary organisations and professional associations in Europe, USA, Australia and Asia. Anthony writes on these issues and has a small counselling, therapy and professional supervision practice. He is a certified facilitator of Holotropic Breathwork.

References

1   M Harner, *The Way of the Shaman*, Bantam, 1980.

2   C Grof; S. Grof, *Beyond Death: The Gates of Consciousness*, Thames & Hudson, 1980.

3   M Eliade, *Shamanism: Archaic Techniques of Ecstacy*, Pantheon, 1964.

    M Harner, *The Way of the Shaman*, Bantam, 1980.

    J Achtenberg, *Imagery in healing: shamanism and modern medicine*, Shambhala, 1985.

    L Le Shan, The Medium, *The Mystic and the Physicist*, Ballantine Books, 1975.

4   J Kornfield, *The Path with Heart: A Guide Through the Perils and Promises of the Spiritual Life*, Bantam, 1993.

5   F Capra, *The Tao of Physics*, Shambala Publications, 1975.

    ———, *The Turning Point*, Simon & Schuster, 1982.

    R. Sheldrake, *A New Science of Life*, J. P. Tarcher, 1981.

    ———, *Seven Experiments That Could Change the World*, Fourth Estate Ltd, 1994.

6   C Jung, *Memories, Dreams, Reflections*, Random House, 1989.

    Moody, R., *Life after Life*, Mockingbird Books, 1975.

    Kübler-Ross, E., *Death – The Final Stage of Growth*, Prentice Hall International Inc, 1975.

    S Grof; J. Halifax, *The Human Encounter with Death*, E. P. Dutton, 1977.

    C Tart, *Out of Body Experiences, in Psychic Explorations* (E. Mitchel and J. White, eds.), Putnam, 1974.

7   Joseph Campbell, *Hero with a Thousand Faces*, World Publishing Co., 1970.

8   C Jung, *The Archetypes and the Collective Unconscious*, Routledge, 1990.

9   C Grof, and S Grof (eds), *Spiritual Emergency*, Jeremy P. Tarcher Inc, 1989.

    Emma Bragdon, *The Call of Spiritual Emergence*, Harper & Row, 1990.

10 O Rank, *The Trauma of Birth*, Hancourt Brace, 1929.

    F Leboyer, *Birth Without Violence*, A. A. Knopf, 1975.

11 S Grof, *LSD Psychotherapy*, Hunter House Inc Publishers, Ponoma CA., 1985.

———, *The Adventure of Self Discovery*, State University of New York Press, 1988.

12 ibid.

13 W Reich, *Character Analysis*, Farrar, Straus & Giroux, 1949.

———, *The Function of the Orgasm*, Meridan, 1970.

14 S Grof, *The Adventure of Self Discovery*, State University of New York Press, 1988, p 167.

15 P Hamel, *Through Music to the Self*, Element, 1978.

Helen Bonny and Savary, *Music and Your Mind*, Harper & Row, 1973.

16 C Grof, *The Thirst for Wholeness*, HarperCollins, 1993, p 15-16.

17 T Sparks, *The Wide Open Door: The Twelve Steps, Spiritual Tradition and the New Psychology*, Hazeldon, 1993.

18 S Grof, The Adventure of Self Discovery, State University of New York Press, Albany, 1988, p196-199.

19 Herbert Benson, *The Relaxation Response*, Collins, 1975.

Joan Borysenko, *Minding the Body, Mending the Mind*, Addison Wesley, 1987.

20 Kylea Taylor, *The Breathwork Experience: Exploration and Healing in Nonordinary States of Consciousness*, Hanford Mead Publishers, 1994.

Further Reading

Achterberg, J., *Imagery in Healing: Shamanism and Modern Medicine*, Shambhala, 1985.

Benson, Herbert, *The Relaxation Response*, Collins, 1975.

Boadella, D., *Lifestreams: An Introduction to Biosynthesis*, Routledge& Kegan Paul, 1987.

Bonny, H and Savary, *Music and Your Mind*, Harper & Row, 1973.

Borysenko, Joan, *Minding the Body, Mending the Mind*, Addison Wesley, 1987.

Bragdon, Emma, *The Call of Spiritual Emergence*, Harper & Row, 1990.

Bremner, J.; Hillin, A., *Sexuality, Young People and Care*, Russel House Publishing Ltd, 1994.

Campbell, Joseph, *Hero with a Thousand Faces*, World Publishing Co., 1970.

———, *Myths to Live By*, Viking Penguin Inc., 1972.

Capra, Fritjof, *The Tao of Physics*, Shambala Publications, 1975.

———, *The Turning Point*, Simon & Schuster, 1982.

Conger, J., *Jung and Reich: The Body as Shadow*, North Atlantic Books, 1988.

Eliade, M., *Shamanism: Archaic Techniques of Ecstacy*, Pantheon, 1964.

Grof, Christina, *The Thirst for Wholeness*, HarperCollins, 1993.

———; Grof, S., *The Stormy Search for the Self*, Jeremy P. Tarcher, 1990.

———, ———, *Beyond Death: The Gates of Consciousness*, Thames & Hudson, 1980.

———, ———, (eds), *Spiritual Emergency*, Jeremy P. Tarcher Inc, 1989.

Grof, Stan, *The Holotropic Mind*, Harper, 1992.

———, *The Adventure of Self Discovery*, State University of New York Press, 1988.

———, *LSD Psychotherapy*, Hunter House Inc Publishers, 1985.

———, (ed), *Ancient Wisdom and Modern Science*, State University of New York Press, 1984.

———; Halifax, Joan, *The Human Encounter with Death*, E. P. Dutton, 1977.

Hamel, P., *Through Music to the Self*, Element, 1978.

Harner, M., *The Way of the Shaman*, Bantam, 1980.

Jung, C., *Memories, Dreams, Reflections*, Random House, 1989.

———, *The Archetypes and the Collective Unconscious*, Routledge, 1990.

———, *Man and His Symbols*, Arkana, 1964.

Kornfield, J., *The Path with Heart: A Guide Through the Perils and Promises of the Spiritual Life*, Bantam, 1993.

Kübler-Ross, E., *Death -The Final Stage of Growth*, Prentice Hall International Inc, 1975.

Kurtz, R., *Body-Centered Psychotherapy: The Hakomi Method*, LifeRhythm, 1990.

———; Prestera, H., *The Body Reveals*, Harper & Row, 1976.

Leboyer, F., *Birth Without Violence*, A A Knopf, 1975.

Le Shan, L., *The Medium, The Mystic and the Physicist*, Ballantine Books, 1975.

———, *You Can Fight for Your Life: Emotional Factors in the Causation of Cancer*, Evans, 1977.

Lowen, A., *Bioenergetics*, Penguin, 1976.

Maslow, A., *Towards a Psychology of Being*, Van Nostrand Reinhold, 1968.

Moody, R., *Life after Life,* Mockingbird Books, 1975.

———, *Reflections on Life After Life*, Mockingbird Books, Atlanta GA, 1977.

Oyle, I., *Time Space and the Mind*, Celestial Arts, 1976.

Rank, O., *The Trauma of Birth*, Hancourt Brace, 1929.

Reich, W., *Character Analysis*, Farrar, Straus & Giroux, 1949.

———, *The Function of the Orgasm*, Meridan, 1970.

Schaef, A., *When Society Becomes an Addict*, Harper & Row, 1987.

———; Fassel, D., *The Addictive Organisation*, Harper & Row Publishers Inc., 1988.

Sheldrake, R., *A New Science of Life*, Grafton Books, 1983.

———, *Seven Experiments That Could Change the World*, Fourth Estate Ltd, 1994.

Sparks, T., *The Wide Open Door: The Twelve Steps, Spiritual Tradition and the New Psychology*, Hazeldon, 1993.

Tart, C., *Out of Body Experiences, in Psychic Explorations* (E. Mitchel and J White, eds.), Putnam, 1974.

Taylor, Kylea, *The Breathwork Experience: Exploration and Healing in Nonordinary States of Consciousness*, Hanford Mead Publishers, 1994.

Vaughan, F., *The Inward Arc: Healing and Wholeness in Psychotherapy and Spirituality*, Shambala, 1985.

Walsh, R & Vaughan, F., *Beyond Ego: Transpersonal Dimensions in Psychology*, J P Tarcher, 1980.

Resources

Rosie Manton
Lower Small Farm
Pecket Well
Hebden Bridge
W. Yorks, HX7 8RF
Tel. 01422 843501

*(There are currently only a handful of certified facilitators in the UK.
Details of workshops in England can be obtained from Rosie Manton)*

Transpersonal Psychotherapy Group
59 Waterloo Lane
Dublin 4
Ireland
Tel. (353 1) 668 5282

*(Details of workshops in Ireland can be obtained
from this organisation)*

Grof Transpersonal Training
20 Sunnyside Avenue
A-314, Mill Valley
CA 94941, USA
Tel. (415) 383-8779
Fax (415) 383-0965

*(This organisation will supply details of certified facilitators worldwide
and details of its training programme)*

Spiritual Emergence Network (SEN)
c/o Institute for Transpersonal Psychology
250 Oak Grove Avenue
Menlo Park, CA, 94025
USA

*(SEN provides information on therapists who
recognise this phenomenon, conferences and a newsletter)*

Homoeopathy
by Eva Tombs-Heirman

The highest ideal of therapy is to restore health rapidly, gently, permanently; to remove and destroy the whole disease in the shortest, surest, least harmful way, according to clearly comprehensible principles.

— Samuel Hahnemann

This is the guideline given by Samuel Hahnemann, the father of homoeopathy. Hahnemann (1755–1843) was a medical doctor, chemist and linguist in Meissen, Germany. He discovered, quite by chance, while translating a Scottish medical book, that ingesting small quantities of chincona bark (the herb used at that time for treating malaria) was making him suffer the symptoms of malaria. This spurred him to do further research and with the help of his family, his colleagues, his students and his patients, he found out that it was possible to overcome the symptoms of malaria using smaller and smaller doses of chincona bark. He discovered that it was not necessary to use the crude tincture but that chincona bark extract worked even better when it was highly dilute. This had the added advantage of preventing the side effects caused by the original medicine. This was the beginning of a life's work which created a comprehensive system of medicine with its own unique concepts and principles.

In 1810 Hahnemann published *The Organon* which is still today regarded as the major textbook for classical homoeopathy. It is a tribute to a man who has significantly influenced health care in the last 200 years.

The Principles of Homoeopathy

The Law of Similars

The basic law of homoeopathy is 'let like be cured with like' (similia similibus curentur). A substance which can cause certain symptoms can also cure them. For instance coffee in homoeopathic preparation can be used to treat insomnia.

Provings

Hahnemann set out a system of establishing 'symptom pictures' of remedies. He did this by testing medicinal substances on healthy individuals and meticulously collating the results. These tests are called 'provings'.

Provings can also occur accidentally when a substance is ingested and causes symptoms. A whole range of poisonous substances are well documented through their toxicology records, for example foxglove, snake venom, belladonna.

New provings are undertaken by homoeopaths all over the world in the form of double-blind trials. The resulting symptoms on all levels – physical, emotional and mental are recorded for each participant and collated to formulate the emerging symptom picture. New substances are continuously tested and listed in the *materia medica* books. New remedies include pollutants, vaccines and synthetic substances.

Materia Medica

All proven remedies are listed in the materia medica, giving all the details of the symptom picture as discovered in the provings. Clinical experience over the years will refine the picture and add symptoms which were cured by the remedy in many different cases.

Repertory

The repertory is an A – Z of all symptoms mentioned in the materia medica. It makes possible cross-referencing of the symptom and indicated remedies, and is therefore an important tool for homoeopaths when prescribing a remedy. Nowadays many homoeopaths work with computer programmes of these repertories to determine the appropriate remedy for their patient. Even though this makes the work much easier it cannot replace the clinical skill, intuition, creativity and often 'detective work' of the homoeopath. Choosing the correct remedy lies in the choice and prioritising of the presenting symptoms and the personality of the patient.

Single Remedy

Complex Homoeopathy

The classical homoeopath will only give one remedy at a time. If several remedies were to be given together, the vital force of the patient might become overstimulated and the therapy would thereby be doing the patient a disservice in the long run. The prescribing of multiple remedies (as in complex homoeopathy) is in some ways much easier – one of the remedies in the mixture is likely to be correct. But it is an unnecessarily crude method, which does not leave the person's immune system stronger and more resistant to disease.

Minimum Dose

It is a principle of homoeopathy to interfere as little as possible with the natural attempts of the body's own healing powers. Hence the principle of the minimum dose. This implies that the minimum amount of medicine necessary to stimulate a cure is the right amount.

Hahnemann's main reason for reducing the concentration of the substances he used as medicines was to reduce the poisoning effects of the drugs. During his research, he discovered that the more work he did on making the remedies more dilute, the more potent the remedies became as a cure. This is the process known as potentisation: a step-by-step process of dilution and succussion.

Potency

Hahnemann potentised all his remedies by hand. If a substance was water soluble he would dissolve it in water, and shake it a set number of times; then he would bang the vial hard on his leather bible. He would add more water to a small measured amount of this liquid and go through this process again. He would continue with this process until he had attained the desired dilution and potency.

Nowadays homoeopathic pharmacies use machines to do this work, although many of the lower potencies, up to 30c, are still made by hand.

Methods for diluting the 'mother tincture' vary in different countries. The mother tincture is arrived at by steeping the substance (plant, mineral, animal or synthetic in origin) in alcohol or water for a period of time and then straining it. In the case of an insoluble substance the remedy is made by grinding the starting substance in a mortar and pestle with sugar or milk.

The number of the homoeopathic remedy reflects the number of times it has been diluted. The letter, for example X, C, D, CH, refer to the proportions of the dilution as in Nat Mur 6X.

In the decimal scale, 9 parts of alcohol are mixed with 1 part of mother tincture and shaken vigorously. In the centesimal scale, 99 parts of alcohol are used for every 1 part of mother tincture.

The Whole Person

Presenting symptoms are only one aspect of the whole picture of the patient. It is important for the homoeopath to get as much information as possible about the patient on all levels (physical, emotional, spiritual).

Symptoms-oriented prescribing is only indicated in first aid situations. It is always preferable to 'take the case' and find the remedy which matches the whole patient – to be able to arrive at 'the similimum'. Therefore the first consultation with a homoeopath is often likened to an autobiography. It takes into consideration the chronological development from childhood, many different aspects of the patient's life seemingly quite unrelated to the presenting problem, as well as a detailed description of the presenting problem, including any factors which may aggravate or alleviate the symptoms.

Constitution and Susceptibility

All people are different. Some have a strong constitution from birth and retain it throughout their lives. Others weaken markedly for various reasons as time goes on. Serious shocks or periods of mental, emotional or physical strain can take their toll on people's general health and well-being, making them more susceptible to disease.

Classical homoeopaths will often focus on the underlying constitution rather than the presenting problems. This is a powerful way of healing and strengthening the damaged immune system and thereby decreasing susceptibility to disease.

Vital Force

The concept of the vital force (or life energy) is crucial in homoeopathy. The organism is seen as a self-regulating system with innate mechanisms to maintain equilibrium (homoeostasis) and compensate for stresses or imbalances. The vital force may produce symptoms in the effort to counteract an imbalance – for instance a fever to fight an infection. The homoeopathic remedies will stimulate the vital force and therefore support the body's self-healing mechanism.

Acute and Chronic Diseases

Naturopathy
Herbalism
Aromatherapy

Acute disease is characterised by three stages: incubation, acute phase and convalescence. Many minor ailments and childhood illnesses fall in this category. In most cases, acute episodes can quite correctly be called a 'healing crisis', and the best thing to do is to let it happen. This is where conscientious nursing care becomes essential. The traditional home remedies are of great value in looking after the patient with an acute illness. Herbal teas, poultices, natural oils and low potency homoeopathic remedies are all useful and of comfort to the patient. In the busy world of instant cure and no days off work, this whole area of health care is often overlooked. Acute illnesses are aborted; fevers are suppressed; headaches are removed. The cumulative effect of all this suppression may well be chronic ill health. A classical homoeopath will try to help patients to bear their acute ailments with the least amount of suffering and the most positive effect for the health and well-being of their vital force.

Chronic disease is more deep-seated. It develops over time, often unnoticed for an extended period and leads eventually to a general deterioration of health. While orthodox medicine treats the presenting symptoms to alleviate suffering, homoeopathy will encourage a process of healing that sometimes may bring to the surface illnesses which had been suppressed in the past. Sometimes it may be necessary for patients to go through profound changes in their lives. Such change can be assisted and supported through the homoeopathic process.

The Laws of Cure

Constantine Hering, the father of American homoeopathy, described the process of cure, as he observed it in many years of practice, as progressing in a specific way:

◆ *from the inside out*: from the deepest parts of the body to the surface. This often means that a threatening situation progresses to a less dangerous symptom, for example asthma symptoms subside and eczema erupts.

◆ *from the top down*: symptoms clear from the head downwards. This is particularly easy to observe in the case of eczema, where the skin rash will 'drop off' the body.

◆ *from the present to the past*: healing will progress in reverse chronological order. As the presenting symptom is cured older layers of disease may reappear and be healed as well.

The Practice of Homoeopathy

Often people come to a homoeopath because they have tried conventional medicine and have not been able to find the help they wanted.

The First Consultation

The homoeopath takes a full and detailed case history, noticing all indications as to the patient's state of mind and being. Some patients find it easy to speak about themselves, while with others, the information has to be elicited with sensitivity and perseverance. Some people have what seem to be trivial symptoms which cause them tremendous trouble, while others live with a high degree of pain and yet are able to cope.

Homoeopaths are renowned for asking seemingly odd questions, such as: 'Do you perspire on the exposed parts of your body, or under your clothes?' or 'Does sympathy annoy you or comfort you?' or 'Are your symptoms better or worse in wet weather?' The answers to these questions can give the practitioner the clue required in order to select the right remedy. The art in homoeopathy is in the listening. In addition, the homoeopath may ask to touch the person's hand, to see if it is cold or warm, damp or dry, soft or hard. There are many subtle signs that can be observed: for instance colour, thickness and quality of hair, and tone, pitch and volume of voice. The aim is to get an accurate, objective picture of the patient's state of health. The practitioner will then look for a remedy picture that matches the person's whole picture. When clear about the remedy, they will give the patient the homoeopathic remedy directly. A follow-up appointment is necessary to review the effects of the remedy.

Most homoeopaths also make themselves available for consultation by telephone, when they can do acute prescribing for their patients; offer advice to midwives on all types of problems concerning their mothers and babies; are available for long-standing patients who are presenting a new symptom; or advise travellers who want information on remedies to replace vaccinations or malaria tablets. There are many situations that do not require the full consultation and classical case taking. Most homoeopaths are willing and able to be flexible.

Follow-up Consultations

The frequency of return visits depends entirely on the case in question. If the case is classically chronic, the second visit will usually occur between six weeks and two months after the initial consultation. If the remedy has worked well, it is quite possible that nothing more will be given at the second visit. If the patient improved but the improvement didn't hold, the same remedy may be prescribed again, perhaps in a higher potency. If improvement did not occur as expected, perhaps a different remedy is called for.

During an acute illness patients often need a lot of support, and a daily or weekly visit is appropriate. The remedy picture can change rapidly, and patients need to be in frequent contact, so they can be given the appropriate remedies and advice. Frequent contact by telephone, sometimes several times a day, is crucial in such situations.

Combining Homoeopathy with Other Therapies

Massage
Flower Essences

In general, it is not advised for a patient receiving homoeopathy to have other treatments at the same time, unless specifically recommended by the practitioner. Mixing therapies can confuse the symptom picture. It has been known for a massage or a Bach flower remedy to completely reverse or halt progress when combined unadvisedly. However, there are some cases where adjunct treatment is beneficial to the overall progression towards better health, but it is important to discuss this with the practitioner before taking any action.

Other Uses of Homoeopathy

Homoeopathy is also used on a large scale in the biodynamic agricultural movement because it increases resistance to disease and improves the quality of the crop and the structure of the soil. It is used very successfully with animals.

Using Homoeopathy for Self-Help

As first aid, homoeopathy is invaluable. Many homoeopaths run first aid classes at adult education centres or at other venues. For some people such a class gives a tremendous boost of confidence, enabling a degree of self-help which frees the person and their family from unnecessary medical drugs, such as antibiotics or painkillers. While it is important not to be negligent and to keep a sensible perspective on what is treatable at home by an unqualified person, most of the time the parent or friend knows when medical or professional help is required. The patient can be treated homoeopathically in the interim.

When home prescribing it is advised to use only the lower potencies, those 30C and below. A remedy should not be repeated for longer than three days. If there is no improvement in that time, either the wrong remedy is being used, or the case is too complicated for home treatment. Taking a homoeopathic remedy repeatedly over a long period of time constitutes a proving, that is, the patient will start to show the symptoms of the remedy rather than of the illness. In an acute situation relief is often felt immediately, in which case the remedy should not be repeated. Often only one tablet suffices. First aid treatment will not cure chronic illness, but pain and distress can be alleviated with homoeopathic remedies.

Research

All these claims have been thoroughly tested and researched. Many research papers are published and are readily available.

The homoeopathic hospitals in Britain also carry out their own research. The Glasgow Homoeopathic Hospital published a paper in 1994 comparing homoeopathic remedies with orthodox treatment, and placebo and no treatment, a double-blind trial. They were researching treatments for asthma. Homoeopathic treatment did better in these trials than the three others.[1]

Training

Fully qualified professional homoeopaths are usually graduates of colleges of homoeopathy which have been approved by the Society of Homoeopaths. They will have passed the tests and criteria as regards competence and suitability, and are bound by a code of ethics laid down by the society. The study of homoeopathy in these colleges lasts a minimum of four years. Successful students earns a licence to practise. At first licentiate homoeopaths practise under the supervision of an experienced homoeopath. After a period of time and a set number of cases, they can then apply for registration with the society. This second phase usually takes about two years. If they are successful, they can then write the letters RSHom. after their name and call themselves a registered homoeopath.

Case Study

Fiona was 39 when she first came for a consultation, suffering from recurrent anaemia. This problem had persisted for several years, and she was regularly prescribed ferrous sulphate by her GP, which worked for a while but did not cure the problem.

She always lost a great deal of blood during her periods, which had started when she was eleven. They were heavy, long (8-9 days) and painful. The periods started slowly, the flow increasing until it was very heavy around the fifth day. By this time she felt so tired that she described the feeling as: 'my legs hardly hold me up'. She suffered quite a lot of premenstrual symptoms as well, such as tightness in the breasts, bad temper and headaches. She had undergone gynaecological investigations, which revealed fibroids. Her GP put her on progesterone, which she was taking from day 15-25. She also had a history of sinus pain. The sinuses have been called the womb of the head as, empirically, homoeopathic remedies that have a special action on the womb are often the same remedies that support the sinuses.

Fiona slept well. She seemed a very controlled person. She was well presented but utterly devoid of any colour. She looked exhausted and drained. Her hair was lank and colourless, although neat and tidy from the hairdresser. She wore quite a bit of make-up which didn't seem to make her look any more colourful. She gave me all information easily and freely.

She has two children, a girl of 13 and a boy aged 9. They were both born by caesarean section and she was unable to breast-feed either of them. She has a difficult relationship with her daughter. They have a lot of arguments; sometimes they don't speak to each other for days. These difficulties, which are beyond the normal problems one would expect with a thirteen year old, often indicate a problem in the mother/daughter relationship, common in patients with menstrual or womb problems.

Asked about the relationship with her own mother, it was revealed that she left home (a small industrial town) as soon as she left school and has never been back, having broken off all relations with her mother. She was quite hard on her mother, who she felt didn't understand her and didn't appreciate her talents: 'She was only a housewife.' From the way she talked it became clear that this was the centre of the case.

In contrast to her conventional appearance, her profession was surprising. She worked as a singer/songwriter and had a business writing and producing musicals. She was successful and worked hard. When she came for the first time, she was in charge of a large production of a musical she had written, including the rehearsing, the staging and costumes. She employed a musician to help her with the transposing of music and to generally assist her, but he always let her down and she often had to redo his work.

She was married to an accountant. She talked quite a bit about her frustration in the marriage. She found it difficult to put up with his lack of emotion and his unresponsiveness. After the first consultation, the assessment was of a talented, artistic person who had become hardened in her personal striving for achievement and success.

Two tablets of Natrum Muriaticum 10M were prescribed and she was advised to take a mineral complex daily as a food supplement. It is interesting to note that a hardening or a mineralisation on the emotional level seemed to have caused a demineralisation in the body as indicated by the limp hair, the pastiness of her skin, the general weakness and exhaustion. She mentioned she was on a low fat diet because she was health conscious. She seemed thin on the top part of her body but heavier on the thighs; this is the typical weight distribution associated with the remedy Natrum Muriaticum. On a subtle energy level, there was not enough light in her body. The plant world is filled with living light and some of it can be absorbed by eating vegetables and fruits; therefore she should follow a diet rich in raw vegetables. It was suggested she stop taking the progesterone and the iron as they would interfere with the healing process. Taking patients off medication should only be done in co-operation with the prescribing doctor, but in this case there was no reason to stay on them as there was no danger to her health in stopping them.

Eight weeks later, at the second consultation, she reported that her period had come after 25 days. It started slowly and then became heavy, as before. But she was not so totally exhausted during the period this time. She felt it was more under control and she could still function. Her piles (which she hadn't mentioned before) were not bothering her. She had difficulty motivating herself. She had sacked her assistant. She had made contact with her mother and their relationship was improving. She was much more relaxed. She complained of a metallic taste in her mouth.

Nat Mur was indicated but in a higher potency, 50M, 1 tablet.

Eight weeks later the third consultation took place. The previous two periods had been fine. The period she had just finished was exhausting. She had a cold with a lot of catarrh. She was feeling 'emotionally heavy'. She had been working very hard on the musical, and had eaten a lot of things 'she shouldn't have', coffee and chocolate bars, to keep her going. The metallic taste in her mouth was gone. Her energy and motivation were high. Her relationship with her mother was *improving: they were seeing each other and communicating. She had a confrontation with her husband, which he found quite shocking. It changed the relationship, but she felt it to be 'more on an even and honest footing'. The most striking point about this third consultation was the change in her appearance. She had a short haircut and her clothes were completely different – bright red, orange and green. She now looked like the artist that she was.*

No remedy was prescribed. The previous remedy was clearly working, requiring more time to bring its effects to the fullest.

Three months later, she reported that her periods were fluctuating, sometimes coming too early. She had some flooding for two to three days. The flow was partly pale and partly clotted. Professionally things were going very well. She had a lot of energy. She had no recurrent anaemia. Her sinuses were bothering her a lot. It felt much better for fresh air. She often felt bloated, like bursting.

Sabina 30 was given, three tablets in one day, only once. Also garlic capsules were advised, to support the clearing out of the sinuses.

The fifth consultation took place two months later. Her periods had settled and were now fine and her legs no longer felt weak during her period. She usually had cold hands but they could get very hot sometimes too. She had continuing sinus problems with tension headaches. She was eating well. She was feeling very creative and learning how to communicate with her daughter, and learning to appreciate her good qualities.

Sepia 30 was prescribed, to be taken three times in one day only.

She was fine for a whole year after this. A year following the last consultation she came back for one visit because she was feeling a little like she did previously. One dose of Sepia was given and she has been fine since.

Biography

Eva Tombs-Heirman, RSHom, was born in Holland and attended the Rudolf Steiner School in the Hague, later studying eurythmy. She lived in the United States, from 1962 till 1972 where she studied medical sciences at the University of Chicago. In 1972 she came to live in Scotland where she was a restaurateur for a few years before spending two years sailing the oceans of the world on a small yacht. For a while she ran a dress design business, completed a science course with the Open University, got married and had three children.

In 1982 she discovered the homoeopathy college in Newcastle. She graduated from the college in 1986 by which time she had also given birth to three more children. Since then she has worked as a classical homoeopath in Edinburgh, Scotland, with a specific interest in mothers and babies.

References

1   David Reilly et al., *Is Evidence for Homoeopathy reproducible,* Lancet, 1994; 334 (Dec 10): 1601-6.

Further Reading

Coulter, Harris, *Divided Legacy: A History of the Schism in Medical thought,* North Atlantic Books, 1973.

———, *Homoeopathic Science and Modern Medicine: The Physics of Healing with Microdoses,* North Atlantic Books, 1987.

Hahneman, S., *The Organon of Medicine,* Victor Gollancz, 1983.

Lockie, A & Geddes N., *The Complete Guide to Homoeopathy,* Southern Book Pub, 1995.

O'Neill, V A, *Overview of the literature on homoeopathy*, Complementary Medical Research, 1988; 3: 1, 55-69.

Reilly, David; Taylor, Morag, *The difficulty with homoeopathy: a brief review of principles, methods and research*, Complementary Medical Research, 1988; 3: 1, 70-8.

———, et al., *Is homoeopathy a placebo responce?*, Lancet, 1986; 2: 8512, 881-5.

Vithoulkas, George, *Homoeopathy: Medicine of the New Man*, Thorsons, 1985.

———, *The Science of Homoeopathy*, Thorsons, 1986.

Resources

The Society of Homoeopaths
2 Artizan Road
Northamptom NN1 4HU
Tel. 01604-21400

The Faculty of Homoeopathy
2 Powis Place
London WC1N 3HT
Tel. 0171-837 9469

The British Homoeopathic Dental Assocation
The Alternative Practice
2B Franklin Rd
Watford WD1 1QD
Tel. 01923-233 336

The British Association of Homoeopathic
Veterinary Surgeons
Alternative Veterinary Medicine Centre
Chinham House
Stanford-in-the-Vale
Faringdon
Oxon SN7 8NQ
Tel. 01367-710 324/710 475

The British Association of Homoeopathic Chiropodists
134 Montrose Ave
Edgware
Middx HA8 ODR
Tel. 0181-959 5421

Homoeopathic NHS Hospitals:

Cotham Hill
Cotham
Bristol BS6 6JU
Tel. 0117-973 1231

1000 Great Western Road
Glasgow G12 0NR
Tel. 0141-211 1600

Great Ormond Street
London WC1N 3HR
Tel. 0171-837 8833

Mossley Hill Hospital
Park Avenue
Liverpool L18 8BJ
Tel. 0151-733 4020

Church Road
Tunbridge Wells
Kent
Tel. 01892-542 977

Hypnotherapy

by Sue Washington

A developing child, before the age of ten, has little or no ability to rationalise. Experiences which are particularly difficult cannot be processed, so the body shuts off the feelings which arise at times like this, to protect the child. These incidents become 'frozen in time' and can cause, in adulthood, physical illness or emotional over-reaction to different stimuli and situations. The mind may recognise an over-reaction but at an emotional level little can be done to prevent it. Someone who has an anxiety state may know that it is illogical to be frightened of, say, going outside but may be gripped by such strong feelings that stepping over the threshold causes panic. When there is conflict between the intellect and emotion, these underlying issues should be resolved. Hypnotherapy is one way of working towards resolution.

There are many misconceptions about hypnotherapy. There is the popular image of the hypnotist as a man with a strong, magnetic personality and piercing eyes, endowed with a supernatural power to take over and dominate the minds of others. Once in the trance, the subject is seen as being reduced to a mere puppet with no will of their own, who obeys every command of the hypnotist without knowing what they are doing.

The concept of an individual having power over anyone in this way quite naturally engenders fear. The dread of losing consciousness is further emphasised by the medical, dental or stage hypnotist who uses the words 'sleep' and 'wake up' at the beginning and end of the hypnotic session. This suggestion of sleep is an unhappy legacy from a Dr James Braid who practised medicine in Manchester in the nineteenth century. In 1841, Dr Braid attended a demonstration of animal-magnetism (Mesmerism) which was conducted by a Swiss magnetist, La Fontaine. Braid started using magnetism on his patients with some degree of success. One day he realised that none of his patients was mesmerised but entered what he characterised as a therapeutic sleep. He took the Greek word 'hypnos' which means sleep, and called the therapy 'hypnotism'. For a time he was satisfied with this term until patients told him that they could hear every word that he was saying. They agreed that they were so physically relaxed that they might appear to be asleep, but mentally they were awake and alert. Braid tried to change the name, but it was too late. It had already entered the language.

Dr Braid was correct in his latter assessment, for no one goes to sleep when they are in hypnosis. Instead it can be defined as an altered state of awareness where the gates to the unconscious mind are open to a greater or lesser degree. There are three things necessary to enter the hypnotic state. The first is that the client/patient must have their attention fixed on something – this can be a spot on the ceiling, repetition of a word or action, the flickering of a candle flame or the classical image of the hypnotist's pendulum.

The second factor necessary is monotony. The client can be asked to focus on the internal repetition of a word, like 'calm', a standard meditation mantra. The hypnotist will usually talk in a monotonous voice.

The third requirement is hypoventilation, i.e. that after a few deep breaths, breathing becomes quite shallow.

Case History

Jane was in her sixties and had suffered irritable bowel syndrome. Much evidence about hypnosis says that it is useful in a case like this.[1] A large number of people have been helped by being taught to relax and feel their gut calming down. Often, though, the hypnotherapist needs to go deeper than this. With Jane I used a visualisation technique to ask her to remember a time in the past when things had been difficult for her. Her mind returned to a time when aged four she had to go into hospital for an adenoids operation. Jane came from a loving home and had never been away before. She remembered the nurse standing at the other side of the ward. Jane wanted to go to the toilet and attracted the nurse's attention. But the nurse came over and rebuked her for making a fuss, did not listen to her and did not let her say what she wanted. As a result, Jane dirtied herself and experienced guilt, shame, embarrassment, anxiety, resentment and confusion. During our session it was important that Jane was able to resolve some of these feelings by allowing her adult mind to process the memories. She did this excellently and over the next three or four visits made many adjustments. Within a short period of time she was able to lead as normal a life as anyone else.

The Practice of Hypnotherapy

During a hypnotherapy session the client is normally seen alone. Occasionally group sessions can be used for people who want help with relaxation, stopping smoking or losing weight.

During an individual session the therapist will spend quite a lot of time listening to the client about the problem they are presenting. The therapist may explain how they work, and their model of how the patient's mind works. At this session the therapist should also discuss how long they expect the treatment to last. A fairly usual working contract is six sessions. This ideally takes place weekly but once the patient has been seen a few times this interval can increase to fortnightly or even monthly sessions.

Hypnotherapy can be useful in many cases. Anything the World Health Organisation lists as being psychosomatic in origin may well be helped, for example migraine, asthma, some kinds of arthritis, ulcers, as well as anxiety states and phobias. It can also be helpful with pain relief, marital problems, sleep problems and so on, as well as smoking, slimming and self-esteem issues.

The writer of one of the most widely used textbooks in classical hypnosis techniques was the late Dr John Hartland. Hartland claims that 60% of patients attending psychiatric hospital as outpatients can be helped by using his technique of suggesting that the patient feels more calm, relaxed and confident.[2] The basis of this technique is still widely used today and a great deal of benefit can be gained by the use of gentle suggestion and relaxation techniques.

Visualisation

Visualisation is widely used by hypnotherapists. There are many forms this may take. The therapist may use words to ask the client to 'paint a picture' in their mind's eye of something relaxing, a beautiful garden or a beach. A development of this may be a visualisation to clear negativity, such as diving into a bottomless pit or into a deep ocean, to locate the deep pain, anxiety or whatever and bring it to the surface where it can be carried away by the wind, or evaporated into clouds, whatever seems appropriate to the client. This technique has been used to great effect by Gerry Jampolski,[3] who took a group of youngsters with inoperable brain tumours, and worked with them with a technique popularised by the Simontons.[4] Each child was asked to visualise the 'bad' cancer cells in their brains. Images were often space invaders or strangely shaped beings from imaginary planets. The youngsters used their own antidote to take bits off these invaders. It would seem that the body has a special healing substance which is activated by such exercises, called a beta-endorphine, which lies dormant in the dorsal horn of the spinal column. It seems that by visually focusing on the destruction of the negative forces within, this innate healing mechanism is activated and used to destroy the inoperable brain tumours. The children all lived much longer than had been predicted.

In my own practice I have seen remarkable results from applying self-healing visualisations. For instance a woman with deep joint inflammation reduced her pain level so much in just one session that she was able to halve her intake of anti-inflammatory drugs.

Cautions

If the presenting symptom is a message from a larger problem then the hypnotherapist will not benefit the patient by removing the messenger. If this does happen, it has been known for patients to develop another illness, as the unconscious mind struggles to find another symptom to replace the habitual one. The underlying issues of conflict need to be resolved before the hypnotic session may be given with great benefit, to help the client be more calm and relaxed by using direct suggestion into the unconscious mind.

Hypnosis cannot be used as a truth drug. I regularly receive calls from anxious wives or husbands fearing their spouses are having an affair and wanting me to hypnotise them to find out the truth. Hypnosis cannot be used in this way. The client/patient can lie just as successfully under hypnosis as at any other time.

In the past few years there has been controversy over the subject of false memory syndrome. This purports that some patients have been encouraged to think untrue things about their past.[5] While not commenting on individual cases, I personally support the view that it is possible for false traumas to be 'uncovered' by a therapist or counsellor. Regular supervision, where the practitioner discusses cases with other colleagues, can prevent them from falling into this trap.

Multidisciplinary Co-operation

A hypnotic state can be achieved spontaneously. Children sitting in front of a school blackboard may drift off into a 'daydream'. In other situations, it can have potentially serious consequences, as for example when driving, as the motorist listens to the monotonous sound of his car engine and wheels.

Training

Hypnotherapy is, as yet, unregulated, which will hopefully change within the next few years. Until then, anyone may call him or herself a hypnotherapist. However, there are good training courses available, and the Institute for Complementary Medicine has a list of hypnotherapy training organisations. The training should include communication skills, skills using hypnotic techniques and psychodynamics. The National Council of Psychotherapists also has a hypnotherapy register. One of the best ways of finding a good hypnotherapist is by personal recommendation.

Research

The Hypnotherapy Unit of the Southern Manchester University Hospital has worked with irritable bowel syndrome for many years. Their research includes patients who suffer from debilitating symptoms – approximately 25% were permanently off work because of their gastro-intestinal condition. The quality of life of these patients has been greatly reduced. For the last twelve years researchers have demonstrated the beneficial effect of hypnotherapy in the treatment of IBS, which was sustained over long periods of time and enabled patients to return to work.[6]

Case History

Ann was a woman in her mid-forties with two grown up children and one teenager. Her presenting complaint was that she wasn't really enjoying her sex life. From the waist down she told me her body felt 'black'. Long since divorced, she lived with a partner, relatively happily, in Scotland.

Ann had a strong reaction when we used the 'child within' technique. I asked her to remember a time when something happened to her as a younger person that was difficult to handle. It took her only a second or two to have a memory of being eleven years old. She was asleep in bed with her two younger brothers. The baby-sitters, two older children, were downstairs. Mother, an alcoholic, and father had gone out for a drink. Unbeknown to Ann, their two caretakers had found a bottle of alcohol, drunk it and passed out. The children upstairs were unprotected.

Ann awoke with a man's hands around her throat. She could only gurgle. He was kneeling on her middle and groping her private parts. She could not understand why the baby-sitters did not hear the struggle from downstairs and come up. Her arms were free and she woke her brothers. The man ran away. They were able to identify him later to the police and he was given a prison term for attempted murder. However, since that time Ann felt dead and black from the waist down. During our session she was able to heal her feelings which had been locked inside, and comfort this smaller child who had been unprotected in a horrific situation. After that one session, she reported that she was 50% better. She had also lost a stone in weight.

A Hypnotherapy Technique – The Magic Garden

The following technique can be used in a session, or recorded onto a cassette and played whenever relaxation is required:

'Close your eyes and picture a garden. Imagine an English country garden, with a high wall round it, trees and creepers growing over the wall, tall flowers in front of it in a border, smaller flowers in the middle and the smallest flowers at the front of the border and then at your feet, tiny flowers in the grass, packed closely together. Feel the warmth of the sun on your head and on your back and smell the sweet scent of flowers. The sun is shining, the sky is as blue as blue can be and all around is an atmosphere of peace and calm and tranquillity.

There are insects, too; little buzzing things, big fat bees, pretty butterflies, and if you're very lucky maybe a dragonfly, translucent wings and beautiful iridescent body. Birds are twittering about the garden with their coloured plumage and sweet songs... lawns, little paths, flowering shrubs, and somewhere water is tumbling...

Now go to the end of the garden where the tall trees are. Tied to the tree with a big stout rope is a big lighter-than-air balloon floating in the air, and swinging from the bottom of it a large empty box hovering about six inches above the ground. It's a very special box. It can contain things that you want rid of. Now look inside yourself and see if there's anything there you'd rather be without. You don't have to say what it is, but if there's anything in there you would be better off without just NOD to let me know... (wait for a nod or pause)... fine. Take it, and push it out into the box and nod to tell me when you've done it... (wait for a nod). (Repeat until there is nothing left. Wait for patient's acknowledgement that they have finished.)

Fine. Next untie the thick rope that holds down the balloon. The balloon will lift the box up, higher and higher, higher and higher. Higher and higher until it gets to the top of the tallest tree. Do you see that? Lighter and lighter and higher and higher until it is as small as the nail on your little finger, do you see that?... Lighter and lighter and higher and higher until it disappears in a dot and the sky is clear. Eventually the balloon will burn up in the atmosphere and the contents of your box will be left in (for example Arizona). (Arizona) has been here for millions of years and your few things will not hurt it, but leaving them (in Arizona) will make you feel better.

Return to the flower garden and find yourself somewhere pleasant and peaceful to be... just sit, or lie, and allow the space inside yourself where the unwanted stuff has left, to fill up with the pleasant smells, sounds and sensations of the magic garden.

In a moment I'm going to count from 1-5 and say, "Open your eyes" and you will open your eyes feeling wonderful on all levels.'

Biography

Sue Washington MSc, BA, Cert Ed, DHP, MCAP, BRCP (H), has worked in the field of hypno/psychotherapy for 28 years and is the principal of Centre Training School of Hypnotherapy and Psychotherapy which trains in various locations throughout the United Kingdom. In 1984 she founded and ran Liverpool Holistic Health Centre. Sue has spent time working in the pain management unit at Liverpool's Walton Hospital. She has recently completed a master's degree from Liverpool University. She and her husband live with a teenage son and three cats. Her main hobby is gardening.

References

1   L A Houghton; D Heyman; P J Whorwell, *Symptomatology, quality of life and economic features of irritable bowel syndrome and the effect of hypnotherapy*, Alimentary Pharmacology and Therapeutics, 1996; 10: 91-5.

2   J Hartland, *Medical and Dental Hypnosis*, Ballière Tindall, 1971.

3   G Jampolski, *Love is Letting Go of Fear*, Celestial Arts, 1979.

4   O C Simonton; S Simonton; J Creighton, *Getting well again*, JP Tarcher, 1978.

5   Goldstein, Eleanor; Farmer, Kevin, *True Stories of False Memories*, SIRS, Florida, 1993.

6   P J Whorwell; A Prior; EB Faragher, *Controlled trial of hypnotherapy in the treatment of severe refractory irritable bowel syndrome*, Lancet, 1984; II: 1232-1234.

    P J Whorwell; A Prior; S M Colgan, *Hypnotherapy in severe irritable bowel syndrome: further experience*, Gut, 1987; 28: 423-425.

    L A Houghton; D Heyman; P J Whorwell, *Symptomatology, quality of life and economic features of irritable bowel syndrome and the effect of hypnotherapy*, Alimentary Pharmacology and Therapeutics, 1996; 10: 91-5.

Further Reading

Colgan S M.; Faragher E B.; Whorwell P J., *A controlled trial of hypnotherapy in relapse prevention of duodenal ulceration*, Lancet, 1988; 1: 1299-1300.

Cotanch, P.; Hockenbury, M.; Herman, S., *Self-hypnosis as antiemetic therapy in children receiving chemotherapy*, Oncology Nursing Forum, 1985; 12: 4, 41-6.

Elman, Dave, *Hypnotherapy*, Westwood Publ., 1984.

Freeman, R M et al., *Randomised trial of self-hypnosis for analgesia in labour*, BMJ, 1986; 292: 657-8.

Haley, Jay, *Uncommon Therapy*, WW Norton, 1987.

Hartland J, *Medical and Dental Hypnosis*, Ballière Tindall, 1971.

Jampolski, G G, *Love is Letting Go of Fear*, Celestial Arts, 1979.

Lever, R., *Hypnotherapy for Everyone*, Penguin, 1988.

Markham, U., *Hypnosis*, Macdonald Optima, 1987.

————, *Hypnosis Regression Therapy*, Piatkus, 1991.

Prior A, Colgan S M, Whorwell P J., *Changes in Rectal Sensitivity Following Hypnotherapy for Irritable Bowel Syndrome*, Gut, 1990; 31: 896-898.

Read, N W (ed), *Irritable Bowel Syndrome*, Blackwell Scientific Publications, 1991.

Shine, Betty, *Mind to Mind*, Corgi, 1990.

Walker, Leslie, *Hypnosis with cancer patients*, Am J Prevent Psychiatry & Neuro, 1992; 3: 3, 42-9.

Whorwell P J., *Hypnosis and the Gastrointestinal System*, British Journal of Hospital Medicine, 1991; 45: 27-29.

Whorwell P J.; Houghton L A; Taylor F.; Maxton D G., *Physiological effects of emotion: assessment via hypnosis*, Lancet, 1992; 2: 69-72.

Young, P., *Personal Change Through Self-Hypnosis*, Angus and Robertson, 1987.

Resources

Association of Professional Therapists (APT)
57 The Spinney
Sidcup
Kent DA14 5NE
Tel. 0181- 308 0249

Association of Qualified Curative Hypnotherapists
16 Station Road
Cheadle Hulme
Cheshire SK8 5AE

British Hypnotherapy Association
67 Upper Berkeley Street
London W1H 7DH
Tel. 0171- 723 4443

British Society of Clinical Hypnotherapists
229a Sussex Gardens
Lancaster Gate
London W2 2RL
Tel. 0171- 402 9037

British Society of Medical and Dental Hypnosis
17 Keppel View Road
Kimberworth
Rotherham
South Yorks S61 2AR
Tel. 01709-554 5580

Central Register of Advanced Hypnotherapists (CRAH)
28 Finsbury Park Road
London N4 2JX

Corporation of Advanced Hypnotherapy
P O Box 70
Southport PR8 3JB
Tel. 01704-576 285

Register of Approved Gastro-intestinal Psychotherapists and Hypnotherapists
Holistic Resources
Cribden House
Rossendale General Hospital
Rossendale
Lancs BB4 6NE
Tel. 01706-240 080

National Council of Psychotherapists and Hypnotherapy Register
24 Rickmansworth Road
Watford
Herts WD1 7HT
Tel. 01923-227 772

Standing Committee for Hypnotherapy
Regent's College
Inner Circle
London NW1 4NS
Tel. 0171-486 0141

The National College of Hypnosis and Psychotherapy
12 Cross Street
Nelson
Lancs BB9 7EN
Tel. 01282-699 378

Iridology

by Peter and Angela Bradbury

The iris of the eye is a complex structure of the body providing a microchip of information. Whereas an ophthalmologist or medical doctor will look inside the eye to see the vascular system exposed on the retina, an iridologist will look at the external nerve endings which make up the iris. Over 2800 nerve fibres, all of which are connected to the brain via the hypothalamus, represent the conditions of all structures in the organism through an optic-neural reflex. Indeed, the iris fibres in the foetus are originally part of the brain and extend out on the iris stalk as development progresses.

Iridology is a safe, non-invasive and inexpensive method of diagnostic analysis. It can be integrated with both orthodox and complementary medicine. Iridology is a universal language, common to all living beings. It monitors the fluctuations between disease and health. As the bodily tissues become less inflamed or toxic, the iris registers the treatment response and the healing process.

Historical Background

Iridology is an old science. In 1000 BC the Chaldeans of Babylonia carved into stone slabs depictions of the iris and its optic-neuro reflex connections with the rest of the body. Records show that Hippocrates, Philostratus and the medical school of Saterno practised iridology. Later, seventeenth, eighteenth and nineteenth century records also contained notes and works on iris markings and their significance, such as Dr Philippus Meyens's book *Chiromatica Medica*, which was published in Dresden in 1670, and Christian Haertels's *De Oculo et Signo* (The Eye and its Signs), published in Göttingen in 1786. One of the better known early European charts linked with the modern revival of iridology was developed by Ignatz von Peczely (1826-1911), a Hungarian physician and surgeon. When he was eleven years old, he accidentally broke the leg of an owl which had instinctively fought against being captured by the boy. Master von Peczely noticed a black mark appearing in the owl's large iris as victor and captive glared at each other. Then, as von Peczely nursed the owl back to recovery, and during the years of their continued, more voluntary friendship, he noticed and correlated his findings and observations, a practice he continued years later whilst practising medicine and surgery.[1] One of his followers, the American

Bernard Jensen, trained in iridology under allopathic doctors such as H. E. Lane, Henry Lindlahr, the champion of 'the healing crises' and F. W. Collins whose two-volume work *The Diagnosis of Disease by Observation of the Eye* was published in 1919. These great pioneers made good use of the access they had to autopsy and surgery to confirm their iridological diagnoses.[2]

At more or less the same time as von Peczely, other physicians in various parts of the world were making similar studies and gaining virtually identical findings, quite independently. Today, with the more detailed, complex charts produced by the Germans Josef Deck, Theodor Kriege and Joseph Angerer, the American Bernard Jensen, and others, an ever wider spectrum of information revealed by the irides are still being discovered.[3]

Theoretical Base

An in-depth analysis of the iris provides a blueprint of one's genetic and constitutional strengths and weaknesses. It also pinpoints congestive and irritative conditions, degenerative processes and various interactions between organs, spinal impingements and pathways of disease. It can be used to help explain to patients how their problems have developed and what constitutes the root cause.

The iris does not reveal specific pathological diseases by name but rather the conditions within, which could collectively manifest in a defined illness. It provides an indication of the root causes of patients' problems. It is also a key to preventative medicine, to correct living habits in mind, body and spirit, revealing conditions within before they manifest without.

The Practice of Iridology

Iridologists normally take the details from the patient's eyes and do a thorough analysis of the various bodily functions before discussing the patient's symptoms and medical history. The iris can reveal a liver dysfunction or congestion, but it does not specifically reveal a diagnosis such as jaundice. To reach a specific diagnosis, the patient's symptoms are equally important. Jaundice can have different pathological causes. It is a putting together of all the information which narrows down the diagnosis to specifics and indicates the correct treatments. Hence, the necessity for every iridologist to have an excellent knowledge of and training in anatomy and physiology.

At the authors' clinic, most of the patients come after orthodox tests have been unable to provide an identifiable diagnosis. This is reassuring as it can then be assumed that the iris findings are not so much pathologically sinister as lowering, insidious conditions, which collectively have reduced the quality of life or created debilitating symptoms.

Iridology is like map-reading. The iris is divided into segments, with the head and brain zone at the top, the legs at the bottom, the stomach and gastro-intestinal tract taking up a third of the iris from the centre, and all the other organs, glands and limbs located in their various neural pathway zones. The left iris reflects the left side of the body, the left kidney and lung, the spleen, etc. and the right iris reflects the right side of the body, the liver status, etc. Most people understand the mechanics of a reflexologist who works on the nerve endings in the feet, hands and even head, picking out the sensitive points which might indicate a disorder. However, an iridologist, although similarly working with nerve endings, is looking at an overall picture of all the bodily systems and their interactions. To exemplify further, a reflexologist, when working on the nerves in the big toe, which extend down from the pituitary gland, can identify a 'disturbance' to the gland and, with stimulation, gain proof of a reaction or response (for example the patient may suddenly break out into a sweat or feel a tingling in the cranial/pituitary zone) but the reflexologist will not have any idea of what is specifically wrong. An iridologist, on the other hand, is looking at a 'picture'. The iris will reveal inherent weaknesses, lymphatic or tumour congestions, toxic infiltrations via the blood from the gastro-intestinal tract, other possibly related endocrine activities and any spinal impingements on the nerve impulses to the pituitary. All this is vital information if the correct therapy is to be administered.

Reflexology

For example, if a patient has a congested liver, the most effective treatment is to administer 'milk thistle' as it is the richest source of silymarin. However, if the nerve supply from the spine to the liver is impinged, and if the intestines are overloaded with fermenting gases and toxins, the assault on the liver from the damaging effects of the methane, hydrogen, nitrogen, etc. renders a cure or reversal impossible. A holistic approach, including osteopathic manipulation and intestinal detoxification therapy as well as the essential dietary regulations would, altogether, complement the benefits of the remedial herbal therapy and assist in achieving a true cure. All these relevant factors are revealed to the iridologist. Explaining the findings to the patient raises the spirits, not just because of the knowledge and understanding, but because the way the thorough analysis makes the relevant treatments obvious.

Osteopathy
Colonic Irrigation
Nutritional Therapy
Herbalism
Naturopathy

Case studies

A 36-year-old woman was suffering from amenorrhoea, where stress was assumed to be the cause as she had recently divorced. Herbal and homoeopathic treatments achieved nothing. Through iridology it was possible to ascertain that nerve impingement was the root cause. I recommended she see an osteopath and the day following her treatment, her periods recommenced. The patient's trust in the iridology diagnosis was the only criterion that sent her to the osteopath for she had no head or neck pains or discomfort.

Another rather dramatic case was a woman, 69, on the verge of blindness in her right eye, who came to see us as she was reluctant to accept surgical removal of the eye, despite being in great pain. She related her symptoms only as far as her localised eye problems were concerned. Surprisingly, there were no negative markings in the irides in either of the eye zones, which somewhat mystified us. There were distinctive signs of a blood sugar imbalance, however, and a tendency towards diabetes but the patient suffered no symptoms of hypoglycaemia, high thirst or frequent urination. Nevertheless, she was given a urine sugar test, which was negative. The only symptom remotely related to diabetes that we managed to ascertain was numbness to the big toe. Fortunately, the patient herself was exceptionally bright and our references to eye symptoms related to diabetes led her to get a book from the library on the subject. By the time she had finished reading it, she was convinced she was diabetic and went to her doctor. He did a blood sugar test immediately and was so concerned at the results he put her straight into intensive care. Soon afterwards, her daughter decided to learn iridology.

Training

Medical research in America and in Europe, particularly in Russia and Germany, including autopsy correlation of findings, has established greater acceptance of iridology and it is part of the curriculum at the Faculty of Medicine at the University of Paris Nord. At the Holistic Health Consultancy and College, this analytical tool has proved invaluable. In some instances further laboratory or medical tests have been recommended where the need for specific naming of the disease state, such as a possible cancerous condition, prompts modern medical attention and identification.

Iridologists are analysts and diagnosticians but only within the realms of complementary terminology unless they are already allopathic doctors. In this country, there are only two schools affiliated with the Institute of Complementary Medicine – the Holistic Health College and the UK College of Clinical Iridologists. Both follow a very high code of ethics which includes the following criteria on diagnosis, as laid out by the ICM:

> *'Medical Diagnosis: the complementary practitioner will need to assess the case from different criteria and no attempt should be made to describe a complementary diagnosis in allopathic terms unless the practitioner is so qualified. An iridologist is qualified to make a medical diagnosis which might indicate inflammation or morbid congestion in certain areas, but it may be outside their competence to put an allopathic medical name to the condition.'*

The Holistic Health Consultancy and College in London, run by the authors, established a training programme in 1993 as a two-year correspondence course in iridology and natural therapeutics, with anatomy and physiology, as well as in-depth nutrition, herbal medicine, naturopathy and a basic grounding in homoeopathy. We also run the Guild of Naturopathic Iridologists with a register only open to fully qualified iridologists who have at least one recognised therapeutic qualification as well as professional insurance.

Conclusion

As Hippocrates said, 'For every organic disorder, there is an organic treatment.' He also said, 'Look well to the spine for the cause of disease.' Therefore, all therapists, no matter how they treat or what they prescribe, whether they be counsellors, herbalists, nutritionists, homoeopaths or doctors, could enhance their talents with the analytical tool of iridology, cutting out the guesswork and achieving speedier results with more precision.

Biography

Peter Bradbury is a medical herbalist and his wife Angela is a homoeopath, nutritionist and naturopath. Despite being the daughter of a medical consultant and her own homoeopathic training, Angela nearly died in 1978 through colossal misdiagnosis. It was soon afterwards that she met her future husband Peter, who, looking deeply into her eyes, commented on her chronic lymphatic congestion. Romantic disappointment was quickly replaced by the excitement of pinpointing the basis of all her ailments in seconds. They studied iridology together in Cambridge. They established the Holistic Health Consultancy and College in 1983.

References

1   Von Peczely, *Discoveries in the Realms of Nature & the Art of Healing*, published 1880.

Emil Schlegel, *The Eye-Diagnosis of V. Peczely*, published 1886.

2   Bernard Jensen, *Iridology – The Science and Practice in the Healing Arts*, Vol. 2, Bernhard Jensen, 1982.

Henry Edward Lane, *Diagnosis From The Eye*, 1904. Published as a *Scientific Essay for the Public and Medical profession*. The title page defined Iridology as *A new art for diagnosing with perfect certainty from the Iris of the eye the normal and abnormal conditions of the organism in general and of the different organs in particular*.

Henry Lindlahr, *Iridiagnosis and Other Diagnostic Methods*, published 1919.

3   Josef Deck, *Principles of Iris Diagnosis*, Ettlingen, 1980.

——, *Differentiation of Iris Markings*, Ettlingen, 1980.

Theodor Kriege, *Fundamental Basis of Irisdiagnosis*, L. N. Fowler & Co. Ltd., 1969

Joseph Angerer, *Textbook of Eye Diagnosis*, Institute for Research into Iris Studies Pty. Ltd., 1987.

Bernard Jensen, op cit.

Further Reading

Hall, Dorothy, *Iridology*, Viking O'Neil, 1989.

Jackson, Adam, *Iridology: A Guide to Iris Analysis and Preventive Health Care*, Optima, 1992.

Jensen, Bernard, *Iridology: The Science and Practice in the Healing Arts*, Vol. 2, Bernhard Jensen, 1982.

Kriege, Theodor, *Fundamental Basis of Irisdiagnosis*, L. N. Fowler & Co. Ltd., 1969

Resources

British Society of Iridologists
998 Wimborne Road
Bournemouth
Dorset BH9 2DE
Tel. 01202-518 078

International Association of Clinical Iridologists
855 Finchley Road
London NW11 8LX
Tel. 0181-458 7781

International Federation of Iridologists
Hayes Corner
South Cheriton
Templecombe
Somerset BA8 0BR

Guild of Naturopathic Iridologists
94 Grosvenor Road
London SW1V 3LF
Tel. 0171-834 3579

(The Guild holds a list of qualified iridologists)

UK College of Iris Analysis
12 Upper Station Road
Radlett
Herts WD7 8BX
Tel. 01923-857670

Holistic Health Consultancy and College
94 Grosvenor Road,
London SW1V 3LF
Tel. 0171-834 3579

Kinesiology
by Lori Forsyth

Historical Background

Like many complementary therapies, kinesiology was created from one person's inspiration. This foundation has since been built upon and researched to form a body of valuable information with applications in many areas such as education, nutrition and personal growth.

George Goodheart is an American chiropractor who started his first investigations into what has become known as kinesiology in the 1960s. For some time he had been testing the strength of muscles as used in conventional neurological testing, before and after making spinal adjustments, to see if there was a discernible difference in relative strength. It was Goodheart's observation that before a spinal adjustment, the muscles seemed frequently to succumb under his manual pressure, but once the adjustment had been completed successfully, the muscles relating to the adjusted segment could resist quite easily.

In one particular case, he had a patient whose muscles did not seem to remain strong, even when Goodheart was sure he had completed the relevant spinal adjustment. While he considered his next action, he massaged the patient's muscles, concentrating on points which the patient reported as sore. This, to his surprise, strengthened the muscles which had, minutes before, tested weak. Goodheart wanted to know why. His research led him to discover reflex points all over the body, the massage of which appeared to strengthen weak muscles. These, he discovered, were already known as Chapman's reflexes,[1] and are now widely known by kinesiologists as neuro-lymphatic points. This also led him to refine his testing method, applying it to investigations beyond the direct neurological context.

His study of muscles which were quite healthy but which tested weak in certain conditions led him to observe that a weak muscle was frequently paired with a muscle which was in spasm. The accepted wisdom was that massaging a spastic muscle was the way to alleviate the spasm, but Goodheart noticed that if he strengthened the weak muscle in the opposing pair, using the neuro-lymphatic points, the tense muscle came back into normal alignment. His analogy was, if a swing door is operated by two springs and one goes slack, the other spring will automatically tighten. Massaging the tight spring will do nothing to bring the door back into alignment – it is the weak spring which needs attention. Goodheart's task was twofold: to find out why muscles tested weak, and to find out how to strengthen them, thereby bringing the body back into alignment.

As he experimented, the two primary factors he came across which cause muscles to test weak, in addition to structural misalignment, are nutrition and emotional disturbances. This made clear to him that he was dealing with an information system beyond the muscular-neurological connection. He therefore investigated acupuncture, and came to an understanding that each muscle in the body is related to an energy meridian. He found that testing muscles can demonstrate whether the energy in a meridian is blocked or free flowing, so while not being as detailed as an acupuncture pulse reading, muscle testing could give valuable and accurate information as to the overall picture of meridian energy flows through the body. As each meridian relates to an internal organ, he deduced that muscles have a relationship with the organs in the body and that specific muscle weaknesses can, if they persist, be an indication of organ dysfunction which would require further medical investigations.

Acupuncture

He found he could strengthen muscles by massaging points on the acupuncture meridians to free the flow of energy, by improving nutrition, alleviating emotional stress and correcting musculo-skeletal misalignments.

The synthesis of these two strands of research – that which causes muscles to test weak, and how to strengthen them – soon became a system which Goodheart called 'applied kinesiology', kinesiology being the study of the movement of muscles. It was greeted enthusiastically by other chiropractors and in 1973 the International College of Applied Kinesiology was founded.

Theoretical Base

Kinesiology is a holistic therapy, assessing the individual in relation to three main areas:

1   the physical body and structure,

2   the chemical and nutritional element,

3   the emotional and mental aspects.

For a person to manifest good health, all these aspects need to be functioning in an integrated way. For example, a client presenting with recurring migraine headaches may have a spinal misalignment or food allergies or may be under considerable stress, and in many cases there may be a combination of causes. Through kinesiology muscle testing, the areas needing attention can be revealed, prioritised and treated in order to resolve the situation and clear the migraines.

The muscle test which is the core of all kinesiology systems has become a specific technique. There are approximately 650 voluntary muscles in the body, of which about 40 or 50 are used regularly for testing in kinesiology. When a muscle is tested, it is placed in a contracted position and pressure is applied firmly but gently to see if the muscle can hold that position when stressed manually. Although the kinesiologist will use the terms 'weak' and 'strong' to refer to the results of the test, it is not in fact muscular strength that is being assessed. If the muscle 'tests weak', there is something impairing the muscular response. It is the job of the kinesiologist to determine the cause of the imbalance, be it structural, nutritional or emotional, and to use the appropriate correction technique to put it right.

Other than testing specific muscles for specific weaknesses relating to meridians or organs, situations arise where a general indicator is used to give feedback about immediate energy responses of the body to different stimuli, such as foods and thoughts. For this purpose, generally the extended arm is used and this is called the 'indicator muscle'.

Touch For Health (TFH)

This system was put together by John Thie, a colleague of George Goodheart, who was motivated by a strong belief in self-help. He wanted to make available to the general public enough of the techniques of applied kinesiology so they could participate in their own health care rather than having to visit a practitioner all the time. The TFH synthesis, which is taught in a series of week-end workshops, contains much of the basic information about kinesiology: how to muscle test, which muscles are related to which meridians, how the meridian system works and how to give a full 'body balance' – assessing and correcting energy flows throughout the person's physical system so that their own self-regulating process is given the best chance possible to create and maintain good health. Dramatic improvements occur in the health of the family and friends of those who use the simple techniques learned in Touch For Health.

In Touch For Health, muscle testing is used with great effect and accuracy for nutritional testing. This involves testing for food allergies or sensitivities usually by placing a small amount of the suspected food on the patient's body and checking the muscles relating to the stomach, small intestine and large intestine meridians. If there is a weakness in any muscle, the inference is that that food has a deleterious effect on the body. Foods are not always long-term allergies, and muscle testing can be used to determine how long the person needs to avoid a food, if it is simply an acute sensitivity. Nutritional deficiencies are checked to determine how much of a food supplement is required and for how long it needs to be taken to redress balance in the system.

In Touch For Health, techniques for addressing emotional disturbances are taught, known as ESR which stands for 'emotional stress release'. As a demonstration, an individual is asked to think of a situation which is causing them distress, and this is confirmed by the indicator muscle testing weak as they focus on the area of upset. The ESR technique involves holding the forehead lightly with fingertip pressure and inviting the person to continue thinking through the problem until it 'becomes lighter' or maybe even stops feeling like a problem. Sometimes they may take as long as 20 minutes, but more commonly a few minutes is enough to defuse the stress. The completion of the treatment is confirmed by rechecking the indicator muscle as the subject is focused on. Consistently, the muscle tests strong after application of the ESR technique, which usually results in the person finding some creative solution to the problem.

Correction Procedures

Areas of the body known as neuro-lymphatic points which relate to internal organs, acupuncture meridians and specific muscles are massaged. This helps stimulate the lymphatic system. A clear flowing lymph system is essential to good health, helping the body to fight infection and cleansing it of certain toxins.

Neuro-vascular holding points were discovered in the 1930s by another chiropractor, Dr Terence Bennett.[2] These points, located mainly on the head, influence the flow of blood to specific organs and structures and have a strengthening effect on specific muscles which test weak. These points are held lightly for a few minutes and often a 'capillary pulse' is sensed under the fingertips which feels erratic when first contacted but subsides into a steady beat as these points are held. Most people find this extremely relaxing. An example of neuro-vascular points are those used in the ESR technique.

Meridians can be activated to strengthen a weak muscle by brushing one's fingers along the pathway of the meridian. In cases where the muscle does not respond, a more intensive procedure is to use acupressure points which are located on the hands and feet, holding them with a light touch for a few minutes. This usually produces instant strengthening of any weak muscle by stimulating the body's energy system via the meridians.

Other Systems

Touch For Health was designed for the lay person. However, many people with professional backgrounds in education or health care have taken the course, applied the techniques of muscle testing and integrated it into their area or expertise. Others have developed a synergy between kinesiology and their original discipline. A brief mention of three of these is given below, from a range of more than a dozen.

◆ *Educational Kinesiology* is concerned with dyslexia and learning difficulties and uses muscle testing to determine, amongst other things, whether the block is in the visual or auditory brain centres, and whether the problem lies with reading aloud, reading silently or comprehending that which is written. Each problem has a specific correction and Edu-K, as it is known for short, is extremely effective in clearing dyslexia and in assisting both children and adults to learn more effectively and easily.

◆ *Creative Kinesiology* was developed by a couple who were trained in acupuncture and bioenergetic psychology before coming to kinesiology. Their system reflects these interests and concentrates on working with subtle energies to increase well-being.

*Acupuncture
Bioenergetic Analysis*

◆ *Health Kinesiology* focuses on disturbances brought about by environmental (especially geopathic and electromagnetic), psychological and physical stresses. Founded by Dr Jimmy Scott, a professor in physiological psychology, it has a particularly extensive analysis of psychological factors and uses muscle checking mostly to 'ask the body questions'.

Debate

The term used above – 'asking the body questions' – is one which provokes controversy in kinesiology circles. There is an ongoing debate about whether muscle checking can be used only to give information related to the individual's immediate physical and psychological condition or whether it can be used as a method of dowsing, to ascertain answers to questions of an unlimited range.

*Dowsing
Radionics*

There are strong arguments on both sides, which in general reflect the dichotomy of rationalism versus intuition. Those who trust in the intuitive faculties of the human mind see muscle checking as a way of accessing that which can be known by each one of us if we are focused and have our minds clear of as many preconceptions as possible. The opposing argument is that these methods are unscientific and unreliable, and again there is evidence that in the wrong hands, this can certainly be true. The practitioner who is not totally detached or who is inexperienced may indeed founder if using an intuitive approach. In the long run, both clients and practitioners will select a way of working in kinesiology with which they are most comfortable.

Training

For those wishing to become professional kinesiologists, the TFH synthesis still provides the core of the foundation training course. Following from that there is a course in basic applied kinesiology which has been taken from the chiropractic syllabus and adapted for non-manipulative therapists. From there, a trainee therapist can follow their preferences and learn in depth from whichever branch of kinesiology most attracts them.

Since the spread of kinesiology took place via Touch For Health, which was designed for non-professionals, its development has not been monitored by a professional governing body. The International College of Applied Kinesiology, which has operated for at least two decades, only accepts chiropractors for membership, which excludes most of those practising kinesiology in Britain. In recent years, therefore, it became necessary to create an organisation to lay down standards for accreditation, training and professional practice for the many hundreds of people using kinesiology, either on its own or in conjunction with other modalities. The Kinesiology Federation was founded in 1991 to fulfil this need and is currently the umbrella organisation which recognises and monitors all branches and systems of kinesiology in the UK.

My Practice

My primary interest has always been how the mind and emotions affect the body. I use the method of 'asking the body questions' which I have found to be accurate if applied under certain conditions – I must be centred, unattached, in balance and very aware of the wording of the question I am asking. This method is well suited to investigating the link between past trauma and present dis-ease. Using muscle checking and working from lists of possibilities, as well as using my intuition, I aim to pinpoint whichever of the life experiences of the client are a causative factor in the client's current state of poor health. Through memory retrieval, conscious cognition and the application of flower remedies, affirmations or some other form of gentle intervention, the client begins to release some of the constricted trauma from the past which in turn frequently shifts the presenting physical symptom.

Flower Essences
Affirmations

Acupuncture
Polarity Therapy

Recently a new system of kinesiology has been developed which takes the effectiveness of the process a quantum leap further. This system is called 'Holographic Repatterning' and has been developed by an Englishwoman, Chloe Wordsworth, whose background was in acupuncture, polarity therapy and educational kinesiology.

Holographic Repatterning has as its starting point a recognition that vibrational resonance is the core of all health and disease. Humans have a wide vibrational range. When a trauma occurs, it gets lodged at a low level of resonance which is characterised by fear or anger or whatever survival response is triggered at the time and this resonance is returned to whenever a situation is experienced which restimulates the original trauma and the response to it. Whatever level the vibration, people attract and are attracted to those things and people which are vibrating at the same level, so frequently the low level is reinforced and a vicious circle is perpetuated.

Wordsworth's system aims to help clients shift vibration, re-establishing an appropriately high resonance. She uses muscle checking as the tool to uncover the cause of the stuck energy and to determine the correction required to make a shift in vibration. A very functional six-step process takes the practitioner and client through a maze of unconscious patterns to discover the precise psychological blocks, beliefs and negative choices by which the client is being limited and prevented from moving forwards. In addition it locates which chakras and meridians are being stressed and what needs to be done to correct their resonance.

Correction is usually by the application of light through a colour filter torch or sound through specially designed tuning forks, which 'repattern' the client's energy and restore their natural optimal vibrational resonance in relation to the issues they are working through. It is an effective system for accelerating change and helping people move into new ways of relating to themselves, others and the world.

Colour Therapy
Sound Therapy

Case Histories

A teenage boy who was finding it hard to get along with his co-workers in the warehouse where he was employed was sent to me by his parents. He had been threatened with dismissal and they wondered if Holographic Repatterning could do anything to change his negative, defensive and rude way of relating to others. After three sessions he was congratulated by his boss for being helpful and co-operative. Several of his other team members commented that he was a 'changed person'. For me, the significant aspect of the case was that the boy himself made no conscious effort to overcome any personal reactions. Having been released from his constricted energy patterns, he simply perceived and responded to experiences in a different, more harmonious way.

A woman of 42, who was attending community council meetings on a regular basis, was finding them distressing because she felt herself unable to contribute her opinions and so returned home after each meeting with an intense headache. The one session we did together on this issue identified a pattern that was laid down in childhood whereby her father invalidated her for sharing any opinion which was at odds with those of her older brothers. We cleared this imprint and the next week she attended a council meeting, spoke eloquently in opposition to the motion being proposed and returned home feeling good about herself. Again, it is significant that she acted in this way without any sense of mustering her courage to speak out. She reported to me that it was while she was part way through her speech that she realised what she was doing and that she felt quite comfortable doing it.

A 36-year-old woman was finding it hard to make friends after moving to a new town. Every time she thought she had connected well with someone, they argued or she was rejected in some way. We did three sessions on this, during which it came to light that because of her difficult relationship with her mother in childhood, she had very little inner commitment to having intimate relationships with others. Therefore, although her conscious mind craved friends, her unconscious patterns sabotaged any attempt she made to form real bonds of intimacy. We cleared this pattern and three months later she telephoned me to say she had just given a birthday dinner party for twenty people; everyone had a wonderful time and declared it the event of the year.

Biography

Lori Forsyth, BA in comparative literature, trained in kinesiology in 1982. Publisher of *The Directory of Holistic Health Care in the Highlands and Islands of Scotland* and *The Vegetarian Guide to the Scottish Highlands and Islands*, author of *Journey into Healing*, (Balnain Books, 1993). Qualified practitioner and teacher of Holographic Repatterning.

References

1   C Owens, *An Endocrine Interpretation of Chapman's Reflexes*, The Academy of Applied Osteopathy, 1963.

2   Terence Bennett, *Dynamics of Correction of Abnormal Function*, Ralph Martin, 1977.

Further Reading

Andrews, Elizabeth, *Muscle Management*, Thorsons, 1991.

Barhydt, Elizabeth, *Accurate Muscle Testing for Foods and Supplements*, Loving Life, 1992.

Benham, Charles, *Optimum Health Balance*, OHB, 1991.

Butler, Brian, *Kinesiology Balanced Health*, Task Publications, 1990.

Dennison, Paul, *EduK for Kids*, Edu-Kinesthetics, 1987.

Dewe, Bruce, *Professional Kinesiology Practitioner*, PKP Workshops, 1990-3.

Diamond, John, *Your Body Doesn't Lie*, Warner, 1980.

Holdway, Ann, *Kinesiology*, Element Health Essentials, 1995.

LaTourelle, Maggie, *Introductory Guide to Kinesiology*, Thorsons, 1992.

Scott, Jimmy, *Cure Your Own Allergies*, Health Kinesiology Publications, 1988.

Stokes, Gordon, *One Brain*, Three in One Concepts, 1984.

Thie, John, *Touch For Health*, TFH Enterprises, 1973.

Valentine, Tom, *Applied Kinesiology*, Thorsons, 1985.

Walther, David, *Applied Kinesiology*, System DC Pueblo, 1981.

Resources

The Kinesiology Federation
P O Box 2891
London SW19 1ZB

International College of Applied Kinesiology (ICAK Europe)
54 East Street
Andover
Hants
SP10 1EF
Tel/Fax. 01264 339512

Association for Systematic Kinesiology (ASK)
39 Browns Road
Surbiton
Surrey
KT5 8ST
Tel. 0181 399 3215

Holographic Repatterning Association
Wordsworth Productions Inc
P O Box 6504
Scottsdale AZ 85261
USA

Holographic Repatterning Association (UK)
34 Matlock Road
Reading
Berks
RG4 7BS
Tel. 0118 947 0385

Laughter Medicine
by Patch Adams with Lori Forsyth

Humour is an antidote to all ills. The late Norman Cousins wrote eloquently about having laughed himself back to health after suffering from a serious chronic disease.[1] The experience had such an impact that he changed careers late in life to help bring this information to the health care profession. Jokes seemed so important to Sigmund Freud that he wrote a book on the subject.[2] But we don't need professionals to tell us about the magnetism of laughter – with great insight we call a funny person 'the life and soul of the party'.

Psychological Therapies Counselling

Theoretical Base

Although humour itself is difficult to evaluate, the response to humour – laughter – can be studied quite readily. Research has shown that laughter increases the secretion of the natural chemicals, catecholamines and endorphins, that make people feel good. It also decreases cortisol secretion and lowers the sedimentation rate, which implies a stimulated immune response.[3] Oxygenation of the blood increases and residual air in the lungs decreases. Heart rate initially speeds up and blood pressure rises, then the arteries relax, causing heart rate and blood pressure to lower. Skin temperature rises as a result of the increased peripheral circulation. Thus, laughter appears to have a positive effect on many cardiovascular and respiratory problems.[4] In addition, laughter has superb muscle relaxant qualities.[5] Muscle physiologists have shown that anxiety and muscle relaxation cannot occur at the same time and that the relaxation response after a hearty laugh can last up to 45 minutes.

Relaxation Therapy

The Practice of Humour as Therapy

Bringing humour into a medical setting must be a joint decision by administration and staff. The most important elements of bedside manner are not medical knowledge or skill but the qualities inherent in fun and love. Once the medical establishment has agreed to accept more humour, people at all levels of employment will be willing to take steps in this direction.

Some hospitals have begun the process already. At Duke University Hospital in Durham, North Carolina, humour carts deliver videos, cartoon and humour books, juggling equipment, toys and games. Dekalb Hospital near Atlanta has created a lively room for romping. Of course, carts and rooms do not make humour; here the volunteer becomes the key. The clowns of the Big Apple Circus in New York City have created Clown Care Units which visit children's hospitals on a regular basis to bring joy and assist with patient care. The wonderful, positive feedback by staff, patients and their families keeps this programme alive.

Humour therapy can include a loud bow-tie, singing on the ward, word play, cartoons put up around the hospital, even inviting comedians to come into the hospital.

The Association of Therapeutic Humor[6] is creating a resource centre with information about humour and about people who practise it as a therapy.

Cautions

One note of caution: some feel humour can be harmful in some situations, especially in psychotherapy. I would certainly suggest humour that is not racist or sexist. I recommend becoming quite close to your patients first and have them be sure of your tenderness and sincerity, so that if a funny situation or joke hurts someone, you can simply apologise. It behoves the medical history taker to make an exploration into the patient's sense of humour.

The Gesundheit Institute

We at Gesundheit are building the first silly hospital, where the entire context will be geared to fun and play. Gesundheit Institute is the dream of a growing number of people, an experiment in holistic medical care based on the belief that the health of the individual cannot be separated from the health of the family, the community and the world. We have taken the most expensive service in America, medical care, and given it away for free. We are now building a facility in West Virginia that embodies this philosophy: a free, home-style hospital and health centre, open to anyone from anywhere. We want this centre to be a health care model, not necessarily to be copied by others but to stimulate caregivers and hospitals to develop an ideal medical approach for their communities.

One of the most important tenets of our philosophy is that health is based on happiness – from hugging and clowning around to finding joy in family and friends, satisfaction in work and ecstasy in nature and the arts. For us, healing is not only prescribing medicine and therapies but working together and sharing in a spirit of joy and co-operation. Much more than simply a medical centre, the Gesundheit hospital will be a microcosm of life, integrating medical care with arts and crafts, performing arts, education, nature, farming, recreation, friendship and fun.

My Personal Story

I was born an army brat and moved from place to place, learning to make friends quickly but being a verbal troublemaker in school, questioning the rules and acting like the class clown. When I was 16, my father died and the three years that followed were the most tumultuous in my life. I was suffering but couldn't express my feelings. By the time I was 19 I had been hospitalised twice with stomach ulcers, and soon afterwards I attempted suicide and was admitted to a mental hospital. My two-week stay there was the turning point of my life. The people who had the greatest impact on my recovery were not doctors but my family and friends and especially my roommate, Rudy.

Rudy lived in an unfathomable abyss of failure and despair. When friends came to visit me, I realised how good it felt, but nobody ever came to visit Rudy. He told me about loneliness I had never dreamed existed and that made my pain seem trivial by comparison. For the first time in my adult life, I empathised with another person.

Talking to Rudy, I realised the importance of love and the people who loved me. I had been surrounded by love but had not let it affect me. I perceived a deep personal truth: I needed to be open to receive love. Without it I was not a strong person. And I realised that if I continued living as I had been – without tender, human love – I would end up like Rudy.

That moment was a spiritual awakening to the power of love. After ten or twelve days in hospital I signed out against medical advice. I was a soul in pain, not insane. Hospitalisation had forced me to formulate a philosophy about happiness. A new experience began that affects the way I am today: I became, for want of a better word, a student of life, of happy life.

After leaving the hospital I knew I wanted to perform some service and decided to go into medicine. While waiting to be admitted to university, I worked in an office as a filing clerk. It was considered to be horrible work: joyless, boring and dull. I decided to change all that. My fellow file clerk, Louis, had dropped out of college temporarily. From the very first day, we decided to makes the files a 'happening' and egged each other on. One day, when anybody asked us for a file, we replied in a high-mass Gregorian chant 'Which file do you wa-ant?' Another day we arrived for work in gorilla suits. Louis was my partner in fun and we gave each other the courage to be goofy in public. This early foray into the world of humour and fun encouraged me to expand and get better at it. I could always find an audience and I discovered that fun is as important as love and life. Nurtured by levity and love, I blossomed. I defeated all my demons and became the person I am today. My self-confidence, love of wisdom and desire to change the world were rooted in that brief period, from late 1963 to the end of 1964, when I climbed out of despair to rebirth.

Medical school might have been a tragedy, but from the outset I resisted the pressure to squeeze us students into a mould that to me seemed inhumane. Hospital staff were not trained to work together as teams to relieve suffering. Doctors supposedly knew all the answers and ordered others around, often rudely. The doctor was seen as the hero who saves the patient, with no room for humility or mistakes. This is dangerous thinking which puts everyone under pressure. No wonder joylessness prevailed, not only in the hospital but in the classroom as well.

I determined to learn about medicine but avoid making my medical school experience a misery as many of my colleagues were doing. The best fun I had was interacting with the patients. I rebelled against grand rounds and the impersonality of ten strangers in white coats trooping into a sick person's room. I discovered that if I entered a hospital room and was vibrant and smiley, the patients would immediately perk up. I was free to talk to them, cry with them, massage them, comfort them, joke with them and inject some exuberance and fun into their lives.

The patients loved it. The nurses loved it. My fellow students were another story: some loved it and some hated it. Many felt threatened by me. A hospital is supposed to be very serious: people were suffering and dying, and doctors should be solemn. I didn't want that. Sometimes, of course, solemnity was entirely appropriate but most of the time it was not.

During the same period I spent 15 hours a week at the Free Clinic in the poorer part of town. Here medicine was practised with the sole intent of relieving suffering – on a shoestring budget. This offered me the ideal environment in which to experiment with humour and see whether it could help others. One day I wore a fire hat and a red rubber nose to work and discovered that my nuttiness did not diminish the respect or trust of the patients. In fact, it seemed to enhance these feelings. Humour helped me become closer to many of the patients. I spent lots of time with them and the closeness that resulted was indistinguishable from friendship. This was the context in which I wanted to work and provided one of the models for what I wanted to do with my medical career.

It did not take me long to realise that if I had dreams about improving health care, I would have to carry them out myself. My mind was ablaze with alternatives. A group-communal situation seemed the most promising approach. But I knew of no models in America for a therapeutic medical community that put humanism first. I set up my practice at home in Arlington, Virginia, in a three-bedroom house I shared with some like-minded friends, three of whom were doctors, where we could express freely our ideals of loving patients and using humour and fun as therapy. This first communal experiment grew into years of practising medicine from our home, a caring environment where play and shared experiences were as important as the medical treatments.

The dream started with an abstraction of wanting to give service and evolved through different forms into a bold new proposal for health care delivery. The model had no name at first; not until 1979 did we name it the Gesundheit Institute. We chose the name because in the USA it makes people laugh (it is what is said to someone who has just sneezed) and thus become open to healing and because, literally translated, gesundheit means 'good health'.

In the twelve years we saw patients during the pilot phase of Gesundheit Institute, we had many opportunities to explore the relationship between humour and medicine. Although we greatly appreciated casual humour, it seemed imperative that we deliberately incorporate it into our day-to-day lives to prevent an atmosphere of agony or despair. Some of this humour came from a stream of jokes that the patients and staff brought with them. However, jokes die quickly, and we found that for an atmosphere of humour to thrive, we had to live funny.

We learned first to develop an air of trust and love, because spontaneous humour can be offensive, and we wanted it to be taken in the spirit of trying. (Cautious people are rarely funny.) It soon became clear that silliness was a potent force in keeping the staff together as friends. And I, as a physician, began to see the potent medicinal effect of humour on diseases of all kinds. Laughter is the white noise of happiness. Comic relief is a major way for happy folk to dissipate pain. In a healthier world, humour would be a way of life. People would be funny as a rule, not an exception.

A Model for the Future

The field of humour in medicine cries out for more investigation. The goal of the medical clown is not to hurt people or belittle suffering but to bring fun to those who are suffering. The nature of deep suffering demands some fun as an antidote.

The silly hospital at Gesundheit is a model health care facility based on this pilot project and on years of subsequent study. The time for such a model is long overdue. Gesundheit is designed as a total community. Our goals are to transform the traditional distinction between doctor and patient by creating an acute-care facility that is both a 40-bed hospital for patients and a home for 40 full-time carers and their families. We will offer a wide choice of allopathic and alternative healing techniques, and integrate medical care with agriculture, crafts, performing arts, education, social services, friendship and fun. We hope it will become a teaching institution for health care professionals, from medical and nursing students to hospital administrators. It will demonstrate that an individual in not a lone organism but part of a family, community and world, all of which are in need of assistance and love. Gesundheit Institute will operate out of deep concern for the quality of people's lives in a world dominated by the values inherent in power and greed.

We are still raising funds to put our dream into reality but are not far off now. We have a 310-acre plot in the West Virginia hills and enough volunteers to build and staff three such hospitals. I spend much of my time giving lectures and presentations around the world, raising not only funds, but awareness of the issues involved in putting care back into health care.

I have reached the conclusion that humour is vital in healing the problems of individuals, communities and societies. I have been a street clown for 30 years and have tried to make my own life silly, not as that word is currently used, but in terms of its original meaning. 'Silly' originally meant good, happy, blessed, fortunate, kind and cheerful in many different languages. No other attribute has been more important.

Biography

Dr Hunter (Patch) Adams is a medical doctor, professional clown and social activist. He founded the Gesundheit Institute in Virginia, USA and is presently lecturing worldwide to fundraise for a 40-bed 'silly hospital' in rural West Virginia.

References

1   Norman Cousins, *Anatomy of an Illness*, WW Norton and Co., 1979.

2   Sigmund Freud, *Jokes and Their Relationship to the Unconscious*, WW Norton and Co., 1964.

3   L S Berk, et al., *Neuroendocrine and stress hormone changes during mirthful laughter*, The American Journal of Medical Sciences, Vol 296, No7, December 1989.

4   W F Fry Jr.; C Rader, *The respiratory components of mirthful laughter*, Journal of Biological Psychology, 1977; 19: 35-50.

5   H A Paskind, *Effect of laughter on muscle tone*, Archives of Neurology and Psychiatry, 1932; 23: 623-628.

Further Reading

Adams, Patch, *Gesundheit*, (3rd ed.), Healing Arts Press, 1993.

Bergson, H., *Laughter, an Essay on the Meaning of the Comic*, Macmillan, 1911.

Bokun, Branko, *Humour Therapy*, Vita Books, 1986.

Brill, A A., *The Mechanism of Wit and Humour in Normal and Psychopathic States*, Psychiatric Quarterly, 1940; 14: 731-49.

Brody, M W., *The Meaning of Laughter*, Psychoanalytic Quarterly, 1950; 19: 192-201.

Coser, R L., *Some Social Functions of Laughter: A Study of Humour in a Hospital Setting*, Human Relations, 1959; 12: 171-182.

Cousins, Norman, *Anatomy of an Illness*, WW Norton and Co., 1979.

Fairbanks, Douglas, *Laugh and Live*, Britton Publishing Co., 1917.

Fry, W F Jn.; Salameh, W A (eds.) *Advances in Humour and Psychotherapy*, Professional Resource Press, 1993.

Holden, Robert, *Laughter is the Best Medicine*, Thorsons, 1993.

————, *Stress Busters*, Thorsons, 1992.

————, *Living Wonderfully*, Aquarian Press, 1994.

Klein, Allen, *The Healing Power of Humour*, Jeremy Tarcher, 1989.

Metcalf, C W.; Felible, R., *Lighten Up*, Addison Wesley Publishing Co., 1992.

Wooten, P. (ed.) *Heart, Humour and Healing*, Commune-A-Key Publishing, Mt. Shasta, 1994.

Resources

Europe:

Robert Holden
29 Linkside Avenue
Oxford OX2 8JE
Tel/Fax. 01865-58417

Caroline Simonds
Le Rire Medecin
75 Avenue Parmentier
75009 Paris, France
Tel. 01-42583991
(French version of clown care units)

Dhyan Sutorius MD
Secretariat of the Centre in Favour of Laughter
Jupiter 1008
1115 TX Duivendrecht
Holland
Tel. 020-690028

Lex Van Someren
Batstangveien 81
3200 Sanderfjord
Norway
Tel. 034-59644
(The Mystic Clown, teacher of workshops)

USA:

Patch Adams, MD,
6877 Washington Blvd
Arlington, VA 22213
Tel. (703) 525-8169
(Physician, clown, lecturer, workshops and performances)

Michael Christensen
Clown Care Unit Big Apple Circus
35 W 35th Street
NY 10001
Tel. (212) 268-2500
(Clowns who visit paediatric wards)

Leslie Gibson RN
The Comedy Connection
323 Jeffords Street
Clearwater, FL34617
Tel. (813) 462-7842
(Lectures and creates hospital humour carts)

Art Gliner
Humour Communications
8902 Maine Avenue
Silver Spring MD 20910
Tel. (301) 588-3561
(Lectures/workshops)

Eric de Bont
Bont's Adventures in Clown Arts
Pardoestheater
Postbus 419
6800 AK Arnheim
The Netherlands
(Centre for learning clown arts)

Annette Goodheart
P O Box 40297
Santa Barbara CA 93103
Tel. (805) 966-4725
(Laughter therapist, lectures and workshops)

Joel Goodman
The Humour Project
179 Spring Street
Box L
Saratoga Springs, NY 12866
(Quarterly newsletter 'Laughing Matters', lectures, workshops, annual humour conference)

International Humour Institute
32362 Saddle Mt Road
Westlake Village CA 91361
Tel. (818) 879-9085

International Laughter Society
16000 Glen Una Drive
Los Gatos CA 95030
Tel. (408) 354-3456

Massage
by Sue Jenkins

History

Massage is not new. It is probably as old as humankind. It is something we all do instinctively; even animals groom each other and lick their wounds. Human beings rub painful areas of their bodies to 'make it better'.

> *Massage can be an expression of love and caring, as well as a means of healing body, mind and spirit. Massage is the art of giving and receiving touch. Warmth, comfort, pleasure and safety are communicated through the hands. With gentle, rhythmical touch the whole person is contacted through the body. The gentle movements over the skin and muscles invite the body tissue to let go of its tension and strain, and to experience deep relaxation.*[1]

There is an early mention of massage in a Chinese book of about 2700 BC which states that 'Early morning effleurage (stroking) with the palm of the hand, after the night's sleep, when the blood is rested and the tempers relaxed, protects against colds, keeps the organs supple and prevents minor ailments.' In the *Nei-Ching, the Yellow Emperor's Classic of Internal Medicine* it is written that the 'people of the centre are kept healthy with diet and massage'.[2]

It was part of the Ayurvedic system of healing in ancient India: 'Massage reduces fat, strengthens the muscles and firms the skin.'[3]

In ancient Greece and Rome it was used before and after sport, during convalescence, after bathing and for the treatment of various medical conditions. Julius Caesar had daily massage to relieve neuralgia.[4]

In the fifth century BC the Greek physician Hippocrates called massage *anatripsis* and said that every physician should be experienced in rubbing... 'for rubbing can bind a joint that is too loose, and loosen a joint that is too rigid'. Others called it tripsis, friction, manipulation, rubbing or shampooing. The word 'massage' probably comes from the Arabic word *masah*, which means to stroke with the hand.[5]

Galen, physician to the Roman Emperor from AD 131-210, wrote much about massage, which he categorised as firm, gentle and moderate. He directed that the strokes and circuits of the hands should be of many sorts, in order that as far as possible all the muscle fibres should be rubbed in every direction. He also wrote that 'massage eliminates the waste products of nutrition and the poisons of fatigue'.[6]

In the eleventh century, Avicenna, the Arab philosopher and physician, thought that the object of massage was 'to disperse the effete matters found in the muscles and not expelled by exercise'.

The Middle Ages seem to have seen a decline in both bathing and massage. But in 1566 there is a story that Mary, Queen of Scots, who was considered dead after contracting typhus, was revived by vigorous massage from her physician, Dr News. An Italian botanist, Alpinus, helped to reinstate massage, after experiencing it in Egypt. A contemporary report states in 1593 that 'perfectly masséed, one feels completely regenerated, a feeling of extreme comfort pervades the whole system, the chest expands and we breathe with pleasure; the blood circulates with ease and we have a sensation as if freed from an enormous load; we experience a suppleness and lightness until then unknown'.

Per Henrik Ling (1776–1839), a Swedish professor, doctor and poet, developed Swedish massage, combining Greek, Chinese, Egyptian and Roman techniques. He set up a school in Stockholm in 1814 to teach massage and gymnastics, based on scientific principles. He classified treatments as passive or gymnastic and as pressure, friction, percussion, vibration or rotation and his techniques are still taught today as Swedish massage.[7]

By the end of the nineteenth century massage was a popular medical treatment, used by eminent doctors, but also by 'houses of ill repute' to advertise their activities. In 1894 in London, as a response to this denigration of their profession, a group of female masseuses formed the Society of Trained Masseurs. This eventually became the Chartered Society of Physiotherapists.

During World War I massage was used in the treatment of nerve injury and shellshock, but the use of electrical equipment for stimulation gradually became more fashionable. Human massage was considered a pampering luxury instead of a form of health care, providing therapeutic effects and the caring, personal touch of another human being.

In 1972 George Downing published his *Massage Book*, combining some of the Swedish techniques with a more intuitive approach, as practised at Esalen in the USA. This was instrumental in leading to renewed interest in massage in particular and in other forms of bodywork, such as shiatsu, Rolfing, Postural Integration and others, and is still a valuable tool for the beginner.

Shiatsu
Postural Integration
Rolfing

Theoretical Base

Massage works with the body's regenerative capacity, promoting the self-healing ability of each individual. It may be used prophylactically as well as to aid or speed recovery from illness. The sense of touch is registered by the largest and most sensitive organ in the body – the skin. In the developing embryo the skin arises from the same cell layer as the nervous system and so may be thought of as the external part of that system.

The sense of touch is the first sense to become functional in the embryo, suggesting how fundamentally massage can affect the body. Massage and touch are a primary means of communication – healing the divisions within and between people, reducing the isolation, loneliness and pain and creating harmony, balance and oneness, enabling people to grow in love, compassion and understanding.

Physiologically massage works on muscles, ligaments and tendons and affects the circulation of the blood and lymph. It oxygenates and nourishes every cell in the body, aids detoxification by speeding up the elimination of waste products by the lymphatic system and helps to cleanse the skin. It may affect haemoglobin levels. It can be used on specific areas of the body according to need (remedial or Swedish massage) or over the whole body to relax and reduce stress. It is thought that it may aid the production of endorphins – the body's natural painkillers – and encephalin, which reduces pain and produces a feeling of well-being. In this way it may lessen the need for excessive medication. Other psychological effects are also felt – deep relaxation, increased vitality and awareness, improved co-ordination, sleep and body image, and a feeling of being cared for. The masseur also receives benefit – like stroking a cat, massage produces a soothing effect and a subsequent lowering of blood pressure.[8]

The practitioner can only invite the body to relax – not force it. Sometimes it takes several treatments for the body to let go completely. However, some clients are very responsive and relax almost at once. Sometimes rapport with the therapist is immediate and at other times it only comes gradually as the client learns to trust and relax.

Massage can be used to prevent or heal many everyday illnesses that derive from the stress and strain of modern life, in which one easily becomes out of touch with the body.[9] It may help in cases of insomnia, fatigue, headache, backache, constipation and muscular cramps, but it is not a substitute for seeking medical advice, especially when symptoms persist or recur frequently.

General Techniques

There are six categories of massage strokes:

◆ *Effleurage* (stroking) is a surface stroke usually done gently over large areas of the body to accustom the recipient to the touch, to assess the state of the recipient's body, to relax, to assist venous return and lymphatic drainage, to stretch muscles, and to connect different parts of the body on an energetic level. It is used at the beginning and end of a treatment and is usually carried out with the whole of the hand.

◆ *Petrissage* (kneading) consists of variations of picking up and squeezing muscles. Its general function is to 'milk' the muscles of waste products and promote circulation. It increases tone and efficiency and is used on large muscles and fatty tissue. Different techniques include picking up, squeezing, rolling, kneading and wringing. The whole hand may be used or only the fingers.

◆ *Friction* massages deeper tissue layers. It consists of small circular movements carried out with thumbs, tips of fingers, heel of the hand or loose fist, moving tissue against bone. Friction leads to increased blood supply, relieves pain and loosens and mobilises muscles and joints. It relieves muscle cramps and stiffness due to overuse, breaks down adhesions, relieves constipation, conditions joints and muscles, and relaxes and energises the spine.

◆ *Compression* (also known as pressure) is applied to acupressure, reflex or trigger points to relieve pain or affect organs some distance away from the area worked on.

Shiatsu

◆ *Tapotement* (percussion) stimulates and invigorates and includes clapping/cupping, hacking/chopping, slapping/patting, tapping, beating, pounding, drumming and plucking/pinching.

◆ *Vibration* (shaking) is used after friction or tapotement to tone or check for release of muscles. It also stimulates circulation, promotes glandular activity and relieves constipation.

The Practice of Massage

A full body massage may last up to two hours. Some forms of massage use oils or powder and require the client to be naked; others allow the client to remain clothed. Some techniques are best performed on a table, others on the floor. The comfort of both giver and recipient is paramount. At the first appointment, the therapist will take a medical history and may not necessarily carry out a massage.

Although it is beneficial to have a problem area massaged, a full body massage is far more relaxing, physically, mentally and emotionally and does more to balance the energy flows in the body. Sometimes it is not possible to carry out full body massage, due to time constraints or to the client being incapacitated in some way, possibly in a hospital bed. In the first instance it is probably better to concentrate on one part of the body – back, face or feet, for example (and if one subscribes to the Eastern concepts of energy flow and meridians, one can affect the whole body by working on certain meridians and acupressure points). In the second instance one must work with whatever parts of the body are accessible. In all cases the practitioner should only work on those areas which the client is happy to have massaged: relaxation will not be attained if the client or therapist is in any way uncomfortable. Therapists are advised not to give massage if they are emotionally or physically out of balance as their tensions may be communicated to the recipient.

Aromatherapy
Osteopathy
Chiropractic
Yoga

Massage works well on its own, but especially well with essential oils (aromatherapy), and before and after osteopathy or chiropractic (to relax and tone muscles). It may be used alongside most other therapies. As an all-round body, mind and spirit maintenance, massage and yoga, in my opinion, are a combination that cannot be bettered. Aerobic exercise and gentle muscle stretching are among the benefits of these techniques used together. Almost anyone, from an infant to a grandparent, can benefit from and enjoy massage.

Contraindications

Massage carries many benefits (as previously listed under types of strokes), but there are some instances when it is best not employed, especially not by a well-meaning amateur:

◆ Within two hours of the recipient having eaten a heavy meal.

◆ When the masseur is unwell, fatigued or upset.

◆ When the recipient is suffering from any of the following conditions: high temperature or fever; infectious conditions; nausea; undiagnosed pain; cancer or suspected cancer; heart conditions, for example angina.

◆ One should not massage directly over varicose veins, which may cause damage to delicate blood vessels; or over bruises, cuts, wounds or recent scars, which could be opened again; inflammation or skin problems, which may be made worse by spreading them; fresh sprains or swellings; or over undiagnosed lumps, where the possibly malignant cells could be spread through the lymphatic system.

Training

Many different people practise massage. Some are trained in it, some are not and some are trained in it as part of another therapy (for example aromatherapy).

There are many different schools of massage and it would be impossible to pick one type as providing the right training. Individuals must look at the syllabus and decide what is right for themselves. Training should include a thorough grounding in anatomy and physiology, as well as practical training in massage techniques. Anyone with a degree of common sense will be able to help friends and family with simple massage techniques, which can be picked up intuitively, found in books or learned in a short course. It is useful to remember the old saying of Hippocrates: 'First do no harm.'

Research

In the 1920s in Philadelphia, research was carried out on rats to investigate the effects of touch. Those who had this treatment showed faster growth rates, better immunity to disease and higher fertility, as well as being less affected by stress. Between 1910 and 1935 Drs Chapman, Knox and Brennemann carried out studies of babies in institutions, and later studies examined the effect of massage on preterm infants. Early death, and physical and emotional disturbances were linked to too little tactile stimulation.[10]

There is currently much research being done into the efficacy of massage, particularly in the realms of cancer and palliative care. In one of the studies patients reported a significant reduction in anxiety levels and improvements in physical and emotional symptoms. All subjects deemed massage a positive experience; the benefits were found to be cumulative and helpful in relaxation after three or four sessions.[11]

Biography

Sue Jenkins has a BA and postgraduate certificate in education. After several years in teaching, she trained as an aromatherapist with the London School of Aromatherapy in 1988 and in 1989 went into practice in Fife, Scotland where she also studied for the school's advanced diploma. She moved to Aberdeenshire with her family in 1993 and now practices from home and at the Findhorn Foundation.

She has taught aromatherapy for the LSA since 1990 and is principal of the Edinburgh School of Holistic Aromatherapy. A member of the IFA, ISPA, RQA and ICM she works for the unification of the therapy, towards consistently high standards in training and research and is involved with building links with the medical profession. She gives talks, workshops and lectures on aromatherapy and related subjects.

In practice her main interests lie in immune system functioning, pregnancy and childbirth and in the psychospiritual aspects of aromatherapy. At home she enjoys walking, dancing, music, swimming and gardening as well as trying to develop a more environmentally friendly and holistic lifestyle.

References

1   Patricia McNamara, *Massage for people with cancer*, Wandsworth Cancer Support Centre, P O Box 17, 20-22 York Rd., London SW11 3QE, 1994.

2   Ni Maoshing, *The Yellow Emperor's Classic of Medicine, an exploratory translation*, Shambhala, 1995.

3   Ayurveda books of wisdom.

4   Ouida West, *The Magic of Massage*, Hastings House, 1990.

5   Clare Maxwell-Hudson, *The Complete Book of Massage*, Dorling Kindersley, 1988.

6   ibid.

7   Frances Tappan, *Healing Massage Techniques: Healing, Classic and Emerging Methods*, Appleton & Lange, 1988.

8   ibid.

    Clare Maxwell-Hudson, *The Complete Book of Massage*, Dorling Kindersley, 1988.

9   *Massage Bavara*, Connections Magazine, Glasgow.

10 F Hammett (1920) research on rats to investigate the effects of touch.

11   The Centre for Cancer and Palliative Care Studies, *An evaluation of the use of massage and massage with the addition of essential oils on the well-being of cancer patients*, 1995.

Further Reading

Barr J S & Taslitz N., *The Influence of back massage on autonomic functions*, Physical therapy, 1970; 50: 1679-91.

Claire, Thomas, *Bodywork*, William Morrow & Co., 1995.

Downing, George, *The Massage Book*, Penguin, 1974.

Ferrell-Torry A T & Glick O J., *The use of therapeutic massage & nursing intervention to modify anxiety and the perception of cancer pain*, Cancer Nursing, 1983; 26: 2, 93-101.

Fraser J & Ross- Kerr J., *Psychophysiological effects of back massage on elderly institutionalised patients*, Journal of Advanced Nursing, 1993; 18: 238-45.

Lacroix, Nitya, *Massage for Total Relaxation*, Dorling Kindersley, 1991.

Lidell, Lucinda, *The Book of Massage*, Ebury Press, 1992.

Longworth J C D., *Psychophysiological effects of slow stroke back massage in normotensive females*, Advances in Nursing Science, 1982; July: 44-61.

Maxwell-Hudson, Clare, *The Complete Book of Massage*, Dorling Kindersley, 1988.

Rankin-Box, Denise, *The Nurses Handbook of Complementary Therapies*, Churchill Livingston, 1995.

Tappan, Frances, *Healing Massage Techniques: Healing, Classic and Emerging Methods*, Appleton & Lange, 1988.

Resources

The British Massage Therapy Council
Greenbank House
65a Adelphi Street
Preston
Lancs PR1 7BH
Tel. 01772- 881 063

The Association of Massage Practitioners
101 Bounds Green Road
London N22 4DF

The Association of Physical and Natural Therapists
12 Cottage Road
Stanford in the Vale
Oxon SN7 8HX
Tel. 01367-710 159

Natural Therapies Database UK
47, Ashby Avenue
Chessington
Surrey KT9 2BT

(This organisation carries a data base on massage and bodywork research)

The Clare Maxwell Hudson School of Massage
87 Dartmouth Road
London NW2
Tel. 0181-450 6494

The London College of Massage
5-6 Newman Passage
London W1P 3PF

The Northern Institute of Massage
100 Waterloo Road
Blackpool
Lancs FY4 1 AW
Tel. 01253-403548

Medical Assistance Program

by Christine Wallace

The Medical Assistance Program (MAP) is a self-healing technique, designed to be used by anyone, to work towards health and balance on a physical, emotional, mental and spiritual basis. It presupposes the existence of other levels of form from which humans can receive guidance and practical help from intelligent beings committed to furthering the evolution of consciousness of humankind. It was developed by the intuitive Machaelle Small Wright in the 1980s. She has been a pioneer in working with nature intelligences with whom she has co-created a garden called Perelandra in Virginia, USA.

MAP grew out of Small Wright's extensive research into 'nature'. In Small Wright's definition, nature is the consciousness which supplies order, organisation and life vitality. Small Wright's aim has been to develop a working partnership between humans and nature, based on the principles of co-creation.

> *Co-creative science is qualitatively different from the science we know because it integrates the involutionary input of nature (order, organisation, life vitality/action) with the evolutionary dynamic of man (direction and purpose). Until now, science has been essentially evolutionary. Co-creative science is therefore not a linear advance over present-day science but it is qualitatively unique. It was developed de novo in the sense that it is not derived from contemporary science. It employs different methodologies and obtains information from sources with which contemporary science has never worked.*[1]

Understanding co-creativity in relation to human evolution or one's personal health does not require extensive study or research into science or medicine. All that is required is sincerity, commitment, an open mind and a willingness to make use of the information and methods which Small Wright has collated. While this chapter gives a brief introduction to the method and principles of MAP, it is important to read the full instructions given by Small Wright before attempting to engage in the programme.

How it Started

Chiropractic

Small Wright's first experience that it was possible to receive medical help from another level, was personal. She was having trouble with her structural alignment, and attending a chiropractic clinic to receive extensive adjustments, once or twice a month. Among other symptoms, she was suffering intense headaches. After a year and a half, the most pressing issue of head pain was resolved and the visits discontinued. When the head pains reappeared a year later, in 1984, Small Wright turned to the White Brotherhood, to ask if they could help with this problem. She intuitively began to receive instructions. She was told to lie down, open a coning (a term explained in the book, *MAP*), and she would receive help. Following these and other instructions, in less than an hour, the head pains cleared. Surprised and inspired, she wanted to know if this was a technique that could be used by others. Told that it was, she began to work with the White Brotherhood medical unit and nature intelligences to create and give form to a system which could be communicated to others and which has become known as the Medical Assistance Program (MAP). As a result, many thousands of people are discovering that MAP can help in very practical ways to overcome problems or increase health and well-being.

The Practice of MAP

MAP can be used for physical or emotional problems of any kind. It requires openness, a willingness to commit oneself to following the steps of the programme, and time. A session takes 40 minutes and there is a routine for opening the connection and a timetable for scheduling sessions.[2]

The Medical Assistance Program involves working with a team of White Brotherhood physicians and medical experts and nature. Each person who chooses to work with MAP connects with their own personal team. The first session requires the person to lie still for one hour to allow themselves to be scanned energetically, to identify the energy patterns on all levels and to be matched with the appropriate medical team. In this first session the person will also 'receive' the name they will thereafter use each time they want to communicate with their personal MAP team.

Kinesiology Dowsing

One problem that had to be overcome in order to make MAP accessible to anyone was that of communication between the human and the medical team. The solution was to use the simple kinesiology technique of self muscle checking, whereby one can receive yes/no answers to questions. This works on a principle similar to that of dowsing: the question is posed mentally and the tool of choice (in this case a finger muscle, but it could be a pendulum or a dowsing rod) is used to amplify the response which is projected through the body's electrical system.

Opening a 'Coning'

Opening a coning is the core of the MAP procedure. Small Wright describes coning as 'a balanced vortex of conscious energy'. A 'four-point coning', which is used in any MAP session, includes four elements which are required for the balance to be established and maintained throughout the healing session. So when a coning is opened, one is working within a protected space with energies that create a balance between the human soul and nature. The simplest way to explain it is as a conference call. Working within a coning establishes the framework in which the healing occurs. It creates not only the team but also the 'room' in which the team meets. When a coning is activated only those team members who are a part of the work are invited to be present. The coning is created and activated by the human team member. Only those with whom that person seeks connection will be included.[3]

> *The keystone of MAP is its coning. It is set up to assure a perfect balance between the involution dynamic (nature) and the evolution dynamic (the White Brotherhood and you). The evolution dynamic supplies the purpose and definition to any thing or action. The involution dynamic (nature) supplies the matter, means and action for achieving evolution's purpose and definition. The human soul is the force behind the evolution dynamic. Nature is the force behind involution. In health, the evolution dynamic comes from one's soul. It is from our soul that we receive the impulses that define our direction and our purpose. It is the soul that gives the necessary data to nature for all that is physically required for a human to fully operate within a given lifetime. Nature then supplies our body according to these soul-directed specifications. This also means that nature is the engineer of the human body and, like any good engineer, nature knows how it is supposed to work and how to fix it if it isn't working correctly.[4]*

MAP is a truly co-creative effort; the team will not perform any treatment which is not requested. Therefore, the person's awareness and ability to describe his health issues determines the degree of intervention they receive. So having opened a coning, the person then needs to outline in detail the presenting problems and the relationship perceived between the symptoms and the physical, emotional, mental and spiritual levels and causes. This will indicate to the MAP team precisely what the person is ready to work on.

Perelandra Flower Essences

A powerful way of using MAP is to combine it with the Perelandra flower essences. Perelandra is the name of Small Wright's home and the flower essences were developed by Small Wright in the 1980s.[5] By incorporating the use of flower essences into the MAP session the results of the work done will be stabilised within two hours as opposed to up to 24 hours. It is also suggested that one makes up an 'emergency

Flower Essences

trauma solution' (ETS) by muscle checking which essences are required to produce a personally effective trauma remedy. Within a family, a personalised ETS will be needed for each member. The ETS should be easily available and used for the first 20 minutes following any trauma, whether physical or emotional.

Other Healing Systems and MAP

It is possible for a MAP coning to be used by any health practitioner to enhance and develop their system or modality. In this case it is recommended that the practitioner has worked personally with the basic MAP programme for at least five months before moving on to requesting a professional MAP team. The practitioners are not connected to their personal health team for the work but to a separate team focused on their area of health care. The team will not be working with the client but with the practitioner to expand and shift his health care practices to new Aquarian dynamics.

A Personal Experience

I have been using the MAP for two years as part of my own personal routine of self-development and healing. What I have found particularly helpful about using the MAP programme is that it is immediately accessible whatever time of day or night I need help and for whatever reason. If I am able to identify and articulate the problem then I have immediate access to help. Another important consideration is financial. For the price of a book and the time and commitment to put this system into practice I have been able to move through some major issues in my life, without spending hundreds of pounds on therapy. Many of the issues I have been addressing have been of an emotional nature and have also affected my general physical health and energy levels.

Starting with MAP was a natural progression for me as I already felt confident about self muscle checking, having used it for several years, and was practised at making and holding connections with other planes of intelligence and energy forms. Whenever I am feeling unsettled or off colour, I use muscle checking to find out if I need to do a MAP session. Usually I get a positive answer although occasionally I find I need to meditate or be outside in nature rather than have a MAP session. During some periods of time in the last two years I have needed sessions daily for maybe a week and then nothing for two or three weeks. I am currently in a phase of averaging one or two sessions a week, working mainly on relationship issues. Also, before embarking on writing this chapter I used a MAP session to deal with the specific emotional blockage I had around writing it.

I usually do my MAP sessions lying down as I find it easier to concentrate and stay focused if I am relaxed. I try to stay alert during the session, but sometimes I do fall asleep. Apparently this can happen if the team wants to get the intellectual part of a person out of the way while they work. If I do fall asleep, I will often wake up precisely at the end of the 40-minute session, ready to close the coning.

Last Christmas a flu virus went rampant in our household. Family and visitors started to succumb one by one and as I usually respond badly to such infections, I was anxious. I opened a coning with my MAP team and told them that I did not want to catch this virus. In the event, I didn't. I had sore kidneys; I was very tired (nine invalids in the house may have had something to do with that), but I remained upright and functioning. However, in April I succumbed to a flu virus myself which was intensely debilitating and protracted. I did use MAP but for various reasons I did not resolve this particular problem with MAP alone. I resorted to my homoeopath and then my allopathic doctor during the third and fourth weeks of illness. Any system is only as good as its user and I had slipped into a position where I was not clear about what was going on and had deteriorated physically and emotionally to a point where I no longer cared or had the resources to work at pulling myself out of it. Within four months I believe I finally worked through all the complexities that I was unable or unwilling to deal with earlier. This is an example of how MAP can be used in conjunction with other health care systems.

Since then Small Wright's book, Perelandra Microbial Balancing Program Manual has been published, which outlines how to bring microbes, including viruses, into balance in the body rather than just attempting to kill them off.[6] In the future I will have more tools at my disposal to deal with such a debilitating infection.

Recently, I experienced a pain in the chest resulting from a pulled muscle. I was in so much pain that laughing or coughing was excruciating and at nights I woke every time I moved. I did a total of three MAP sessions over a week and although the area was still slightly tender to pressure it no longer affected my lifestyle in any way. The issues surrounding this particular problem took a lot of deep thought and I received several insights in the course of the week, each of which helped me to move deeper into the core issue once I had identified it. That is the crux of the success of MAP; developing a clearer insight into what is happening on the physical, emotional, mental and spiritual levels of one's being. The more I do and the longer I have been working with MAP the better I become at identifying the issues behind each problem as it presents itself.

My partnership with my MAP team is an ongoing learning situation and as I continue to explore and develop this system the more I discover.

It is important that anyone using MAP has the information contained in the book, *MAP: The Co-Creative White Brotherhood Medical Assistance Program*, by Machaelle Small Wright. For more information, write to: Perelandra Ltd., P O Box 3603, Warrenton, VA 20188, USA.

Biography

Christine Wallace has lived on the west coast of Scotland, running a smallholding and home-educating her three children, for the past 20 years. Her interest in healing and self-care has led her to take courses in massage, intuitive awareness, dowsing and meditation. She is especially interested in working with nature for personal and planetary healing.

References

1   Albert Schatz, PhD., *Preface to Medical Assistance Program*, 2nd Edition, Perelandra, 1994.

2   Machaelle Small Wright, *MAP: The Co-Creative White Brotherhood Medical Assistance Program*, Perelandra Ltd, 1990.

3   See p227–228, op cit.

4   ibid., p227–228.

5   Machaelle Small Wright, *Flower Essences, Reordering our understanding and approach to illness and health*, Perelandra Ltd., 1988.

6   Machaelle Small Wright, *Perelandra Microbial Balancing Program Manual*, Perelandra, 1996.

Further Reading

Small Wright, Machaelle, *Behaving As If the God In All Life Mattered*, Perelandra Ltd., 1983.

———, *Garden Workbook I – A Complete Guide to Gardening With Nature Intelligences*, Perelandra Ltd., 1987.

———, *Garden Workbook II – Co-Creative Energy Processes for Gardening*, Agriculture and Life, Perelandra Ltd., 1990.

———, *Flower Essences, Reordering our understanding and approach to illness and health*, Perelandra Ltd., 1988.

———, *Perelandra Microbial Balancing Program Manual*, Perelandra Ltd., 1996.

Resources

Perelandra, Ltd.
Box 3603
Warrenton, VA 20188
USA
Tel. (540) 937 2153
Fax. (540) 937 3360
email: email@perelandra-ltd.com

Metamorphic Technique
by Barbara Hummel

The word *metamorphosis* comes from the Greek and means transformation. As can be observed in nature, the blueprint for the butterfly is held within the cellular make-up of the initial life form of the caterpillar. The blueprint for the oak tree is already part of the seed which is an acorn. So it can be assumed that human beings carry the blueprint for their transformed state – their potential. They are simply waiting for a catalyst to set the process in motion. For some, this may be contact with the Metamorphic Technique.

History

The founder of the technique was Robert St John, a naturopath who worked in England with handicapped children in the 1960s. He started to use reflexology with the children and noticed that, while it helped considerably with certain symptoms, it did not cure the main problems. Working mostly with Down's syndrome children, St John deduced that the cause that had created their problems occurred some time during their development in the womb. He searched for a zone on the feet which could be related to the gestation period. After considering the fact that a foetus develops from 'head to tail' (cranio-caudal), which is manifested in the spine, he came to form his theory that the spine itself reflects the time period of gestation. The occiput, with its own (foot) reflex at the first joint on the big toe, stands for conception, while the coccyx, with its reflex at the heel, reflects the birth. This initial form of the technique he called 'prenatal therapy'.

Reflexology

St John started working on the reflex zone of the spine on the feet of Down's syndrome children and noticed dramatic changes in them. But he also found that these changes were not permanent, that the patterns seemed too strong to break. So he determined to develop his theories further. There are reflex points for the spine also on the head and hands and he began to work on these points, as well as those on the feet. He viewed the feet as the principle of moving, the hands as the principle of doing and the head as the principle of thinking. This holistic approach towards his patients was fully effective and from then on the changes were permanent: the old patterns did not return once they were gone. He now changed the name to 'Metamorphic Technique', because a metamorphosis is a transformative process which does not contain the possibility of moving backwards (the butterfly cannot become the caterpillar again).

Theoretical Background

Down's syndrome occurs when, very early in the gestation period, chromosome 21 is created three times in each cell-nucleus instead of twice – a genetic fault. There are some recorded cases of Down's syndrome children, who have had sessions in the Metamorphic Technique regularly from a very early stage, who, while they still show some physical signs of Trisomy 21, do not have any intellectual setback.[1]

St John named the two basic behavioural structures he found in people the *afferent* and the *efferent* pattern. The afferent is the one that is receptive (like the nerves leading to the brain which take in information about the outer world), the efferent the one that is responsive (like the nerves which make muscles work). People's behaviour lies somewhere in the middle of these two extremes and can become imbalanced towards either end of the spectrum. Down's syndrome represents an extreme form of imbalance in the efferent pattern because these people seem to lack awareness but are very responsive. The opposite pattern is represented by autism where the patients seem to have a rich inner world but are unresponsive. The Metamorphic Technique can bring people more into balance.

Gaston Saint-Pierre was a pupil of Robert St John who took this work further and spread it throughout the world. His interpretation of how the Metamorphic Technique works was that it seems to loosen the structure of linear time, bringing the gestation period into the present, so that the energies that became blocked then can move in the way they need to – guided by the inner life-force of the person – and bring about transformation.

The Practice of the Metamorphic Technique

As the technique has developed into a practice which is quite widely available, various principles in addition to the actual techniques have become important. The primary principle is that the practitioner's role is one of non-interference. Practitioners facilitate rather than manipulate the path of the life-force. Practitioners do not concentrate on symptoms or on finding a diagnosis; nor do they try to give any solutions to problems, but use the time of the session simply for being there as a catalyst, knowing and accepting that the life-force of the person receiving the session is powerful, appropriate and able to do the work to bring about the transformative changes required.

In this way, the Metamorphic Technique is not seen as a therapy or massage by the practitioners who use it, but rather as a unique tool for self-realisation or transformation.

The actual work of transforming (sometimes resulting in health) occurs as the gentle touch on the feet, hands and head acts as a catalyst for the life-force of the person receiving the session. The practitioner does not give actively but is there for the other person to draw from. This contact helps the life-force to do the wonderful work of transformation in a direction the innate intelligence of the person sees as 'right'. To extend a metaphor used earlier, the earth, which is the catalyst for the acorn, does not give, but is there to loosen the structure and the seedling can draw from it what is needed.

Sometimes dramatic transformations are seen, sometimes none at all. This is not what concerns the practitioner. When a caterpillar with a broken leg transforms into a butterfly, the broken leg is of no further importance. The detachment of the practitioner, which is not always easy to achieve, allows the life-force more freedom to do the work and makes the method safe.

The Metamorphic Technique is a tool that can safely be used by people without any medical background, on themselves or others. It is easily taught in one session. It is ideal for sharing with friends or relatives and between parents and children. It is very accessible and very simple. Nevertheless, people all over the world who have experienced the Metamorphic Technique affirm that their lives have never been the same after they stepped onto the metamorphic path.

A Metamorphic Session

A normal session lasts about an hour. The person receiving treatment can either lie or sit, as long as they are comfortable. The practitioner will sit at right angles to the person, deliberately avoiding a face to face position in order to support the principle of non-interference in the process. Usually practitioners take the feet or hands of the person on their lap with a cloth or cushion between, while they do the massage. The person receiving treatment can decide at any time to end the session; the practitioner will respect the recipient's wishes at all times. The practitioner will gently touch or stroke the reflex zone of the spine on the feet (which is along the inner arch of the foot), then work along the spinal zone of both hands (at the thumb) and will finally work on the head. There is sometimes a feeling of ticklishness for the recipient. This usually stops very soon, but if it does not, the practitioner can cease touching them, and can work off the body instead.

The usual timing is 20 minutes for each foot, 5 minutes for each hand and 10 minutes for the head. No relaxation afterwards is needed, but if the person wishes to, then it should be possible.

There is no specified time interval between sessions, but it is advisable for someone leading a normal working life not to have more than one session per week. This is to ensure that there are not too many demands put on the energy system and that the recipient can continue to function healthily while engaged in the transformation process. Children or people who for some reason do not work can accept as many sessions as feels right for them. Sessions can be given by anyone who is willing to do 'the gentle touch', no matter what their training is, but practitioners should understand the importance of detachment. They need to hold onto the awareness that it is not their work that guides the process. If there is a financial exchange for the session, it is the time that is being paid for, not the results.

If one is treating oneself, or exchanges with the same person on an ongoing basis, it is advisable to get one session in four from someone else to avoid an energy-trapping circle. When sessions are exchanged between friends or in a group, it is not necessary to concentrate solely on the technique. Talking or even reading a book is quite permissible – the process will unfold anyway.

Anyone can receive sessions, no matter what symptoms are present. The practitioner should be responsive to non-verbal signals in people who are unable to express their needs in any other way, for example if a baby pulls back its feet to indicate the end of a session. People who are in therapy because of addiction problems should be told that the transformation process sometimes leads them into regressional patterns; for example they might start drinking again. But experience has demonstrated that there is no danger in this; it can be part of the process of solving the addiction at base.

The Metamorphic Technique can be received together with all therapies; it does not disturb their effectiveness. Very often, people find the particular treatment they require through the metamorphic path.

Because of the paradigm of detachment it is not advisable that the same practitioner works with the same client using the Metamorphic Technique and any therapy in the same period of time.

My Personal Experience

My first contact with the technique was through a friend who gave me a session while we were sitting in front of a fire in winter. It was a very relaxing experience and I slept very deeply afterwards.

Reflexology

Soon after, having studied reflexology, I decided to take part in a Metamorphic Technique workshop. I got a headache and an enormous tiredness came over me, but it felt totally right at the time. I got a very clear understanding of the power of the technique by seeing the results of the other participants as well as my own.

I would advise anyone to take part in one of these workshops, even if they have no interest in becoming a practitioner. Seeing how the Metamorphic Technique catalyses transformations is very motivating and moving. I am personally convinced that my life would have been totally different without it. Since then I seem to meet the right people at the right time without any effort; or if I have to go through a period of chaos, it usually feels right in the end. I made good use of the technique during my pregnancies and labour with my three children. They were all born totally naturally and without any complications. They are all very lively.

Working in groups with the technique is, for me, most rewarding. Not only do I receive sessions from others, but everyone gets to see how effective it is for every participant.

Testimonials Regarding the Metamorphic Technique

The Metamorphic Technique has been used quite widely in institutions concerned with the welfare of disturbed children and other 'problem' members of society. The following are testimonials from doctors or heads of institutions who have witnessed the effects of the technique on those for whom they are responsible.[2]

> *I was introduced to the Metamorphic Technique some four years ago. Since then I have seen the remarkable changes which have taken place in patients generally regarded by the medical profession as 'incurables' – especially in the fields of mental health. I am now currently engaged in research in the Metamorphic Technique and have had some most encouraging results to date.*
>
> — Dr R.S. Durrant MD LCSP
> Heatherlea Educational Unit (ESN)

> *I have personally received metamorphic treatment, so as to experience its value at first hand; I have in addition observed its effects on severely mentally handicapped people (young and old) who reside at Leytonstone House. I can confirm that it has a very soothing and calming effect on the nervous system and I was particularly impressed at the excellent rapport which the practitioners were able to establish with those undergoing this form of treatment. Since, generally speaking, mentally handicapped individuals receive far too little rewarding stimulation, I regard metamorphic therapy as being especially applicable and useful for such individuals.*
>
> — Dr D A MacSweeney
> Consultant psychiatrist, Leytonstone House
> Senior lecturer and Hon. consultant in mental handicap,
> The London Hospital Medical College

> *As a medical doctor, my initial reactions to the claims made for this treatment were sceptical ones, since I have difficulty in understanding how such treatment can work, when it accords with no known physiological principles known to the Western mind. Having said this, my reactions*

have had to be modified by having seen the effects it has had upon individuals well known to me. These include a teen-age girl with clinically proven glandular fever, whose recovery from this debilitating disease was rapid and free of sequelae. At the same time there was a dramatic improvement of her hand eczema. Reflecting upon this and other experiences, I feel that what I have seen goes beyond any placebo effect; neither can it be related solely to the personality of the therapist who carried out the massage... Clearly something of a healing nature has been operating and I would therefore consider it important that this means of therapy, its nature and effects, should be confirmed and investigated further.

— Dr P.H. Tatham MA MB BCh

Blaisdon Hall is a special boarding school for 55 emotionally disturbed boys aged from ten to sixteen. For the past year, [two practitioners of the Metamorphic Technique] have treated boys with a wide range of problems; from angry, hostile boys to pathologically indecisive, withdrawn boys, others who are unintegrated and some victims of early maternal deprivation... The apparently simple, direct form of metamorphic treatment appealed immediately to our boys. Instead of dismissing it as 'way out' or 'weird', they all come readily and willingly; there are always two or three boys waiting to begin treatment... All the boys who have experienced the Metamorphic Technique have benefited from it. The results speak for themselves: they go far beyond what anyone may expect. In certain of our boys, we have seen dramatic change for the better. From my own experience, I am convinced that the Metamorphic Techniques can and does achieve good, beneficial results with emotionally disturbed boys..

— Fr J. Pilling MA
Psychiatric Social Worker

Raddery is a school for 30 disturbed and disturbing children from all over Scotland. For the last four years, we have happily and productively utilised the Metamorphic Technique... I am quite sure in my own mind that participating in the technique has been of some assistance to our very difficult children. That they could contemplate it in the beginning was remarkable and yet succeeding pupils have retained an interest and fervour for it over the four years...

— David Dean
Principal of Raddery School

Biography

Barbara Hummel was born in 1962 in Munich, Germany. She trained as a physiotherapist, reflexologist and yoga teacher and worked for 11 years in hospitals as well as in private practice. She is also the mother of three daughters. She learned the Metamorphic Technique in 1985 from two different teachers, both direct pupils of Robert Saint John and also from Gaston Saint Pierre. She organised workshops for Gaston Saint Pierre in Bavaria and acted as translator for him. She is a member of the Metamorphic Association, living in Scotland since August 1995.

References

1   Robert St John, *Prenatal Therapy and the Retarded Child*, Robert St John, Norfolk 1976.

2   reprinted with the kind permission of the Metamorphic Association.

Further Reading

St. John, Robert, *The Prenatal Therapy and the Retarded Child*, Robert St John, 1976.

St. Pierre, Gaston; Shapiro, Debbie, *The Metamorphic Technique, Principles and Practice*, Element, 1982.

St. Pierre, Gaston; d'Arcy Thompson, Barbara, *Fundamentals of the Metamorphic Technique* (Short Guide), available from the Metamorphic Association, London.

The Journal of the Metamorphic Association.

Resources

Books, videos, tapes and the journal, as well as addresses of members and practitioners and the schedule of workshops given by Gaston-St. Pierre are available from:

The Metamorphic Association London
67 Ritherdon Road
London SW17 8QE
Tel/Fax. 0181 672 5951

*(The Metamorphic Association prints out
a list of practitioners every four months)*

Naturopathy

by Keki Sidhwa

♣

Health and Wellness as the Focus of Health Care

Naturopathy is the science of healing based on the principle of co-operation with those natural laws of life already working within as well as outside the body – a re-establishment of the harmonious relationship between human beings and the earth on which they depend for their sustenance. In order to be healthy the primordial requisites of life have to be met in full. These include adequate rest and sleep; exposure to fresh air, sunshine and warmth; the ingestion of wholesome food derived from wholesome soil, providing the body with the nutrients it requires; exercise in sufficient quantity, including aerobic, to build strength and flexibility; mental and emotional poise to meet the stresses and strains of life; freedom to express opinions rather than their curtailment by the established norms of a particular society; and faith in the capability of the body to renew and repair and rejuvenate if sufficient time and patience are bestowed by the ailing person.

Naturopathy does not deny the presence of bacteria and viruses, but believes they are only secondary factors. The discussion whether the environment or the pathogen is the determining factor is as old as the discovery of microbes in the nineteenth century. It is reported that even Louis Pasteur, the famous bacteriologist, declared, 'The pathogen is nothing. The terrain is everything.'[1]

Rudolph Virchow, the father of modern pathology, emphasised the need to consider environmental causes of health, not simply the microbes.[2] In 1957 Prof. René Dubos, a microbiologist, admitted that the 'soil' in which these germs thrive is more important than the germs per se.[3]

Historical Background

The practice of naturopathy goes back a long way. The Persian, Babylonian and Greek traditions and the Hindu *vedas* and yoga *sutras* all expressed some of the basic precepts of naturopathy. The Greek Aesculapian temples were devised to heal the human organism by hygienic measures. In ancient times, human beings depended on fasting and praying to get well. They rested, and since the body has the innate power to heal and repair, they got well.

Modern day naturopathy came into being more or less simultaneously in Europe and America. In Germany and Austria a tradition of nature cure started with Vincenz Priessnitz (1799–1851), a simple but observant farmer, who founded a healing establishment in Grafenberg, based on the use of water, air, diet and exercise. He took his patients back to nature, to the woods, the streams and open fields, and treated them with the natural elements and prescribed a diet of unadulterated foods. He was followed by various other well-known unorthodox healers like Johannes Schroth (1798–1856), an Austrian, who developed a treatment for chronic diseases based on a rigorous diet, including fasting and physical applications such as wet packs and poultices; Sebastian Kneipp (1821–1897), better known as Father Kneipp, a Bavarian, who became famous for his hydrotherapy cures; Arnold Rickli (1823–1907), who established a light and air sanatorium (atmospheric cures) in Austria in 1848; and Louis Kuhne (circa 1823–1907) of Leipzig, who wrote in 1891 *The New Science of Healing*, a work on the basic principles in natural healing. Kuhne is the founder and first master of naturopathy.

The history of naturopathy was not, however, made only in Europe. Long before the Europeans, Dr Isaac Jennings (1788–1874) of the USA, a qualified medical doctor, decided in 1820 to give up prescribing drugs for his patients when he stumbled by chance on the precept that it is the body (the living organism) that heals and that the drugs only disguise the symptoms. He was influenced by Sylvester Graham, a Presbyterian preacher, who created the Graham bread, which is still known today. Dr Jennings founded the movement called hygienism, derived from Hygeia the Greek goddess of health. He also coined the word orthopathy, that is, right action on the part of the body when it has an acute inflammatory disease.

Dr Jennings was really the forerunner of the modern day natural hygiene movement. His fame spread far and wide in the USA and many other doctors followed in his footsteps. One of them, Dr John Tilden, was originally a practising medical doctor in Denver, Colorado, who turned to dietetics and nutrition, formulating his theory of 'auto-intoxication' and 'toxaemia'. One of the major proponents of natural hygiene in the twentieth century was Dr Herbert Shelton[4], who died aged 90 in 1985. In Britain there were Stanley Lief, an American-trained naturopathic and chiropractic physician, who founded Champney's Health Farm near London, and James Thomson, the founder of the Kingston Clinic in Edinburgh.

Nutritional Therapy

These pioneers relied on fasting or restricting the food consumption of their acute and chronically ill patients. They believed in plenty of sleep and rest; moderate daily activities; sunbaths; air baths; relaxation; massage; hydrotherapy to give relief (not cure) and comfort; manipulation, where structural integrity had to be maintained (by osteopathic or chiropractic means); psychological counselling and re-education of patients to motivate them by example and education to live a healthier lifestyle in order to prevent disease and maintain optimum health.

Relaxation Therapy
Massage
Osteopathy
Chiropractic
Counselling

Theoretical Background

Naturopathy, which used to be known as *nature cure* in Britain, recognises three primary life requirements of the physical cells of the human body:

◆ The cells must have enough inherent nerve energy to function.

◆ The cells need to be provided with the nutrients which they require.

◆ There is a need for drainage, that is, discharging the waste matter which each cell manufactures in the process of functioning.

It therefore follows that the causes of bodily disease stem from disruption in one of these primary life requirements:

◆ Lowered vitality or enervation due to overwork, overindulgence or overstimulation, poisonous drugs, ill-advised surgical operations, mental shock or emotional strain.

◆ Abnormal composition of blood and lymph due to improper diet, especially living mainly on refined foods, too much fat, sugar, salt or stimulants and lack of organic mineral salts. In the last decade neurobiologists and immunologists have amassed much research pointing to a link between the brain and the immune system.[5] Wrong thinking and lack of emotional poise breeds anxiety, neurosis and tension which deplete the body of its vitality and nerve energy.

◆ Due to the above factors the body becomes toxic – what Dr John Tilden called toxaemia[6] and modern day researchers call accumulation of free radicals.

Naturopathy recognises that disease symptoms are a means whereby the body expresses its discomfort at the inharmonious functioning of the cells, tissues and organs and that most acute diseases, for example colds, fever, inflammation, boils and skin eruptions are the means by which the body tries to establish homoeostasis within the living organism by elimination of toxaemia.

Naturopathy believes that the healing power is resident in the living organism and that each cell is equipped to deal with this toxaemic load. Thus naturopathy postulates that the suppression of every acute disease symptom by drugs, sera, vaccines and certain surgical procedures like removal of tonsils or adenoids, prepares the body for more chronic disease in the future. Acute disease, and inflammation, is a process manufactured by the body to correct body chemistry and establish normality. When this process is interfered with or suppressed by various means, the body will continue to attempt to complete the process of self-cleansing. This process is stimulated even more by suppressive chemicals, which are alien to the body. After a few attempts the body gets tired and debilitated, as acute disease is a process which consumes vitality. When the body has reached such a stage where it can no longer nurture up enough energy and vitality to have a vigorous self-cleansing, then it has reached the stage of chronic disease.

Almost all acute diseases are self-limiting by nature; the body repairs and rejuvenates in spite of the abuse of the living organism, but repeated abuse renders the body irreparable. Even then the natural hygiene mode of living can prolong life and make it more comfortable as in the case of cancer, severe arthritis and other degenerative diseases.

We all need the primordial requisites of life (rest and sleep; sound nutrition; physical activity; sun and air baths; cleanliness and sanitary habits; freedom from worry, fear, anxiety and negative thinking). People who put these principles into practice will help themselves to heal. It is self-evident that if people stop doing the things that make them ill, they will start to get well. Frequently a simple change in eating habits can make a dramatic difference: avoiding stimulants and denatured, processed, packaged, pasteurised or microwaved foods and eating moderately of fresh fruits and vegetables, wholegrains, nuts and seeds and some low fat dairy products.

Missing a meal now and again to experience what real hunger means rather than eating from habit, practising daily exercises which involve some aerobic and strength-building activities, securing more sleep and rest, learning to control emotional outbursts – all these can assist the body to put itself right. These practices will then reduce the amounts of drugs required, which in turn will increase people's health dramatically. Research now shows that over 35% of illnesses are due to so-called side effects of drugs. While I am not advocating that people should take into their own hands the decision to stop all medications, I am convinced that putting the natural hygiene concepts into practice will enable a lot of people to come off the drugs on which they have become dependent, for example tranquillisers, antidepressants and antibiotics.

The Practice of Naturopathy

Since naturopathy is basically a science of healthful living, my approach to my patient is educational. During an hour-long consultation, I not only try to assess the signs and symptoms of the disease process going on in the body, but try to find out what brought it all about and what the patient has been doing to eradicate the problem.

Medical History and Examination

In the consultation I try to find out the health of the mother when she conceived the patient and subsequently during the birth; whether the patient was breast or bottle fed, vaccinated or not, given drugs in early life, how childhood diseases were treated and whether drug therapy was applied. Many chronic ill-health problems stem from such procedures, that is, from the suppression of acute diseases such as fever, boils, sore throats, flu and other infectious diseases by treating the symptoms with drugs, sera, vaccines, tonics, etc.

Preconceptual Care

After this preliminary investigation, I approach the patient regarding the present day mode of life. How much sleep and rest they secure daily, any time for actual unwinding and relaxation, both mental and physical. I ascertain their posture – sitting, standing and walking. I give them a physical examination using palpation; auscultation; touch; monitoring of pulse, heart rate, blood pressure, weight; and occasionally blood tests, when I consider it necessary. I am also a qualified osteopath and bring my osteopathic skills to ascertain any structural misalignment in joints and the spine.

Osteopathy

Nutrition

Nutritional Therapy

Nutrition is the key to good health, and the next step is to find out the kind of fare that my patients are having daily for breakfast, lunch and dinner and snacks. Today it is widely recognised that living on junk foods produces ill health. The nutritional value of such foods is so poor that they do not provide the immune system with the nutrients it requires to cope with water, soil and air pollution. Such foods lack the natural enzymes, vitamins and minerals essential to each cell. Sugar, salt and fat added to manufactured food overload the body with these substances which are not part of natural food. In naturopathy the emphasis is on the quality of the food we put into our digestive tract rather than the quantity. I also enquire of my patients whether they are smokers (active or passive) and whether they drink alcohol, and if so, how often and how much.

The duty of a natural hygiene practitioner, as I call myself, is to teach people how to maintain and preserve their health, if necessary by changing their lifestyle. Food is the building block and we emphasise to our patients the value of eschewing all 'foodless foods' and beverages such as tea, coffee, alcohol and soda drinks, in favour of fresh fruits and raw salads, cooked vegetables (steamed or stir-fried), whole grains, pulses, nuts and seeds. I recommend a minimum of dairy products, since most of our dairy foods are now made with homogenised and pasteurised milk. These processes de-naturise an originally wholesome and nutritious food. I cajole and encourage my patients to adopt a vegetarian diet and have been advocating this for more than four decades.

My views on nutrition are now echoed by Dr Neil Barnard, President of the Physicians' Committee for Responsible Medicine, which represents 3500 US medical doctors. He says, 'The major dietary change is to avoid animal products: not just beef, but also chicken, fish, eggs and dairy products'. Dr Barnard believes that animal protein is a major cause of degenerative diseases and animal fat consumption lowers the immune system.

Exercise and Environment

Apart from food and drink, I enquire whether my patient is allocating enough time to fresh air and sunshine to counterbalance the stuffy atmosphere in most workplaces and homes. My next investigation is to assess how much physical activity and exercise they practise. It has been shown by modern research that exercise, whether it be sport, swimming, weight training, jogging, brisk walking or cycling, contributes to helping the immune system to remain intact and build health, mentally and physically.[7]

Today naturopathy is so fragmented that I prefer to call myself a natural hygienist. Natural hygiene, which has been called 'the purest form of naturopathy', does not concentrate only on physical means but pays a good deal of attention to the mental, emotional and spiritual aspirations of the patient. It is indeed a holistic approach to ill-health. My stance is that while modalities such as massage, hydrotherapy, reflexology, acupuncture, etc. can be useful to alleviate pain and bring relief, they must be secondary to removing the basic cause of ill-health, which is our pattern of living.

Massage
Reflexology
Acupuncture

I see patients either once a week or once a fortnight, not to treat diseases, but to monitor their progress and motivate them further to lead a more disciplined life. Since naturopathy is all-embracing it can be used in all circumstances for both acute and chronic ill-health. Of course, there are circumstances where outside intervention is needed and should be applied, as in certain medical and surgical emergencies. Even in such life-threatening situations, the basic principles of natural hygiene will help enormously to get the living organism (our human body) on a sound footing of health and vigour. Natural hygiene does not deny the progress that modern technology has made in life-threatening situations, especially in the field of surgery. But most naturopaths believe that the aftercare of such patients, when based on natural hygiene principles, will ensure a quicker rate of recovery, as I myself have witnessed on numerous occasions.

A real naturopath is seldom popular since people do not like changing their lifestyle or pattern of living. Most people are looking for a remedy and so will prefer to go to an orthodox medical professional rather than to a naturopath. The whole art of naturopathy is counselling, in order to find out what individuals are doing in their lives and then correct and balance it. A natural hygiene practitioner has to be a guide, philosopher and friend. It has been my life's work to raise awareness of the fact that health care is self-care, so that people can take up the cudgels against all the vested interests that are threatening their health. I feel that unless we do that we are going to get more degenerative diseases, more ill-health and more suffering and death than we have ever seen.

I remember being at the Bronx Zoo in New York many years ago. There was a sign saying 'Come and see the most dangerous animal on earth' – and there was a cage with a mirror in it, reflecting those who came to look. It stuck in my mind. Human beings are sick today because we have endangered our health by polluting the earth, the water, the air we breathe and the food we eat, and by adopting a lifestyle based on greed, violence and non-awareness of our spiritual selves. Unless a healthy human existence is made possible, we will still only be scratching the surface when we just use modalities to treat symptoms. We have to teach people that prevention is better than cure.

Training

In America there are various colleges and institutions where students undergo training of four to five years in anatomy, physiology, biochemistry, diagnosis, dietetics, fasting, the use of water for relief, and counselling, to equip them to care for their patients. John Bastyr College in Seattle now has a course in natural hygiene methods; there is a college in Portland and other smaller establishments, as well as the International Association of Professional Natural Hygienists, which certifies people in training to supervise fasts.

In Britain there is the British College of Naturopathy founded by Stanley Lief with a full-time four year course. Here students are taught anatomy, physiology, biochemistry, diagnosis, principles and practice of naturopathy, manipulative skills, etc.

Research

That naturopathy works efficiently in helping people to get well is empirically ascertained by hundreds of thousands who have drastically changed their lifestyle and are now healthier and happier human beings. What naturopathic and natural hygienist pioneers preached and thought over 150 years ago is now being echoed by modern research into the questions of diet, of sleep and rest, of the elimination of free radicals by fasting, and of activity and exercise in obesity, heart and circulatory problems.

Fasting – A Cornerstone of Naturopathy

Fasting is defined as abstinence from all food and drink except water for a specific period of time, usually for therapeutic or religious reasons. The history of fasting goes back thousands of years. Almost all great religious leaders fasted. Hippocrates and the ancient Greeks prescribed fasting for their ill patients in the Aesculapian Temples.

During the fast the body sustains metabolism by extracting nutrients from the non-essential tissues (adipose tissue, digestive enzymes, muscle contractile fibres and glycolytic enzymes). This process does not compromise the vital organs – the heart, lungs, liver, kidneys – and the brain and nerves, or deplete the mineral and vitamin status.[8]

Fasting and starvation are not synonymous. Starvation begins when, during fasting, all the reserves are used up.

Fasting is physiological rest. It enables the body to repair, rejuvenate and detoxify through various channels of elimination. During the fast it is advisable to secure adequate physical, mental, emotional and sensory rest, so that the body can use the energy for healing and repair work. Fasting means 'downing tools': bed rest, very little reading or watching TV or listening to music. It is important to have sensory rest, to close the eyes and relax completely. During the fast the body uses this conservation of energy for more useful purposes such as heightening the sense of taste, smell, hearing and visual clarity, and detoxifying the liver, lungs and digestive tract of the accumulated debris. Awareness and creativity can become heightened. Pythagoras, the Greek philosopher, fasted for 40 days before he took his University of Alexandria exams and would advise his students to do the same. Having myself fasted several times in my life I can verify the experience. Over 25,000 patients over a period of 43 years have fasted under my supervision, from 3 to 4 days at a time up to 62 days, and I can truly say that this kind of rest afforded to the body enables it to repair and rejuvenate in a way that no other method can.

During the fast there may be some symptoms such as light-headedness, mild palpitation, nausea or vomiting, headaches, rise in temperature, backaches, sore throats, etc. But these soon disappear as the fast continues. However, natural hygiene practitioners have always suggested that a prolonged fast of more than five days should be done under competent supervision in hygienic surroundings where fresh air, peace and quiet, and mental and emotional support are provided. Distilled water is the ideal to drink – otherwise purified water or Malvern water should be used, because Malvern is the water with the least inorganic mineral salts in it.

The chemistry of the body changes during the fast, especially blood chemistry. This has been monitored with blood tests in many studies.[9] It is advisable to prepare for a fast by going on a diet of fresh fruit for one to two days beforehand to avoid withdrawal symptoms. Most people would be able to carry out a short fast of two to four days in their own home, but I prefer that they read one or two books on the subject before they do. Longer fasts and fasts for people with serious illnesses should only be undertaken under competent supervision.

During a fast there is a definite rejuvenance.[10] Wounds heal faster, hormones balance out,[11] inflammation subsides and all vital organs – liver, heart, lungs, kidneys and digestion – have improved function. During the fast, the cytoplasm of the cell decreases to maintain nourishment, but the nuclei of the cells retain their size. M. Kunde, a professor at Chicago University, wrote: 'It becomes evident that where the initial weight was reduced by 45% and subsequently restored by normal diet, approximately one half of the restored body is made up of new protoplasm. In this there is rejuvenescence.'[12] On 18 May 1933, one of the physicians attending Mahatma Gandhi during his fast reported that on the tenth day of the fast, 'despite his 64 years, from a physiological point of view, the Indian leader is as healthy as a man of 40'.

Toxins are rapidly discharged from the system while a person fasts. This was observed in a study of PCB poisoned patients in Taiwan in 1984.[13]

Fasts can be broken with fresh raw fruits in small quantities, for example three or four small meals, or with fresh raw fruit and vegetable juices, about 40 ounces per day divided into four or five glasses. After very long fasts it is better to break the fast with diluted juices.

Almost all chronic and acute diseases are benefited by fasting. Numerous studies have been undertaken in diseases including patients with diabetes,[14] obesity,[15] epilepsy[16] and rheumatoid arthritis.[17] In my own experiences patients with long-standing digestive and metabolic disturbances, and those with food intolerance and allergy will benefit greatly after a fast. Long fasts, in particular, have helped many to overcome their various addictions to tea, coffee, alcohol, tobacco, salt, sugar and strong spices. However, people with diabetes, history of tachycardia, fibrillation, heart block and various kidney diseases should abstain from fasting unless well monitored.[18]

Transcendental Meditation

The most common mistake made while fasting is to be active instead of resting. Watching a lot of TV or reading can also be counter-productive. Fear of fasting can be avoided by preparatory reading, so that all negative emotions are excluded and fasting is done with a positive attitude. Fasting goes hand in hand with prayer or meditation and this is a useful way of being connected to one's own divinity. Another common mistake is to break the fast with concentrated foods which can lead to oedema. Post-fasting nutrition is very important otherwise most of the benefits will be undone. How you live after the fast is as important as the fast itself. A yearly fast is advisable, or three or four fasts per year of three to four days. It could save a life when everything else has failed.

Biography

Keki Sidhwa was born in Bombay, India. After studying at Bombay University, he graduated from the Edinburgh College of Natural Therapeutics and the British College of Naturopathy and Osteopathy. He has been in private practice since 1952 and is the co-founder and president of the British Natural Hygiene Society, ex-president of the International Association of Hygienic Physicians, and the founder and director of Shalimar Health Home, where he has helped over 25, 000 people using hygienic precepts. He has lectured extensively in Europe, India, America and Britain where he now resides. He is editor of the magazine *The Hygienist*, now in its 36th year, and the author of several books.

References

1   J E Pizzorno; M T Murray, *A Textbook of Natural Medicine, Vol I+II*, John Bastyr College Publications, 1987.

2   G Rosen, *From Medical Police to Social Medicine,* Science History Publications, 1974.

3   R Dubos, *Mirage of Health*, Harper & Row, 1957.

4   H M Shelton, *Fasting Can Save your Life*, Natural Hygiene Press, 1964.

———, *Fasting for Renewal of Life*, Natural Hygiene Press, 1978.

———, *The Science and Fine Art of Fasting*, Natural Hygiene Press, 1978.

5   The recent science of psychoneuroimmunology (PNI) has a large number of interesting publications of which we can only list a few here:

R Ader; N Cohen; D Felten (eds), *Brain, Behaviour and Immunity*, Academic Press, 1990 This is a journal that covers regularly research in PNI.

S Cohen; D A J Tyrrell; A. P. Smith, *Psychological stress and susceptibility to the common cold*, N Engl J Med, 1991; 325: 606-12.

6   John Tilden's papers were largely published 1915-1925.

7   E Fuller, *The role of exercise in relief of stress*, in R Eliot (ed) Stress and the Heart, Futura, 1974.

J H Griest, MH Klein, R R Eischens, J W Faris, *Running as a treatment for non-psychotic depression*, Behavioral Medicine, 6, 19-24.

J D Brown, *Staying fit and staying well: physical fitness as moderator of life stress*, J of Personality and Social Psychology, 1991; 60: 555-61.

8   A Keys; J Brozek; A Henschel, et al., *The biology of human starvation*, Vol 1&2, University of Minnesota Press, 1950.

9   N Ende, *Starvation studies with special reference to cholesterol*, Am J Clin Nutr, 1962, 11: 270-80.

A M Uden; L Trang; N Venizelos; J Palmblad, *Neutrophil function and clinical performances after total fasting in patients with rheumataoid arthritis*, Ann Rheum Dis, 1983, 42: 45-51.

10   G Hoeffel; M Moriarty, *The effects of fasting on metabolism*, Am J Dis Child, 1924, 28: 16-24.

11   V R Young; N S Scrimshaw, *The physiology of starvation*, Sci Am, 1971, 225: 4: 14-21.

I Z Beitins; A Barkan; A Kiblanski, et al., *Hormonal responses to short term fasting in post menopausal women*, L Clin Metab, 1985, 60: 1120-6.

12   M Kunde, *The after effects of prolonged fasting*, J Metab Research, 1923.

R Weindruch; R Walford, *The Retardation of Aging by Dietary Restriction*, Charles Thomas, 1988.

L Chaitow, *Natural Life Extension*, Thorsons, 1992.

13   M Imamura; T Tung, *A trial of fasting cure for PCB poisoned patients of Taiwan*, Am J In Med., 1984, 5: 147-53.

14   Guelpa, *Starvation and purgation in the relief of diabetes*, Br Med J, 1910; ii: 1050-51.

F M Allen, *Prolonged fasting in diabetes*, Am J Med Sci, 1915, 150: 480-5.

15   W L Bloom, *Fasting as an introduction to the treatment of obesity*, Metabolism, 1959, 8: 214-20.

E J Drenick; ME Swenseid; WH Blahd; S Tuttle, *Prolonged starvation as a treatment for severe obesity*, JAMA, 1964, 187: 100-5.

18   W G Lennox; S Cobb, *Studies in epilepsy*, Arch Neurol Psych, 1928; 20: 711-79.

19   T Sundquist; F Lindstrom; K Magnusson; L Skoldstam, *Influence of fasting on intestinal permeability and disease activity in patients with rheumatoid arthritis shows normalisation during fasting*, Scan J Rheumatol, 1982, 11: 33-8.

G F Kroker; R M Stroud; R Marshall, et al., *Fasting and rheumatoid arthritis: a multicentre study*, Clin Ecology, 1984, 2: 3: 137-44.

20   F Norbury, *Contraindications to longterm fasting*, JAMA, 1964, i: 1378-9.

A Burton, *A fasting too long*, Health Science, 1979, 2: 144-6.

Further Reading

Benjamin, Harry, *Everybody's Guide to Nature Cure*, Thorsons, 1983.

Campbell, A. (ed), *Natural Health Handbook*, Burlington, 1991.

Chaitow, Leon, *Body/Mind Purification Program*, Simon and Schuster, 1990.

Diamond, Harvey and Marilyn, *Fit for Life*, (I) Bantam, 1987; (II) Warner Books, 1993.

Lindlahr, Henry, *Philosophy of Natural Therapeutics*, CW Daniel, 1981.

———, *Practice of Natural Therapeutics*, CW Daniel, 1975.

Loomis, Evarts, *Healing for Everyone*, DeVorss & Co., 1975.

Murray, Michael; Pizzorno, Joseph, *Encyclopedia of Natural Medicine*, Macdonald Optima, 1990.

Newman Turner, R., *Naturopathic Medicine: Treating the Whole Person*, Thorsons, 1990.

Oswald, J A, Shelton, H M, *Fasting for the Health of It*, Nationwide Press, 1983

Pizzorno, Joseph; Murray, Michael, *A Textbook of Natural Medicine*, Vol I+II, John Bastyr College Publications, 1987.

Salloum, Trevor, *Fasting Signs and Symptoms – A Clinical Guide*, Buckeye Naturopathic Press, 1992.

Salloum, Trevor; Burton, A., *A Therapeutic Fasting Textbook of Natural Medicine* (eds J Pizzorno, M Murray), Bastyr University Press, 1989.

Shelton, Herbert, *Fasting Can Save Your Life*, Natural Hygiene Press, 1964.

———, *Fasting for Renewal of Life*, Natural Hygiene Press, 1978.

———, *The Science and Fine Art of Fasting*, Natural Hygiene Press, 1978.

———, *The Hygienic System*, Natural Hygiene Press, 1971.

Sidhwa, Keki, *The Quintessence of Natural Living for Health and Happiness*, British Natural Hygiene Society, 1994.

———, *Medical Drugs on Trial – Verdict Guilty*, American Natural Hygiene Society, 1976.

Siegel, Bernie, *Love, Medicine and Miracles*, Arrow Books, 1990.

————, *Peace, Love and Healing*, Arrow Books, 1991.

Simonton, Carl; Matthews-Simonton, Stephanie; Creighton, James, *Getting Well Again: A step-by Step Guide to Overcoming Cancer for Patients and Their Families*, Bantam, 1986.

Trattler, Ross, *Better Health Through Natural Healing*, Thorsons, 1987.

Wilhelmi-Buchinger, Maria, *Fasting: The Buchinger Method*, C W Daniel Co., 1986.

Resources

British Natural Hygiene Society
c/o Shalimar
3 Harold Grove
Finton-on-Sea
Essex CO13 9BD
Tel. 01255-672823

British Naturopathic and Osteopathic Association
Frazer House
6 Netherall Gardens
London NW3 5RR
Tel. 01458-840 072

General Council and Register of Naturopaths
Goswell House
2 Goswell Road
Street
Somerset BA16 0JG
Tel. 01458-840 072

Incorporated Society of Registered Naturopaths
The Coach House
293 Gilmerton Road
Liberton
Edinburgh EH16 5UQ
Tel. 0131-664 3435

British College of Naturopathy
6 Netherhall Gardens,
London NW3 6RR
Tel. 0191-435 6464

USA:

International Association of Professional Natural Hygienists
c/o Mark Huberrman
204 Stambough Building
Youngstown, OH 44503

National College of Naturopathic Medicine
11231 SE Market Street
Portland, Oregon 97216
Tel. (503)255-4860

John Bastyr University
144 NE 54th
Seattle WA, 98105
Tel. (206) 523 9585

Neuro-Linguistic Programming (NLP)
by Magdalena Mihm

Perceptions Determine Reality

One autumn afternoon I stood at the edge of a bay gazing at the wondrous sight before me. The sun was low in the sky and its beautiful striations cast reflections of vivid reds and pinks in the mirroring water below. Against the sky was the silhouette of a forest and the shadowy outlines of silent birds darted in the slight breeze. The sea was calm, rocking the seagulls gathered on its surface and whispering quietly as it lapped the sand beneath me.

In contrast, behind me cars droned by, a motor bike with its shrill engine crescendoed as it passed, vibrating the ground beneath it. Workmen were drilling the road, their mechanical tools pounding the hard tar. Trucks thundered in the distance and, in the sky, jet fighters from the nearby air base ripped through the air, painfully assaulting my eardrums.

If I had been deaf this would have seemed like the most beautiful place on earth. If I had been blind it would have seemed horrific. One of the fundamental beliefs of NLP is that it is easier to change your perception of reality than reality itself.

Explanation of Terms

To understand NLP, it is useful to define the words:

◆ *Neuro*: relates to how information is taken in through the senses and how the brain processes this information. Utilising this knowledge of how the brain functions and using methods to interrupt dysfunctional patterns, quick changes can be facilitated.

◆ *Linguistic*: refers to how one's understanding of 'reality' is expressed through language and how, in turn, the language influences the experience of reality. For instance, saying 'I can't do this' or saying ' I can't do this yet' conveys two very different messages.

◆ *Programming*: addresses becoming consciously aware of the above processes and learning to use them for one's benefit.

Another key word in NLP is *modelling*. Learning a new skill is achieved most effectively from somebody who demonstrates it. Modelling means observing very closely how highly skilled people do what they do, finding out all the essential details and mentally identifying with them, asking oneself what it is they see, hear, say and feel internally and externally. NLP teaches techniques to do this.

Short History of NLP

NLP began in the early 70s, as a modelling process. Richard Bandler, a mathematician, and John Grinder, a linguist, were intrigued by the fact that some psychotherapists, such as Fritz Perls, Virginia Satir and Milton Erickson, were so strikingly successful while others were not.

Gestalt Therapy
Family Therapy

Fritz Perls developed Gestalt therapy, opening up a holistic view of people and emphasising the importance of role play in psychotherapy. He worked with the tool of bringing past experience into the present, processing it while staying aware of the internal reactions and exploring them in the moment. Virginia Satir was famous for her therapeutic work with families and couples and her extraordinary communication skills. She encouraged her clients to become aware of any omissions, distortions and generalisations in their communication and thereby helped them create more fulfilling relationships. Milton Erickson was a master in addressing and working with the unconscious mind. He deliberately used a vague language in his hypnotic work, so that his clients could relate to the images based on their own experience. His outstanding accomplishment in renewing hypnotherapy paved the way for a well-established therapy form which continues to fascinate and inspire thousands of practitioners.

Hypnotherapy

Bandler and Grinder observed these therapists intensively for a long period of time, listening to audio tapes and observing them working with clients in order to discover patterns they used. They modelled these therapists so that they could learn and so teach the patterns they used to other people.

What these outstanding therapists had in common was the ability to create rapport with their clients. They had outstanding communication skills and were able to 'pace' their clients' own reality. *Pacing* means using the same language, responding to and mirroring the client's representation of reality. Pacing can happen through matching the other person's body movement, breathing, language – predicates and syntax for example. It is then possible to lead the person into new experience. The more one can perceive about the components of people's reality, the more one knows about how to listen and the more successful one will be in communication and in creating rapport with others.

Some Principles of NLP

Psychotherapy

NLP is not a therapy: it is a way of maximising communication. NLP can therefore be applied in psychotherapy, health care, education, business, performing arts and in any field of work which involves communication.

Emphasis is laid on learning to rely on one's own resources. Using the metaphor of a map, the first step is to get an overview of the map, where one is at the moment (structure of the problem), where one wants to go (the goal) and how to get there (the path). NLP teaches how to read the map, so it can be used over and over without referring to a professional for help.

NLP addresses what it considers to be the different levels of processing which occur in the brain (see table 1).

Spirituality	Who else?
Identity	Who?
Belief/Values	Why?
Capabilities	How?
Environment	When?/Where?

Table 1: Levels of processing

These are referred to as the logical levels. A change in behaviour is more likely to occur when the working of the brain is understood and its different levels are addressed.

To bring about change on any level, one operates at the level above it. That means one changes environment through behaviour. No one can change behaviour unless they have the capabilities to do so. Becoming capable may require a belief in one's capabilities, and in order to look at beliefs and change them one has to be at the level above, which is the level of identity. Beyond identity (the level beyond ego) is the level which is out of control and beyond personal power – the level of spirituality.

Presupposition

A term which is important in NLP is *presupposition*. A presupposition is the assumption that something is true. Unconsciously everybody presupposes things in their everyday lives. For example, if someone asks, 'How can I help you?', he is presupposing firstly that you want help and secondly that he can help you. Another presupposition is 'Behind every behaviour is a positive intention'. Integrating this into clients' beliefs can help them to stop fighting against parts of themselves they find difficult to accept and can therefore create a sense of inner peace and harmony.

This may lead to a reduction in judging others, to understanding that they are just doing the best they can.

Sub-Modalities

People's maps of reality are made of *VAKOG*: Visual pictures, Auditory sounds, Kinaesthetic feelings, Olfactory smells and Gustatory tastes. These are called *sub-modalities*. The reality is represented internally through images, sounds and feelings.

Internal pictures, or images, vary, and depending on what size, colour, location, focus or shape they have, the emotional response can be very different. Sounds can vary in pitch, clarity, volume, location and speed. Feelings can differ in location, pressure, extent and intensity.

Usually people are not aware of the existence of these internal pictures, but when they recognise them, most find it easy to change them. The distinction between associated and dissociated pictures is an important one. In an associated picture people experience an event through their own senses, whereas in a dissociated picture, they sense themselves experiencing the event. The emotional response to associated pictures is stronger than to dissociated pictures. People with a fear of spiders, for example, are afraid to imagine spiders but can often manage to imagine themselves looking at spiders.

This knowledge is applied in the 'fast phobia method' which creates a double dissociation by encouraging clients to visualise a picture of themselves watching themselves watching a video of the event in which they experienced the phobia the first time. The second stage then is to step into the video and run it backwards, which changes the meaning of the event, as you do when you say a sentence backwards.

Case History: The Fast Phobia Method

I was talking to my friend G. on the phone to arrange a time for us to meet. My newly acquired caged bird started to call loudly in the background. 'Oh no! I am terrified of birds,' my friend said; 'I'm sorry, I don't think I want to come to your house after all. I have a phobia of birds.'

'No problem,' I assured her, 'we can do a phobia method and within ten minutes your phobia will be gone!'

My friend was very sceptical at first, but said she would give it a try. When she arrived at my house, she was not able to go near the bird, even when it was in its cage. Just seeing the bird terrified her and made her skin turn pale and her hands sweaty. I took her to my treatment room and did the phobia method. Here are parts of a transcript of that single session with G.:

MM: *Please remember the first time you experienced fear of birds. Can you tell me about the situation?*

G: *Oh yes, I remember it clearly, it was horrible. I was eight years old and went into my room and there was this bird, fluttering about, banging against the walls and it couldn't find the open window. I was so frightened, I screamed. My mother came into the room and she couldn't do anything either. Finally the bird found the window by chance and escaped. Ever since I have been scared of birds. But not only of birds, of feathers as well. That means I don't enjoy being outdoors, no walking, no cycling or sitting in gardens because everywhere there could be birds or feathers. It really makes life miserable.*

G. was pale and shaking, she looked very frightened and I could see her phobic response. Now it was important to get her out of this state.

MM: *Well, this must have been a very frightening experience indeed. But now you are here in my room. Look around, here you are safe, aren't you?*

G: *Yes, it is OK now.*

We made a few jokes and when she was feeling comfortable again we could proceed. The next step was for her to think about this situation without re-experiencing the fearful feelings. To make this possible, she needed to gain distance in her pictures. This is done by creating a picture in which she sees herself two times removed; that is, she sees herself sitting in a cinema watching herself on a screen going through the experience. The picture should be in black and white.

MM: *Now imagine yourself sitting in a cinema looking at yourself from the projection booth. Can you see that?*

G.: *It is really very difficult for me to make clear pictures.*

MM.: *That is OK, just imagine yourself in the cinema. Get the feeling of what it feels like to be sitting in a cinema watching a film.*

G.: *It is not easy but I can get a sense of it.*

MM: *OK. Now you see yourself sitting in a cinema looking from the projection booth, and on the screen you see yourself in black and white.*

G: *Well, it's quite difficult. But I've got a sense of it.*

MM: *Now here is what you do: you watch yourself sitting in a cinema watching yourself on a black and white screen going through that experience you had as a child with the bird. Go from the beginning to the end. Take all the time you need and tell me when you're done.*

G: *OK.*

MM: *How do you feel?*

G.:   *I feel quite scared, but not so bad as before.*

MM: *That is OK. Now I want you to step inside the picture, turn the picture into colour, and run the film backwards very rapidly, as if you are rewinding the film, from the end to the beginning.*

Because it was so difficult for G. to create clear pictures, we had to go through this process several times before she could do it feeling safe and comfortable. After the fifth time she experienced no discomfort at all and she had no experience of fear when thinking of a bird. We went to the kitchen where my bird started to call, and G. went to the cage and not only looked at and heard the bird without fear, but actually opened the cage and took the bird in her hands.

My friend told me later that overcoming this phobia had changed the quality of her life. She was now able to enjoy sitting outside a cafe observing the birds picking up the bread crumbs she threw to them, hearing them twitter and admiring their liveliness.

Reframing

A client came to see me and mentioned casually that he was very nervous about a journey abroad he was making in three weeks' time. 'Oh,' I said to him, 'you are nervous beforehand, so that you do not need to be nervous during the journey.' He looked at me startled. Some time afterwards he told me that his nervousness had ceased and he had not been nervous before journeys ever since.

In another case a client wanted to be 'connected better to his feelings' but was afraid of the reaction of his family and friends, that they might not understand him any more. I suggested that he see himself as a model for others. He accepted this suggestion and felt free of a limitation that did not suit him any more.

What I did in the first case was to change the client's frame of time: it was not so bad to be nervous before a journey as long as he was not nervous during the journey. This might not make sense to the conscious mind, but obviously it did to his unconscious mind. In the second case I changed the frame of meaning, turning the client's fear of rejection to his being a model for others. This process is called *reframing*, which means changing the frame of either meaning or time.

Fairy tales and teachings often use reframing. Being rich is usually regarded as comfortable and desirable. But Jesus said in the New Testament: 'How hard it is for the rich to enter the kingdom of God. It is easier for a camel to through the eye of a needle than for a rich man to enter the kingdom of God.' (Mark 10:23-25) This is an example of 'negative' reframing because Jesus has turned the positives of being rich into limitations.

A theme often found in fairy tales is that of three brothers, the youngest of whom is stupid and too soft-hearted. However, this naivety and weakness often turns out to be the reason for his ability to rescue his older brothers, who, for all their cleverness, get themselves into trouble. Here, attributes which appear to be negative are reframed into positives. Although reframing does not necessarily solve a problem by itself, it can be very effective and can be applied conversationally, which makes it a useful technique in any context.

Anchoring

An anchor is a physical, conscious or unconscious response to an external stimulus. For example, looking at a photograph of one's children, one might respond with an emotion such as love, in which case the photograph is a conscious anchor for the emotional state of love. On the other hand, if somebody resembles a disliked teacher from the past, the same previous emotional response might be triggered unconsciously. This would be an unconscious anchor. In therapy, anchoring can be a very useful technique.

Case History: Anchoring

I was once working with a client who came to see me urgently because she couldn't swallow. She had choked four weeks previously while eating chocolate and had developed an infection in her throat. After the infection cleared up she could not swallow food any more, although fluids were all right. 'It is as if my body cannot remember how to swallow any more,' she explained. She had eaten nothing for two weeks.

I used an anchoring process to remind her body how to swallow. I told her to remember a situation in which she enjoyed eating and drinking. When I perceived that she was in touch with a strong memory, I touched her left knee thereby anchoring this memory in her body. I removed my hand and let her think of her present situation and anchored this on her right knee. Then I touched her left knee for a while and then, leaving my hand on her left knee, touched her right knee simultaneously in order to overlap her negative response to her present situation with her positive memory. After that she felt comfortable thinking of her present situation and to her utter surprise was able to eat a biscuit. I recommended that she touch her left knee while eating for the next few days. I phoned her up a few weeks later and she was still eating without any problems.

Anchors are very powerful and can be created intentionally to provide another resource which can be accessed when needed.

Applications of NLP

NLP is a flexible tool tailored to each client's individual needs, with different problems requiring different approaches.

Past Life Therapy

Time line therapy utilises the way people experience time and could take a client back as far as past lives. The *re-imprinting process* heals past traumas and difficult family constellations. There is a process designed to turn limitations into 'core states' of love, peace or light. Working with *sub-modalities* changes what people do with their internal pictures, sounds and feelings. Whatever techniques are used, clients will be reminded that they already have the resources they need. Every NLP session can be an adventure of its own.

NLP has a wide range of applications. People can learn to overcome phobias, allergies, anxieties, compulsions, addictions, past and present traumas, depression, stress, learning difficulties or shyness. There are techniques to enhance positive qualities such as increasing creativity, health and well-being, strategy building, decision making, leadership skills, clarifying goals and much more. NLP is not only psychotherapy but a valuable resource for self-development.

Although NLP is becoming more widespread it is still not well known. However, as people are faced with increasing challenges to cope with changes not only in the immediate environment but in work situations and political and ecological circumstances, they are increasingly in need of tools to create and maintain quality of life. NLP is certainly a tool which can help in achieving remarkable outcomes and as its value becomes more recognised, demand will increase. I believe and hope that one day NLP principles will be part of everyday life and a way of thinking and acting for our own benefit, as well as for that of our neighbours.

Appendix: Three Useful NLP Techniques

The Fast Phobia Method

Select a phobia or a traumatic experience:

1 Imagine yourself in a cinema and see yourself on a small black and white screen doing something neutral.

2 Step outside and behind yourself so that you can see yourself twice. You see yourself watching yourself on the screen.

3 Now see yourself as in a movie going through the experience you chose to work on.

4 Now step out of the movie and turn it into a still picture. Step back into the picture and turn it into colour. Then run the film backwards, very fast.

5   Now think of this event again. If you can think of it comfortably without any reaction or fear, the exercise is complete. If not, repeat the process as often as you need to, until any fear has disappeared.

Six Step Reframing

A technique called 'six step reframing' separates intentions from behaviours and is like building a bridge to an unconscious process. The six steps are:

1   Identify an unwanted behaviour: this could be any behaviour that prevents you from acting in a desired way.

2   Contact the part that generates the identified behaviour by using internal dialogue to ask: 'Is the part of me that generates the unwanted behaviour willing to communicate with me?' Pay attention to any response, which could be in pictures, sounds, words or feelings.

3   Separate intention from behaviour by asking: 'What are you trying to do for me?'

4   Find three new ways of satisfying the intention by accessing your creative part and having it generate three new more satisfying ways to accomplish the intention.

5   Ask the original part if it is willing to accept the new choices and the responsibility for generating them when needed. If it does not agree to the new choices, continue to work with the creative part and come up with better ones.

6   Make an integrity check by asking if any part objects to the negotiations that have taken place.

Anchoring Resourceful States

1   Identify the situation where you want to be more resourceful.

2   Identify the particular resource you want, for example inner power, confidence, motivation, etc.

3   Find an occasion in your life when you had that resource.

4   Select the anchors you are going to use from something you can see, hear or feel. (For example touch your knee, rub your little finger, etc.)

5   In your imagination step into another location and put yourself back into the experience of that resourceful state. Re-experience it again as strongly as you can. When it has peaked, step out of it.

6   Re-experience your resourceful state again and as it comes up to peak, connect the anchors.

7   Test the association by firing the anchors and confirming that you do go into this state. If not satisfied, repeat step 6.

Biography

Magdalena Mihm holds a BA in social work and a BA (Hons) in education. She was born in Italy and lived most of her life in Germany where she worked as a social worker and adult educator. For 15 years she has been involved in the field of psychotherapy and complementary medicine, and has studied psychoanalysis and trained in bioenergetic and client-centred psychotherapy. She is an NLP master practitioner. She is also trained in accelerated learning, and educational and other forms of kinesiology and hypnotherapy. She uses an integration of different techniques in her ongoing work as trainer and therapist and she has been living in the North of Scotland for the past eight years with her two sons.

Further Reading

Andreas, Connie-Ray & Steve, *Heart of the Mind*, Real People Press, 1989.

———, ———, *Change your Mind – and keep the Change*, Real People Press, 1987.

Andreas, Connie-Ray with Tamara Andreas, *Core Transformation*, Real People Press, 1994.

Bandler, Richard, *Using your Brain for a CHANGE*, Real People Press, 1985.

———; Grinder, John, *Frogs into Princes*, Eden Grove, 1990.

———; ———, *Reframing: Neuro-Linguistic Programming and the Transformation of Meaning*, Real People Press, 1983.

Cameron-Bandler, Leslie, *Solutions*, Real People Press, 1985.

Chomsky, Noam, *Syntactic Structures*, The MIT Press, 1957.

———, *Aspects of the Theory of Syntax*, The MIT Press, 1965.

Dilts, Robert, *Applications of NLP*, Meta Pub., 1983.

———, *Changing Belief Systems with NLP*, Meta Publications, 1990.

———; Hallbom, Tim; Smith, Suzi, *Beliefs: Pathways to Health and Well-being*, Metamorphous Press, 1990.

Erickson, S., *My Voice Will Go With You: The Teaching Tales of Milton H. Erickson, MD*, W W Norton, 1991.

Haley, J., *On Milton H. Erickson*, Brunner/Mazel Inc., 1993.

———, *Uncommon Therapy: Psychiatric Techniques of Milton H. Erickson*, WW Norton, 1968.

Jackson, Don D., *Communication, Family and Marriage*, Science and Behavior Books, 1968.

———, *Therapy, Communication and Change*, Science and Behavior Books, 1968.

James, Tad, Woodsmall Wyaltt, *Time Line Therapy and the Basis of Personality*, Meta Publications, 1988.

Lankton, Stephen R., *Practical Magic: The clinical Application of Neuro-Linguistic Programming*, Aquarian Press, 1979.

O'Connor, Joseph; Seymour John, *Introducing Neuro-Lingusitic Programming: The New Psychology of Personal Excellence*, Aquarian, 1993.

Perls, Fritz, *The Gestalt Approach, Eyewitness to Therapy*, Science and Behavior Books, 1989.

Robbins, Anthony, *Unlimited Power*, Simon & Schuster, 1989.

Satir, Virginia, *Conjoint Family Therapy*, Souvenir Press, 1978.

———, *Peoplemaking*, Science & Behavior, 1988.

Watzlawick, Paul; Beavin, J.; Jackson, D, *Pragmatics of Human Communications*, WW Norton, 1967.

———, Weakland, John; Frisch, Richard, *Change*, WW Norton, 1974

———; Beavin, J.; Jackson, Don D., *Pragmatics of Human Communication*, WW Norton, 1980.

Resources

The Association for Neuro-Linguistic Programming (ANLP) provides information – publications, training programmes and services provided by its members to all who are interested in NLP. It publishes a magazine 'Rapport' four times a year, which is also available for non-members. The ANLP – Psychotherapy and Counselling Section is recognised by the United Kingdom Council of Psychotherapy (UKCP)

Association for NLP (ANLP)
48 Corser Street
Old Swinford
Stourbridge
West Midlands PY8 2DQ

Nutritional Therapy

compiled by Cornelia Featherstone

You Are What You Eat

The importance of nutrition is widely recognised and there are many different sciences applying themselves to the subject. However, the importance of nutrition on human health has not found entry into the curricula of medical schools and therefore nutrition, apart from dietetics, is one of the areas delegated to the complementary field.

The wide variety of nutritional approaches is testimony to the fact that there is no one right approach to nutrition, or if there is, it has not been defined yet. Some basic agreements have been reached as to what constitutes a healthy diet, but in the arena of healing intervention through diet there are many, even diametrically opposed, approaches on offer. This leads to confusion for the public and contributes to the lack of acceptance of nutritional therapy by the medical profession.

Naturopathy

Good diet is an essential component of health care and disease care. In health, a good diet allows the maintenance and enhancement of a state of well-being. In disease, diet can become a powerful intervention to counteract deficiencies or to support the body and the immune system by supplying high quality 'building blocks' which are essential for regaining health.

Nutrition in Health

The basic constituents of a healthy diet are, ideally:

◆ plenty of fresh fruits, vegetables, unrefined grains;

◆ only a moderate intake of fat, sugar, salt and protein;

◆ all produce organically grown without the use of artificial fertilisers or pest control;

◆ the less pre-processed food the better, and if processed foods are eaten, they should be carefully selected, having read the list of ingredients to identify, and avoid, preservatives and food additives which may be harmful;

◆ variety in the diet, achieved, for instance, by eating locally grown produce in season (the fact that tomatoes and strawberries are available all year round is a recent development in human history);

◆ food should be prepared with love and respect, and eaten in a relaxed and nourishing environment.

The Food Groups

The importance of plenty of fresh fruit, vegetables, and unrefined grains is widely recognised. They supply vitamins, minerals and trace elements which are essential for a myriad of processes in the body, especially for the immune system. They provide fibre to ensure smooth peristalsis in the intestines. The health-conscious cook uses herbs and condiments to enhance the flavour of food and refrains from using sugar, salt or chemical flavour enhancers.

◆ **Fats** have long been recognised as major etiologic factors for obesity and certain cancers (breast cancer, endometrial cancers[1]). Saturated fatty acids, in particular, are blamed for high cholesterol levels and increased arteriosclerotic degeneration. Rancid or overheated fats are considered carcinogenic and are best avoided. Animal fats are best reduced and replaced by cold-pressed vegetable oils with high levels of unsaturated fatty acids (for example olive oil).

◆ **Sugar**, especially refined sugar, has become one of the most widely suffered addictions with deleterious effects ranging from allergies and intolerance to hypoglycaemia and diabetes. Sugar has been implicated as a major contributing factor in hyperactivity and attention deficit in children. Considering its effects on the central nervous system and the body's metabolism, sugar ought to be called a drug and be treated with due caution.[2] Sugar stimulates insulin secretion from the pancreas. In some people blood sugar levels swing between extremes causing symptoms of hypoglycaemia which includes dizziness, faintness and irritability.

◆ **Salt** intake has been linked with high blood pressure[3] and therefore has to be considered one of the central causes of the vast increase in cardiovascular diseases. Empirically, it can be observed that sugar and salt consumption are correlated – a salty meal is completed with a sweet dessert; over-indulgence in sweets may trigger craving for pickles. Both sugar and salt consumption result in an overstimulation of taste buds in the first instance, but in the long run lead to a dulling of the sense of taste. After avoiding salt and sugar for an extended period of time, many different nuances of taste can be experienced; for instance an onion's sweetness will enhance a savoury meal and herbs will enrich and deepen the flavour.

◆ **Meat** consumption is connected with many degenerative diseases. It was known since ancient times that over-indulgence in meat can lead to the painful condition of gout. If, in previous times, the concern about meat was its contamination with parasites, nowadays this is outweighed by the threat of chemical contamination with drugs used in animal husbandry (including hormones and antibiotics) and chemicals used in fertilisation and pest control. The etiology of decreased male fertility is still debated but it may well be connected with oestrogen contamination in foods.[4] Study results confirm that a vegetarian diet leads to a reduction in premature mortality due to cancer and possibly ischaemic heart disease. The protective effects of a vegetarian diet – 40% for cancer mortality and 20% for total mortality – are large.[5]

If meat is a component of the diet it should be a condiment to the rest of the meal. Best meat sources are from the wild – venison, rabbit, fowl. Organic supplies of lean white meat are next best. Red meat, particularly if it has been produced on a large scale by the agricultural industry, must be considered a health hazard. This is especially true after the BSE contamination and its likely connection with Creutzfeldt-Jacob Disease.[6]

◆ **Coffee, tea and alcohol** can be called the poisons of civilisation. These are substances which are addictive, and have potentially deleterious effects on the body (caffeine contributes to raised blood pressure, increased muscular tone and adrenalin levels; alcohol to liver disease and neurotoxicity). Used in small measures they could be considered a special treat. Consumed on a daily basis and in large dosages they are certainly detrimental to health.

Alcohol is a highly addictive, soporific drug which is socially sanctioned and causes tremendous hardship for the individuals afflicted by alcoholism and their families. 'Alcohol is a solvent – it dissolves relationships, employment contracts, bank accounts and personalities.'[7]

Twelve Steps Programme

Fluids

The importance of sufficient hydration cannot be overemphasised. Some experts claim that with the consumption of eight glasses of water daily, many degenerative illnesses, as well as their acute presentations can be prevented or treated.[8] It is important that fluid is not only consumed as tea or coffee, as the body requires fluids to excrete some of the chemicals present in tea/coffee, often leaving it with a net deficit of water. Plain water is most desirable, provided that it is pure.

Additives

Preservatives, artificial colours and flavours as well as flavour enhancers have become a standard item on the menu of modern day cuisine. It has been known for many years that these create significant side effects for large numbers of people, ranging from allergic reactions (for example asthma and skin irritation), to hyperactivity, gastr-ointestinal symptoms (vomiting, abdominal pains, diarrhoea), neurological disorders (vertigo, migraine) and cancer.[9] If buying a processed food which contains additives is unavoidable, it is crucial to be selective, reading the packaging and choosing only products containing the least dangerous chemical, ideally well tried substances with a track record of many decades. It is always important to ask the question: 'Is there food in this poison?' before deciding to eat food which contains additives.[10]

Variety

A varied diet is the best way to guarantee sufficient ingestion of all the different nutritional elements required by the body. In addition to creating interesting menus for the whole family, this is also the best guard against developing food sensitivities should the gut integrity or the immune system be impaired. The motto of a rotation diet is 'never eat the same ingredient three times a day!' If this were to be applied to common ingredients used frequently, such as sugar, dairy produce and wheat, the diet of a nation would change dramatically. Choosing to live by this rule can become an adventure in finding ever new ways of combining ingredients, which may include learning from previous generations to recapture how they used different food stuffs.

Eating in season is one way to achieve this objective even though it may take some re-adaptation in a culture where everything, even strawberries, are available all year round.

Preparing and Enjoying Food

Food is more than the chemical constituents it contains. Gourmets the world over know that preparation with the essential ingredients of love of food and care for those who will eat it makes all the difference. The presentation of the meal is also significant, as is the atmosphere in which the food is consumed. An attractive, peaceful environment which allows the food to be ingested in a contemplative, appreciative manner will increase the benefits gained many fold.

The Ecological Implications of Diet

A healthy diet affects not only human health but also the ecological health of the land. The described healthy diet is not only healthy for the individual but also for the planet. Eating organic, locally grown food, in season, is the best recipe for low ecological impact. No poison will be mixed in the earth, transport energy is low and no energy is used for preservation (such as freezing). This is important to note as it is only too easy to buy an organic piece of fruit which has been shipped around the planet in cold store. In this very process more energy will have been used up than is actually contained in the fruit itself. Organically grown food, locally produced and consumed when it is fresh and unprocessed, spares the earth and builds community.

The ecological impact of the coffee and tea plantations in many third world countries has been the tremendous loss of intact natural environments, and the use of agricultural chemicals is a source of poisoning to land and people.[11]

From an ecological point of view it is important to consider that one kilogram of meat requires the consumption of ten kilograms of plant protein. This is the reason why 95% of all agricultural land in the UK is given over to animal and animal food production rather than to the production of foods for humans.[12] On a global scale this contributes directly to a significant loss of rainforests for the creation of cattle pasture. Considering that there is still famine in the world, the overconsumption of complex protein could be argued to be immoral.

The ideal of eating local produce promotes the potential of building community. Although for a primarily urban population this can only remain a fantasy, it is important to acknowledge the pleasure it can bring if consumers know the people who have grown the food or if they know the animals who have given the milk or eggs. Projects of community-supported agriculture are excellent examples for this, where a farm is supported by a group of shareholders who contribute labour and an annual subscription in exchange for farm produce which is often organically grown.

Nutrition in Disease Care

The role of nutrition in the disease process has been described in numerous instances. Sir Richard Doll attributes 35% of all cancers to dietary factors.[13] The role of diet as significant contributing factor has been established for the majority of causes of death in modern society: cardiovascular disease, diabetes, obesity, hypertension, diverticulosis, and, of course, cancer.

Nutritional therapy works with four basic principles:

◆ detoxification of the body;

◆ correction of vitamin and mineral imbalances;

◆ restoration of healthy digestion;

◆ the development of a positive attitude of self-care – the need for an individual to make nourishing choices in relation to diet.

Detoxification

Ridding the body of accumulated toxins is the first step towards enabling the innate healing forces to be fully activated. Detoxification is therefore often the first step in nutritional therapy. This can be achieved gradually over a long period of time or more vigorously through a well-designed programme of fasting or mono-diet. Fasting has been practised, for physical as well as spiritual reasons, since ancient times in

Naturopathy

many cultures and is described in all old scriptures. There are many variations of fasting programmes: some using fresh juices; others prescribing a certain amount of exercise; some advocate rest and retreat whilst others offer a group experience for support. Mono-diets of rice, or grapes, or apples, are also designed to excrete toxins whilst consuming only the one particular type of food for several days. Detoxification does not necessarily involve heroic deeds or violent purgings; it is best done as a gentle and co-ordinated attempt at 'spring cleaning' the whole body. At least as much attention has to be given to the process of coming off the fast or mono-diet as to the detoxifying itself, in order not to jeopardise all that has been achieved.

Nutritional Supplementation

The use of vitamins and minerals as food supplements is important to correct imbalances and to provide the body with the building blocks required for optimal functioning. The assessment of imbalances is done by clinical assessment, as well as by laboratory testing of blood, sweat and/or hair samples. Nutritional supplementation becomes necessary if the body does not get all the required nutrients from the diet or if the demand is increased so that it cannot be met by the diet. It is debated whether a healthy person requires any supplementation. The spectrum of answers stretches from the assumption that a normal diet will supply everything needed to the assertion of the need to take all available vitamins and minerals in large doses. The right answer probably lies in between.

The modern human being is exposed to many demands and stresses, including impoverished soils after centuries of intense agriculture, increased pollution of air and water, artificial light potentially for 24 hours a day, and electromagnetic and noise pollution. These are very different demands on the body than those experienced by our ancestors in the Stone Age, yet genetically our bodies have only changed a small percentage since then. Therefore the requirements for a diet designed to maintain and enhance health will optimally include some degree of supplementation. This is particularly important at specific stages in life such as pregnancy, lactation, growth spurts, puberty, menopause and old age.

Some vitamins and supplements are also used as medication to treat certain conditions. Especially vitamin C has been used in large dosages (up to 50g a day) in cases of cancer or AIDS.[14]

Intestinal Health

The healthy function of the gastro-intestinal tract is essential for the optimal absorption of nutrients and therefore an obvious prerequisite for health and well-being. Gut health is affected in many situations, most commonly through the widespread use of antibiotics which causes a temporary imbalance in the gut flora (dysbiosis), which in some cases does not get restored to its optimal proportions of the different bacterial and fungal species. One such condition is candidiasis, which in the last decade has taken on epidemic proportions, resulting in a complex symptom picture including lack of energy, digestive problems, food sensitivities, acne and headaches.[15]

The effects of stress on the functioning of the intestines are commonly experienced, for example diarrhoea just before exams or stomach cramps caused by unresolved conflicts. Chronic stress plays an essential role in many gut-related illnesses: ulcer disease, irritable bowel syndrome, colitis.

The restoration of the physiological, healthy function of the gastro-intestinal tract is therefore crucial in nutritional therapy. Different preparations for restoring the normal acidity of the stomach, the enzyme activity of pancreas, liver function and bile excretion are used according to the needs of the individual patient. The gut flora are replenished with preparations containing mixtures of bacteria which will help the physiological balance in the flora to be re-established and to suppress pathogenic bacteria or mycotic organisms, such as yeasts. Gut flora restoration can either be achieved through oral application or through 'implants' during colonic hydrotherapy treatments. If oral preparations are used, it is important to ascertain that the preparation contains sufficient amounts of live bacteria, which are in a presentation ensuring that they are protected from the stomach acid, and which are capable of implanting themselves in the intestinal lumen.

Colonic Irrigation

Apart from supplementing the physiological elements of the gastro-intestinal tract, it is crucial to address underlying factors such as stress. Cognitive-behavioural therapy, psychosomatic medicine, stress management, gut-related hypnotherapy – all have their place in the restoration of gut health.

*Counselling
Stress Management
Hypnotherapy*

Self-Care

Optimal nourishment of the body is rarely the highest priority when people prepare to take in food and drink. More often than not, social convention, emotional comfort, convenience or neurotic patterns determine the content and context of eating. In order to establish a sustainable modification of diet, patients have to gain sufficient insight into the unconscious patterns which determine their eating habits and have to develop a commitment to self-care which will allow them to make healthy choices on a daily basis. The commitment to self-care is proportional to self-esteem and self-empowerment and therefore, in most cases, a lifelong process which can be measured tangibly in the daily relationship to food and nourishment.

Examples of Remedial Diets

The Gerson Diet

Dr Max Gerson advocated a diet to treat cancer.[16] He believed that cancer was a multifactorial degenerative disease. He considered that the modern diet is too far removed from nature and that people's intake of denaturalised food exceeds the body's ability to cope with and process it. Overuse of artificial and chemical fertilisers and pesticides in the soil, the over-refining and over-processing of packaged foods and poor cooking methods are major causative problems.

The basis of the diet is in detoxification and stimulation of the elimination organs, especially the liver. This is achieved by ingesting freshly prepared juices from fruits and vegetables with a particular emphasis on green juices, such as wheat grass. Raw liver juice is recognised as the best source of the components which build the blood. Coffee enemas are used to stimulate the liver and aid the excretion of toxic material from the body.

This diet should not be attempted without professional supervision and monitoring.

Food Combining

Various people have championed this way of eating, the most renowned being Dr Hay, from whence comes the name the 'Hay Diet'.[17] This diet is based on the assertion that since the body uses different enzymes to break down carbohydrates and proteins, eating these two food types separately ensures maximum efficiency in digestion. Emphasis is also given to the acid/alkali balance in different foods, recommending that more alkali foods are eaten overall than those which reduce to acid components when digested. The diet is of benefit especially in obesity, food allergies, poor digestion (heartburn, IBS, constipation, etc.) and many remarkable results have been reported. Charts are available to guide anyone wishing to attempt this diet.

The Feingold Diet

Dr Ben Feingold suggested a diet to combat hyperactivity in children and allergies in people of all ages, with sometimes dramatically positive results. The two main groups of food to avoid are, firstly, those which contain synthetic and artificial colours, flavours and other products regulated by E numbers in Britain, and, secondly, those fruits and vegetables which contain salicylates – a naturally occurring group of chemicals. These include almonds, apples, cherries, cucumbers, grapes, oranges, peaches and plums among others.

Eliminating all products from these two groups of foods can relieve symptoms. After a period of six weeks when improvement has been noted, it may be possible to reintroduce some of the fruits and vegetables which contain salicylates, but it is recommended that artificial colourings and flavourings be removed from the diet permanently.[18]

Macrobiotics

Macrobiotics is not just a diet but a way of life encompassing all dimensions of living. Translated, the word means 'long life' and describes a concept of living in harmony with nature, eating a simple, balanced diet and living to an active old age. In the late nineteenth and early twentieth century macrobiotics experienced a revival originating in Japan. Macrobiotics today is a synthesis of Eastern and Western influences.

The philosophy affects all areas of life as represented in the following questions:

◆ Did I eat today in harmony with my environment?

◆ Did I think of my parents, relatives, teachers, and elders with love and respect?

◆ Did I happily greet everyone today and express an interest in their life?

◆ Did I contemplate the sky, the trees and the flowers and marvel at the wonders of nature?

◆ Did I perform my tasks faithfully and thereby contribute to a more peaceful world?[19]

Macrobiotics promotes the principles of a naturally balanced diet, which takes into account differing climatic and geographical considerations, and the age, gender, activity level and personal needs of the individual. These principles include:

◆ Harmony with the evolutionary order – whole grains evolved parallel with the human species and should therefore form the major part of the diet. Animal food is eaten only as a supplement, and therefore does not upset the delicate balance of nature at any level, the most harmonious ratio being one part animal food to seven parts vegetable food. Any animal food which is taken should be from those species which are most removed from humans, such as fish and shellfish.

◆ Harmony with universal dietary tradition – ethnic food consists largely of cooked whole grains, beans and vegetables; this is true for indigenous cultures the world over.

◆ Harmony with ecological order – foods should originate in the geographical area in which a person lives. Eating imported foods from regions with a different climate can lead to loss of natural immunity to diseases in the local environment and chronic imbalance.

◆ Harmony with the changing seasons – foods should be eaten in season and the preparation of food should reflect the seasonal conditions; for example in colder weather, longer cooking times are appropriate, as is the reduced intake of raw salads and fruits.

◆ Harmony with individual differences – using food to balance individual disharmonies, for example if one has a yin temperament, eating yang foods can bring balance and harmony to the person.

References

1   Bal & Forrester, *Chronic Diseases Control Branch*, Cancer, 1993; 72 (3 Suppl): 1005-10.

Holm et al., *Treatment failure and dietary habits in women with breast cancer*, Journal of National Cancer Institute, 1993; 85: 1.

D I Gregorio, *Dietary fat consumption and survival among women with brreast cancer*, Journal of National Cancer Institute 1986; 75: 1, 37-41.

2   William Dufty, *Sugar Blues*, Warner, 1975.

J Yudkin, *Pure White and Deadly: Problem of Sugar*, Penguin, 1988.

Nancy Appleton, *Lick the Sugar Habit*, Avery Pub., 1988.

3   Paul Elliot, et al., *Intersalt revisited: further anyses of 24 hour sodium excretion and blood pressure within and across populations*, BMJ, 1996; 312: 1249-53.

Richard L Hanneman, *Intersalt: hypertension rise with age revisited; and two commentaries*, BMJ, 1996; 312: 1283-9.

4   Stewart Irvine et al., *Evidence of deteriorating semen quality in the United Kingdom: birth cohort study in 577 men in Scotland over 11 years*, BMJ, 1996; 312: 467-71.

R M Sharpe, N E Skakkebaek, *Are oestrogens involved in falling sperm counts and discorders of the male reproductive tract?*, Lancet, 1993; 341: 1392-5.

Ministry of Environment and Energy, Denmark, *Male reproductive health and environmental chemicals with estrogenic effects*, Danish Environmental Protection Agency, Copenhagen, 1995.

5   Margaret Thorogood, et al., *Risk of death from cancer and ischaemic heart disease in meat and non-meat eaters*, BMJ, 1994; 308: 1667-70.

6   Anon, *Creutzfeldt-Jakob disease and bovine spongiform encephalopathy: any connection?*, BMJ, 1995; 311: 1415-21.

7   Dr med. Dubenhorst, Ulm, Germany.

8   Batmanghelidj, Dr F., *Your Body's Many Cries for Water: Body Thirst Signals and Damages of Dehydration*, Global Health Solutions, 1994.

9   Maurice Hansen, *E for Additives. The Complete E Number Guide*, Thorsons, 1984.

Foresight, *Findout*, Foresight, Godalming, 1986 – a small pocket translator for E numbers.

10 Viktoras Kulvinskas, *Survival into the 21st century*, Omangod Press, 1975, p12-4.

11 R Tucker, *Five Hundred Years of Tropical Forest Exploitation in Head*, S. and Heinzman, R (eds.) *Lessons of the Rainforest*, Sierra Club Books, 1990, pp39-52.

M Collins (ed), *The Last Rainforests*, Mitchell Beazley, 1990, p144.

N Dudley, *The Death of Trees*, Pluto Press, 1985, p80.

12 K Jannaway, *Abundant Living*, Movement for Compassionate Living, Leatherhead, 1991.

G Yates, *Food: Need, Greed & Myopia*, Earthright Publishing, 1986.

13 Prof Sir Richard Doll, R Peto, *Causes of Cancer*, OUP, 1981.

14 A Hanck (ed), *Vitamin C: New Clinical Applications in Immunology*, Lipid Metabolism and Cancer, Huber Verlag, 1982.

15 Jane McWhirter, *The Practical Guide to Candida, and UK Directory of Practitioners*, All Hallows House Foundation, 1995.

Leon Chaitow, *Candida Albicans*, Could Yeast be your Problem, Thorsons, 1996.

Orian Truss, *The Missing Diagnosis*, The Missing Diagnosis Inc., 1983.

16 Max Gerson, *A Cancer Therapy*, Gerson Institute, 1986.

17 Diamond, Harvey and Marilyn, *Fit for Life*, Bantam, 1987.

Doris Grant, *Food Combining for Health*, Thorsons, 1991.

18 Ben Feingold; Helene Feingold, *The Feingold Cookbook for Hyperactive Children, and Others with Problems Associated with Food Additives and Salicylates*, Random House, 1979

19 Michio Kushi, *The Cancer Prevention Diet*, Thorsons, 1984.

Further Reading

Ballentine, Rudolph, *Diet & Nutrition*, The Himalayan International Institute, 1978.

Davies, S.; Stewart, A., *Nutritional Medicine*, Pan, 1987.

Diamond, Harvey and Marilyn, *Fit for Life*, (I) Bantam, 1987; (II) Warner Books, 1993.

Feingold, Ben and Helene, *The Feingold Cookbook for Hyperactive Children, and Others with Problems Associated with Food Additives and Salicylates*, Random House, 1979

Gawler, Ian, *You can Conquer Cancer*, Hill of Content Publishing Co., 1984.

Gerson, Max, *A Cancer Therapy*, Gerson Institute, 1986.

Goodman, Sandra, *Nutrition and Cancer – State of the Art*, Green Library, 1995.

Grant D.; Joice, J., *Food Combining for Health*, Thorsons, 1991.

Hansen, Maurice, *E for Additives. The Complete E Number Guide*, Thorsons, 1984.

Lewith, George, *Allergy and Intolerance*, Green Print, 1992.

Kushi, Michio, *The Book of Macrobiotics*, Japan Publications, 1986.

———, *The Cancer Prevention Diet*, Thorsons, 1984.

Lappé, Frances, *Diet for a Small Planet – 20th Anniversary Edition*, Ballantine Books, 1991.

Mayes, A., *The Dictionary of Nutritional Health*, Thorsons, 1986.

Minchin, M., *Food for Thought*, Alma Productions, 1982.

Pitchford, Paul, *Healing with Whole Foods*, North Atlantik Books, 1993.

Robbins, John, *Diet for a New America*, Stillpoint 1987.

Shils, Maurice E.; Young, Vernon R., *Modern Nutrition in Health and Disease*, Lea & Febiger, 1988.

Wright, Brian and Celia, *Nutrition Handbook*, Green Library, 1996.

Journal of Nutritional Medicine, published by the British Society for Nutritional Medicine.

Resources

British Society for Nutritional Medicine
P O Box 28
Totton
Southampton SO40 22A

The Institute for Optimum Nutrition
Blades Court
Deodar Road
London SW15 2NU
Tel. 0181-877 9993

Society for the Promotion of Nutritional Therapy
P O Box 47
Heathfield
East Sussex TN21 8ZX
Tel. 01435-867 007

College of Nutritional Medicine
Eastbank
New Church Road
Smithills
Greater Manchester BL1 5QP
Tel. 01884-255 059

Dr Lawrence Plaskett Nutritional Medicine College
23 Chapel Street
Camelford
Cornwall PL32 9PJ
Tel. 01840-212 782

Osteopathy
by Hilary Dewey

Osteopathy is a well-established approach to health care which is complementary to, and supportive of, orthodox medicine. It is based on a system of clinical diagnosis and manual treatment which is now recognised by the British Medical Association.

Osteopathy is a safe, natural form of treatment with a caring approach to patients' individual needs, treating the person as a whole. It is concerned with the interrelationship between the musculo-skeletal system and the whole function of the body. Many things can alter the body framework, such as congenital and developmental abnormality, injury, disease states, habitual misuse or overuse, and osteopaths treat the variety of conditions that occur as a result, such as pain in the low back, hips, shoulders or neck; sports injuries; arthritic pain and headaches. By noting alterations in structure or function of the body the osteopath is able to interpret patterns of aches and pains and other health problems that might appear unconnected and analyse how the condition has arisen and what can be done to help.

Osteopaths work with their hands using a variety of treatment techniques. These may include soft tissue stretching; rhythmic, gentle, passive joint movements; or high-velocity thrust techniques (often described as a 'clicking' or 'popping') to improve the mobility and range of movement of a joint. Gentle release techniques are used when treating children or elderly patients. Osteopaths are taught to identify conditions where osteopathic treatment may not be appropriate. A full case history will always be taken prior to treatment to help the osteopath make the correct diagnosis.

Historical Development

The founder of the science of osteopathy was an American physician called Andrew Taylor Still, who was born in 1828 in Virginia. His father was a physician and a Methodist minister. From an early age he decided to follow in his father's footsteps by studying medicine. After graduating from a college of physicians and surgeons in Kansas City, he began practising with his father in Missouri. In those days medicine was rough and primitive. Ether and chloroform were the only anaesthetics. Dr Still served in the Union Army as a surgeon, where he was performing crude surgery and prescribing newly discovered and often poisonous medicines. This experience led him to a detailed study of anatomy and physiology.

In 1874 the state of Missouri was stricken by a 'plague', an epidemic now known to have been a form of viral meningitis. Three of his children died from this disease. With all his medical knowledge he could do nothing to save them. In his grief he began to question the way medical science was developing in America. He started looking for the causative factors of illness and in time came to adopt the principle that disease was caused by an alteration in the structure of the body which in turn caused an alteration in the function. He regarded the skeleton as more than just the physical framework of the body, since it provides not only attachment for muscles but also protection for the vital organs. Therefore, the skeletal alignment must be considered in any attempt to maintain good health. Dr Still called his new system of medicine 'osteopathy' because it was based on the bony framework (*osteon* means bone in Greek). Thus osteopathy began, and is taught today, more than a hundred years later, based on the same principle, that 'structure governs function'. Dr Still set out to reform medical practice by founding the first school of osteopathy in Kirksville, Missouri. His first student graduated in 1893.

Osteopathy was brought to Britain by John Martin Littlejohn, a Scottish academic who emigrated to the USA in 1892 at the age of 27. He consulted Dr Still for a medical problem and was so impressed by the treatment that he decided to study under him. He gained his diploma of osteopathy in 1900 and went on to found the second school of osteopathy, in Chicago, before returning to Britain in 1913, where he developed plans to establish the British School of Osteopathy.

Training

The first British School of Osteopathy was opened in London in 1917, and the syllabus used was based on the American system. The profession grew until in 1980 larger premises were needed and now the British School of Osteopathy is situated near Trafalgar Square and the building is named after Martin Littlejohn.

Today, the course at the British School of Osteopathy involves four years of full-time study. Students graduate with a diploma or a BSc degree. In the same building is a clinic where over 1000 patients are treated each week. The patron of the school is the Princess Royal. There are currently over 2000 osteopaths working in the UK and there are now four recognised independent schools offering training for osteopathy to the required standard.

From the earliest days in Britain, osteopaths have sought recognition by Parliament for their work and practice. In the 1930s bills to regulate the practice of osteopathy were submitted to Parliament but were not debated. The General Council and Register of Osteopaths was set up in 1936, so that the public would be able to distinguish between trained and untrained practitioners. The council has worked to set and enforce standards of training and an ethical code of practice. In 1993, statutory recognition was at last achieved with the passing of the Osteopaths Act by Parliament. With the implementation of this Act a General Osteopathic Council has been established, which will set standards of training and ethical conduct for the profession. Patients who consult osteopaths are now afforded the same safeguards as when they consult doctors, dentists and other statutory health care professionals.

The Practice of Osteopathy

In order to understand how it is that a simple osteopathic manipulation can often have such dramatic effects, offering relief from pain and increased mobility to people whose own family doctor can only give them painkilling pills and instructions to rest, one has to return to Dr Still's teaching: 'structure governs function'. If bodily structures are damaged or deformed, their function is impaired. Osteopathy works by finding out where the damage is and making simple adjustments to enable repair or healing to occur. This alteration is achieved by working on the neuro-muscular-skeletal system (NMSS) by using soft tissue massage and manipulation of joints.

Diagnosis is made from a combination of history, examination and palpation. When seeing a patient for the first time, the osteopath will take a detailed medical history which identifies the nature of the complaint and assesses any possible contraindications. The osteopath needs to know as much as possible about the patient in order to formulate a treatment plan. The ensuing physical examination confirms the diagnosis. This will include observing the range of movement in different directions, standing, sitting and lying. Palpation forms the third stage of the diagnostic procedure. Osteopaths spend most of their time working with their hands and develop a very refined sense of touch enabling them to assess normal and abnormal tissue states.

The treatment plan depends on the individual, as well as the nature of the complaint. The following techniques are amongst those regularly used.

Soft Tissue Treatment

Massage

This is almost always used. Osteopaths are trained to see and feel the response of tissue as the treatment continues. This is called 'palpatory awareness'. Soft tissue treatment is comparable to massage except that it is targeted to the contracted muscles to induce relaxation and thereby re-establish good blood flow and speed up the elimination of waste products which have built up. Muscle tissue consists of thousands of fibres bound together in bundles. Massage forces movement in the intercellular fluid and blood flow, allowing fresh, oxygenated blood to penetrate the tissues, thus helping to relieve pain and stiffness.

Treatment of Joints

Perhaps the most talked about osteopathic technique is the joint manipulation known as high velocity thrust and described by the layman as 'popping' or 'cracking'. This is not dealing with bones going in or out of place. When an osteopath manipulates a joint, the surfaces separate slightly disturbing the pressure on the capsule surrounding the joint. As this happens minute gas bubbles (CO_2) come out of solution and cause a popping sound. This is not a painful technique for the patient and can give instant relief. The aim of this technique is to stretch the joint capsule; this improves the range of movement of the joint which, in turn, reduces muscle spasm. The effect of this technique can be quite dramatic. Such a manipulation takes only a few seconds of the complete osteopathic treatment, which may take half an hour. Manipulation therefore forms only a small part of a treatment.

Passive Movement and Articulation

These are useful techniques used both to diagnose and treat a problem. The patient's limbs are moved by the osteopath without any effort by the patient. Articulation is a passive technique used to gently stretch the tissues, using the patient's own arms or legs as levers. As with other techniques the response of the tissues is constantly monitored by the osteopath.

Disc Injuries

A large number of patients seeking osteopathic treatment believe that they have 'slipped a disc'. This is still a surprisingly common medical diagnosis when the patient sees the family doctor with acute low back pain. In anatomical terms, discs do not slip. They are held in place with strong fibres and ligaments. Most disc-associated pain is caused by ligamentous damage and muscle spasm. There are many pain sensitive nerve endings in the muscles and ligaments close to the discs, which is why such injuries are painful and incapacitating. If too much pressure is put on the disc, the outer fibres will tear, allowing the jellylike core to be squeezed out. This will cause a bulge known as a disc herniation. If this presses on the nearby nerve, it can trap or pinch it, causing severe pain, numbness or pins and needles down the leg, even as far as the toes.

Most of these more serious back problems can be treated without surgery. Osteopaths can help to relieve the pressure and muscle spasm in the area, allowing the disc to heal itself with the co-operation of the patient. Usually bed-rest at home would be prescribed. If the nerve root pressure is severe and there is danger of persistent damage of nerves to organs which, for instance, may cause loss of bladder control, surgical removal of the disc is indicated. This is very rare and in most cases good osteopathic treatment can prevent the necessity for surgery.

The frequency of treatment is not set. Some acute conditions require only one treatment whereas a chronic ailment would benefit from regular sessions. Usually a further appointment will be made after the initial visit in order that the effect of the treatment given can be assessed. Advice can be given to the patient to help prevent recurrence. The osteopath is usually able to tell the patient at the first consultation how many treatments will be necessary.

A survey of osteopathic practice in the UK revealed that Britain's 2000 osteopaths undertake over 5 million patient consultations a year. Many patients are referred by their doctors. Thus osteopathy is playing an important role in the health care of the nation.

Other Manipulative Therapies

Chiropractic

As well as osteopaths, other professionals use touch and manipulation as part of their work. These include chiropractors, masseurs, some physiotherapists and some physicians and surgeons. The difference between osteopathic manipulation and other kinds lies in basic philosophy, as well as in the actual techniques.

Chiropractic

Of all the professions using manipulation as part of their treatment, modern chiropractic is probably the most similar to modern osteopathy.

Chiropractors believe that sections of the spine can become misaligned and need manipulation to put them back in position. Osteopaths believe that minor displacements are possible but that it is far more common to have a locking or jamming of the joints without any real displacement. Chiropractors tend to use X-rays considerably more than osteopaths, to diagnose badly aligned joints and to suggest which way to direct their corrective thrusts. Osteopaths use X-rays mainly to exclude any serious disease, if suspected. Both professions are trained to consider the body as a whole. Osteopaths place more emphasis on overall posture and body mechanics while chiropractors emphasise very detailed local mechanics. An osteopath will perform a variety of procedures prior to manipulation based on palpatory findings. Some chiropractors first produce a detailed diagnosis based on X-ray findings and then perform a 'thrust' manipulation with the aim of redirecting the vertebrae into a specific direction. The actual manipulative thrusts are similar; though as a general rule, those given by chiropractors will be more forceful than those given by osteopaths.

In the UK chiropractors complete a four-year training, as do osteopaths, after which they receive an American degree entitling them to use the title of Doctor of Chiropractic. Osteopaths now receive a BSc (Ost).

McTimoney Chiropractic

A form of treatment gaining in reputation is McTimoney chiropractic, which is extremely gentle and as a rule does not involve the use of X-rays. McTimoney emphasises a whole body treatment, rather than focusing on a problem area. The school, founded in 1972 by John McTimoney, offers a three-year, part-time training. McTimoney developed a technique for manipulation called the 'toggle recoil', which consists of a light and fast movement – a thrust, torque and recoil – of the hands on a specific part of the bone. It requires accuracy and expertise, and carried out correctly it is usually painless. McTimoney also developed ways of working with animals, and students are trained in this sideline.

Manipulative Physiotherapy

Physiotherapy training is fairly broad based and takes place over a three year period in a general hospital. Unlike osteopaths and chiropractors, physiotherapists' experience is gained by carrying out treatment on hospital patients as prescribed by the doctors. Specialisation comes after the basic training when students take appropriate postgraduate courses in the type of practice that interests them.

Until very recently physiotherapy training did not include medical diagnosis. Physiotherapists were trained to carry out a range of procedures but were prohibited from treating a patient without referral from a doctor. Treatment was mainly exercise, electrotherapy and traction.

In recent years the situation has changed since the development of the Manipulative Association of Chartered Physiotherapists (MACP), which offers postgraduate courses in manipulative therapy.

There have been two major influences on manipulative physiotherapy: the teachings of the English doctor James Cyriax, and those of the Australian teacher of physiotherapy Geoffrey Maitland. Dr Cyriax maintained that all spinal problems are due to minute disc displacements and that vigorous manipulation is necessary to correct them. Cyriax was unfortunately antagonistic towards osteopaths and chiropractors, which did a lot of damage to the relationship between the professions. Geoffrey Maitland's techniques are more widely used today and his teaching has become known as the 'Maitland Method', forming the foundation of most teachings by the MACP. The teaching emphasises safety at all times, based on a set of rules using gradually increasing amounts of force and constant feedback from the patient.

Using Osteopathy in the Treatment of Headaches

One of the most common complaints of a patient seeking medical help is headache. Pain in the head, neck and interscapular area is second only to pain in the low back.

Usually symptomatic relief is given by the doctor, in the form of analgesics plus reassurance that there is no serious underlying cause. A headache does not usually represent a life-threatening disease, though it can be extremely severe and cause the patient much anxiety.

The causes of headaches are numerous but the mechanisms producing the symptoms are relatively few. The brain substance itself is not pain sensitive. Headaches arise from pain-sensitive structures both inside and outside the skull.

Most headaches are due to mechanical faults in the cervical spine causing muscular tension, frequently at the base of the skull. The ache often spreads up into the back of the head, thus giving rise to concurrent neck pain and headache. Slight headaches can even extend to the frontal area and around the eyes.

Sites of pain within the head are most commonly caused by the stretching of blood vessels. Vascular headaches, including migraine, are due to this stretching. Pain in the head may be referred, either from within the head itself, or from the eye, nasal sinuses, the teeth and jaw, or from the chest or abdominal area.

Headaches due to mechanical faults usually respond well to osteopathic treatment. Specific adjustments to an affected joint in the neck may be required to relieve tension. Sometimes gentle massage and manual traction is sufficient. The flow of arterial and venous blood to and through the muscles and tissues will be improved, thus relieving the congestion so frequently associated with headaches. If there are no localised signs of mechanical fault or tension in the neck, further investigations may be necessary to explain the headaches.

Migraine headaches are also very common, and the borderline between tension headaches and migraine is vague. There are several different forms of migraine. Classical migraine gives rise to nausea and vomiting, visual disturbances and unilateral headache. Often there will be a warning of onset, called 'aura', such as a clarity of vision, acute awareness of colour, even hunger or thirst. Migraine is thought to be due to a chemical imbalance but is often accentuated by mechanical faults and muscular tension.

Cranial Osteopathy

Cranio-Sacral Therapy

This is a very specialised form of osteopathic technique following the teaching of Dr William Garner Sutherland. He was a student of Dr Still's at Kirksville in 1895. He studied the skull, finding that there is very slight movement between the eight cranial bones. The brain is surrounded by sheets of tissue known as the meninges, which extend all the way down the vertebral column to the sacrum at the base of the spine. This forms a reciprocal tension mechanism connecting the movement of the skull bones and the sacrum.

An approach to diagnosis and treatment has evolved in which the osteopath's sense of touch is used to identify and correct slight disturbances of tissue mobility and fluid flow, not only in and around the joints of the skull, but throughout the body. Cranial work helps to balance the rhythmical forces in the body by gently guiding and releasing the tensions within the tissues.

The technique is very gentle and relaxing and is used in cases of acute pain of mechanical origin and to help relieve different types of head pain, such as neuralgia, sinusitis and migraine headaches, as well as the pain following blows to the head, whiplash injuries and dental work. Disturbances of balance and tinnitus can sometimes be helped by these techniques, as well as circulation and breathing problems, high blood pressure and stomach ulcers, which may be aggravated by pressure on the nerves in the brain.

Children respond well to the gentle approach offered by this treatment, especially newborn babies suffering from birth traumas and conditions causing distress and anxiety such as colic and constant crying. It is always worth consulting an osteopath specialising in cranial techniques about any child who is causing concern to his parents. Often problems that cannot be given a specific diagnosis can be helped by this form of treatment.

Biography

After leaving school, Hilary Dewey studied nursing at UCH, London. She worked as a staff nurse, completed her training in midwifery and worked as a district nurse before travelling and practising in Canada and Switzerland. In 1980 she underwent her training in osteopathy at the BSO, taking postgraduate courses in cranial osteopathy and osteopathy for sports injuries. She had practices in Henley-on-Thames and Clifton Hampden in Oxfordshire for 11 years before her husband's work brought them to Scotland. Hilary joined the multidisciplinary team at HealthWorks in Forres in 1995. Hilary and her husband have two children adopted from Romania and maintain their links with and support for that country.

Further Reading

Belshaw, C., *Osteopathy – Is it For You?*, Element Books, 1987.

Chaitow, Leon, *Osteopathic Self-Treatment*, Thorsons, 1990.

Giovanna, E L; Schiowitz, S., *An Osteopathic Approach to Diagnosis and Treatment,* J B Lippincott, 1991.

Master, P., *Osteopathy for Everyone*, Penguin, 1988.

Neumann, H D, *Introduction to Manual Medicine*, Springer Verlag, 1989.

Northrup, George, *Osteopathic Medicine: An American Reformation*, American Osteopathic Assoc., 1987.

Sandler, S., *Osteopathy*, Macdonald Optima, 1992.

————., *New Ways to Health: Osteopathy*, Hamlyn, 1989.

Triance, E., *Osteopathy: a Patient's Guide*, Thorsons, 1986.

Trowbridge, Carol, *Andrew Taylor Still – 1828-1917*, Thomas Jefferson University Press, 1991.

A selection of interesting papers recently published:

Aswani, K., *Fund GP study reveals benefits of osteopathy*, Fundholding, 1994; 7 June: 10-8.

Frank, A., *Low back pain*, BMJ, 1993; 306: 901-8.

Kinalski, R., *The comparison of the results of manual therapy versus physiotherapy methods used in the treatment of patients with low back pain syndromes*, Manual Medicine, 1984; 4: 44-6.

MacDonald, R S, *An open controlled assessment of osteopathic manipulation in non-specific low back pain*, Spine 1990; 15: 5, 364-70.

————, *Osteopathic diagnosis of back pain*, Manual Medicine, 1988; 3: 110-3.

Stodolny, J., *Manual Therapy in the treatment of patients with cervical migraine*, Manual Medicine 1989; 4: 2, 49-51.

Szmelsky, A O., *The difference between holistic osteopathic practice and manipulation*, Holistic Medicine, 1990; 5: 2, 67-9.

Thomas, K J., *Use of non-orthodox and conventional care in Britain*, BMJ, 1991; 302: 207-10.

Turk, Z., *Mobilisation of the cervical spine in chronic headaches*, Manual Medicine 1987; 3: 1, 15-17.

Burns and Lyttleton, *Osteopathy on the NHS: one practice's experience*, Complementary Therapies in Medicine, 1994; 2: 200-3.

Cleaky, C.; Fox, J., *Menopausal symptoms: osteopathic intervention*, Complementary Therapies in Medicine, 1994; 2: 181-6.

Koes, B W, et al., *Randomised clinical trial of manipulative therapy and physiotherapy for persistent back and neck complaints: results of one year follow up*, BMJ 1992; 304: 601-5.

Little P., et al., *General Practitioners management of acute back pain: a survey of reported practice compared with clinical guidelines*, BMJ 1996; 312, 485-8.

Peters, Davies and Pietroni, *Musculoskeletal clinic in general practice: study on one year's referrals*, British Journal of General Practice, 1994; 44: 25-28.

Pringle, M.; Tyreman, S., *Study of 500 patients attending an osteopathic practice*, British Journal of General Practice 1993; 43: 15-18.

Shekelle, P G; Adams, A H; Chassim, M R; Hurwitz, E L; Brook, R H., *Spinal Manipulation for low back pain*, A Int Med, 1992; 117: 590-8.

Resources

The Osteopathic Information Service and General Council and Register of Osteopaths
P O Box 2074
Reading
Berkshire
RG1 4YR
Tel. 01734-512 051

(This organisation provides information regarding the profession, the schools and the governing bodies.)

Accredited schools of osteopathy:

The British School of Osteopathy (BSO)
1-4 Suffolk Street
London SW1Y 4HG
Tel. 0171-930 9254

The British College of Naturopathy and Osteopathy (BCNO)
Frazer House
6 Netherhall Gardens
London NW3 5RR
Tel. 0171-435 6464

The European School of Osteopathy (ESO)
104 Tonbridge
Maidstone
Kent
ME16 8SL
Tel. 01622-671558

The London College of Osteopathic Medicine (LCOM)
8-10 Boston Place
London NW1 6QH
Tel. 0171-262 5250

The BCNO, BSO and ESO offer university degrees and at each the undergraduate course is full-time for four years. The BSO offers different pathways through its course including an extended 'learn and you earn' version. The LCOM runs a 13-month course for doctors only.

Maidstone College of Osteopathy
30 Tonbridge Road\Maidstone
Kent ME15 8RT
Tel. 01622-752375

The John Wernham International Academy of Osteopathy
Roodestraat 2
B-3151 Sint-Joris-Weert
Belgium
Tel. (36) 1-647 7695

Postgraduate Course:
Sutherland Cranial College
Morecambe Lodge
Archenfield Road
Ross-on-Wye
HR9 5BB
Tel. 01989-567359

Past Life Therapy
by Judy Hall

The theory underlying Past Life Therapy (PLT), also known as regression therapy, states that what has occurred in the past will affect a person's physical, emotional, mental or spiritual well-being. Where PLT differs from conventional psychotherapy is that the past is seen as extending back to previous lives; in other words, it is based on the principle of reincarnation. In PLT, people re-experience aspects of their past lives.

Psychotherapy

Historical Background

PLT is an ancient technique that has been resurrected in modern times. The Greek philosopher and mathematician Pythagoras (582-507BC) said that he had formerly been Euphorbus, who died from wounds inflicted by Menelaus at the siege of Troy. As Euphorbus he was given a gift – the memory of his soul's transmigrations from life to life and the recollection of what his own soul, and the souls of others, had experienced between death and rebirth.[1]

PLT was used in the temples of Egypt[2] and, as 'soul retrieval', has formed part of the shamanic practices of many native peoples, including North and South American Indians, Tibetans and Hunas. Hypnotic regression to past lives is an ancient yogic technique. At the beginning of this century the Hindu sage Ramakrishna regressed his disciple Vivekanada into a trance, so that he could remember who he was before his present birth. What he remembered confirmed that he was to be Ramakrishna's successor.

The modern Western therapeutic use of past lives began with the rediscovery of altered states of consciousness by Franz Anton Mesmer (1734-1815) but it was not until the beginning of the twentieth century that Lieutenant Colonel Albert de Rochas hypnotised 19 people and took them back to what appeared to be past lives. By the middle of the century many hypnotists were regressing people to other lives. There was often great reluctance on the part of the hypnotists, and many of them steadfastly refused to believe in the validity of what their clients were experiencing. Dr Alexander Cannon, an Englishman who was knighted for scientific achievement, regressed more than a thousand people to other lives. He accepted the existence of past lives only when the weight of the case history evidence he had collected over many years

Hypnotherapy

*Psychological
Therapies*

became overwhelming. Before that 'the theory of reincarnation was a nightmare' to him.[3] He would argue with his subjects whilst they were in trance that they could not possibly be experiencing another life (a most untherapeutic practice). Eventually, however, he declared that psychoanalysis did not benefit the majority of people because the root cause of their problems lay in previous lives. It was the marriage of altered states, such as hypnosis, with psychotherapeutic techniques and the esoteric doctrine of reincarnation that gave birth to PLT as it is practised at the end of the twentieth century. No one person can be said to have developed the therapy. Indeed, many of the people who practise it came to it independently.[4] Nowadays, it is used by hypnotherapists, psychotherapists and complementary therapists from a wide range of disciplines.

Theoretical Base

The theoretical base for PLT is, on the one hand, extremely simple: it is possible to reframe the past to create healing in the present. But, on the other hand, it is a complex process which presupposes that a human being is not merely a physical body but a Gordian knot of energy fields. Each of these fields can affect the others. With the exception of the physical, these fields are not confined by the boundaries of time.

PLT differs from conventional psychotherapies in that it is conducted in an altered state of consciousness in which past, present and future coexist simultaneously. PLT works with subtle energy bodies[5] and the human soul or spirit, an eternal aspect of consciousness, which can move beyond and between physical death carrying with it the imprint of former lives. There is now considerable evidence in support of this theory.[6] Many past life therapists believe that this soul or spirit is in the process of evolving, learning and growing as it moves through different lives. PLT is, therefore, a spiritually based therapy. It is firmly grounded in the here and now. It does not exist merely to prove the concept of other lives. Its objective is to improve the client's quality of life in present time through making conscious the contents of the unconscious and restoring the memory of events or emotions which have created blockages or traumas in the past, and which have then been carried over, via the subtle energy bodies, to the present life.

The root cause of a problem may be an event in one life, or a repetition, through several lives, creating a pattern. In recognising, experiencing and releasing from past life events or patterns, the past is healed and the root cause no longer resonates in the present life. The dis-ease is no longer manifested.

Application of Past Life Therapy

In my own practice I have seen some dramatic improvements in health and well-being after therapy, and other practitioners report the same results.[7] Many people want to enhance their present-life functioning. People often consult a past life therapist after conventional therapy has failed to reveal the cause of a deeply ingrained pattern of behaviour or health problem. Winafred Blake Lucas, the doyenne of American PLT, has identified several short-term results and long-term objectives with which most past life therapists would concur:

◆ Short-term results: alleviation of crises and conflicts, improvement in relationships, and augmentation of the patient's sense of competence and self-worth.

◆ Long-term objectives: acceptance of who one is on every level, leading to a pervasive sense of well-being and comfort with one's place in the skein of life.[8]

PLT may be helpful in conditions such as phobias, irrational fears, chronic anxiety, eating disorders, addictions or sexual difficulties. It can also help when people have problems with physical health, relationships, guilt or family dynamics. In addition it can be used in healing emotional wounds, defusing negative energy patterns, establishing positive change, regaining confidence and self-worth, rewriting lifescripts and connecting to the spiritual dimension of life.

The Practice of Past Life Therapy

There are many forms of PLT, some of which operate in conjunction with other approaches such as bodywork. All past life techniques create an altered state of consciousness, but the induction process varies from guided imagery or hypnosis, to touch or specifically induced emotional tension. The depth of regression (return to the past) may move between a sense of 'watching a film' to a graphic reliving of the experience.[9] The following are some of the techniques used in PLT.

Hypnotic Trance

Hypnosis accesses the subconscious mind. Regression under hypnosis is vivid and the subject may actively experience traumas, dramas and emotions from the past life. Some hypnotherapists believe that simply rerunning a past life is sufficient for change to take place in the present life. Others work at reframing and healing the past life. In hypnosis, the therapist usually retains control of the process. (Not all hypnotherapists work with past lives.)

Hypnotherapy

Active Imagination and Guided Imagery

In active imagination or guided imagery, a deep sense of relaxation is induced and the subject is then taken on a visual journey which leads into past lives. Many therapists use contact with the 'higher self' (the eternal consciousness) to guide the process. Control of the process remains with the subject, and the success of the therapy depends both on the depth of regression achieved, and on the skill of the therapist in directing the healing process.

Christos Technique

A long-established approach, called the Christos technique and used all over the world, combines deep relaxation, induced by rubbing the feet and forehead, with guided imagery. It usually achieves deep regression but the disadvantage can be the length of time taken to reach another life.

Past Life Healing

Past life healing combines elements of regression, guided journeys, soul retrieval and emotional release. It is a graphic reliving of the past life events, combined with clearing away or reframing blockages created in the past. The process is facilitated and guided by the therapist but control remains with the subject.

Bodywork

SHEN Therapy
Shiatsu
Kinesiology
Massage

There are various types of bodywork which will release and heal past lives. SHEN therapy, acupressure, deep tissue massage and kinesiology are just a few of the possibilities. Some bodywork techniques may incidentally trigger past life memories; others deliberately seek to induce memory. Most are concerned with releasing the energy pattern or blockage held in the physical body as a result of past life experience. The clearing can be cathartic or gentle, depending on the technique and the skill of the therapist.

Far Memory

Far memory is one of the oldest techniques for inducing past lives. The practitioner is usually psychic, that is, able to 'see' past lives. Accessing past lives may be via the higher self or through the 'Akashic records': in esoteric terms, this is the knowledge of all that has happened since the beginning of time. In some far memory approaches the therapist will 'see' the relevant lives, and pass this information on to the client. In others, the client will join in the 'seeing' and move into reliving the life. Many psychics have the ability to enter into past lives with their clients and actively work to release the trauma.[10]

A Past Life Therapy Session

After discussing the presenting problems, most therapists start by inducing deep relaxation. Some use a technique whereby key phrases their client has used during discussion of the problem are repeated until the past suddenly surfaces. Or, if an area of the body is painful, this may be used as a lead to the past life. Many therapists will take the journey back through time in stages – seeing the hands of a clock move backwards, for instance. Others use images of doors or tunnels to facilitate entry into the relevant life. Some use commands: 'Go to the time this first happened to you.'

Many therapists take their clients through death and into the between-life state for healing or reframing; others do this as the session progresses, or as a follow-up.

PLT can take anything from one session to perhaps forty or fifty sessions, depending on the problem and the way the therapist works. Sessions may be weekly, monthly or at longer intervals, depending on how much time is required to assimilate material and make changes.

Cautions

PLT is a powerful and intense therapeutic tool. So people who do not want to work deeply with their emotions should avoid this therapy. For people who are gullible and prone to delusions of grandeur, or seeking to prove they were someone important in a past life, this is not an appropriate therapy. Nor is PLT suitable for people with psychiatric problems, except in the hands of a very experienced therapist, who is fully conversant with the problem from the start. It may be helpful in cases of inexplicable depression or addiction but this should be discussed most carefully between client and therapist before commencing work. The ideal would be also to involve the psychiatrist in charge of the case.

Research

Although a great deal of research has gone into 'proving' past lives, much less has, as yet, taken place into the long-term effects of past life healing. It is, in any case, virtually impossible to measure improved quality of life and this is an objective for at least half of those seeking PLT. However, Hazel Denning's research correlating physical healing with altered state work, including past life recovery, showed that, in a five year follow-up, 64% of her sample experienced mild to complete relief.[11]

Case Study

Ann consulted me regarding a phobia. Her phobia had been present since childhood but had been made much worse by an incident a few years previously. Ann's problem was that she could not stand people vomiting. It severely restricted her life. She could not go on holiday, nor could she go out on social occasions with her friends. After all, as she said, drunks vomit. As a child, she had been forced to travel with her younger brother, who was always travel sick. Her parents clearly did not perceive her response as phobic and reinforced her fear. On one occasion she was locked into a room with her brother when he had an upset stomach (her mother believed this would 'cure her'). She learned to shut off what was happening by leaving her body. This involves a state of dissociation, where from the outside the person still looks normal and is physically functioning, but on the inner the mind and psyche have withdrawn to a place outwith the body.

The incident that had reinforced her abhorrence of vomit in her late teens was getting into a car after someone had been sick. She sat down before she realised, and some of the vomit was on her clothes. She went home and scrubbed herself raw.

When I regressed Ann, I asked her to find the incident that had triggered this fear. She found herself on a ship, locked below decks with many other people. It was during a very bad storm. People were terrified they would drown. Everyone but she was seasick, the decks were awash with vomit. Wherever she stepped she trod in it. At first she beat on the door, begging to be let out, but no one came. Exhausted, she huddled in a corner unable to move. Finally, someone was sick down her back. She was unable to cope and left her body. She simply could not stand it any longer. A part her had remained trapped in the incident. Not surprisingly, when locked into the room with her brother in her present life, she repeated the pattern of leaving her body.

We had to reframe the situation. I took her back to the point where she was beating on the door. We had someone open it and let her out. She was taken to another cabin where, despite the stormy sea, she could bathe and change her clothes. Then she went up on deck where the air was clean and fresh. Interestingly, she herself had no fear of drowning and she revelled in the rise and fall of the boat. Finally, it struggled into port and she was able to leave the ship, leaving her fear and the memory behind. She was no longer stuck in that incident. We did some between-life work to heal that incident further and integrate the newly retrieved part of herself before we returned to her traumas as a young child in the present life. Her newly healed self could now offer support to that child shut in the room with her vomiting brother, giving her the understanding the parents had lacked.

She imagined letting herself out of the room, going to a favourite place to play instead. In an inner dialogue, the part of her that had been stuck in that incident agreed to return. She pictured her parents giving her brother a pill to prevent travel sickness before they travelled, and visualised instead a fun-filled time. Gradually her trauma lessened. Finally, we were able to take her to her teenage self and warn her not to get into the car where vomit lay on the seat. Yet another part of herself was stuck here, so this part could be welcomed back. This was as far as we could go in that session, so I brought her back into the present moment.

As she lived a great distance away from me, we were not able to do further sessions, which could possibly have uncovered more of a pattern in other lives. Some months later, however, she told me that she was now able to travel on public transport and had ventured out socially a few times. Each time she felt more confident, more able to cope. Her phobia had lessened to the extent that it no longer controlled her life. With further therapy, she could well overcome the problem totally.

Biography

Judy Hall has been a past life therapist and karmic counsellor for over twenty years. She was trained by the late Christine Hartley, who had fifty years experience in the field. Author of *Principles of Past Life Therapy* and *Menopause Matters: a practical approach to menopause*, co-authored with her partner Dr Robert Jacobs (Element), she utilises a wide variety of approaches in her therapeutic work. Judy runs workshops in past life exploration both in Brltain and abroad and has regressed hundreds of people to other lives. She is currently training therapists in past life therapy techniques.

References

1   Head and Cranston, *Reincarnation – an East West Anthology*, Julian Press, 1961, p. 78.

2   Joan Grant, *Many Lifetimes*, Corgi, 1976, p11ff.

    Judy Hall's personal past life memories.

3   Cannon, Alexander, *The Power Within*, Rider & Co., 1950 quoted in Marcla Moore, Mark Douglas, *Reincarnation, Key to Immortality*, Arcane Publications, p. 73.

4   See, for example, *Brian Weiss: Through Time Into Healing*. Even as late as the 1992, he believed he was developing a new therapy.

5   Judy Hall, *Principles of: Past Life Therapy*, Thorsons, 1996.

6   Moody, Raymond, *Life after Life: The Investigation of a phenomenon – Survival of Bodily Death*, Bantam, 1975.

    Margot Grey, *Return from Death, an Exploration of the Near Death Experience*, 1985.

    Whitton, Joal; Joe Fisher, *Life Between Life*, Warner Books, 1995.

7   Judy Hall, *Principles of: Past Life Therapy*, Thorsons, 1996.

    Roger Woolger, *Other Lives, Other Selves*, Bantam, 1988.

    Winafred Blake Lucas, *Regression Therapy: A Handbook for Professionals*, Deep Forest Press, 1993.

8   Lucas, op cit., p. 5.

9   Judy Hall, *Principles of: Past Life Therapy*, Thorsons, 1996.

    Glen Williston; Judith Johnstone, *Discovering your Past Lives*, Aquarian Press, 1995.

10 Judy Hall, *Principles of: Past Life Therapy*, Thorsons, 1996.

11 Statistically analysed and presented in Association for Past-Life Research and Therapies monograph, *Altered States of Consciousness: A Technique for Healing the Body*. Current research is covered in the Journal of Regression Therapy.

Further Reading

Bache, Christopher, *Life Cycles: Reincarnation and the Web of Life*, Paragon House, 1990.

Fiore, Edith, *You Have Been Here Before*, Ballantine Books, 1978.

Hall, Judy, *Principles of: Past Life Therapy*, Thorsons, 1996.

Hartley, Christine, *A Case for Reincarnation*, Robert Hale, 1972.

Kelsey, Denys and Joan Grant, *Many Lifetimes*, Victor Gollancz, 1969.

Lucas, Winafred Blake, *Regression Therapy: A Handbook for Professionals*, Deep Forest Press, 1993.

Moody, Raymond A, *Coming Back, A Psychiatrist Explores Past Life Journeys*, Bantam, 1990.

Motoyama, Hiroshi, *Karma: Reincarnation*, Piatkus 1992.

Netherton, Morris; Nancy Shiffrin, *Past Lives Therapy*, Ace Books, 1978.

Stevenson, Ian, *Twenty Cases Suggestive of Reincarnation*, VA, USA, University Press of Virginia, 1974.

———, *Children Who Remember Previous Lives: A Question of Reincarnation*, University Press of Virginia, 1987.

Wambach, Helen, *Reliving your Past Lives*, the Psychology of Past Life Regression, Ballantine Books, 1978.

———, *Life Before Life Bantam Books*, 1979.

Weiss, Brian, *Many Lives, Many Masters*, Piatkus, 1988.

———, *Through Time into Health*, Piatkus, l992.

Williston, Glenn; Johnstone, Judith, *Discovering Your Past Lives*, Aquarian Press, 1995.

Woolger, Roger, *Other Lives, Other Selves*, Bantam, 1988.

Journal

Journal of Regression Therapy, from the Association for Past Life Research and Therapy, Riverside, CA, USA.

Resources

Woolger Training Seminars
Briarwood Long Wittenham
Oxford
OX14 4QW

(provides a list of practitioners)

The College of Past Life Healing
118A Regents Park
London
NW1 8XL

Directory of Past Life Therapists and Regressionists
P O Box 26
London
WG2H 9LP

Atkinson-Ball College of Hypnotherapy and
Hypnohealing
P O Box 70
Southport

PR9 8JX

Institute of Clinical Hypnosis
28 Tantallon Road
London
SW12 80G

Association for Past Life Research and Therapy
Journal of Regression Therapy
P O Box 20151
Riverside
CA 92516
USA

Polarity Therapy
by Rosamund J Webster

Historical Background

Polarity therapy is a multidisciplinary approach to health and well-being, developed by Dr Randolph Stone (1890–1981). He was born in Austria but emigrated to the USA with his family when he was 13 years old. He was always interested in health care, and initially studied osteopathy, chiropractic and naturopathy.

Osteopathy
Chiropractic
Naturopathy

Dr Stone practised in Chicago and for over 50 years he researched and studied different systems of health and healing – acupuncture, Ayurvedic medicine, Chinese medicine and yoga, to name a few. In 1948 he published his first book: *The New Energy Concept of the Healing Art*.[1] In later years he spent six months of the year in India, providing a free clinic for 'the hopeless and the helpless' which he considered a fair test for the effectiveness of polarity therapy.

Acupuncture
Traditional Chinese
Medicine
Yoga

Theoretical Base

Polarity therapy is the art and science of stimulating and harmonising the flow of vital energy in the body. This energy is called *prana* or *chi* (also spelled *qi*).

Both modern science and ancient art and philosophy have shown us that the human organism is not just a physical structure but that, like everything else, we consist of energy fields. Illness and disease are the result of blocks in the energy fields. When the energy flow becomes blocked or restricted due to stress, trauma, injury, unresolved emotions, environmental factors, etc., this can result in pain, illness or 'dis-ease'. These energetic states also influence our consciousness, behaviour and health. Understanding them provides opportunity for insight and healing.

Energy comes into the body through air, food, heat and light, physical touch, spiritual experience and love. Some of this energy is used to maintain the organism on all its levels; the rest is given out again through communication, physical work, love, creativity and the expression of emotion, as well as through the excretion of waste.

The theory is based on the premise that everything is made up of five elements: ether, air, fire, water and earth; these elements being governed by the opposing and complementary forces of yin and yang.

◆ **The ether element** governs creativity and personal self-expression. Ether people will be full of inspiration, may be immersed in the arts, and are likely to have strong spiritual aspirations. If they are out of balance in this element, they may be ungrounded and unable to manifest anything in form.

◆ **The air element** governs movement and mental activity. Air type people enjoy the realm of thoughts, concepts and ideas, tend to be fairly detached and can be impersonal. If the air element is out of balance they may be restless, dizzy, anxious, or stuck in old thought patterns.

◆ **The fire element** governs will and personal power. Fire type people are very precise with a keen intellect; they are enthusiastic and warm. If this element is out of balance, it can manifest as a bitter taste in the mouth, a lack of energy and vitality, an inability to have one's needs met or power-hungry and aggressive behaviour.

◆ **The water element** governs pleasure and sexuality. Water type people are very supportive, caring and nurturing; they can be receptive and accepting. If this element is out of balance, one may experience an inability to let go and move on in life, becoming overwhelmed by strong emotions, inhibitions or excesses.

◆ **The earth element** governs survival and the material world. Earth type people are down-to-earth and practical; they have patience and stability. If this element is out of balance, one may become too rigid about routines, lack vision, and find it difficult to be present in the here and now.

The practitioner works to rebalance the whole person by looking at the polarity relationship within the body (positive, negative and neutral) while working the various reflex and pressure points.

The Practice of Polarity Therapy

Polarity is a broad-based approach. A consultation starts with a case history and an energetic diagnosis to determine which elements are out of balance. The practitioner will assess what impact this is having on the client's health and how it expresses in their lifestyle. Depending on what condition the client is suffering from, diet may be discussed and recommendations made. If it is appropriate there may be some cleansing or an individualised detoxification programme. The client may be given some exercises to support the work done in the session. The greater portion of the session is spent doing bodywork, during which the client remains fully clothed. Polarity theory maintains that emotional well-being is a vital part of the work and so time is set aside for talking.

◆ *Polarity bodywork* is an extensive range of techniques and skills used to rebalance and release the blocks of energy in the body. It influences the energy on many different levels. It can work on the musculo-skeletal system, central nervous system and autonomic nervous system, the structural system and the five element system. The therapist will work to release the source of the blocked energy by means of therapeutic bodywork which has its application in soft tissue manipulation; the use of reflex/pressure points and techniques from osteopathy and chiropractic are also to be seen. In the process of release, renewed creativity arises to sustain and integrate body and soul in its search for fulfilment. The bodywork helps the client work with old patterns, educating the body into a new way of being in the world.

Massage
Osteopathy
Chiropractic

◆ *The diet and nutrition component* takes a naturopathic approach. Cleansing diets are seen as an important process in the journey back to complete health, as they aid the elimination of harmful products that may have built up over time. Health is more than just the absence of disease, so emphasis is placed on health-building diets.

Naturopathy
Nutritional Therapy

Polarity therapists are trained to look at food elementally, that is, to look at the type of energy each food carries and how that can create a balance for the individual. (For example, fruits are in the category of the air element; grains and pulses are fire element foods, etc.) For optimum health, foods from each of the elements need to be eaten, but a slightly larger portion from the element pertaining to the individual. Food can be used to balance energies by eating a larger amount of a food of a particular element for a length of time.

◆ *Polarity exercises* have their roots in the yoga system but have been adapted for specific purposes. There are individual exercises to boost and develop specific elements in the body and these are used to support the bodywork done during a session. Dr Stone developed some poses that involve gentle rocking and stretching and others that are quite robust in movement. They all get the energy moving.

Yoga

◆ *Emotional factors* are taken into account. Thoughts and attitudes play a part in how people find themselves in the world. The practitioners are trained in counselling and communication skills. They apply the techniques of active listening and engage in a client-centred approach which seeks to support clients in their progression from illness to health.

Counselling

◆ *The Ayurvedic model of types* is another model used in polarity therapy. The types, known as *doshas*, govern the constitution of a person. The *vata dosha* constitutional type is governed by the air element and, generally, will be thin and talk and move quickly. They are quite creative with alert and active minds. The *pitta dosha* constitutional type is governed by the fire element and will have a strong digestion, large appetite and an intolerance for heat and the sun. They have good comprehension and are quite ambitious. The *kapha dosha* constitution is governed by water and these people have well-developed bodies and slow digestion; they are usually tolerant and calm. The Ayurvedic system of health care is a complex but valuable model for determining imbalance and treatment.

To be effective, a series of between six and ten sessions is recommended. However, if clients have a chronic complaint, they will need more, and even after the presenting condition has cleared up clients may still need to work with the therapist for a longer period.

Polarity should not only be seen from a rehabilitative point of view. It is also effective as a preventative and maintenance form of health care. Polarity works in conjunction with conventional medicine and other forms of alternative therapy. However, it is seldom recommended to receive many different types of therapy at the same time.

Training

Anyone can train in polarity therapy; the main qualities needed are a respect for humanity and a genuine desire to assist jointly in the process of restoring the well-being of others.

The training offered by the International School of Polarity Therapy is 20 weekend workshops over a two-year period or an intensive one-year training, one day a week.

Case History I

Gwen, 30, presented with irritable bowel syndrome from which she had suffered for four years, unable to receive any effective help from allopathic medicine. The pains and spasms in her abdomen, constant diarrhoea or constipation and general fatigue were reducing her quality of life: she could not remember when she felt well.

As a client's case history unfolds, I develop an elemental interpretation of the presenting symptoms. In the application of the five elements, the liver, stomach, small intestine and the process of digestion are all governed by the fire element. The large intestine and the eliminative process are governed by the earth element. In Gwen's case it was clear that these two elements were the primary ones out of balance. Having taken detailed dietary information, I made recommendations about the foods that would be best avoided and the foods that could add variety and breadth to her diet, and I recommended some supplementation. Another aspect of the treatment was bodywork, an area that is of vital importance in the process of health and healing. When the soma has experienced pain and trauma, this needs to be relieved through a rebalancing of the energies, in order that harmony and balance can be restored. This is the uniting of body and soul.

In a matter of days Gwen began to feel better, so in the following treatment I advised a mild cleansing programme. The purpose of this was to remove the toxins and allergens that were still in her system. After she completed the cleanse, she reported that she felt much better and was surprised to find that she was not as short-tempered as she used to be.

After the initial series of treatments, she is greatly improved on all levels, including feeling more empowered: since she is aware that what she eats and drinks affects her health, she is now able to make conscious decisions about her health. She enjoys greater vitality and chooses to continue to have her sessions once a month as a maintenance and preventative measure.

Case History II

Bill, 43, presented with ME. His life had altered drastically from being that of an active family man with a good social life, who held a managerial position, to being on extended sick leave, unable to work, unable even to help at home without becoming exhausted, and because of all this feeling isolated. His GP had said nothing could be done. His condition was very debilitating; Bill was experiencing mental confusion, unexplained pains in the body, headaches and extreme fatigue.

However, Bill was determined to get well and over the weeks experienced definite improvements as a result of the additions to his diet and the effects of the bodywork. As the months went on, cleansing was included and later he was doing well enough to take on a few energy-building exercises, which helped to support the bodywork being done in the sessions, as well as encouraging self-empowerment and self-awareness. Some of the bodywork we did focused on the central nervous system, the lymphatic system, the digestive system, the circulatory system and the eliminative system, which encompassed work on all the elements in turn.

We worked together for over a year but within a few months Bill was able to re-establish his active role in family life. He was able to read and he was free from pain.

During the later months Bill had to make a major decision regarding work. He realised that if his health was not going to be put at risk again, full-time employment was no longer an option. Eventually he came to terms with the fact that there were other creative and imaginative ways of working. At the end of the treatments Bill had recovered from his condition sufficiently well enough to work part-time and enjoy a good quality of life with his family and friends.

Biography

Rosamund Webster is the Director of the International School of Polarity Therapy. Her studies and practice have been in therapies that seek to integrate body, mind, feelings and spirituality. Her past studies include psychotherapy and counselling, yoga, stress management, polarity therapy and Chinese massage. Her work is also integrated with awareness meditation practice developed through her experience in Buddhist spiritual practices. Some of the people who have influenced her work are: Dr Stone, Carl Rogers, Joseph Campbell and Carl Jung. Her work reflects a belief in the self-regulating and healing capacity of the human organism, thus fostering empowerment and self-responsibility.

References

1   Randolph Stone, *The New Energy Concept of the Healing Art*, 1948.

Further Reading

Becker, Robert, *The Body Electric*, Morrow William & Co., 1987.

Brennan, Barbara Ann, *Hands of Light – A Guide of Healing Through the Human Energy Field*, Bantam, 1990.

Brugh Joy, W. M. D., *Joys Way*, Tarcher JP., 1979.

Gerber, Richard, *Vibrational Medicine: New Choices for Healing Ourselves*, Bear & Co., 1988.

Gordon, Richard, *Your Healing Hands*, Wingbow Press, 1984.

Johari, Harish, *Chakras*, Inner Traditions, 1988.

Keleman, Stanley, *Emotional Anatomy*, Center Press, 1986.

Leadbeater, C W., *The Chakras*, Theosophical Publishing House, 1972

Mc Farland, Don, *Body Secrets*, Healing Arts Press, 1988.

Seidman, Maruti, *A Guide to Polarity Therapy: The Gentle Art of Hands-on Healing*, Elan Press, 1991.

Shapiro, Debbie, *The Bodymind Workbook*, Element Books, 1994.

Siegel, Bernie, Peace, *Love and Healing*, Arrow Books, 1991.

Sills, Franklyn, *The Polarity Process*, Element, 1990.

Stone, Dr R., *Polarity Therapy: The Complete and Collected Works – Vols. I+II*, CRCS Publications, 1988.

Resources

International Society of Polarity Therapists
54 Ashford Road
Topsham
Exeter
Devon EX3 0LA
Tel. 01392-877 015

Polarity Therapy Association UK
Monomark House
27 Old Gloucester Street
London WC1N 3XX
Tel. 01483-417 714

Polarity Therapy Educational Trust
The Ashburton Centre
79 East Street
Ashburton
Devon TQ13 7AL
Tel. 01364-652 784

The International School of Polarity Therapy
7 Nunney Close
Cheltenham
Glos GL51 0TU
Tel. 01242-522352

Paul Francis
Energetics Training
22 Dumbarton Road
Lancaster
LA1 3BX
Tel. 01524-67009

Postural Integration
by Sean Doherty

Theoretical Background

Postural Integration (PI) is a style of deep holistic bodywork developed in the United States around 1970. Within PI, deep manipulation of the fascia or soft tissue, breathwork, Reichian techniques, Gestalt, acupressure, bioenergetics and visualisation may all be used at various times to bring about a state of wholeness, which may be defined as a successful, dynamic balance between body and mind. Health exists in the harmonious interplay of energy throughout all aspects of being – physical, emotional, mental and spiritual.

Chiropractic
Osteopathy
Holotropic Breathwork
Rebirthing
Bio-Energetic Analysis
Gestalt Therapy
Traditional Chinese Medicine
Visualisation
Health and Wellness as the Focus for Health Care
Massage, Rolfing
Hypnotherapy
Yoga

Jack Painter, who designed Postural Integration, was a student of psychology and philosophy at Emory University, Atlanta. He became a professor at the University of Miami. His PhD thesis investigated mind/body relationships. Many years of exploration in the therapeutic areas already mentioned, as well as massage, acupuncture, Rolfing, hypnosis and yoga, preceded the creation of Postural Integration as an integrated style for addressing the growth and balance of the whole person. The term 'deep bodywork' is used for this therapeutic form in order to distinguish it from superficial massage styles; PI works with the basic body structure.

The work is designed to release chronic tensions and frustrations that have built up in the body/mind throughout life. These restrictions are referred to as 'armouring'. Armouring occurs when part of the person is afraid of possible pain or confusion. The effect is to distort and desensitise the body and to keep thoughts and feelings corralled within narrow boundaries. These parts of the being resist change and the protective behaviour is generally unconscious. The intention of armouring is protection but the effect in adult life is often restriction. A defence designed to protect a desperate two year old may not fit the needs and capacities of an adult.

Armouring can be observed in the physical posture, and detected in mental attitudes. Thus when rigidly held body postures are 'melted', stuck feelings and thought processes become available to change. While this can happen spontaneously, the practitioner needs to have the skills to support emotional or mental change and to stimulate and facilitate this when necessary.

Postural Integration offers opportunities for relief from a particular symptom or to have one's body straightened and made more flexible. It is also designed to offer a transformational journey where clients can explore, in a therapeutic context, that which is blocking their lives, learning to develop and change on any level of body, mind, emotion and spirit. Effective and lasting deep bodywork is dependent on the active participation of the person looking to change their life. This participation includes giving attention, reporting on sensations and emotions or more usefully expressing them, using the breath fully, making sound, moving with the manipulations, visualising to assist release, and generally providing feedback on how the body/mind is responding and processing the work.

When there is an attempt to hide or control feelings, it is done by restricting breathing, by tensing various muscle groups and by dissociating – not being present to what is occurring. Such efforts to control experience produce physical distortion, rigid neck, rounded shoulders, swayed back, etc. It manifests emotionally and mentally in rigid and repetitive attitudes of mind and behaviours, which are incompatible, exaggerated or diminished in response to current events. There may be lack of eye contact, lack of focus, or other indications of absence of attention and awareness. As the bodyworker uses the deep manipulations to soften and reorganise the soft tissue, awareness is needed of other levels of change taking place. If resistance occurs, the practitioner may need to switch from one work mode to another, following the energetic release, encouraging energy to flow in an easy, balanced way throughout the functions of the body/mind.

The purpose is not to have all clients balanced in a similar way. Individuals are encouraged to find their own optimum, dynamic order, making the most of their unique energy potential. As old patterns of physical and mental rigidity are released, there is a need to integrate this new freedom and flexible energy into everyday life. Old habits can be gradually replaced by authentic behaviour. Old ways are not so much given up as outgrown.

The Practice of Postural Integration

A Postural Integration session begins like most other styles of work, with the therapist making contact and establishing rapport with the client. Some clients like to make a progress report and review their week and they would feel unsatisfied without that; others are ready to begin bodywork at once.

A body reading is taken. This involves the client making a body inventory reporting on body sensations, pains, stresses, also emotions and thought processes, while the bodyworker observes, paying attention to overall posture, muscular tensions and imbalances, skin colour, etc. Between them the client and therapist produce an energy map of the body and detect blockages. Sometimes movements and bio-energetic positions will be used diagnostically or to begin a process of release.

Breathwork is likely to be used at this point, to prepare the client for deep work by ensuring a flow of charge and discharge, a balanced flow of inbreath and outbreath, a rhythmic use of abdominal, diaphragmatic and thoracic breathing. This allows tissue to be manipulated more easily and with less discomfort. Attention will be given to whatever aspect of breathing is neglected in the client.

Using a variety of physical techniques, the therapist will then begin to soften tight fascia, allowing muscles to move more freely. Insensitive, unresponsive tissue can be warmed and enlivened. Acupressure points are often used to assist release. Tight fascia may restrict muscle movement and stick muscles together. When the fascia is relaxed, muscles regain independent movement; for example the head can be turned without using the whole trunk. As tense muscles are released, parts of the skeletal structure can move into a different alignment, reducing wear on joints, allowing easier co-ordination. As tissue becomes less dense and contracted, circulation, lymphatic and nerve functions may improve. Improved energy flow can clear toxins and produce a sense of well-being.

Shiatsu

Throughout these manipulations the client will be encouraged to breathe, move and make sounds that assist release. There may be quiet pauses to integrate a change, to calm a level of excitation or to study what has been achieved.

The client has the right and responsibility to say 'Stop, Go slower', 'Lighten up', 'Go deeper', 'I want more'...; while the bodyworker needs to use good judgement as to how deep, how fast and how much work is likely to be beneficial. At any point during a session, emotional issues may be accessed and when this happens, physical manipulation ceases while emotional work is supported. At other times both physical and emotional release can occur together, often including mental review and integration. Old memories can come up and be given new meaning. In some cases, trance states are used; in others a piece of gestalt resolution technique can seem appropriate. Because the work is deep, a practitioner will usually complete a session with some form of fine energy work. Use is made of acupressure balance and calming points, simple polarity connections and gentle breathwork. This supports clients as they rest and find a new balance at that point on their therapeutic journey.

Polarity Therapy

Training

Postural Integration practitioners are to be found in most countries in Europe, and the work is spreading in the USA, Canada, Mexico, Australia and New Zealand. A three-year training is a minimum requirement for practitioners. Students study supporting therapy styles as part of their course work, so facilitation and fine energy styles may vary somewhat with individual practitioners according to the elective studies that were added to the core training.

Case History I

Peter was an artist in his mid 30s. The skin on his face and torso was heavily scarred from acne and skin rashes he experienced as a child and teenager. He easily suffered from anxiety and depression. He was 6' 3" tall and experienced a lot of tension from the tight, stooped postures he adopted while engaged in his creative work. His legs were slim to the point of being skinny and his chest and back, whilst strong, were tight and rounded. His body was stiff and immobile.

In a series of ten PI sessions, we explored his issues of lack of self-confidence and unassertiveness. We worked at validating him as a person who had created good options for himself in life and had a spirit that remained ready to fight for what he felt was positive for him. Validation of the skills and gifts that he had already developed was interwoven with physical and energetic work. A typical session would involve Peter describing current issues in his life and exploring the thoughts and feelings about these issues, where they lodged in his body and where they were affecting his posture.

Breathing exercises and physical bodywork on his neck, chest and back helped open his posture, allowed him to breathe more freely and eased the ongoing tension created by his work postures. The breathing helped Peter to have more energy. Work on his upper body was physically and energetically connected through his hips, legs and feet to foster a sense of centredness and groundedness. The physical and energy work on his legs helped the tissues soften and fill out, so that he felt more physically substantial and emotionally relaxed. Sometimes he felt tinglings and buzzings in his body as life energy started to enliven his tissues. Other times he would feel and work through repressed emotions of fear, sadness and anger.

PI was a powerful experience for Peter and often enjoyable as he experienced the changes to his body and the effects this was having on him as a person. Both physically and symbolically he felt more at ease in how he moved and how he 'stood' his ground in the world. At the conclusion of his PI work he experienced himself as standing taller, feeling physically and energetically full in himself and yet more relaxed and centred with his sense of humour and enjoyment of life bubbling through. This sense of standing taller was literal as well as subjective.

Peter entered a new relationship towards the end of his series of PI sessions. He felt that the psychological and physical changes he experienced were very supportive in this. He could move beyond his physical and energetic constrictions and truly meet, enjoy and feel stable with his new girlfriend. As he changed his relationship with himself, so new options emerged for him in how he related to others.

Case History II

An impressive case quoted to me during my training was that of a woman of 36 who had a fall which damaged her sacrum, coccyx and sacro-ileac joint. She was told by a hospital consultant that within five years she would be unable to walk and would have to use a wheelchair.

Postural Integration work eased stresses from the accident to her lower back and hips. This was supported by physical work for her whole body to maximise flexibility and quality alignment of her structure so as to minimise strains from elsewhere in her body that would exacerbate the weakness she had been left with in her sacrum. The traumatic shock of the accident was also worked with and the other emotional stresses that threatened to tighten her structure and trigger the pain in her hips. Self-help exercises to encourage flexibility, relaxation and good body alignment gave her skills that she could use between sessions and after her Postural Integration therapy concluded. Twenty years later she is fit, active, not in a wheelchair and continues to enjoy her rich and full life.

Biography

Sean Doherty, after completing a degree in psychology and linguistics, has worked as a therapist since 1981. He has trained in many forms of therapy, specialising in Oriental methods of energy-work and Western approaches to body-psychotherapy. He has trained in Reichian psychotherapy, energetic integration, family therapy and supervision skills, and in postural integration, osteopathy and Chinese, Thai and Swedish massage. He is currently chairperson of the British Massage Therapy Council and former president of the International Council of Postural Integration Trainers. His main interests are in developing the synthesis between Eastern approaches to energy and health and Western approaches to body, mind and spirit.

Further Reading

Bertherat, Therese; Bernstein, Carol, *The Body has its Reasons*, Millennium Books, 1992.

Elsworth Todd, Mabel, *The Thinking Body*, Princeton Book Co., 1980.

Painter, Jack, *Deep Bodywork and Personal Development*, Element Books, 1986.

———, *The Technical Manual of Deep Wholistic Bodywork*, can be obtained from the International Centre for Release and Integration.

Rolf, Ida, *Rolfing and Physical Reality*, Healing Arts Press, 1990.

Resources

Jack Painter
The International Center for Release and Integration
450 Hillside Avenue
Mill Valley
CA 94941
USA

Sean Doherty
3 Woodhouse Cliff
Headingley
Leeds LS6 2HF
Tel/Fax. 0113-278 5601

Ian Holland
26 Ashburton Road
Glasgow G12 OLZ
Tel. 0141-334 5846

Silke Ziehl
c/o The Open Centre
188 Old Street
London EC1V 9FR
Tel. 0181-332 6979

Psychological Therapies Historical Development
by Ulla Sebastian

Historical Background

Psychology is a child of the twentieth century. Its birth and growth reflect the cultural shift from humans simply being part of the collective, guided and ruled by the Christian order of the Middle Ages, to humans responding and reacting as individuals, creators of their own destiny. With the acknowledgment in the latter half of the nineteenth century of the power of the human brain and consciousness, the need arose to understand the make-up and the deeper dynamics of the mind. Psychology, especially in its applied form of psychotherapy, has been the attempt to do this.

Sigmund Freud[1] was the first to undertake systematic expeditions into the jungle of the human unconscious. His was an attempt to free people from the sexually repressive influences of the capitalist-bourgeois society at the turn of the century. In a life span of 83 years, Freud laid the ground for a dynamic understanding of the human mind that has substantially influenced and permeated our culture and science. Being a man of broad education, an adventurer and explorer, a humanist and courageous atheist, he examined the notion that culture and society are of primary importance in forming, impacting and restricting the human mind. He set out to demonstrate how humans re-create that culture through education, religion and art. He was also the first to elaborate in a systematic way how conflict in the human mind, conflict between inner drives and cultural demands, can express itself in neurotic behaviour (such as compulsions or obsessions) or body symptoms (such as hysteric paralysis or blindness). His topographic model of the id, ego and super-ego became standard knowledge in many academic disciplines and the words became part of everyday language. His treatment technique, called psychoanalysis, is still a basic pillar in the health care systems of Western countries although there are many variations nowadays in the setting and duration of the treatment.

His disciples, of whom there have been many, developed his ground-breaking work in many different directions. Most influential, perhaps, was Carl Gustav Jung,[2] a contemporary of Freud's. Jung took Freud's model of the unconscious as a mud of suppressed personal drives and desires, and expanded it to include the concept of the collective unconscious, which could be explored through the medium of dream symbols and archetypes. Alfred Adler[3] shifted the focus from biological determination to interaction, reintegrating the isolated 'I' back into the 'we' of the community. Wilhelm Reich investigated the connection between verbal and body expression and developed the most refined character analytic approach within the analytic movement. His main focus and life work was the research of the make-up and dynamics of the life-energy itself.

Bio-Energetic Analysis

In the first half of this century, the neo-analysts stayed closest to the core of Freud's work. Many of them left Nazi Germany and emigrated to the USA (A. Freud[4], K. Horney[5], E. Fromm[6], H. Marcuse). The confrontation with a new culture brought up questions of how social factors impact the personality structure and how the ego may adapt to new conditions. These questions were similar to those researched by American academic psychologists who were investigating conflict-free ego functions, such as perception, cognition, memory, intelligence and motility (the free flow of energy). With the shift of focus from Freud's ego defence mechanisms to ego functions, the neo-analysts succeeded in integrating psychoanalysis into American academic psychology.

The Social Context

World War II brought about major cultural and socio-economic changes which affected the lives of people the world over. A fast-developing technology was able to produce mass consumer goods and connect people throughout the world via a rapidly expanding communication system. Radio and television became major agents of mass education, influencing people's values on a scale unseen and unheard of. The self-made man, achieving material wealth and social status through his own effort, became the new American hero. Women grasped their chance to liberate themselves from patriarchal structures and to find their own voice and socio-economic power. Mobility became a prerequisite for social achievement and material wealth. Neighbourhoods and family units started to decay, producing a whole generation of 'latch-key' children. Sexuality, which had been suppressed in Freud's lifetime, became a public event, turning the most intimate expression between two partners into a mass stimulation.

In the seventies, social scientists identified the emergence of a new cultural personality type. They described it as someone who was distant, cool, formal, arrogant, shy, but smart. Key factors were a high ability to compete and achieve; an ability to function efficiently; and a focus on social status, success and superficial, sensual satisfaction. The down side was an inability to form intimate relationships; an avoidance of deep inner feelings, spontaneity and subjectivity; personal isolation; lack of contact; emotional impoverishment; and the loss of meaning in life. New psychosocial and clinical problems arose in response to the emerging needs of the culture. Suppression was no longer the central factor of personal suffering as in Freud's time, but was replaced by the split between body and mind, heart and sex, individual and group.

People no longer complained about neurotic symptoms but about inner emptiness, isolation, anxiety and depression. They tried to escape these painful states through alcohol, drugs, pills or workaholism. The occurrence of psychosomatic diseases such as high blood pressure, heart attacks and stomach ulcers and chronic diseases such as cancer, ME and later AIDS, increased considerably. Addiction and co-dependency became key words in psychological literature.

Developments in Medicine and Therapy

New challenges called for new answers. With the decline of religion, physicians were regarded as gods, and psychologists and psychotherapists took the role of the priests, trying to catch that which was disintegrating in the midst of an abundance of material wealth.

Business took on prime importance in the functioning of society and this led to specific cultural demands. The labour force had to keep functioning, and supporting this system became the job of psychologists, social scientists and the medical system.

Behavioural Therapy

Behavioural science and therapy (I.P. Pavlov[7], E.L. Thorndike[8], B.F. Skinner[9], J. Wolpe[10], C.L. Hull[11], H.J. Eysenck[12], A.A. Lazarus[13], A. Ellis[14]) offered an answer to the challenge by dealing with the symptoms that prevented people from working efficiently. Using principles of conditioning and model learning, they developed techniques to alter behavioural problems, especially anxieties and phobias. They expanded their models to look at people's beliefs, thought-forms and the concepts which influence emotions and behaviour, and they successfully helped patients in psychiatric institutions to regain social abilities in dealing with everyday life demands.

Psychosomatic Medicine

Psychosomatic medicine established itself as a separate faculty within medical schools of Western universities. Special clinics were set up, offering medical and psychotherapeutic support in dealing with inner and social conflicts that had found an outlet in physical diseases. In the 1960s and early 1970s it had the potential to become part of the general curriculum essential to all medical disciplines. It represented the upsurge in awareness of the patient as a whole person rather than 'a case'. But by the 1980s it had established itself as a separate speciality, and while it had gained the acceptance and reputation of an academic discipline, it had lost the potential it once seemed to have of influencing all medical interactions.

Psychotherapy

Psychoanalysts realised that there was more to humans than the ego and the mind. The self became the new focus of research, alongside people's demands to improve their self-worth, self-acceptance and self-assertion. Traditional psychoanalysis, the aim of which was to provide a space for self-recognition, proved to be too lengthy, expensive and mind-oriented for the emerging need of the masses for psychosocial and health care. A broad variety of short and middle range psychotherapies started to take its place, helping people to adjust to social reality.

Psychotherapy

Family Therapy

One of the major problems on the social scale as a result of all the factors mentioned previously was the increasing divorce rate in the Western countries reflecting a drastic change in lifelong commitments. Family research had shown that broken and dysfunctional homes were a disposing factor for mental disease and behavioural disorder. The need to support couples and families in holding the unit together inspired a broad variety of family therapies. System theory provided a model to view the whole family as a single unit with its own specific structures and functions, such as expressing a family distortion through making one person into a symptom carrier or scapegoat. The psychoanalytic approach contributed knowledge about the deeper dynamics between the family members, looking at how children are used as partner substitutes or projection screens for the parents' own ideal or negative parts. Behavioural science provided tools to help partners to communicate clearly and to improve sexual pleasure and intimacy.

Family Therapy

Groups in Therapy and Self-Development

Another related problem, especially in the wealthier middle classes, was a growing sense of isolation and loneliness. Humans are group beings. They need the group 'family' to survive when they are born. The decay of families and neighbourhoods combined with an increased inability to contact others from their hearts, left many isolated in their wealthy homes. Group dynamics and group therapies responded to this need and became the major mode of treatment. This satisfied the human need for group bonding, and also put psychotherapy in economic reach of a new sociological group.

Group dynamics (K. Lewin[15]), an application of social psychology, aimed at an improvement of social competence through self–perception and perception of others. This method, still widely used today, practises ways of dialogue with each other and increases the efficiency of individuals and groups. Group therapy embraced a broad spectrum of techniques from analytical group psychotherapy (H. Argelander, A. Heigl-Evers[16]), transactional analysis (E. Berne[17]), role plays, psychodrama (J.L. Moreno[18]) and Gestalt (F. Perls[19]) to encounter groups (C. Rogers[20]) and EST (W. Erhard). In this

Gestalt Therapy

category, which continues to grow and change in response to cultural demands, the common focus is on the way people relate and interact with each other. The therapist or seminar leader can act as a participant observer or take a leading role reflecting upon behaviour and deeper motives, encouraging the expression of feelings, practising new behaviour or improving communication structures. Self-help groups became a big success during the seventies, providing information, hope and a support network for people suffering from addiction, emotional problems and chronic diseases. The best known representative is Alcoholics Anonymous.

Twelve Steps Programme

The group movement received a strong impetus through the human potential movement. This is the third main strand of development in psychological therapies alongside psychoanalysis and behaviourism. Its main representatives, F. Perls (Gestalt) and C. Rogers[21] (client-centred therapy), shifted the focus in the therapeutic scene from adjustment to social reality, to human growth and self-realisation. They saw men and women as intrinsically whole, and therapy as a process of rediscovering or reintegrating the lost or overlaid wholeness. Within the format of group work and individual counselling they helped their participants and clients to re-experience the non-verbal physical and emotional side of being human that had been lost within the technological rationality of the Western world. They were joined in their approach by a broad spectrum of body-oriented therapies such as bioenergetic analysis, radix, Rolfing, Feldenkrais and Janov's primal therapy.[22] Their ethos has permeated much of the conventional psychotherapy in recent years.

Counselling

Bioenergetic Analysis
Rolfing
Feldenkrais

Transpersonal Psychology

During the last 25 years a fourth force has come into being called transpersonal psychology. The transpersonal is the shift from the little self to the transcendent self, from the mind/body consciousness to unity consciousness, where we become aware that we are one with our environment and one with the universe. Transpersonal psychology is a response to the repression of the transcendent in our culture, to the meaninglessness of life. C.G. Jung, the 'father' of the movement, demonstrated through his life that we can move beyond the mind/body identification by using mythological awareness.

Psychosynthesis
Holotropic
Breathwork

In his footsteps have followed a multitude of explorations and methods. One approach is that of psychosynthesis (R. Assagioli[23]) which trains the 'inner witness' to help dis-identify the higher self from all aspects of the personality. Another approach is that of A. Maslow[24] who identified a personality type, named self-actualising, whose aim is to fulfil their life's purpose in pursuit of higher or soul needs. S. Grof[25] created a new map of the unconscious that is related to the birth process and opened with his Holotropic Breathwork an avenue to move into the realms of the unconscious that link us with all life forms. K. Wilber[26] integrated the psychological approaches of the West and the meditation practices of the East into a new scale of development describing the evolution of human consciousness.

Beyond the transpersonal, beyond the realm of psychology, reign the meditation techniques of the East that open awareness to the union of humankind with the formless consciousness that cannot be reached through psychology today. Psychology can, however, help to clear the obstacles that result from individuals being part of a specific family, culture and time, and give them the inner strength and contentment to pursue higher goals.

*Transcendental
Meditation*

Biography

Ulla Sebastian, Dr rer. soc. (social science) trained in psychoanalysis, bioenergetic analysis, group dynamics and group therapy. She is a writer, educator, psychotherapist and trainer for bioenergetic analysis at the German Institute for Bioenergetic Analysis. From 1979 to 1986 she held a professorship in clinical psychology in Germany, training social workers in psychopathology and supervising their work in crisis intervention, with addicts and psychosis. She is also trained in African dance by an African medicine man from Ghana and practises the Healing Tao as taught by Mantak Chia. She has written many books and articles about 'pathways to life', the relationship between the genders and spiritual awakening. In her therapeutic work she helps people to shift basic patterns in their lives so that love, joy and fulfilment become part of their daily activities.

References

1   James Stradey (ed), *Standard Edition of the Complete Psychological Works of Sigmund Freud*, Chatto & Windus, 1975.

2   Jung's work is published in *Collected Works I-XVIII*, Walter, Olten and Freiburg/Br. 19793

3   A Adler, *Praxis und Therapie der Individual Psychologie*, J F Bergmann Verlag, 1922; reprint Fischer, 1972.

4   A Freud, *Normality and Pathology in Childhood*, International University Press, 1965.

5   K Horney, *The Neurotic Personality of our Time*, Routledge, 1951.

6   E Fromm, *Man for Himself*, Routledge, 1949/1971.

7   I P Pavlov, *Conditioned reflexes: An investigation of the physiological activities of the cerebral cortex*, Oxford University Press, 1927.

8   E L Thorndike, *The Fundamentals of Learning*, Teachers College, 1932.

9   B F Skinner, *Science and human behavior*, McMillan, 1953.

10 J Wolpe, *The Practice of Behavior Therapy*, Pergamon, 1969.

11 C L Hull, *Essential of behavior*, Yale University Press, 1951 .

12 H J Eysenck, S Rachman, *The Causes and Cures of Neuroses: an Introduction to Modern Behaviour Therapy Based on Learning Theory and the Principles of Conditioning*, Routledge & Kegan Paul, 1965.

13 A A Lazarus, *Behaviour therapy and beyond*, McGraw-Hill, 1971.

14 A Ellis, *Reason and Emotion in Psychotherapy*, Birch Lane Press, 1994.

15 K Lewin, *Field theory in social science: selected theoretical papers*, Harper & Row, 1951.

16 A Heigl-Evers, *Konzepte der analytischen Gruppentherapie*, Vandenhoek & Ruprecht, 1972.

17 E Berne, *Transactional analysis and psychotherapy*, Grove Press, 1961.

18 J L Moreno, *Psychodrama*, Vol. I, Beacon, 1946/1964.

19 Fritz Perls, *Gestalt therapy verbatim*, Real People Press, 1969.

20 Arthur Burton (ed), *Encounter: The Theory and Practice of Encounter Groups*, Jossey-Bass, 1969.

21 C R Rogers, *On Becoming a Person*, Houghton Mifflin, 1961.

22 A Janov, *The Primal Scream*, G. P. Putnam's Sons, 1970.

23 R Assagioli, *Psychosynthesis*, Viking Press, 1965.

24 A Maslow, *The Farther Reaches of Human Nature*, Viking Press, 1971.

25 S Grof, *Realms of the Human Unconscious*, Viking Press, 1975.

26 K Wilber, *No boundary. Eastern and Western approaches to personal growth*, Shambala, 1981.

Further Reading

General:

Kovel, Joel, *A Complete Guide to Therapy, from Psychoanalysis to Behaviour Modification*, Pelican Books, 1976.

Freud:

Appignanesi, Richard; Zarate, Oskar, *Freud for Beginners*, Icon Books, 1979.

Clark, Ronald W., *Freud, the Man and the Cause*, Jonathan Cape, 1980.

Greenson, Ralph, *The Technique and Practice of Psychoanalysis*, Hogarth Press, 1975.

Storr, Anthony, *Freud, Past Masters*, Open University Press, 1989.

Post-Freudians:

Brown, J A C., *Freud and the Post-Freudians*, Penguin, 1961.

Greenberg, Jay R.; Mitchell, Stephen A., *Object Relations in Psychoanalytic Theory*, Harvard University Press, 1983.

Jung and Jungians:

Fordham, Frieda, *An Introduction to Jung's Psychology*, Penguin Books, 1957.

Hall, Calvin S.; Nordby Vernon J., *A primer of Jungian Psychology*, Penguin Books, 1987.

Hyde, Maggie; McGuiness, Micheal, *Jung for Beginners*, Icon books, 1992.

Stevens, Anthony, *On Jung*, Routledge, 1990.

Humanistic:

Clarkson, P., *Gestalt Counselling in Action*, Sage, 1989.

Lowen, Alexander, *Bioenergetics*, Penguin Books, 1975.

Mearns, D.; Thorne, B., *Person-Centred Counselling in Action*, Sage, 1988.

Perls, Fritz, *Gestalt Therapy Verbatim*, Real People Press, 1969.

Rogers, Carl, *On Becoming a Person*, Houghten Mifflin, 1961.

Sharaf, Myron, *Fury on Earth. A Biography of Wilhelm Reich*, St. Martin's Press, 1983.

Transpersonal:

Grof, Stanislaw, *Beyond the Brain*, Sung Press, 1985.

Maslow, Abraham, *The Farther Reaches of Human Nature*, Viking Press, 1972.

Tart, C., (ed), *Transpersonal Psychologies*, RKP, 1975.

Wilber, Ken, *No Boundary. Eastern and Western Approaches to Personal Growth*, Shambala, 1981.

Wilber, Ken; Engler, J.; Brown, D. P., *Transformations of Consciousness*, Shambala, 1986.

Behavioural and Cognitive Therapy:

Beck, A T., *Cognitive Therapy and the Emotional Disorders*, Pergamon, 1989.

Dryden, Windy, *Rational-Emotive Counselling in Action*, Sage, 1990.

Trower, Peter; Casey, Andrew; Dryden, Windy, *Cognitive-Behavioural Counselling in Action*, Sage, 1991

Psychosynthesis
By Diana Whitmore

Motivation for Seeking Therapy

Freedom from Pain

People seek therapy because they are in pain. Pain in this context is one of the most powerful motivating forces for change. Although seemingly negative, the motivation to become free of pain provides a healthy, energising and life-affirming force for the beginning of therapeutic work. Psychosynthesis maintains that when an individual seeks to enter therapy, there are causative factors lying beneath the immediately obvious symptoms. Problems in life may not simply be distractions to be eliminated, the result of mere inadequacy or psychological wounding from childhood experiences. It may be that problems and obstacles at their deepest level are inherently meaningful, evolutionary, coherent and potentially transformative. Perhaps it is no accident that various conflicts become foreground issues at particular times in our lives. The energy of conflict is the energy of transformation. Old psychological forms die in order for new ones to be born.

The Existential Crisis

Also among those who seek therapy are many who are basically healthy and able to function well, but who experience a sense of dissatisfaction with their current quality of life and long for greater fulfilment. There may be a need, conscious or unconscious, to expand individual identity beyond personal existence. The choice to enter counselling can reflect a life-affirming impulse which transcends the confines of conventional life. A search for meaning, for purpose and a deeper identity leads to this choice. Even a person who appears to be integrated and to live a more or less successful life with many goals achieved can experience times when life loses its lustre and becomes somewhat grey and meaningless. While not deteriorating into neurosis, such a person may positively question issues not previously addressed, such as: 'What am I here for?' 'What is the meaning of my life?' 'What is my place in the world?' 'Is there more to life than this?' These pertinent questions may cause a person to seek therapy.

Counselling

Reframing Pathology: the Creative Use of Pain and Crisis

Psychosynthesis hypothesises a model of emerging purpose which provides a progressive context within which clients can experience themselves and make choices, rather than merely mend brokenness. A client will report many experiences which prompt the psychosynthesis therapist to question what is trying to emerge through these difficulties and what potential for growth is contained within them. If the client is unconsciously seeking a step forward, what might it be? What old behaviour pattern is dying in order for something new to be born? This attitude provides a way of reframing experience, enabling the creative potential within a problem to be actualised.

The Theory and Practice of Psychosynthesis

Psychosynthesis has its roots in psychoanalysis. Before founding psychosynthesis, Dr Roberto Assagioli (1888–1974) was a member of the Freud Society in Zürich in 1910, and together with various other pioneers of the psychoanalytic movement, was among the first to bring psychoanalysis to Italy.

Assagioli likens the three principal stages of psychosynthesis therapy to Dante's *Divine Comedy*: first there is the descent into the inferno, which represents the psychodynamic phase of descent into the lower unconscious; then the journey through purgatory, which resembles working with the client's existential reality; and finally the ascent to paradise, which symbolises exploring the transpersonal dimension of the psyche.

The Past: Assessment of the Unconscious

Psychosynthesis counselling begins by assessing the client's blocks and potentials to allow for a purposeful exploration of the unconscious. In order to reach the roots of psychological complexes, childhood experiences are uncovered with particular regard to the impact they currently have on the client's life. The influence of childhood is multidimensional, often indirect and pervasive. It profoundly affects people's capacity for love and intimacy, for assertion and self-affirmation; it determines their perception of life, and colours their deepest attitudes and values. Unless people are willing to be puppets to the past, neurotic elements must be brought into consciousness and transformed. The first step in psychosynthesis, therefore, is the attainment of a certain level of self-knowledge, enabling clients to move within their inner world with some degree of awareness.

The past, personal history and childhood experiences do not sit quietly in the basement of the psyche. Repression, suppression or denial of feelings create emotional stress. Psychosynthesis works extensively to release the grip of the past and to help people learn to express real but buried feelings in the present. When a natural capacity for expression of feelings is redeemed, emotional health can be re-established. Our perception is also conditioned and coloured by our history. From past experiences, defence mechanisms are formed which preserve the stability of the personality but do so at the expense of distorting reality. They lower anxiety in order to maintain a stable level of functioning. Initially these defences serve their purposes, but later they may restrict quality of life. These loyal soldiers must be acknowledged for how well they served in the past, but then released as obsolete. Psychosynthesis contends that the past may have an even deeper function in determining the quality of adult life. Inner life and world picture may be incongruent with outer life and manifestation, which contributes to a sense of inauthenticity. As a result, the integrity of feeling at home in the world may be lacking. Mentally, too, people's history influences their attitudes, beliefs and philosophies about life. They may, for example, unconsciously believe that people cannot be trusted, or that they will never get their needs met. These basic attitudes will, in turn, condition the image of reality.

The main difference between psychodynamic work with the unconscious and psychosynthetic work is that pyschosynthesis delves into the past in a focused way on particular life issues. Indiscriminate delving into the unconscious is not encouraged. The client's presenting problem will evoke a further exploration into the roots and historical background. The principle in psychosynthesis is for awareness to be expanded into the unconscious regarding an issue in the client's life and then for that awareness to be integrated in a controlled manner. This work with the unconscious will include attention to the dynamics of transference and counter-transference. The transferred childhood pattern, which clients unconsciously live again in their relationship with the therapist, also needs to be addressed.

The Present: Exploration of Subpersonalities and Identity

Experiences which are familiar and repetitious are often to be found in the client's presenting problems. It is as if some uncontrollable force is conditioning both inner and outer experience. Recurring situations, seemingly out of the client's control, result in predictable and limited behavioural responses. Every chronic life pattern has its historical base, its biography, often traumatic, around which many other painful experiences accumulate. Whether positive or negative, the core experience tends to repeat itself again and again, forming a generalised behaviour pattern, which in similar situations evokes similar responses. Eventually the client will perceive their whole world through this psychological system and it will colour vividly their attitudes and expectations.

The memories belonging to such a life pattern will have a similar basic theme and carry a strong emotional charge of the same quality. For example, a pattern of low self-esteem will contain the client's memories of past experiences, of the humiliating and degrading situations that damaged it. These life experiences will form identities, autonomous configurations within the personality, called subpersonalities. They are discrete psychological identities, coexisting as a multitude of lives within one person; each with its own specific behaviour pattern and corresponding self-image, feelings and beliefs. Their unique characteristics form a relatively unified whole. Each of these subpersonalities has an exclusive way of experiencing and responding to life.

People are often different when they are with their children compared to when they are in the workplace; or in certain challenging situations the calm, self-assured demeanour that is on display most of the time is quickly lost. Shifting identifications in this way is often in reaction to the demands of the situation and in response to the unconscious feelings evoked. People are unaware of the expectations from the environment and the demands of their inner world that control them. They are caught in ambivalence, confusion or conflict. These identifications are usually unconscious and largely beyond conscious control. Identifications will change in response to the demands of both inner and outer conditions, much more than to the desire or will. People who identify too closely with any one aspect of their personality will lose accessibility to the rest of their personality. The need is to be free from the limited and dominating behaviour of any one particular identity.

A longer-term goal of psychosynthesis therapy is the fostering of a stable sense of identity. Exploring the unconscious, and working with chronic life patterns and specific identities fosters the recognition that true identity is beyond the contents of consciousness. We all have within us an element which is permanent, consistent and unchanging. Little by little we can acquire an internal point of reference, a centre of identity which is psychologically free, uncluttered and available at will. A goal of psychosynthesis is to detach and free people in order to access more of the personality, resolve conflicts and become more self-determining and autonomous. This will provide access to a wider range of experience and choice. The above, longer-term work of psychosynthesis therapy is not the same as distancing or suppression. People too often live submerged in a particular identity, role or behaviour, lost in an unconscious way of being. Liberating them from an identification does not mean rejecting or abandoning it. On the contrary, to be conscious brings more aliveness.

The Future: The Transpersonal Dimension of Therapy

As previously mentioned, establishing a stable centre of identity and a degree of inner mastery is an aim of psychosynthesis therapy. A balanced emphasis on the development of self-identity provides the psychological stability for an awakening and exploration of the transpersonal domain. The revival of interest in the transpersonal today is triggered by an increasing dissatisfaction with competitive materialism, the pursuit of immediate gratification, as well as by a conscious or unconscious search for different and higher values and activities, a longing for what is sometimes termed 'spirituality'. Few would deny that people are hungry for truth, goodness and beauty, but in our culture, and in psychology, it is difficult to talk about this transpersonal dimension. Spiritual life has become as embarrassing a topic as sexual life was to the Victorians.

Until recently scientific bias has limited Western culture to quantitative and statistical exploration. In spite of accounts of experience of a higher reality found in all ages, there is reluctance to admit the existence or experience of spiritual values. Freud saw the desire for something beyond the personal as neurotic – a regressive tendency to return to the undifferentiated primal unity of the mother's womb – or as a sublimation of drives and instincts. Assagioli criticised Freud for labelling people's higher values and achievements as adaptations of these lower instincts and drives. Assagioli maintained that these higher impulses, desires and motives exist in their own right, develop whether or not the aggressive and sexual drives are satisfied and have their own source – a spiritual centre of identity. Transpersonal work in therapy is not a substitute for psychological work, but rather a vivifying and practical complement. A therapist working in a transpersonal context will be committed to a particular set of assumptions, which are not absolute, but which are useful as working hypotheses.

This may be, for example, that in each of us there exists a spiritual centre of identity, the 'self', which includes the personal dimension, but goes beyond it, and that both the experience and expression of this self fosters growth and well-being. It can be assumed that pain, crisis and pathology are opportunities and challenges for growth and creative steps forward, and are intimately connected with our self-realisation. There is a richness and benefit from identifying a purpose in life which is meaningful and potentially fulfilling. Many therapists would add that spiritual drives are as real, fundamental and indispensable as the basic psychological ones, and that these needs must be met for optimum health. A goal of psychosynthesis is to enable the client to meet physical, emotional, mental and spiritual needs appropriately in accordance with individual temperament. Hence, no one principle, method or technique is correct for everyone. However, it is seen as therapeutically valuable to explore experiences of superconscious content. Transpersonal experiences can arise at any time, often spontaneously and when least expected. There are various modalities through which the contents of the superconscious emerge into consciousness – through intuitive insight into one's problems, through the imagination and images which carry a positive charge, through inspiration and its subsequent creative expression or through illumination which reveals the essential nature of life and its true unity.

The therapist who holds a transpersonal context will use these moments to further clients' work on themselves by responding to these moments and encouraging their elaboration. Consciousness plays a pivotal role in determining the outcome of therapy. Consciousness is both the instrument and the object of change, and the therapist will be less concerned with 'problem solving' than with enhancing the conditions in which clients can address the challenge creatively. The emphasis is upon learning how to deal effectively with problems as they arise, rather than resolving a particular situation in the client's life. Most essentially, working from a transpersonal context means that, regardless of method or technique, the therapist has taken a firm stand for basic human goodness, trusts that the client is fundamentally all right and is willing to accompany the client on the journey to wholeness.

The 'self' can be described as a person's most authentic identity, the deepest experience of being. It can be a conscious experience for some, while for others it may be latent until superconscious experiences stimulate awareness of its existence. Experiences of beauty, of creative intelligence, of illumination, of insight into life, and of altruistic imperatives can awaken the individual to this deeper identity. The yearning for unity or the lack of connection to self or soul can underlie many psychological symptoms: a chronic feeling of isolation; self-destructive behaviours such as alcohol or drug consumption, which dulls reality and creates a false sense of unity; suicidal impulses, which may suggest an unconscious desire to return to security and the primal unity of the womb; existential despair and hopelessness. It is also worth noting that the awakening of the self may also be stimulated by crisis and negative experiences. For one client the death of a loved one stimulated a search for meaning which led her to the experience of the self; another, overwhelmed by a mid-life crisis, found relief through deep acceptance of her being, which altered her priorities and life direction. For an overstressed businessman, the loss of his valued career shocked him into a transcendent experience of his true identity, far beyond his role as a businessman. These insights are often gained through psychospiritual work in therapy. In times of stress or trauma, people in therapy tend to be more open to move towards a wider perspective and a greater sense of proportion.

The Therapeutic Relationship

Working from a transpersonal context also creates a transpersonal element in the relationship between therapist and client – essential for sincere and successful work. The ground on which they stand together is rich with the necessary components for the client to both heal themself and move progressively forward. There is no doubt that the quality of the human relationship has a profound influence on determining the outcome of therapy. Without a 'bifocal vision' – one which sees both the light and the shadow in clients – and without a context which sees clients as more than their pathology, the therapist greatly reduces the effectiveness of the work. Assagioli spoke of the relationship being the very heart of the therapeutic process. He believed that without authentic human relating, trust would not be established between therapist and client and without this essential ingredient little growth was possible. He further elaborated the dangers of both dependency and projection of the sublime without a genuine relationship. The client might remain dependent upon the authority figure of the therapist for answers to problems and guidance towards normative psychological health. Autonomy and a healthy separation from the therapist then become immensely difficult. Projection of the sublime occurs when clients perceive the therapist as more intelligent, more creative, more in possession of all the positive qualities for which they yearn.

Assagioli did not see transference as the centre of gravity around which the therapy revolves in the way that Freud did. The psychosynthesis attitude towards transference is to treat it as it arises, as one of many ways to help clients confront their issues. Psychosynthesis uses active techniques like subpersonality work and guided imagery to access inner child levels in therapeutic work. Erich Fromm said that after all, it is the child in the client who is transferring. Working experientially with parental relationships can also address transference issues. Reliving the re-experienced parental relationships can release past trauma and profoundly affect transference dynamics.

The Interface with Society

Just as treating the symptoms of disease brings relief but does not heal the whole person, therapy without exploring the client's relationship with the larger whole would be limited and unreal. With its emphasis on purpose and meaning, psychosynthesis therapy places a high value on the fact that people do not exist in isolation, but within the context of the larger whole of society and of an intricate network of relationships. Individual identity is not the end-result but leads to a recognition of interdependence and to a more creative response to life. At any time the client may naturally begin to question and want to explore the nature of values and how they choose to relate to their world. This idea is congruent with the hypothesis that, as personal survival, safety and self-esteem needs are fulfilled, the individual will move towards a more universal orientation, a natural expansion of ego boundaries and a desire to make life choices that are consistent with this larger identity.

Biography

Diana Whitmore MAEd is chairperson of the Psychosynthesis and Education Trust, joint chief executive, senior trainer and supervisor in psychosynthesis. Having practised psychosynthesis for over twenty years, she has trained professionals throughout Europe, and consults on research and the development of new projects in psychosynthesis. She is on the UKCP National Register, and is a BAC recognised supervisor and a founding board member of the Association for Accredited Psychospiritual Psychotherapists. Her background includes Didactic Training with Roberto Assagioli, the founder of psychosynthesis. She trained in humanistic psychology and gestalt therapy at the Esalen Institute, California and studied with Dr. George Brown in confluent education at the University of California. She is the author of two books, *Psychosynthesis & Education: A Guide to the Joy of Learning* and *Psychosynthesis Counselling In Action*.

Further Reading

Assagioli, Roberto, *Psychosynthesis: A Manual of Principles and Techniques*, HarperCollins, 1993.

——, *The Act of Will*, HarperCollins, 1994.

——, *Transpersonal Development*, HarperCollins, 1991.

Ferruci, Piero, *What We May Be*, HarperCollins, 1990.

Ferruci, Piero, *Inevitable Grace*, Thorsons, 1990.

Hardy, Jean, *Psychology With a Soul*, Penguin Books, 1989.

Parfitt, Will, *The Elements of Psychosynthesis*, Elements Books, 1994.

Whitmore, Diana, *Psychosynthesis Counselling in Action*, Sage, 1994.

Resources

The Psychosynthesis & Education Trust
92-94 Tooley Street
London Bridge
London SE1 2TH
Tel. 0171-403 2100
Fax. 0171-403 5562

Psychotherapy
by Courtenay Young

Historical and Theoretical Background

Psychotherapy has expanded dramatically over the last 100 years since Sigmund Freud first started developing some principles in psychoanalysis, even though many people still have an image that psychotherapy consists of many sessions of free-associating on a psychoanalyst's couch, subject always to the analyst's interpretations.

*Psychological
Therapies*

There are a number of distinct and different branches of psychotherapy, of which psychoanalysis or psychoanalytically-oriented psychotherapy is just one, and the modern forms are much more eclectic, personal and humane than the prevalent image. The primary theory is still that if the reason why neurotic behaviour originally developed is understood, the behaviour will then change and the trauma at the root of it will dissolve and heal.

A significant development of this type of psychoanalysis is Jungian analysis or *analytical psychotherapy*, based on the work of Carl Jung, which focuses more on the social context, the world view or archetypes and the client's dreams and images, rather than their personal history and childhood traumas.

Very different, and found more frequently in the National Health Service, is *behavioural psychotherapy*. This focuses on ways of changing inappropriate behaviour rather than on the origins of a trauma. A series of behavioural modifications, 'one step at a time', can quite successfully help overcome problems like obsessive compulsions, claustrophobia, agoraphobia, or debilitating fears of many kinds.

Similar in some respects to the above are *systemic psychotherapies*, which tend to focus on particular aspects or areas of work for which reasonably effective systems have been developed. People with sexual problems, family and marital issues or post-traumatic stress patients can fall within this classification or branch of psychotherapy.

Within the field of *humanistic* or *integrative psychotherapies* are found *transactional analysis*, *Gestalt psychotherapy*, *object-relations theories*, *existential psychotherapy*, *psychosynthesis* and many others. These psychotherapies generally consider, as a

*Gestalt Therapy
Psychosynthesis*

basic hypothesis, that the person's mind, body and spirit or soul have a functional integration and each are of equal importance. Furthermore they may all need to be worked with to help the client achieve 'wholeness'.

Bio-Energetic Analysis
Postural Integration
Rolfing

The psychoanalyst classically never touches the client. *Body-oriented psychotherapies* (Reichian, bioenergetic or biodynamic) may actively work with the physical tensions in the body to help release them and thus the earlier psychological traumas that underlie these chronic tensions.

Gestalt Therapy

Emotional expression is considered very important in all these therapies. Gestalt psychotherapies often use an empty chair or a cushion to help focus the client's feelings on an absent person in order to help this expression. By expressing long-held-in feelings, the sought-after emotional release may occur, even though it may be frightening to express them in the first place. 'If I were to get really angry, everyone will hate me' can be a fear that stops any form of self-assertion, constructive criticism, independence of viewpoint etc. to the detriment of the person.

Psychosynthesis

Psychosynthesis might focus on some of the 'subpersonalities' or facets of a person's complex psyche in order to highlight that some aspects of the self have been favoured and developed at the expense of others. It might also help connect the client with their 'higher self' – the wisdom, the overview, the part that relates to that which is greater than the self – in order to help free the person from a limiting perspective of themselves. Much work is done with 'reframing' the client's views, of themselves or others. This is not to say the client is wrong to think their boss is unprincipled or their spouse is despicable, but they may find this perspective unhelpful as they engage in working therapeutically to resolve their difficulties in life. Some psychotherapies take this one stage further and focus on helping to 'reprogram' some of the client's basic working patterns.

More recent developments, like process oriented psychotherapy (POP) which developed out of a combination of Jungian analysis and bodywork, focus on the client's developmental process. The dynamic is more important than the state or position. Indeed they often encourage the client to change position and adopt a different, often opposing viewpoint to help move them forward. Here the classical 'resistance', seen by the analyst as destructive to the progress in therapy, is seen more as an important 'edge' to be crossed over in the process of self-awareness.

Hypnotherapy

There are psychotherapies that base themselves more on hypnosis and hypnotherapy, working with the deep or almost unconscious aspects of the psyche. These can be very helpful for people wishing to stop addictive behaviours like smoking.

In addition there are a number of therapies which do not involve talking as their primary mode, but which are psychotherapeutic in that a release of emotion is achieved, a more positive self-image is encouraged, self-empowerment is sought and deep healing of old traumas or emotional wounds can happen. They may incorporate some aspects of a particular psychotherapy or psychotherapeutic theory. Art therapy and dance and drama therapy are examples.

*Art Therapy
Drama and
Movement Therapy*

Counselling

Generally speaking counselling happens when one person goes to another for advice or help. Counselling is effective in an immediate or ongoing situation and many health professionals, like doctors, nurses, health visitors and social workers practise counselling as a significant aspect of their work. Counselling training is usually much shorter, more focused on the practical or the type of client (drug or alcohol counselling) and less able to deal with the more complex problems or more deeply disturbed clients.

Counselling

Psychiatry

At the other end of the spectrum, psychiatry deals with mental illness or pathology and with people who have deep and long-term problems, often of an organic nature. These are called 'psychoses' and most psychotherapists have been trained to refer psychotic patients to a psychiatrist, though some will work constructively in conjunction with a psychiatrist and with the client possibly taking psychotropic medications to ease their symptoms.

Training and Professional Standards

Psychotherapy is becoming an independent profession in the UK; independent from academic psychology (which dominates in the USA) and independent from psychiatry, which, in some European countries, is seen as the only proper profession to practise psychotherapy. In Britain all aspects of the wide field of psychotherapy are held to be valid, though it is accepted that some are more appropriate to certain situations than others. Experience of other psychotherapies is part of the training and all trainees receive the psychotherapy they are going to practise. High standards are being set and codes of ethics and complaints procedures are coming into force. A good psychotherapist now knows which approach to use in the same way as a good mechanic knows which particular spanner, wrench or tool to use.

The Practice of Psychotherapy

In this self-empowering relationship, the recipient is usually referred to as 'client', since 'patient' implies there is something wrong with them. A psychotherapy session is intended to help the client discover what he or she needs and the role of the psychotherapist is to encourage this. In the process, whatever has been preventing the client from achieving this, is hopefully understood more clearly, worked with and cleared out of the way.

This usually happens through talking. Psychotherapy is in the main a 'talking' therapy. It is also possible to work very differently – with the tensions in the body, with the expression of emotions, with altered states (like a light hypnotic trance), and with drawings, movement, or whatever seems appropriate. I was working with one client who, after a lot of emotional abreaction, shouting, screaming and crying, went to sleep (briefly) in a session. He later reported feeling that this had fulfilled his needs exactly. The peace and quiet and the trust he experienced in another's caring presence was the healing factor.

The setting for the session can contribute to the results. Personally I have a couple of deep, comfortable armchairs in my therapy room. There is a carpet, a divan-type sofa (so that someone can lie down if they need to), some big cushions (and a bat to hit them with if needed), a library of books that clients can borrow, tea-making facilities and a few plants and pictures. The aim is for the client to feel welcome, secure and at ease.

What occurs within this setting is quite unpredictable. As the therapist, I do not dictate what the client should do; we work together with what the client presents. Often, during the course of a session, emotions, feelings and memories are stirred up. Deep, powerful anger of which the client is aware, but is terrified to access or express, might need to be liberated. They fear they may not be able to put things back together again or that their relationships with other people may change irrevocably. Allowing it to come to the surface can change their whole perspective of themselves. At other times the anger may just burst out, sometimes even directed against the therapist. This anger may be preceded or followed by a deep sadness or crying. There can be no expectations of what will happen. Sometimes we talk about a particular issue, explore possibilities, access other ideas, follow threads or themes, make connections, consider the wider influences – the social and political implications. At other times, and usually only after some significant work by the client, there is an indescribable quality of healing grace. These moments are very special. One occasion on which this occurred was when I had been very moved by the client's story and they noticed the tears in my eyes. That someone else was crying, that someone else understood and empathised, was a significant point in their therapy.

Studies are being done and have been done on how effective psychotherapy is. There is strong evidence that it reduces a person's need or dependence on conventional medicine. Other studies can founder on the 'feel-good factor'; it is difficult to evaluate how someone feels better about themself, but most people will not refute that psychotherapy is reasonably effective. It can certainly treat or heal areas that drugs and massages cannot. Deep emotional traumas can distort and warp the personality. The person's facade or their coping mechanisms can become totally inappropriate. A heavily armoured person, for example, defending themself against all possible threat or invasion because of their earlier experiences, needs to change if they decide to get married or enter into a committed relationship. Psychotherapy may be the most effective form of assistance in such a case.

My own personal criterion is to work efficiently and effectively for the client. I try to make myself redundant as quickly as possible. I am also prepared to stay there for as long as it takes.

Application of Psychotherapy: Spiritual Emergence

A phenomenon increasingly being observed is that of people going through a deep transformational process as a result perhaps of some shock or trauma. It might be that the shock is physical – a car accident, an illness, a near-death experience; equally it might be an emotional trauma – discovering one is a survivor of child abuse or that one's life-partner has been dishonest or unfaithful. The transformational process can also occur spontaneously, as a result of a powerful encounter, conversation or thought-process, or a psychic or mystical experience. These events can propel some people into a process of profound change which can encompass a fundamental change of life, direction and belief systems. Some people can integrate this change gracefully, whilst others are not so successful at breaking out of the chrysalis of their old self, developing symptoms which make it obvious that they need help.

The value of psychotherapy in these instances is to affirm the person's process and encourage them to move with the change. Like a nurse who assists someone in their dying process or a midwife who assists at a birth, a psychotherapist has the opportunity to help people in their emerging – their living process. Not only does the individual often need help, counselling and support during parts of this transition, but also some of the symptoms that a person evidences during this process can look very much like psychotic symptoms. If society does not facilitate such transformations with some rite of passage or acknowledge it with respect, the result may be hiding the person away in a mental hospital, if, for example, they think they are hearing the voice of God. I do not think people are becoming increasingly psychotic, but they do seem to be becoming increasingly psychic. The manifestations are often quite similar and can include mystical or psychic experiences, visions and revelations. For example, an elderly lady described her experience:

Since last Christmas I seem to know things that are going to happen before they happen and I get messages telling me what to do and what is happening with other people. I know what people are thinking. My Minister says that I am of the Devil and my women's group at the church say that I am a witch and my husband just doesn't want to know anything about this at all.

Therapists and the community at large need to know how to deal with this. It is only recently that 'spiritual crisis' has been included as one of the possible origins of manic or schizophrenic symptoms in DSM IV (the classificational diagnostic directory used by psychiatrists).

The following case illustrates a client's spiritual emergence:

A medical doctor had an intuitive 'insight' that he should pay more attention to his musical interest and that medicine, which had involved him totally up to that time, would be of less relevance to him. He had been playing in a rock band on occasional weekends and evenings. He was married and had two children. He acted on his insight very enthusiastically, with resulting difficulties in both his professional and home life. The opposition around him possibly exacerbated the situation and he became quite manic for a short period of time. A breakdown was diagnosed and he was 'sectioned' (admitted against his will) into a psychiatric hospital. Having been stabilised on medication, he eventually went back to work as a doctor, but in a more administrative capacity. However his wife began divorce proceedings. He maintained his interest in the music throughout, writing songs for the guitar. Many of the songs had a spiritual component, and seemed to just 'come out from' him. He then met a woman with similar interests and she became his new partner, giving up her high-powered work in a bank to join him and help promote their music. He resigned from his practice and they increased the output, range and standard of their music. They seem happy in this new situation, albeit less financially secure and in less prestigious professional positions.

Holotropic Breathwork

Stanislav Grof, a psychiatrist whose interest lies in the development of human consciousness, described this type of life-change as a spiritual emergence process.[1] In his research he has come to identify a catalogue of experiences common to the spiritual emergence process:

◆ opening to life's myths, where the experience is one involving commonly held archetypes – kings, heroes, gods, the devil, Gaia etc.

◆ shamanic journeys, where the themes are more about birth, death, rebirth and communion with natural elements (rocks, trees, earth etc.)

◆ kundalini awakening, where powerful body energy experiences are part of an often dramatic cleansing process;

◆ episodes of unitive consciousness or peak experiences when the person experiences being at one with the universe or similar states;

◆ near death experiences, when the person, usually during an illness or after a serious accident or operation, experiences dying and then returning to life again;

Past Life Therapy

◆ emergence of karmic patterns, which usually includes the remembering of past life experiences and leads to understanding about present day patterns and relationships;

◆ psychic openings, or the development of a person's 'sixth sense', awareness, especially intuition, healing abilities, astral projection, etc.;

◆ possession states – essentially the taking over of the personality by another entity, but also being affected by one's own or other people's shadow sides;

◆ communication with spirit guides and channelling; these can include channelling information from higher beings or having the experience of being in direct communication with one's spirit guides;

◆ or some synthesis of these forms, as it is frequently the case that more than one of these types are experienced during a spiritual emergence process.

Distinguishing Spiritual Emergence from Psychosis

There are various criteria to distinguish between someone undergoing an emergence process and someone undergoing a psychotic episode. A primary criterion for making the distinction is whether or not the person is capable of seeing what is happening to them as a process, with any of the forms listed above as symptoms of the spiritual emergence. This ability to objectify is crucial, otherwise the person may get lost in the symptomology. The absence of paranoia and the willingness to work with people and therapists is another indication of someone in process, rather than someone in a psychotic state. A major consideration is the presence of other medical conditions which can interfere with the situation (for example diabetes, epilepsy, weak heart) or a long history of psychiatric treatment which can complicate and obscure the working through of the presenting challenges. Someone suffering from any of these conditions may undergo spiritual emergence, but it would have to be treated with additional caution.

Acceptance is the Key

Acceptance of the unfolding process is of primary importance. Western society's fears of mental illness and the social stigma that surrounds it can blind us to some of the possibilities inherent in the process. While psychiatry and the special care that is found in many mental wards and hospitals is valuable and necessary in some cases, a wider framework needs to be provided, where aspects of the process of spiritual emergence and change can be more widely recognised and worked with more creatively. With the growth of 'care in the community', more training for psychotherapists in this area and more general recognition of this as a possibility or an alternative to psychosis is desperately needed. In the same way as views on epilepsy have changed (the 'unmentionable' disease of the nineteenth century) with new forms of treatment, the symptoms of spiritual emergence will become more acceptable and understood.

Case Study

A man of 45 attended a week-long workshop on 'Deep Ecology' where people were encouraged to express the pain and suffering of the earth and animal species in relation to pollution and devastation caused by people. During the workshop he became increasingly distressed, over-identifying with the vanishing species. He stayed up all one night and became quite manic. He was heavily built and very strong. He scared the workshop leader when he fell to his knees and clutched her round the legs as she was taking a walk. 'Tell me how to save the world!' he said. Many people wanted him to be removed from the workshop and placed in a mental hospital. However, the situation was contained and he was given A Sourcebook for Helping People in Spiritual Emergency,[2] *which he read. This enabled him to identify with the process she described. 'Oh I've got that symptom and that one. So that's what is happening to me. O.K. I'm all right then.' It had been his fear that was making him manic. He stayed for a few extra days after the workshop to integrate his experience and then returned home. Since then he has written nine books – self-help books for people in crisis.*

An international group has formed called the 'Spiritual Emergency Network', which acts as a referral service for people requiring counselling or psychotherapy during their process. It was started by the Grofs in 1980 as a response to an increasing incidence of this type of experience.

Conclusion

If there is a new pattern or phase in human evolution happening, that of a more spiritual nature, then there is a need to recognise and prepare for it. In the same way that rites of passage or initiations are created for adulthood, marriage and to some extent death, there is also a need to develop these for spiritual emergence, for however frightening or disturbing these processes may seem, they can be part of a healthy development and need to be recognised as such.

Biography

Courtenay Young is a psychotherapist living and working at the Findhorn Foundation, a spiritual community in the north of Scotland. He is an accredited and registered psychotherapist member of the Association of Humanistic Psychology Practitioners in Britain and of the UK Council for Psychotherapy and of the European Association of Body-Psychotherapy. He is regional co-ordinator for the Spiritual Emergency Network and director of a local charity running projects in conjunction with the social services department and the local Health Trust for people with mental health issues in the community.

References

1   Stan and Christina Grof, *The Stormy Search for the Self,* J P Tarcher, 1990.

2   Emma Bragdon, *A Sourcebook for Helping People in Spiritual Emergency,* Lightening Up Press, 1988.

Further Reading

Bragdon, Emma, *The Call of Spiritual Emergence,* Harper & Row, 1990.

Ferruci, Piero, *What We May Be,* HarperCollins, 1990.

Ferruci, Piero, *Inevitable Grace*, Thorsons, 1990.

Grof, C and Grof, S (eds), *Spiritual Emergency*, Jeremy P. Tarcher Inc, 1989.

Holmes, J., *Psychotherapy – a luxury the NHS cannot afford? – More expensive not to treat*, BMJ, 1994; 309: 1070-2.

———; Lidley, R., *The Values of Psychotherapy*, Oxford University Press, 1989.

Karasu, T., *The psychotherapies: benefits and limitations*, Am J Psychother, 1986; 40: 324-43.

Resources

The Spiritual Emergence Network
603 Mission Street
Santa Cruz, CA 95060-3653
USA
Tel. (408)-426 0941
e-mail: sen@cruzio.com

The contact address in the UK currently is:

Courtenay Young
The Park
Findhorn
Forres
Moray IV36 0TZ
Scotland
Tel. 01309-690251
Fax. 01309-690974
e-mail: cyoung@findhorn.org

Radionics

by Elizabeth Grindley

Theoretical Base

Radionics is a form of energy or vibrational medicine. As energy is not restricted to time and place, treatment with radionics can be done at a distance and does not require the patient's physical presence. The practitioner requires a 'witness' from the patient, usually a small snippet of hair or a blood sample, and using the radiaesthetic faculty and instrumentation they can then discover the imbalances in the patient and 'broadcast' corrective energy patterns. The radiaesthetic faculty in the practitioner is a sensitivity to subtle radiations of varying frequencies and is a form of extrasensory perception.

Basic to radionic theory and practice is the concept that humankind and all life forms share a common ground in that they are submerged in the electromagnetic energy field of the earth. When the electromagnetic field of a particular life form is sufficiently distorted, it will ultimately result in disease of the organism. Accepting that 'all is energy', radionic theory considers physical organs, diseases and remedies as having their own particular frequency or vibration. These factors can be expressed in numerical values which are known in radionics as *rates*, and radionic instruments have calibrated dials on which such rates are set for analysis and treatment purposes. Nowadays the rates are set directly in digital form through a key pad. This is a development from the earlier instruments which used rotary dials to set rates.

Human beings are considered to have physical, etheric, emotional, mental and spiritual dimensions. Dimensions other than the physical are called the subtle bodies. In energy medicine, different forms of matter are each seen as having a unique frequency of vibration. This is compatible with Einstein's concept whereby matter and energy are seen to be the same thing. These vibrations are recognisable at the physical level in modern science as part of the electromagnetic spectrum. At the emotional and mental levels the frequencies of the vibrations are higher and are not readily measurable by scientific means at present.

Radionics amplifies the self-healing capacity, or the natural recuperative processes of the patient. It facilitates a flow of energies between the body's various levels to restore the patient to balance and good health.

Historical Background

The basic principles of radionics were first formulated by an American physician, Dr Albert Abrams.[1] Born in 1863, Dr Abrams graduated from Heidelberg University in Germany with first class honours. He became one of America's leading specialists in diseases of the nervous system, a respected teacher and a writer of medical textbooks. He originated a completely new concept of diagnosis and healing by identifying the unique energy patterns of different diseases – ideas which were far beyond the boundaries of the accepted medical and scientific thinking of the time. The name radionics is derived from the rather wordy title of Abrams's technique which involved *Radi*ation and Electr*onics.*

In 1924, the year of Dr Abrams's death, his basic diagnostic techniques were investigated by a committee of the Royal Society of Medicine headed by Sir Thomas Horder. The committee found Dr Abrams's fundamental proposition to be 'established to a very high degree of probability'. Dr Ruth Drown, an American chiropractor, carried on Abrams's work and added a further dimension to radionics with her discovery that it was possible to treat a patient from a distance, using a blood sample as a link (witness) between patient and practitioner.

Later notable researchers were George Delawarr and subsequently Malcolm Rae. They carried out extensive research into the vibrational rates specific to different diseases, and fine-tuned the instrumentation to facilitate further the identification and treatment of diseases. Delawarr verified the use of a hair sample as a witness.

More recently, in the 1970s and 1980s, a notable radionics practitioner and teacher, David Tansley, integrated Eastern and Western concepts concerning the esoteric aspects of human subtle bodies and linked them to the theory of radionics.[2] The accessibility of his books has made radionic theory available to a much wider audience.

Uses of Radionic Therapy

Many years of experience have shown that, in a wide variety of cases, radionic treatment is effective in alleviating, if not completely eliminating, the physical or psychological effects of diseases, both chronic and acute.[3] Long-standing cases of asthma, hay fever and other allergic diseases have been helped, as have muscular, skeletal, digestive and other problems. Mental illness, hypersensitivity and psychological states often respond well, although not necessarily quickly. Blockages in the flow of the natural health-giving energies caused by stress can also be removed.

Radionic Analysis and Treatment

In order for a treatment in radionics to occur, the patient has to send a snippet of hair to the practitioner to act as a witness or link between the two. The witness provides the focus of attunement between patient and practitioner during analysis and treatment. This link is based on the principles of holography in which, from a vibration and energy viewpoint, a small portion removed from the whole (for example a hair sample removed from the body) reflects the total energy pattern of the whole. The witness maintains a resonant link with the source over time and space. This concept is mirrored in cellular biology where each cell carries a copy of the master DNA blueprint of the body.

When a practitioner accepts a case, as well as providing a hair sample the patient completes a case history giving details of current symptoms, previous medical history and medication taken. Other personal details are sometimes required to complete the picture.

Dowsing

While mentally tuned into the patient, the practitioner poses a series of questions in order to develop a picture of the disturbances or irregularities in the energy patterns of the patient. Feedback of the required information is through the subconscious channel of the mind. Responses in the nervous system of the practitioner's body transform the information into conscious data via motor neurone activity which influences the response of a pendulum held by the practitioner.

From the resultant data, a radionic blueprint of the patient's health is built up and this will include the underlying causes which gave rise to the symptoms reported.

Flower Essences
Colour Therapy
Homoeopathy

Treatment is given by directing corrective energy patterns, determined in a similar way to the analytical data, to the patient via the witness. Instruments are used to set these energy patterns in a coded numeric sequence (rate) or geometric pattern. The patterns may be for organ functioning, subtle bodies, energy patterns of elements, tissue salts, flower remedies, colour, homoeopathic remedies, corrective patterns for psychological states, complementary (antidote) patterns for viruses or other causes of an energy disturbance. Instruments provide an external focus for the radiaesthetic and healing skills of the practitioner. They have no independent function but act as an aid to the practitioner.

A treatment can continue, focusing on different aspects of the disease or using different vibrational remedies, over an extended period of time. During a course of treatment it is very important for the patient to keep in regular contact with the practitioner, as this is found to strengthen the healing link between them.

Applications of Radionics

Investigations into the use of radionics in agriculture and horticulture have been in progress for some time. There are now practitioners who specialise in the treatment of soil and crops and through radionics provide a natural method of weed and pest control.[4]

Animals usually respond well to radionic treatment. The same procedure of analysis and treatment is carried out as with humans. Children have few psychological blocks or conditioning, and generally respond very well to radionic treatment.

Training

The School of Radionics, governed by the Radionic Association, is responsible for the professional training of practitioners. It takes approximately three years of part-time study, with residential study weekends and periodic examinations to become a fully qualified member of the Radionic Association. Weekend introductory courses are held twice-yearly for prospective students and others who may simply wish to further their knowledge of radionics.

The school is currently working on the development of a training structure compatible with national vocational qualifications (NVQ), as part of the care sector consortium (government appointed CSC) work in that direction. This will eventually lead to a national qualification in radionics.

The Radionic Association

The association, which was founded in 1943, has two roles. First, it is the professional society of qualified radionic practitioners. Secondly, it is a society of laypeople interested in radionics who wish to keep in touch with the development of the subject.

The association's aims are to protect and promote the practice of radionics as an honourable and skilled profession, to foster research into the science of radionics, and to provide a clearing house for the collection and dissemination of relevant information.

In addition to publishing the *Radionic Journal*, which is provided free to all members, the association holds an annual weekend conference in the autumn and meetings in London and the provinces; publishes various brochures and monographs; supplies books and other publications about radionics; maintains a library of over 1000 titles from which members may borrow books by post; issues a list of practising members; and handles a large volume of requests for information, literature and general advice about radionics from all over the world.

Biography

Elizabeth Grindley, M. Rad A. is a part-time practitioner of radionics, living at the Findhorn Foundation. She attained a diploma in architecture in 1959 and practised for almost 20 years. Her interest in radionics stemmed from her familial hereditary condition of paralysis which led her to becoming a radionics patient in the early 1960s. She was so helped by the treatment that she trained in radionics and thereafter reduced her architectural workload, so she could focus on radionics as well.

She would like to thank the Radionic Association for permission to quote from material covered by its copyright in Leaflet B @ 6/94 and the *Radionic Journal*.

References

1   Sir James Barr (Ed.), *Abram's Methods of Diagnosis and Treatment*, Heinman 1927.

2   David Tansley, *Radionics and the Subtle Anatomy of Man*, Health Science Press, 1972.

——, *Radionics, Interface with the Ether-Fields*, Health Science Press, 1975.

——, *Radionics, Science or Magic?*, C W Daniel & Co., 1982.

——, *Chakras, Rays and Radionics*, C W Daniel & Co., 1984.

——, *Raiment of Light*, Routledge Kegan Paul, 1984.

——; Aubrey Westlake, *Dimensions of Radionics*, Health Science Press, 1977.

3   B Rubik, *Energy Medicine and the Unifying Concept of Information*, Alternative Therapies 1(1): 34 – 39, 1995.

4   Scofield and Hodges, *Demonstration of a healing effect in a laboratory using a simple plant model*, Journal of Psychical Research 57: 321 – 343, 1991.

Further Reading

Bloomfield, Bob, *Radionics – Tomorrow's Physics?*, Bob Bloomfield, 1984

Davidson, John, *Subtle Energy*, C W Daniel Co., 1987.

Dossey, L., *How Should Alternative Therapies be Evaluated?*, Alternative Therapies 1(2): 6-85, 1995.

Gerber MD., Richard, *Vibrational Medicine*, Bear & Co., 1996.

Russell, Edward, *Report on Radionics, Science of the Future*, C W Daniel Co., 1973.

Tansley, David, *Radionic Healing – Is it for you?*, Element, 1991.

Talbot, Michael, *The Holographic Universe*, Harper Perennial 1991.

Resources

Enquiries for books, publications and membership application forms are welcomed by:

The Secretary
Radionic Association
Baerlein House
Goose Green
Deddington
Banbury
Oxford OX15 OSX
Tel. 01869-338 852

Rebirthing

by Anna Bondzio

As new yoga, rebirthing is not a discipline. It is an inspiration. It is not teaching a person how to breathe, it is the intuitive and gentle act of learning how to breathe from the breath itself. It is connecting the inhale with the exhale in a relaxed, intuitive rhythm until the inner breath, which is the spirit and source of breath itself, is merged with air – the outer breath.

— Leonard Orr, founder of Rebirthing[1]

Leonard Orr, a businessman who worked as a staff trainer for Werner Erhard's 'EST' seminars, developed rebirthing or 'conscious connected breathing' in the mid-1970s in the USA. It is a technique which has since benefited thousands of people.

The breath plays a primary role in cleansing and purifying our body systems. Most of the metabolic toxins and wastes of our body are released through the breath. Only 3% of total body wastes are eliminated via defecation, 7% via urination and 20% via our skin. If people are not breathing properly, they are not ridding themselves of toxins and wastes at the same speed as they are taking them in. The body is gradually polluted which then leads to upset and disease. At the same time the quality of breathing affects blood oxygenation and therefore the rate at which the body builds and maintains healthy tissue and its functions. It is a limitless source of vitality and aliveness, available at any time.

It is surprising to observe that most people are not breathing effectively most of the time. The air is usually pulled in with a short gasp, then held for a while until a long exhale is again followed by a pause before the next gasp.

The technique of *conscious connected breathing* means learning to breathe in a circular way with no pause between the inhale and exhale and no holding of air. The outbreath should be effortless rather than forcing and pushing, and the inbreath more a willingness to open up and receive. This can be a hard thing for people to do: to let go of control, to surrender to their own rhythm of breath and life.

Leonard Orr started his research on breathing with 'wet rebirthing'. His purpose was to stimulate memories of the womb. To this end, he asked people to breathe while in warm water. This usually took place in redwood hot tubs (plentiful in California) with a snorkel, so that those breathing could be completely submerged in warm (102°F) water to simulate the womb. This practice developed over years of his own experimentation, breathing in his own hot baths and saunas. He found there always came a time when he wanted to stop breathing and/or leave, and choosing to continue was effective in enabling him to go into deep feelings and memories.

Holotropic Breathwork

Those being rebirthed became so restimulated by the combination of the safety of being held in the water by a rebirther (one who has cleared their own birth trauma and has been trained to assist others) while consciously connecting with the breath, and with the womb-temperature water, that within a few minutes many became paralysed with fear and had to be assisted out and placed on dry towels to continue more easily with the breathing cycle.

In this way it was discovered that the connected breathing in the presence of a trained rebirther, without being in water, was enough to trigger off a session. Indeed, after a number of 'dry' rebirthing sessions (the number varied with the degree of birth trauma of each individual), 'wet' rebirthing stood a better chance of being experienced as useful, powerful, even enjoyable or ecstatic rather than terrifying. Following a number of wet rebirths, another stage may be experienced through cold water rebirthing, which involves breathing continuously while entering cold water extremely slowly. Whereas hot water tends to restimulate womb or birth memories, cold water tends to bring to consciousness material associated with death. Clients will go into material only as deeply as they feel safe, depending on the clarity, training and experience of the rebirther and the depth of the trust that has been built up in the relationship.

Theory and Practice of Rebirthing

The client lies down in order to relax as much as possible. A safe and undisturbed environment is needed to create a space where the individual feels safe enough to express and process whatever comes up in the breathing session.

As rebirthing has spread over the last 20 years, many different approaches have been developed by different people. Although the conscious connected breathing is the common denominator, the emphasis may be on different aspects. One important development is working with pregnant women, with the aim of supporting them to empower themselves in their delivery process and to help mother and baby to make birth an enjoyable, blissful experience, so that the negative cycle is not perpetuated.

*Psychotherapy
Postural Integration
Rolfing*

Rebirthing can be done in groups or individually, as dry rebirthing, or as wet rebirthing in either hot or cold water. It can be used as part of the psychotherapeutic process, as part of bodywork treatment, or as a purification of body and mind. Breathing is also an aspect of the spiritual path, and rebirthing can assist in clearing the channels for this process.

Rebirthing can be done by anyone. It addresses all levels of being – physical, emotional, mental and spiritual. It can be done on one's own, but because most people have to relearn a healthy breathing pattern, the presence and support of a trained rebirther is strongly recommended in the beginning. Ten to twenty sessions are recommended. It is advisable to stay with a guide at least until the client has experienced what is called a 'breath release'. This is the moment when there is a spontaneous memory of the first breath into consciousness. It happens when the client feels safe enough to let go completely. Many people have deep spiritual or mystical experiences at this point when they finally have surrendered to themselves and breath is flowing freely again. They often encounter an intense feeling of joy and pleasure in being alive. This is a turning point, the breath mechanism is transformed. After this a person will know when their breathing is inhibited and be able to correct it.

Obviously, rebirthing is a very personal experience. As clients experience the breath release, they bring into consciousness not only the memories but also the beliefs and decisions created at the moment of the first breath. Their perceptions, even before birth, form their impressions about the world, life and safety. Many of these impressions are negative. These early experiences form the basis of their approach to life and often need re-evaluating or transforming.

Many people experienced trauma of some kind before, during or after birth. They may have struggled through the birth channel, or been forced out by forceps which scrunched and twisted the head. They may have come out breech or have shared their mother's anaesthetic in the process. Emotionally they may have experienced terror, fear or loneliness, being separated from the mother who was the source of life and well-being. Many felt unloved or rejected for being the wrong sex according to the expectations of the parents. It may have been the physical pain of drawing the first breath or the shock of being exposed to a lower temperature than they were used to; or to glaring light, or of having the umbilical cord cut too quickly by the obstetrician. A frequent experience was receiving a good smack to get the breath going.

Whatever were the conditions of birth, the perception of it makes a huge impact on the psyche and determines personal life patterns, emotional, mental and physical. With rebirthing, clients have not only the chance to relive their past but also to examine decisions made then. With this information consciously recognised, they can evaluate if they feel blocked and hampered by these beliefs in present time and can choose to decide differently. They can release and heal traumas and hurts, which may run or unconsciously impact their everyday lives.

A Personal Experience

I first heard about rebirthing ten years ago. I was told it would help me to relax, release tension, heal my anxiety attacks, headaches and even my skin problems. It sounded like an all-round cure and too good to be true, but I was at a point where I would have tried anything.

I was lucky to find a rebirthing practitioner who totally accepted my state and situation. As I started to breathe in a circular way, as I had been instructed, my fears manifested instantly in hyperventilation. I was told that this occurs when a person forces the breath out and blows off CO_2 excessively. As a result I felt breathless, gasped in more air and pushed out even harder, which increased the problem. When CO_2 in the body decreases, a condition known as alkalosis develops which is characterised by tetany and muscular spasm and can cause intense pain.[2] In my first sessions I experienced excruciating pain in my joints, especially my jaws and I was convinced that I never would get enough air again to survive. It was like travelling on the breath back to my early childhood.

Being a 'child of the war', fear was a prevalent emotion, transmitted from mother to developing foetus, and I was able to feel this fear very tangibly in my rebirthing session. My mother had been on her own with my two older sisters when she was pregnant with me. I remembered the moment of my birth in very fearful surroundings with an uncertain future.

Breathing through this 'video' of my birth, I saw myself clearly making the decision that life is not safe. Being in a body is not safe and I need to be in control, since mother herself is afraid.

My first reaction to these threatening and unpleasant memories was the impulse to get rid of them as fast as I could by trying to push them out through my breath, which then initiated the hyperventilation. As I gradually accepted my past, I was able to relax more and follow the instructions of my rebirther who reminded me to surrender my exhale. The more I relaxed, the faster the condition of hyperventilation subsided. Deep breathing without forcing the exhale was the key.

Through my own personal growth and spiritual awakening, I started to train as a rebirthing practitioner.

Case Study

The following case study was kindly provided by Lee Preisler, founder of the British Rebirth Society and Director of the Holistic Rebirthing Institute.

Counselling

In 1992 I worked with a male client aged 28, for about nine months. He had moved through a series of sessions dealing with a challenging relationship and also his difficulty focusing on his work. Breathing sessions, combined with counselling, helped him to contact and work through repressed emotions, leading to recognising and responding to his own present needs. Four years later, with a decent career and a solid marriage for support, he was back to learn how to take charge effectively of his own life and development. He continued to feel that something vital was missing from within. It was as if he was searching for a special key or formula that would then reveal the solution or fix everything in his life. We did some deep work with feelings concerning his family and his fears regarding groups of men and men in authority.

On the day of one appointment he met me at the door, out-of-breath, almost wheezing, although he hadn't been running and had given up smoking six months previously. He was obviously upset, and explained that anger, which he had held in check all these years, was now spilling over into all walks of his life and beginning to cause havoc. He was worried that he might lose all his friends. I suggested that he lie down and simply continue breathing, and after briefly protesting how difficult it was, he did just that. He lay turned away from me for all but the last part of the session (unusual but obviously helpful for him), and spent over an hour breathing furiously, but with lots of pauses. It was almost as if he was coming up to something and then backing off just before it arrived. Finally there was an intense release of emotions. I intuitively wanted to respond to an unspoken 'I need you', but felt an equally strong 'Don't touch me', so I merely covered him with a soft blanket because he was shaking all over (although it looked and felt more like a response to fear than cold) and to remind him of my presence. He later glanced over at me with such fear in his eyes that I knew whatever he had found had been buried deep.

After a while when it felt appropriate I carefully placed a hand on the small of his back and urged him to stay in touch with the experience and his feelings. He said, 'I remember it, but I can't believe it.' He said that he had been raped at age eleven by a teacher at his new school. Able to do nothing, terrified and told he must be silent, he did the only thing he could do. He 'left', that is split off from his feelings of himself but at such a price that it will take him some time still to reclaim a sense of wholeness in himself. There are innumerable advantages in remembering and learning to care for his 'inner' eleven-year-old, reclaiming his power from that teacher, and making conscious an entire area of his psyche to own again that which was damaged, out of reach and affecting him adversely.

He is now aware of the material that his anger was protecting him from, and many other bits of the puzzle are finally and naturally beginning to fall into place for him. We are continuing to use the breathing, as it is helping him to integrate memories and feelings into his life. The breakthrough session was a result of his determination and rebirthing, which he had learned to use to his advantage. This case study shows that rebirthing is as effective in bringing to consciousness traumas from childhood as those from infancy and birth itself.

Biography

Anna Bondzio, born 1942 in Germany, has raised three children. She worked as an artist and teacher. In 1984 she moved to the Findhorn Foundation and trained in group facilitation, personal growth and psychosynthesis counselling. She took a rebirther training in London 1989 with Binnie Dansby, a master rebirther. She facilitates single sessions as well as group rebirthing. She returned to live in Germany in March 1996 and there offers rebirthing and counselling.

References

1   Sondra Ray, *Celebration of Breath*, Celestial Arts, 1984.

2   W N Gardner; C Bass, *Hyperventilation in clinical practice*, British Journal of Hospital Medicine, 1989; 41: 73-81.

     Elizabeth A Holloway, *The role of the physiotherapist in the treatment of hyperventilation*, in B Timmons; R Ley, *Behavioural and psychological approaches to breathing disorders*, Plenum Press, 1994.

Further Reading

Hendricks, Gay and Kathlyn, *Radiance!*, Wingbow Press, 1991.

Leboyer, Frederik, *Birth Without Violence*, Cedar, 1991.

Leonard, Jim; Laut, Phil, *Rebirthing: The Science of Enjoying All of Your Life*, Celestial Arts, 1983.

Minett, Gunnel, *Breath and Spirit: Rebirthing as a Healing Technique*, Aquarian, 1994.

Orr, Leonard; Ray, Sondra, *Rebirthing in the New Age*, Celestial Arts, 1983.

Ray, Sondra, *Ideal Birth*, Celestial Arts, 1984.

———, *Celebration of Breath*, Celestial Arts, 1984.

———; Mandel, Bob, *Birth and Relationships*, Celestial Arts, 1987.

Sisson, Colin, *Rebirthing Made Easy*, Total Press, 1987.

Resources

The British Rebirth Society
22 Rossall Road
Lytham St Annes
Lancs FY8 4ES
Tel. 01253-739 107

Reflexology
by Brian Young

Reflexology is based on the theory that there are invisible zones running vertically through the body, and stimulation of a particular zone by massaging the corresponding part of the foot will affect all parts of the body within that zone. The reflexes for a particular organ or problem area lie within one of the zones, which has a corresponding location on the foot. This area on the foot is massaged gently using the thumbs or fingers, and in turn the organ is affected for the better.

Metamorphic Technique

As all parts of the body are represented on the feet, this means the whole body can be treated in one session. Alternatively the practitioner can treat similar reflexes on the hands, the face, the ears or the abdomen, if, for example, the client has injured or painful feet.

Historical Development

Reflexology has existed for many years in various guises. The oldest reference to it comes from ancient Egypt. In Saqqara there is a pictogram in the tomb of the physician Ankmahor dated between 2500 and 2330 BC, showing two people having their feet attended to. Present-day reflexology dates from research done in Europe and Britain by an American physician called Dr William Fitzgerald[1] who specialised in ear, nose and throat problems. One of his colleagues, Dr Joseph Riley, had an assistant called Eunice Ingham who was a physiotherapist. She became known as the 'mother' of modern reflexology, because of her untiring work in bringing it to the attention of the general public in America. A nurse from England, Doreen Bayly, studied in the USA with Eunice Ingham, and she in turn brought her knowledge back to Britain, founding the Bayly School in the 1960s. Now there are many schools throughout Britain offering tuition to practitioner level.

Theoretical Base

The hypothesis of reflexology is that invisible energy lines (the zones) act as a matrix or blueprint for the physical body. If the energy within the body is blocked in any way, it will lead to disease, manifesting in all the variations of illness. Conversely, physical illness will eventually affect the energy blueprint. By massaging the energy zones and reflexes, the body can be helped to return to a state of balance, or homoeostasis. It has been noted that after surgery some amputees feel that they still have both limbs, and this may be a result of the energy blueprint still being present. There are various names for this energy: *chi, ki* or *prana* in the East and subtle-body energy or bio-energy in the West are amongst the most common. It is separate from the central nervous system, and the energy travels more slowly around the body than blood or lymph. Clients often claim that they can feel 'energy' or heat moving around during treatments.

The Practice of Reflexology

Clients are encouraged to wear loose comfortable clothing, which helps with the process of relaxation. Some practitioners use a treatment couch, such as a portable massage table, or, if treatment takes place in the home of the client, an ordinary settee or armchair is adequate, with the client's feet up on a support, at a working height which is comfortable for the practitioner. Quietness and privacy, with no interruptions, are essential for treatment. A case history is taken and when the client is comfortable and relaxed, treatment begins.

Massage

Over the course of about one hour, the feet will be treated by the practitioner's fingers or thumbs gently pressing on the reflex points. Some reflexologists use talcum powder as a skin lubricant to enable the thumbs and fingers to move across the skin more smoothly. Others use various oils, and others nothing at all. One reason reflexology is more than just a foot massage is that the practitioner is feeling and pressing specific points to see if it provokes a reaction from the client. This may manifest in different ways: as a sharp sensation; a mild pain; or momentary acute pain. The experienced practitioner quickly develops a sense of how hard or softly to press. Too much pressure causes discomfort at the expense of the client's state of calmness and relaxation; too little pressure renders the treatment less effective. The feet are systematically worked on from top to bottom. There is a variance amongst reflexologists as to whether the feet should be treated one at a time, or back and forth from one to the other, left foot first, right foot first, or by systems (the endocrine system reflexes, the lymphatics and so on). My personal experience is that it seems to make little or no difference, but that doing one foot at a time is less disruptive for the client, and hence more relaxing. This way the foot not being worked on can be wrapped in a warm towel, or the sock left on.

The number of treatments needed varies from person to person, depending on the nature of the complaint. There seems to be a correlation between the length of time the sufferer has had a particular complaint and the amount of time it takes to bring about a significant improvement. Sometimes clients will experience a 'healing crisis' or healing reaction, when they might feel marginally worse after the first treatment, or extremely tired. This is caused by the body clearing toxins via the lymphatic system and excreting them through the kidneys and bladder. The side-effects of this necessary purging of toxins can be minimised by drinking plenty of water after treatments, in order to flush out the kidneys. Mostly, though, clients feel in a relaxed and pleasant state after each treatment. 'Like walking on air' is a frequent comment.

Many reflexologists combine their treatment with, for example, flower essences, Reiki or aromatherapy. Basic instruction on a properly balanced diet may also be given, and referrals to other therapists, will be given where it is felt that this may be more appropriate for the client than reflexology. It has been noticed that homoeopathy works well in conjunction with reflexology, and that where there are back problems, the reflexes on the feet indicate the areas needing attention by an osteopath or chiropractor. Chinese meridian theory (as used in acupuncture and acupressure) is incorporated into the treatment by some practitioners, utilising the fact that most of the meridians start or end on either the hands or feet. This offers a good combination of the Western and Eastern traditions.

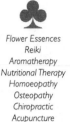

Flower Essences
Reiki
Aromatherapy
Nutritional Therapy
Homoeopathy
Osteopathy
Chiropractic
Acupuncture
Traditional Chinese Medicine

Reflexology is a holistic treatment, taking account of body, mind and spirit, which implies that there is no condition that cannot be helped in some way, contraindications excluded. However, certain ailments do respond more readily than others, and the circulatory system, the endocrine system, the digestive system and the autonomic nervous system respond very well indeed. This covers a lot of the more common ailments afflicting people nowadays, such as stress disorders, food sensitivities and allergies, headaches and sleeping problems. However, as with other complementary therapies, reflexology should not be seen as a cure for all aches and pains, but rather as a part of the clients' own progress towards full health, helping them fulfil their potential. Most people find they can be helped to some degree – their pain is eased, or the problem clears up enough to make it bearable, while in some cases there is a full remission of symptoms. Reflexology also works well for busy people who are tired or overstressed, as a session is very relaxing, and provides a one-hour break from the pressures of modern living.

While it is true that the whole body is treated during a session, reflexology can work well for specific ailments. For example in the case of kidney or bladder problems, such as a urinary tract infection, the appropriate reflexes on both feet would be given extra attention during the treatment. In addition, the reflexes for the circulatory and lymphatic systems would be worked on, to tone the system and help with the elimination of toxins, and the digestive system, to help encourage peristalsis. Clients would of course be advised to see their GP if they had not already done so, as this form of treatment is complementary and not alternative to standard medical practice. In the case of urinary calculi (kidney stones), massaging the reflexes can encourage the tubules to dilate and thereby ease the passage of the stones, and treatment to the parathyroid reflex would be indicated in case there is hyperactivity, causing too much calcium to be released to the bloodstream.

Contraindications

There is currently a debate amongst reflexologists as to whether there are any contraindications for treatment. It is generally held that to be on the safe side, lighter treatments or none at all should apply for the following conditions: heart disorders, acute infectious diseases, fevers, shingles, pre- and post-surgery, malignant melanoma, first trimester of pregnancy, unmedicated high blood pressure, any inflammatory condition of vascular or lymphatic origin, and for anyone on multiple medications.

Training

My advice is to use a practitioner who belongs to a recognised professional body, i.e. one which complies with or exceeds the recommended training requirements of the BCMA (British Complementary Medicine Association). To be attached to a professional body means that the practitioner has attended a course and passed the examinations of an accredited school. The most famous of these in Britain is probably the Bayly School in London or the Scottish School of Reflexology.

Examples of Conditions Treated

Hypertension

Relaxation Therapy

A woman, aged 50, suffered from raised blood pressure for which she was being prescribed Captopril by her doctor. She identified stress at work as the cause of her condition. Over a period of nine weeks I worked on the reflexes for her circulatory system (heart, spleen, and lymphatics) and on the reflexes to the adrenal glands and the diaphragm. Tenderness of the reflexes diminished over time, and with instructions for breathing exercises to help with relaxation, her condition improved to the point of her being able to come off medication after consulting her doctor again.

Sleeping Difficulties/Stress/Ulcers

A man of 39 was a light sleeper who suffered from nervous anxiety. He also had problems with indigestion and was being treated for a stomach ulcer. In addition, he felt he had a bladder problem as he had to urinate two or three times a night. In treatment, special attention was given to the reflexes for the diaphragm to aid with relaxation, the stomach and intestines to help with his digestion, and the bladder and prostate reflexes. After four or five treatments he was able to sleep all night undisturbed. When we discussed his indigestion, he told me he eats sandwiches whilst driving between jobs. He was reluctant to alter this habit, although I explained to him how this might adversely affect the adrenal glands and the autonomic nervous system. So he continued with his prescribed medication for the ulcer, and this was his choice. People sometimes need the obvious to be pointed out to them, and after that it's up to them whether they wish to begin the healing process, or to cling to old patterns.

Neck and Shoulder Pains

A·woman of 56 was being treated for iron-deficiency anaemia, but had come to me about her neck and shoulder pains caused, she thought, by rheumatism. The left shoulder reflex showed sensitivity, as did the reflexes for the neck, adrenals and gall bladder. I gave her basic dietary advice to cut down on sugar, refined flour and red meat and to eat fish or fowl instead. She was also fond of salt, and drank lots of tea. She had to cut down drastically on both. To compensate for the possible loss of iron in her new regime I encouraged her to eat more greens, which had been lacking in her diet. She also suffered from night cramps in her feet, which cleared up after three treatments to her parathyroid reflex, coupled with a suggestion to take calcium/magnesium tablets or dolomite. After five sessions she said she felt much improved, the pain in her shoulder had eased, and she had more zest. She continued taking iron tablets from the doctor; 'to be on the safe side,' she said.

Sinusitis

A man of 68 had stomach and abdomen pains, which were at times acute. In addition, his sinuses were inflamed and gave him extreme discomfort. These conditions, although relatively minor from a medical point of view, were a source of much discomfort in his daily life as an active pensioner. I found most parts of the spine reflex to be sensitive at the first treatment, but this did not continue. The abdominal pains were kept at bay for increasingly long periods after each session, until they disappeared completely after four weeks. I suspected them to be caused by an energy blockage somewhere on the spine. His sinus reflexes did not show up right away, as often happens, but on the third visit. Then with the usual stimulation to the toes, his body seemed to respond almost instantly, causing his legs to jump involuntarily. Thereafter he had no more problems with his sinuses. A follow-up phone call three months later found him still free of symptoms and very grateful.

ME

A young man who was very fit and active, and by his own description a high achiever in sports, has suffered from ME (myalgic encephalomyelitis) for several years and when I saw him, was unable to hold down a job. Amongst ME sufferers there seems to be a tendency to strive too hard or expend too much energy in trying to achieve impossible goals. This client undertook a long course of treatments over twelve weeks. Almost all of his reflexes were inflamed and tender, but especially the thyroid, neck, sinuses, testes, prostate and lymph/groin. The treatment stimulated the organs of elimination and the cervical area of the spinal cord. This latter reflex improved over the period, as did the reflex for the lumbar spine. The client was largely chair-bound and had developed back problems as a result. After several treatments his symptoms were eased. There was much elimination from the sinuses after most sessions, which left him feeling clearer headed, and his energy levels improved considerably, but not totally. Reflexology, while not necessarily bringing about a cure for his ME, was helping to keep his very inactive body stimulated, to keep the systems of elimination working, and the lymph and circulation moving as best they could. This aspect of reflexology is important for the comfort and well-being of the long-term patient and the bedridden.

Conclusion

Reflexology's ability to normalise all bodily functions and systems, to help bring about homoeostasis, and to relax the client generally is perhaps its greatest contribution to the human condition, together with the sensitive practitioner's encouragement of clients to heal themselves, to take the first steps on the road to self-healing. As the Chinese proverb states, 'Rather light a candle than complain about the darkness'.

Biography

Brian C Young GSSR lives and practises in Forres, Morayshire. From Glasgow originally, he has lived in the north-east of Scotland for 20 years. Having once had a career in television with the local TV station and later as a freelance director, he has been interested in the healing arts for many years, and incorporates into his reflexology treatments his knowledge of Chinese meridian theory, reiki, spiritual healing, Findhorn flower essences, and intuition. He is a graduate of the Scottish School of Reflexology and a member of the Scottish Institute of Reflexology.

References

1   William Fitzgerald with Dr. Edwin Bowers, *Zone Therapy*, published 1917.

    William Fitzgerald with Dr. Joseph Riley, *Zone Therapy Simplified*, published 1919.

Further Reading

Bayly, Doreen E., *Reflexology Today*, Thorsons, 1982.

Dougans, Inge with Ellis, Suzanne, *The Art of Reflexology, A Step-By-Step Guide, A Totally New Approach Using the Chinese Meridian Theory*, Element, 1992.

Gillanders, Ann, *Reflexology*, A Step-By-Step Guide, Gaia Books Ltd., 1995.

Gore, A., *Reflexology*, Macdonald Optima, 1990.

Hall, Nicola, *Reflexology – A Patient's Guide*, Thorsons, 1986.

———, *Reflexology, A Way To Better Health*, Gateway Books, 1988.

———, *Reflexology for Women*, Thorsons, 1994.

Reed Gach, Michael, *Acupressure, How to Cure Common Ailments The Natural Way*, Piatkus, 1992.

Stormer, Chris, *Reflexology, The Definitive Guide*, Headway/Hodder & Stoughton, 1995.

Resources

British Reflexology Association
Monks Orchard
Whitbourne
Worcester WR6 5RB
Tel 01886-821207

Association of Reflexologists
27 Old Gloucester Street
London WC1N 3XX
Tel 01892-512 612

Reflexologists' Society
Bannerdown Cottage
Bashley Cross Roads
New Milton
Hants BH25 8SY
Tel. 01425-618 000

International Institute of Reflexology
15 Hatfield Close
Tonbridge
Kent TN10 4JP
Tel. 01732-350 629

Scottish Institute of Reflexology
The Secretary
D A Grant
14 Tyney Road
Paisley PA1 3EY
Tel. 0141-883 1887

Institute for Complementary Medicine
P O Box 194
London SE16 1QZ
Tel 0171-237 5165

British Complementary Medicine Association
39 Prestbury Road
Pittville
Cheltenham
GL52 2PT

The Bayly School of Reflexology
Monks Orchard
Whitbourne
Worcester WR6 5RB
Tel 01886-21207

The Scottish School of Reflexology
2 Wheatfield Road
Ayr
KA7 2XB
Tel 01292-287 142

International Council for Reflexology
4311 Stockton Boulevard
Sacramento CA 95820
USA

Reiki

by June Woods

The History of Reiki

Reiki was discovered in the last century by Dr Mikao Usui. He was the principal of a Christian boys' school in Japan. He was also a minister and delivered sermons on Sundays. One of the older pupils asked him if he really believed what was written in the Bible. His reply was that he had faith in what it said. The student then asked if he believed in the method Jesus used for healing, and if so could he demonstrate it. Dr Usui could not comply with this request. This prompted him to take time out from teaching to go on a quest to see if he could find the information himself.

After studying many other religions and philosophies at a university in Chicago, he was no nearer to finding the 'formula' that Jesus had left. So he returned to Japan and spent several years in a Buddhist monastery studying Buddha's teachings. But the monks there did not share his interests. They told him they were only concerned with the happiness of the spirit and how to gain peace of mind, as the body is merely a temporary vehicle and therefore they left the caretaking of the physical body to doctors and medicine.

Dr Usui then spent time studying the Chinese *sutras*. Once again he found very little so he learned Sanskrit in order to study the Tibetan sutras. Here he found symbols that he felt might be close to the knowledge he was seeking. He undertook a fast, hoping to receive through prayer and meditation a vision which would explain it all. With just a container of water he journeyed to Mount Kurayama in Japan. He climbed the mountain until he found a place near a stream and by a pine tree. Here he gathered 21 stones and placed them around him.

Each day at dawn he removed one stone, before entering into meditation and studying the sutras. On the dawning of the twenty-first day at the darkest of dark, as he finished his meditation, he saw a great flashing light moving towards him very fast. Bracing himself, he felt the light strike him on the brow, in the place known as the third eye. He fell back, almost unconscious.

As dawn began to break he awoke and looked around him. Millions of bubbles of all colours of the rainbow were dancing before him. Next he saw the sacred symbols and was told how to use them. He was given the procedure for the sacred initiation ceremony for each of the Reiki degrees, I, II, and III – the master level.

Now he could infill and enfold his life with this energy and teach others. The sacred life-force energy would be available to all those who wished to open as vehicles for transmitting the light and way of being.

On leaving the mountain, feeling energised and happy, in his haste he stubbed his toe and it bled badly. Putting his hands around it and using the Reiki energy, he immediately healed it. When he reached the inn on his descent he ordered a big Japanese breakfast. The innkeeper advised against this as he knew Mikao had fasted for 21 days. But Dr Usui assured him that his body system was renewed and could enjoy it – and he did, blessing the food.

The innkeeper's granddaughter, who served him, had a very swollen face due to a bad tooth. He placed his hands around it and she was immediately relieved of the pain and the swelling abated. These three 'little miracles' were proof to Dr Usui that this healing energy existed and could be channelled to all.

He began by working with beggars, hoping to help them lead better lives. After spending seven years in an asylum treating many illnesses, he noticed several of the beggars who were supposedly healed kept returning for more treatment. When questioned, they replied that to work was too much effort and it was preferable to go begging. Dr Usui was shaken by this and realised that he needed to teach people gratitude for receiving the healing energy. So he devised the ethical principles of Reiki:

> *Just for today do not worry.*
> *Just for today do not anger.*
> *Honour your parents, teachers and elders.*
> *Earn your living honestly.*
> *Show gratitude to everything.*

He began to travel around teaching and sharing this knowledge. On his death Dr Usui was buried in a Kyoto temple. It is said his grave was honoured by the Emperor of Japan.

Dr Chijiro Hyashi worked very closely with Dr Usui and became the second grand master. He ran a private Reiki clinic in Tokyo until 1940, where severe cases could receive ongoing treatment from the many practitioners there, often having group therapy. The effects of World War II and the death of Dr Hyashi in 1941 put an end to this clinic.

Reiki Today

Hawayo Takata had been a student of Dr Hyashi for some five years, having received Reiki treatment from him. Literally hearing words from her subconscious mind saying that an operation she was just about to have was not necessary, she asked the surgeon if he knew how she could receive some other cure. He recommended Hyashi to her. Hawayo Takata and Hyashi's wife were the first two women to be initiated as masters. Takata succeeded him as the grand master in 1941. Living and working in Hawaii, she began to train Reiki masters herself when in her seventies. On her death in 1980, Takata left 22 Reiki masters in Canada and USA.

Shortly before she died, Takata and some other Reiki masters founded the American Reiki Association, which was to organise and co-ordinate the passing on of the knowledge of Reiki.

Today other organisations have been formed. One is the Reiki Alliance founded in 1981 by Phyllis Lee Furumoto, the granddaughter of Hawayo Takata and the present grand master. Phyllis and 21 other masters formed this as a non-profit-making organisation registered in the USA. In 1987 about 100 Reiki masters, some in Europe, were members of the Alliance. The Reiki Alliance takes a spiritual approach to the spreading of Reiki and uses the traditional teachings. They rarely advertise, knowing those who are drawn to them will use this method of teaching.

The American International Reiki Association, Inc. (AIRA) was founded in 1982 by Dr Barbara Weber Ray. She had been trained by Hawayo Takata to convey the knowledge involved in the attainment of the master grade. The AIRA has been concerned with the scientific aspects of Reiki, and is well publicised. It is very active in running public events, conferences and symposiums.

Many other organisations have grown through these original groups, leading to much research and experimentation on methods. Reiki Outreach International was founded in 1990 by Mary McFadyen for the purpose of creating a worldwide network of Reiki practitioners who are united in service to humanity and planet earth and to link in daily or whenever possible to specific world situations and crises.

Training

Often it is because people have received a treatment themselves and benefited from it that they become interested in learning Reiki, intrigued by what seems to be a very gentle but powerful experience.

Although the universal life energy – Reiki – is available to all, there is a special sacred ceremony – an initiation – that has been honoured and passed down through Dr Usui to the present grand master, Phyllis Furumoto. Phyllis and the 21 other masters each in their turn have trained others who now teach and train the recipients who are used as channels for the universal life energy.

Reiki I is usually taught to groups of between four and twelve, over two days. The history and energy is explained and the placement of hands and positions in relation to the organs and joints is demonstrated. Medical knowledge is not required; even children can learn how to receive and transmit this energy. A certificate is awarded which enables students to share Reiki, practising on self or friends, relatives, animals or plants to build up confidence.

Reiki II again is usually a two-day event, and involves the learning of three symbols and the Japanese words that describe them. The first is the universal, all encompassing symbol, the second is the mental symbol and the third is the absent/distant healing symbol. People are asked to honour these symbols and not to reveal them to others who have not completed the Reiki II degree. Learning the symbols and words seems to enhance the healing energy to a more powerful vibration.

If students feel that a greater commitment can be embraced, a period of training is arranged to attain grade III – master level. Written answers are submitted to questions posed by their master/teacher, including questions as to the manner and reason for their wanting to take the step, which is total life commitment to honour and live the Reiki energy in all aspects of their physical incarnation. If the answers are acceptable, then the ceremony of initiation proceeds, in which the healing knowledge and Reiki energy is sealed into the crown, hands and heart chakras of the student. This is a sacred ceremony and is performed privately, with only the master and student present. The recipient receives with eyes closed that which they most need as the energy flows into their whole being. The ceremony is very special and holds much meaning for the serious student of Reiki. Following this initiation, students are monitored and supported by the master/teacher as they learn the process of initiating and teaching other individuals and workshop groups.

The word 'master' is given as an honorary title which is earned through study and a commitment to live Reiki in all aspects of life. It is attained in the same manner as any exam or degree in any subject or profession.

Students do not pay for the enlightenment and knowledge. What they agree to pay for is the time, the expenses, the certificate and all the various material factors that are involved. Basic amounts are generally mutually agreed upon. Variations can be arranged to suit different financial situations.

The Practice of Reiki

Although Reiki can be used in all types of situations, to enjoy a full session of 1 to 1½ hours is most beneficial. Reiki can also be used in combination with other therapies, especially those working with touch, and will enhance the practitioner's effectiveness.

A comfortable, relaxing space is required which is warm and quiet. The clients start by lying on their backs, then turn onto their stomachs, while the therapist proceeds to touch them using appropriate Reiki hand positions. Usually after a few minutes relaxation gently enters as the energy begins to flow. The practitioner works from the head down the trunk to the coccyx, then balances the chakras into the heart centre, revitalising the energy.

Reiki treatment can help release emotion and stress; it can amplify and balance energy and increase awareness. It works on the causal level of disease, creates relaxation in the physical body and can reverse processes which hasten ageing.

Often childhood or archetypal traumas are brought into focus. The memory is awakened as a joint or organ that has been 'holding on to something' is ready to be released and healed. In these cases it is good if the recipient can have several sessions within a short period of time. In some cases, the body undergoes a healing crisis when symptoms can occur or be exacerbated, for example sweating, loose bowels, excess water retention and so on.

If people come for specific ailments or injuries, they often find that other parts of the body are healed, conditions that they have been so used to they have stopped noticing, until they realise they are gone.

Reiki can speed recovery from operations, accidents and injuries of all kinds. The only time it is not advisable straight away is if bones are broken and need to be set and realigned or if there is a deep, bleeding wound which needs cleaning. This is because the Reiki energy may encourage the body to start healing before the wound has been cleaned or the bone set in place. In these cases, Reiki should only be used on the energy over the auric field.

Reiki does not always invite complete cure, and in cases of terminal illness it can bring gentle relief for the soul as it prepares to leave the physical plane. Reiki practitioners do not invoke or visualise results; it is entirely up to the recipients how much energy they wish to receive, or not, as the case may be.

Practitioners always benefit from a Reiki session also, as they channel the energy for the recipient. Practitioners are not using their own personal energy, but the universal creative life-force which is abundantly available. Once a person is attuned to become a Reiki channel, concentrated life energy will flow through their hands of its own accord and this ability will remain for the rest of their lives.

Biography

June Woods has always been intuitive. She was a civil servant for many years, supporting and raising a family of three. When she was 45 she started attending spiritualist church meetings and became involved in various forms of healing. She was initiated in January 1992 as a Reiki master. She now lives and works in the Findhorn Foundation Community.

Further Reading

Arnold, L E., Nevius, S., *The Reiki Handbook*, PSI Press, 1982.

Baginski, B J.; Sharamon, S., *Reiki – Universal Life Energy*, Life Rhythm Publication, 1988.

Brown, F., *Living Reiki: Takata's Teachings*, Life Rhythm Publications, 1992.

Burack, M., *Reiki – Healing Yourself and Others*, LoRo Productions, 1995.

Haberly, H., *Reiki: Hawayo Takata's story*, Blue Mountain, 1990.

Horan, Paula, *Empowerment through Reiki*, Lotus Light Publications, 1990.

Müller, B.; Günther, H., *A Complete Book of Reiki Healing*, Life Rhythm Publication, 1995.

Resources

Reiki Association of Great Britain
Cornbrook Bridge House
Clee Hill
Ludlow
Shropshire SY8 3QQ
Tel/Fax. 01584-890 284

The Reiki Alliance
P O Box 5327
Eugene OR 95705
USA

Reiki Touch Masters Foundation, Inc.
P O Box 571785
Houston. TX 77057
USA

The Center for Spiritual Development
917 Woodcrest Drive
Royal Oak MI 48067
USA

The Radiance Technique Assoc. International, Inc.
4 Embarcadero Center Suite
5123, San Francisco CA 94111
USA

Mary McFadyen
Reiki Outreach International
P O Box 609
Fair Oaks, CA 95628
USA
Tel. (916) 863-1500
Fax. (916) 863-6464

Reiki Outreach International sends information monthly about which areas are in most need. Also how to adopt children, such as the Romanian orphanage children, so they can receive regular Reiki healing. A news sheet is sent out twice a year.

Relaxation Therapy

by Beverly Feinberg-Moss

Everybody knows what relaxation is, but most people have forgotten how to do it. That relaxation is important for health is not in dispute: increasingly in modern medicine doctors prescribe relaxation therapy – on its own or as an adjunct to holistic and orthodox medical treatment – for a very long list of symptoms The list includes such problems as head, back and stomach aches, insomnia, angina and coronary heart disease, herpes, asthma, ulcerative colitis, trauma injury, premenstrual and menopause symptoms, infertility, skin disorders, cancer, diabetes, MS, hypertension and others.[1] Relaxation therapy is also advised for certain psychiatric diagnoses, for example anxiety, panic attacks, attention deficit, substance abuse and post-traumatic stress disorders, as well as many illnesses for which no diagnosis or treatment is known. Relaxation therapy has widespread use and demonstrated results: if it were a pill, we would probably all take one daily.

Historical and Theoretical Background

The Application of Holism in Health Care

Common sense tells us that the mind, emotions, body and spirit are united. To try to separate them for scientific or medical purposes has been a problematical development in twentieth century medicine, which nonetheless has brought us many marvellous advances. This tendency in health care to divide attention between the mind and body, to ignore the spirit and resist an integrated treatment, is now phasing out. The paradigm shift is clearly taking hold, as evidenced in the new science of behavioural medicine, which has achieved a mind/body integration, although only after a battle.

The two main tools of behavioural medicine that have been instrumental in achieving the integration are relaxation therapy and psychoneuroimmunology (PNI). Behavioural medicine is a flourishing field of research and practice, encompassing PNI research and numerous creative applications of mind/body therapies, in which some form of relaxation therapy typically features. The arrival of the technology which permits the study of intercellular brain behaviour has resulted in rapid and intriguing advances in PNI which explains how cognitions, hormones and biochemical messengers (called neurotransmitters) regulate mood and affect the immune system.

Relaxation therapy has theoretical and historical links with meditation and the psychospiritual science of the breath with its role in calming the mind and in promoting the experience of the inner self. It is also linked with psychosomatic medicine and medical psychology which historically have been concerned with the impact of psychological factors on health and illness – the effect of emotions, conflicts, tension and attitudes; the particular meaning a person may give to symptoms as well as the predisposition, onset and course of disease in the individual. In both behavioural medicine and relaxation therapy, non-judgemental attention is given to real or imagined symptoms and to the tendency in some patients toward somatisation (preferring to focus on physical complaints rather than addressing the underlying psychological issues).

Extensive experimental research literature supports the benefits of relaxation therapy on measures of physiological and psychological change. The pioneering studies of Harvard cardiologist Herbert Benson, MD, on meditating Tibetan Buddhist monks and on hypertensive patients practising Transcendental Meditation, produced documentation of the physiological changes accompanying meditative states and demonstrated the power of the mind over the body.[2] Benson risked his scientific respectability by introducing the 'relaxation response' (RR) treatment into mainstream medicine via his Harvard Medical School hospital cardiology practice in the early 1970s. Subsequently in the United States, with Benson's leadership, hospital-based and independent 'mind/body clinics' and stress management programmes have proliferated as an outgrowth of RR training, which is essentially a simple meditation breathing technique couched in the language of behaviour modification and without any religious overtones. Together with the work of many others, notably Hans Selye, Candace Pert and Edmund Jacobson, the field of behavioural medicine has been established.[3]

Transcendental Meditation

Stress Management

The conceptual cornerstone of relaxation therapy is the body's 'fight-flight response'. This phenomenon was perhaps first described at the turn of the century by Harvard physiologist Dr Walter Cannon as the 'emergency response'. The term refers to an innate protective survival mechanism linking the mind and body, whereby the brain, registering stress or danger, alerts the body through a sequence of biochemical signals to fight or flee. We experience this response as the familiar surge of adrenalin or the feeling of being trapped when excited, stressed, angered or frightened.

What happens physiologically is a complex chain reaction. It starts when the brain's hypothalamus registers danger or stress and triggers the secretion of a series of neurotransmitters around the body, which travel to the pituitary gland and the adrenal glands, then course through the body's five major systems – cardiovascular, musculo-skeletal, gastro-intestinal, neurological and endocrine/immune systems – causing a cascade of responses enabling the body to react physically to the perceived stressor.

When the body is thus aroused, one of the two alternate branches of the autonomic (involuntary) nervous system – the sympathetic branch – is activated. The other branch – the parasympathetic (maintenance) branch – simultaneously shuts down. The fight-flight reaction is most often an overreaction, unwarranted, and therefore a waste of energy. Whether it is triggered by acute or chronic stress, positive or negative stressors, the fight-flight response wreaks havoc on all five major systems, and weakens the immune system. The Canadian endocrinologist Hans Selye wrote the classic work describing the harmful effects of 'eustress' and distress in 1956, *The Stress of Life*.[4]

Vulnerability to the common cold, and more serious illness, is well documented in anxiety-provoking situations like exams, or emotional crises like divorce. Holmes and Rahe's 'life events scale' lists various social adjustments and major life changes both good and bad (for example new job or job loss, marriage or divorce, childbirth or death) which, over time, in close succession, often predict illness.[5]

Another area of behavioural medicine research has identified what is called coronary-prone behaviour, specific personality traits of impatience and hostility, labelled 'type A personality', which are highly associated with coronary heart disease. Psychologist Suzanne Kobassa tracked health and illness in hundreds of business people over several years to determine what made the difference.[6] She attributed health to a cluster of cognitive behaviours she called stress-hardiness, now referred to as the three Cs, the attitudes of challenge, commitment and control.

Neuro Linguistic Programming

Stress-hardy people see problems as challenges; they value commitment to community or relationships; and they perceive control rather than helplessness in difficult situations through their ability to choose a positive internal perspective rather than succumb to external infringements on their freedom. The key here is perspective, or what is called in psychology 'cognitive reframing'. In relaxation therapy this is a critical skill to learn, as not only life events but also one's inner appraisal bring on stress. To cultivate and maintain stress-hardy attitudes one has to take time to step back and reflect, to calm the mind and body, to relax.

The notion of relaxing may seem simple enough but, in fact, it is as internally complex as its antithesis, the fight-flight response. By focusing on the breathing pattern the relaxation response allows the body to shift out of the arousal state of the fight-flight response regulated by the sympathetic nervous system, to the opposite state regulated by the parasympathetic nervous system, thus breaking the anxiety cycle, and calming the mind and body. It is like shifting from high gear to coasting.

The depth of theory supporting relaxation therapy and the relaxation response originates in the ancient psychospiritual teachings of Indian, Tibetan, Chinese, Judeo-Christian, Polynesian and other traditions, which instruct how significant the breath is in stilling the mind, finding inner peace, securing a sense of inner self/observer and attaining wisdom or expanded consciousness. Over millennia these diverse traditions have taught that quality of life and health can be cultivated by the pursuit of meditation. For many patients relaxation therapy is the beginning of the inner adventure of meditation.

The Practice of Relaxation

The relaxation response exercise is very easy to do. Benson states four requirements: a quiet place, a focus word or phrase, a receptive, passive attitude, and a comfortable, symmetrical, upright posture (except for treatment of insomnia or chronic pain when lying down may be preferable).[7] It should be noted that no equipment is needed except a headset if one chooses to use an audio cassette. I personally add a fifth requirement: a commitment to one's self, a priority in one's life to take time to relax. This is not easy for people to do; they have good excuses. However if one does not do the exercise, there will be no benefits. Start with five minutes daily of sitting quietly. In our relaxation therapy courses we follow Benson's recommendation of 10-20 minutes, twice daily. The more regularly one practises, the better one functions under stress. If one manages a half-hour daily, preferably in the morning upon waking, one experiences greater benefits. A relaxation exercise can bring immediate symptomatic relief. In daily irritations, like telephone stress, one finds oneself using a brief version for on-the-spot composure. Although at times physical or mental benefits may not be apparent, the negative effects are noticed if one ceases to do it regularly, like a pain that is forgotten until it reappears. This is the experience of many people.

In a sense, relaxation is an ideal state. The word derives from the Latin *laxus* meaning 'loose', 'open'. It implies a state of looseness, flexibility, a flow of energy, a sense of inner connection or wholeness, an ease within oneself and in the world. Regular practice brings the deeper levels of relaxation, an inner state of trust and stillness that is akin to meditation.

Any number of techniques are used together in relaxation therapy and stress management programmes: biofeedback, autogenics, flotation tanks, music, yoga, caring for pets, hypnosis, guided imagery and visualisation, sensory awareness, nutrition, cardiovascular exercise, etc., but the principal techniques are Benson's *relaxation response* (RR)[8] and Jacobson's *progressive muscle relaxation* (PMR).[9]

Autogenic Training
Yoga
Hypnotherapy
Visualisation
Nutritional Therapy

The Relaxation Response

The RR exercise calls for focusing one's attention on the internal process of rhythmical abdominal breathing. Starting with a long oral exhalation to empty the lungs of all stale air, one co-ordinates the inbreath with a mental focus, such as silently repeating a reassuring word (for example 'yes'), phrase ('I am safe') or peaceful image (the beach) while also experiencing the sensations of relaxing and letting go with each outbreath. In RR usually a nasal inbreath and an oral outbreath are recommended with a sigh-like outbreath. As the breath becomes slower and deeper, one begins to notice the space between breaths and the expanding moment of stillness at the bottom of each outbreath. One becomes aware of the ever-present state of inner peace and thus slips into the healing space of the inner self.

When the mind observes the breath and accompanying sensations, the RR is physiologically reinforced. This is the antidote to the fight-flight response. Placing a hand on the heart may also be comforting. When the mind strays from the focus on the breath or word, and the noisy chatter intrudes from the ongoing stream of consciousness, the instruction is gently to bring the attention back to observing the breath. A non-judgemental, non-critical receptive attitude is fostered, permissively allowing whatever happens without seeking results. Just doing the exercise is the goal. No further expectations are relevant. Obviously any notion of striving would be counterproductive.

A common pattern of breathing associated with the fight-flight response in chronically stressed people centres in the chest and is shallow, similar to panting. In contrast, RR depends on the natural, innate deep breathing pattern called abdominal, diaphragmatic or yogic breathing. This can be observed in babies and sleeping adults. In relaxation therapy it is often necessary to teach this technique anew to patients for whom it may initially feel strange and awkward. However, it is introduced gradually into the RR exercise because the goal is not to strain to get it right, but to focus on the pleasant, comfortable sensations of breathing, allowing whatever happens. Abdominal breathing can be practised at whim until it becomes quite natural again. Often people don't realise how a sinus condition, eye glasses, or tight jeans, belt or collar can be factors in shallow chest breathing.

Progressive Muscle Relaxation

Colour Therapy
Sound Therapy
Visualisation

Progressive muscle relaxation (PMR) is a more active, energetic exercise. The breath is co-ordinated with the contraction and release of specific muscle groups, heightening tension on the inbreath with the contrasting sensation of release on the outbreath. The process may start with the feet or the head (for grounding) and work sequentially through every part of the body with care for any areas of pain. As with RR, specific effects can be elicited through the psychomotor impact of visual, auditory or kinaesthetic imagery. Examples are a chosen colour or light; sounds and images of the ocean or of a clear deep lake; an open window or mountain air (for asthma); a baby's cheek or a soothing caress (for skin or itching); a warm or cool temperature state (for headaches or chronic pain). Counting is also helpful with PMR, emphasising the middle pause and contraction before the outbreath.

Indications

PMR seems preferable for discharging pent up energy, for people who are restless, agitated or angry. RR is contraindicated for people with major depression who have difficulty in directing attention away from depressive thoughts. In marital and sexual counselling, relaxation therapy can improve communication and listening. With simple phobias, obsessive thinking, obsessive/compulsive disorder or nervous tics, both RR and PMR techniques can be useful. With trauma sufferers, the techniques are useful at some stages of recovery to reclaim body sensation and dispel numbing. Because the relaxed mind may recall repressed memories, these exercises are not indicated when uncovering trauma material may destabilise a patient. The boundless calm of RR may feel like emptiness or void, which scares some people. It is clear that relaxation therapy is best learned in a therapeutic setting.

Self-help books and audio and video tapes give instruction in various relaxation techniques.[10] These are excellent as an introduction. However, it is undoubtedly better to learn these techniques with a therapist or a group. People hardly realise the extent of tension, numbing and contraction they are used to tolerating, and how such tight holding of their bodies stems from a real need to protect and defend. To experience the state of relaxation with a teacher who models that state, and who can help in working through blocks and difficulties, is by far the most effective method. Supervision helps maintain the essential daily practice as do group experiences and feedback.

Whatever one chooses from the wonderful array of health-promoting and health-restoring options, the benefits are magnified if one is relaxed. By contrast, benefits can shrink if tension is extreme. Moreover, when a person is genuinely relaxed, chances for overall health improve. Costly and time-consuming treatments and appointments may be reduced.

Research

Benson's research in the early 1970s on Transcendental Meditation represents some of the earliest studies in this field.[11] Now volumes of well-designed experimental research on the effects of relaxation therapy on diverse conditions and populations demonstrate strong support for benefits on physiological, behavioural, psychological and self-report measures. The following studies are representative of current research.[12]

◆ A Harvard study showed the efficacy of preoperative relaxation therapy, administered personally as well as by video-tape to cardiac surgery patients, in pre- and post-surgery measures of pain, sleep, medication use and length of stay.[13]

◆ RR has been shown to reduce hot flushes in menopausal women, and a recent study also demonstrated its benefits in reducing the intensity and frequency of chemotherapy Tamoxifen-induced hot flushes in breast cancer patients, thus increasing their compliance with chemotherapy.[14]

◆ Stress-reducing relaxation strategies have been found to enhance immune function for a variety of conditions. Relaxation therapy (specifically a PMR stretching exercise) was found to increase immune function significantly as tested by the secretion of salivary immunoglobulin in facial pain patients when contrasted with patients resting quietly for the same time period.[15] Relaxation therapy patients also reported feeling less sad.

◆ Brain activity measured by electroencephalogram (EEG) showed that healthy adults in both a breathing exercise and a meditation/imagery group had increased intercortical connectivity as contrasted with adults in a relaxing music group.[16]

Case Study

A straightforward, short-term case involved Jane, a quiet, attractive, tearful 29 year-old woman. Recently married, Jane was referred by her physician because of chronic head, jaw, neck and facial pain. Otherwise healthy, she had slightly injured her neck and back three years earlier. It had happened in a boating accident where she had felt socially pressured and inadequate to participate with her boyfriend and his friends. After several different physicians and two years of chiropractic, her back was better but she was suffering almost daily from a debilitating pressure in her head and jaw, for which there were no neurological findings. For the last year she was taking Klonopin daily, a psychiatric medication prescribed by her physician to relieve anxiety and depression. She felt disappointed in herself and unhappy about gaining some weight. She had recently been laid off from a good job, but was being paid and would teach school in the autumn. The pressure bothered her more when she felt she should be relaxing, that is, at night, at weekends and during the holidays. Her childhood and family of origin were unsymptomatic and she had no previous psychiatric history.

After hearing her story, we discussed the comprehensive questionnaires she had completed on psychiatric and physiological/behavioural symptoms (including her pessimism and feelings of self-blame, her positive marital relationship, her alcohol use, and eating and sleep habits). She wrote out her treatment aims which were to gain relief from the pain, and self-confidence. We contracted for a nine-session therapy to suit her insurance. I recommended she read Joan Borysenko's book, Minding the Body. Mending the Mind.[15]

We did the RR in the third session for about 15 minutes, eyes closed, sitting comfortably upright, with the back well supported. In the exercise I ask patients to put their left hand on their belly and their right hand on their chest while breathing normally to see which hand moves. Her right hand moved, indicating the shallow chest breath associated with hyper-arousal and the fight-flight response. Most of the activity in breathing under stress takes place in the chest. In the relaxation response, the breath centres in the diaphragm or abdomen, first emptying all stale air (CO_2) from the abdomen and lungs, then allowing the greater inflow of oxygen into the abdomen as if inflating a balloon. This RR breath pattern is innate. Only under chronic stress do we become habituated to shallow breathing. Surprisingly most adults have difficulty at first in unlearning this shallow breathing pattern, and relearning the natural breathing pattern. When asleep we do it naturally. In relaxation therapy the priority is to feel comfortable. Changing the breathing pattern is not the goal, so it is introduced gradually according to the individual's inclination. As one becomes more habituated to being relaxed, deeper breathing becomes automatic.

Jane felt very tired when she came into the sessions, and energised when she left. At home she was practising the RR 20 minutes daily in the morning. She was feeling better after the first week, but said it was hard to sit and do nothing. She felt well enough to decrease her Klonopin medication (with her physician's approval).

We did the PMR exercise in the fourth session. She described the jaw pain and the pressure in her head as puffing up like it was going to explode. She said it got worse when she thought about its coming on, and it did not bother her when she was too busy to think of it. In sessions three and four she talked about obsessive thinking over her husband's former secret friendship with his ex-long-term girlfriend. Jane had never spoken up to him about this, feeling at the same time both deceived and that she was making more of it than it was. She was symptom-free by session five. She said the audio RR tape I make for clients was helping.

We talked about worrying, and the mind traps section of the Borysenko book, 'Outwitting the Dirty Tricks Department of the Mind'. In session six Jane retold the story of her boating experience in detail, including the insecurity she felt among her then boyfriend's college friends (she had not finished college); she also spoke about being too quiet compared to her more socially outgoing sisters and about feeling inadequate.

By session seven Jane was doing RR every day for 20 minutes; she had no symptoms but was still puzzled and ruminating about not knowing what was wrong with her. We did a guided imagery exercise where she would find her inner wisdom, starting and ending at her kitchen table and going to a treasure chest in the cellar where she found a purple scarf, her favourite colour since childhood. It symbolised peace. The scarf told her that the pain came from different sources: that she took things too seriously; she was too sensitive, and didn't have self-confidence. It said, 'You know there are many positive things. You don't feel it or see them. You should. You need to let things go from the past and don't dwell on them and think people are judging you all the time. These are the things that get you worked up and anxious.' Jane was not impressed with this experience. She felt more peaceful but she thought it was silly for a scarf to talk.

In session eight she said she thought she knew what the problem was and stated several insights about herself. We talked about the coincidence that her inner wisdom had given her the silly talking scarf as a symbol, and how she tended to take things too seriously. We discussed her pattern of contact and withdrawal, and her need to protect her sensitivity. We mentioned the value of being quiet.

Her last session, the ninth, took place two months after the start of treatment, as planned. Jane said she had noticed head pressure very slightly at night after a week of substitute teaching. She was doing the RR five times weekly for 20 minutes with the audio tape which helped her focus. She continued to reduce her medication. I have had no further contact with her in the three months since therapy ended.

This is an example of a reasonably successful short-term therapy. The patient gained insight into her personality dynamics and interpersonal difficulties. She clearly recognised her need to speak up with her husband and under social pressure. She learned to relax using the relaxation therapy tools and she experienced relief and improvement in a chronic pain condition that had been resistant to other treatments. She made reasonable progress in her two goals of gaining self-confidence and relief from head pressure.

Biography

Beverly (Besmer) Feinberg-Moss, PhD, a licensed health psychologist, holds a doctoral degree in clinical/developmental psychology from the University of Sussex, with doctoral research on mental imagery strategies and psychosynthesis. Completing a post-doctoral internship at Harvard Medical School in the Behavioural Medicine Mind/Body Clinic supervised by Herbert Benson, MD and Joan Borysenko, PhD, she has directed mind/body programmes in hospital, medical, work and educational settings. She holds master's degrees from Stanford University and the University of California, Santa Barbara, and a bachelor's degree from Cornell University (NY) Her interest in holistic medicine grows out of 30 years of meditation and clinical practice. She currently lives and practises in Salem, MA., USA.

References

1   Andrew Weil, Natural Heath, *Natural Medicine*, Houghton Mifflin, 1990.

2   Hans Selye, *The Stress of Life*, McGraw-Hill, 1956, p 527.

3   ibid. p 458.

    Joan Borysenko, *Minding the Body, Mending the Mind*, Addison Wesley, 1987, p 124.

    Herbert Benson, *The Relaxation Response*, Avon Books, 1975, p 458.

4   ibid.

5   T H Holmes; R H Rahe, *Schedule of Significant Recent Life Events*, Journal of Psychosomatic Research, 1967; 11: 213-8.

6   Suzanne Kobassa, *The Hardy Personality: Toward a Social Psychology or Stress and Health*, in *Social Psychology of Health and Illness*, GS Sanders; J Suls, Erlbaum (eds), 1982.

7   Herbert Benson, op cit., p 27.

8   ibid.

9   Edmund Jacobson, *Progressive Relaxation*, University of Chicago Press, Chicago, 1938. Variations of the RR exercise are found in such comprehensive health guides as physician Andrew Weil's *Natural Health, Natural Medicine,* Houghton Mifflin, 1990, and British acupuncturist Edith Just's *The Truth about Your Health*, T W M Publ., Pangbourne, Berks, 1996.

10 Joan Borysenko, *Minding the Body, Mending the Mind*, Addison Wesley, 1987.

11 H Benson; R K Wallace, *Decreased drug abuse with Transcendental Meditation: A study of 1861 subjects*, in C J D Zarafonetis (ed), *Drug abuse-proceedings of the international conference*, Lea and Febiger, 1972: 369-76.

    H Benson, *Transcendental meditation – science or cult?*, JAMA, 1974; 227: 807.

12 reported at the 1995 16th Annual Scientific Sessions of the Society of Behavioral Medicine (USA).

13   E Stuart; M. Baim; A Casey; J Irvin; P.Zuttermeister; H Benson; A Domar, *A comparison of preoperative personal versus videotaped relaxation response instruction in cardiac surgery patients*, Annals of Behavioral Medicine, 1995; 17: 130.

14   J Irvin; R Friedman; D Mills; A Domar, *The use of relaxation training to reduce the frequency and intensity of Tamoxifen-induced hot flashes*, Annals of Behavioral Medicine, 1995; l 7: 176.

15   J J Sherman; C R Carlson; J McCubbin; J Wilson, *The effect of relaxation on salivary immunoglobulin A in facial pain patients*, Annals of Behavioral Medicine, 1995; 17: 82.

16   T Kato, *Neurophysiological correlates of relaxation, a coherence analysis of electroencephalogram (EEG)*, Annals of Behavioral Medicine, 1995; 17: 173.

17   Joan Borysenko, op cit.

Further Reading

Ader, R.; Cohen N., *Psychoneuroimmunology: Conditioning and Stress*, Annual Review of Psychology, 1993; 44: 53-85.

Benson, Herbert, *The Relaxation Response*, Avon Books, 1975.

Borysenko, Joan, *Minding the Body, Mending the Mind*, Addison Wesley, 1987.

Charlesworth, Edward A; Nathan, Ronald G., *Stress Management, A Comprehensive Guide to Wellness*, Ballantine Books, 1982.

Irvin, J.; Friedman R.; Mills, D.; Domar, A., *The use of relaxation training to reduce the frequency and intensity of Tamoxifen-induced hot flashes*, Annals of Behavioral Medicine, 1995; 17: 176.

Jacobson, Edmund, *Progressive Relaxation*, University of Chicago Press, 1938.

Just, Edith, *The Truth about Your Health*, TWM Publ., 1996.

Kato, T., *Neurophysiological correlates of relaxation, a coherence analysis of electroencephalogram (EEG)*, Annals of Behavioral Medicine, 1995; 17: 173.

Maier, S F.; Watkins, L R.; Fleshner, M., *Psychoneuroimmunology, the interface between behavior, brain and immunity*, American Psychologist, 1994; 49: 1004-17.

Selye, Hans, *The Stress of Life*, McGraw-Hill, 1956.

Sherman, J J.; Carlson, C. R.; McCubbin J; Wilson, J., *The effect of relaxation on salivary immunoglobulin A in facial pain patients*, Annals of Behavioral Medicine, 1995; 17: 82.

Siegel, Bernie S., *Love, Medicine and Miracles*, Harper & Row, 1986.

Stuart, E.; Baim, M.; Casey, A.; Irvin, J.; Zuttermeister, P.; Benson, H.; Domar, A., *A comparison of preoperative personal versus videotaped relaxation response instruction in cardiac surgery patients*, Annals of Behavioral Medicine, 1995; 17: 130.

Weil, Andrew, *Natural Heath, Natural Medicine*, Houghton Mifflin, 1990.

Annals of Behavioral Medicine, 1995; 17(suppl.), *Proceedings of the Society of Behavioral Medicine's Sixteenth Annual Scientific Sessions*.

Resources

Society of Behavioral Medicine
103 South Adams Street
Rockville, MD 20850
USA
Tel. (301) 251 2790
Fax. (301) 279 4749

Rolfing: Structural Integration
by Kathy Webster Bates

General Introduction

Some individuals may perceive their losing fight with gravity as a sharp pain in their back...others as a constant fatigue...those over 40 may call it old age. And yet all these signals may be pointing to a single problem... they are off balance. They are at war with gravity.

— Dr Ida Rolf, PhD[1]

The major segments of our bodies – the head, shoulder, chest, hips, knees and feet – are as a vertical stack of child's building blocks. As long as the structure is correctly aligned, all is well. If, however, any part is out of balance – due to physical injury, emotional stress, or simply poor postural habits – the structure becomes unstable.

Instead of muscles performing their natural function of coming into action when required, some will be used constantly, in holding up the structure. Eventually, they lose their elasticity; adhesions develop in the connective tissues and energy is lost as the body adjusts to coping with supporting itself in a new, out-of-kilter arrangement. Gravity, instead of reinforcing balance and integration of the body, is now the cause of stress.

Rolfing, or structural integration, is a method of manipulating the connective tissue of the body in order to realign its structure.

Theoretical Background

Connective tissue, according to Dr Rolf, the biochemist who developed the technique, holds the body together. She believed it to be the most important structural component of the body. The connective tissue, or fascia, forms a continuous malleable web directly under the skin. Deeper levels of the tissue envelop each muscle fibre, internal organ, bone and muscle grouping. If the body becomes injured, this connective tissue shortens and thickens to provide extra support to the troubled area. A sprained left ankle, for example, quickly becomes immobilised by acute pain and swelling. Most of the body's weight will now be carried by the right leg, causing a noticeable limp. Subtle changes gradually occur: the hip tilts a little to the right; the left shoulder is carried higher; and the head automatically moves to the left. Twinges of discomfort may be experienced in the lower back and/or neck area. Even this comparatively minor injury can create a long-lasting effect on the entire body, simply due to the resulting imbalances.

In this manner, our bodies 'remember' all our physical injuries that may be long forgotten mentally: a lengthy forceps delivery; a frightening fall from the highchair; a violent whiplash acquired en route to school, for example. Totally individual physical patterns develop during our lives, due to the myriad of events that literally shape our bodies. From early childhood, environmental factors can affect our vulnerable structure – cumbersome nappies, ill-fitting shoes, poorly designed school furniture. Children are talented mimics and will often copy the physical mannerisms and gait of a parent. As we mature, daily occupational tasks may contribute to structural imbalances and stress.

Just as damaging is our physical response to emotional events. Emotional stress often manifests itself physically, so that descriptions of our feeling states are a standard part of our vocabulary. Some examples are: 'shouldering the burden', 'tense with rage', 'cringing with fear'. These physical and emotional stresses can result in a catalogue of side effects ranging from general fatigue to specific aches and pains.

The process of allowing the body to straighten and balance itself through a series of Rolf sessions establishes an order in the body that affects physical, mental, emotional and spiritual levels.

Historical Background

The art of structural integration represents the life's work of Dr Ida Rolf. Born in New York in 1896, Ida Rolf received her PhD in biochemistry from Columbia University and furthered her knowledge of the body through her scientific work in organic chemistry at the Rockefeller Institute.

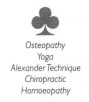

Osteopathy
Yoga
Alexander Technique
Chiropractic
Homoeopathy

Dr Rolf became anxious to discover solutions to personal and family problems. Medical treatment at that time was proving inadequate. This quest led to years of investigating techniques which explored body function, including osteopathy, yoga, the Alexander Technique, chiropractic and homoeopathy. These systems, together with her scientific work, guided her to a deep understanding of structural order.

A sequence of work emerged, later to become known as structural integration, or Rolfing. For the next 30 years, until her death, Dr Rolf devoted herself to developing the technique, and creating training programmes. Although the method of structural integration has been formally taught for over 25 years, tremendous care is taken to ensure that Dr Rolf's teachings remain clear and undiluted.

The Practice of Rolfing

Many thousands of people, from the very young to the elderly, discover Rolfing to be extremely beneficial. The technique is no substitute for medical help when needed and sessions are not offered to the acutely unwell or frail. If the Rolf practitioner is in any doubt, medical advice is always sought.

During its infancy, Rolfing unfortunately became known as a rather painful process. Over the decades, however, Rolfers have developed a much more gentle, sensitive technique. When working on those areas of the body which are inevitably tight, such as the neck and shoulders, a client may feel momentary discomfort, which is soon replaced by a newly discovered freedom of movement.

Rolfing has proved significantly successful in helping a wide variety of conditions. Perhaps the most common is long-standing pain and fatigue brought about by poor postural habits or structure imbalance. The technique is frequently used by athletes, dancers and actors to enhance their performance. People come to Rolfing to regain that feeling of lightness and flexibility they remember once having. Children respond beautifully to the work, and Rolfing can greatly help their growing bodies to develop in a co-ordinated, balanced manner.

The results of Rolfing are varied. People generally report feeling lighter and freer, with a higher level of energy. In 'after ten session' photographs of people who have been Rolfed, they appear leaner, lighter and longer. Many clients do, literally, measure taller. People report breathing more fully, rediscovering their waistlines, becoming less stolid and more agile, feeling as if their joints have been oiled and that they have much more energy.

The Rolf sessions are conducted one-to-one. Together, the client and practitioner work toward establishing a trusting, relaxed relationship. This is a process both parties embark upon, with the client fully participating, and being in control of the work. Each of the carefully designed series of ten sessions lasts approximately one hour. The initial appointment is inevitably longer, as client and Rolfer share pertinent information. Although most people favour booking weekly appointments, sessions are always scheduled to suit each individual.

After the case history has been taken, the Rolfer will discuss the client's immediate postural concerns. Rolfers are trained to 'see' the body's structural organisation, and the clients are observed in their underwear, so that particular areas of imbalance can be identified. Clients are photographed – front, back and both side views – to document initial alignment. These pictures often offer valuable revelations to the clients, as they view themselves for the first time from the perspective of alignment. At the conclusion of the ten sessions, a further series of photographs is taken to record the physical changes.

With the client lying on a massage table, the Rolfer begins to use his of her hands to gently apply pressure or energy to areas of constricted connective tissue. The client may be asked to 'breathe' into the area being worked with and sometimes to make synchronised movements.

This combination of applied energy and synchronised response frees and repositions the connective tissue and aligns the body's structure. Different areas of the body are worked with to bring about certain changes. Each session builds on the last, and prepares the body for the next, so that the results are cumulative. Although the ten Rolf sessions follow a methodical pattern, each is tailor-made to the individual's particular structure.

Rolfing combines comfortably with many other therapies in bringing the body toward a more centred place, physically and emotionally. Because the Rolf technique is concerned with movement, it is compatible with almost all exercise disciplines. It is also significantly beneficial in resolving unfinished emotional issues, which are characterised in the postural attitudes and chronic holding patterns of the body. Gentle pressure on connective tissue can release long-held memories stored in them, and this may trigger emotional release. Occasionally people will experience emotions such as grief or anger during the session or at a later point in time, when they are ready to integrate the experience. The Rolfer will assist them in their process with counselling skills or, if indicated, refer them.

Training

Choose a job you love, and you'll never have to work a day in your life.

— Confucius

Two schools, both based in Boulder, Colorado, USA, offer training classes in structural integration. Teachers also run courses in Australia, Brazil and Europe. The classes are small, to maximise individual attention, and the entire training typically takes three or four years to complete. As yet, training classes have not been held in the UK.

The training requires a background of careful preparation in body, mind and spirit, and aspiring Rolfers are drawn from many varied careers. They are trained in detailed anatomy and physiology as well as extensive experience with hands-on manipulative work, and a high degree of psychological and empathetic skills.

Once qualified, practitioners of structural integration develop their own practices – with the ongoing support of the established worldwide Rolf community. Rolfers have the opportunity of attending scheduled continuing education workshops. Regional and annual meetings also provide further educational experience and fellowship.

Research

Research into the efficacy of structural integration has been conducted on an ongoing basis for many years, primarily in the United States. Information concerning specific research studies can be obtained by contacting the two training schools in Boulder, Colorado, USA.

Personal Approach to Rolfing

Prior to becoming a Rolfer, I worked for many years in a residential treatment centre for emotionally disturbed children. It was my observation that although many of these children benefited from their stay, proving more able to express their emotions and developing a greater degree of self-confidence, their physical appearance seemed to remain 'stuck', continuing to display the initial aggression or cowering fear which characterised their personal history on admittance.

One memorable afternoon, a fellow colleague arrived for work seemingly walking on air with shining bright eyes. He looked taller, calmer and certainly lighter on his feet. 'I've been Rolfed!' he announced. When the general hilarity subsided, I was intrigued to learn more.

The logic of the theory and methodology of Rolfing made sense to me. It seemed a perfect way of allowing our emotional and physical bodies to become more integrated – more 'up-to-date'. The holding patterns of our bodies, as described by Ida Rolf, explained the phenomena I had noticed in the disturbed children. Within a few weeks I had embarked upon the lengthy training to become a Rolfer myself.

Eighteen years later, almost all those with whom I trained continue to practise Rolfing. This speaks volumes, as I have heard that in most trainings in complementary therapies, only one third of students go on to become practitioners. Because of the prerequisite stipulation that prospective candidates be over 26 years old, each Rolfer brings previous skills and experiences into their work. Many refine their techniques and develop specialist applications. Some train to join the school's teaching faculty.

Each Rolfer develops their own individual style of work, though the primary intentions and goals remain unaltered. My own personal approach is one of gentleness and calm supportiveness.

Rolfing's potential to benefit so many people in differing situations is, in my experience, limitless.

Biography

Kathy Webster Bates studied child psychology, counselling and family therapy in Toronto, Canada, and worked for many years with emotionally disturbed children and their families. Kathy completed her training in Rolfing at the Rolf Institute, Boulder, Colorado, USA in 1979. She is also qualified as a remedial massage therapist from the Canadian School of Massage and Hydrotherapy. Kathy developed a Rolfing practice in London and Sussex before moving to Aberdeenshire with her young family. Although there are many hundreds of practitioners of structural integration worldwide, Kathy is currently the only one in Scotland.

Further Reading

Anson, Brian, *Rolfing - Stories of Personal Empowerment*, Heartland Personal Growth Press, 1992.

Feitus, Rosemary, *Ida Rolf Talks About Rolfing and Physical Reality*, Harper & Row, 1978.

Rolf, Ida P., *Rolfing - The Integration of Human Structures*, Harper & Row, 1978.

———, *Structural Integration: Gravity, an Unexplained Factor in a More Human Use of Human Beings*, Rolf Institute, 1979.

———, *Structural Integration: A Contribution to the Understanding of Stress*, Confinia Psychiatrica 16.69.79., Rolf Institute, 1973.

Spiegal, Rosie, *Yoga for Rolfers: Rolf Movement, Teachers and their Clients*, Rolf Institute, 1987.

Resources

Two schools teach Dr. Rolf's method of Structural Integration. Information can be obtained regarding training programmes, further details and literature and copies of their International Directory of qualified Practitioners.

Guild for Structural Integration
P O Box 1559
Boulder, CO 80306
USA
Tel. (303) 447-0122, (800) 447-0150

The Rolf Institute
International Headquarters
205, Canyon Boulevard
Boulder, CO 80302
USA
Tel. (303) 449-5903, (800) 530-8875
Fax. (303) 449-5978

For information regarding Rolf practitioners
in Britain, please contact:

Jennie Crewsdon
49 Charlwood Street
London SW1 2VDR
England
Tel. 0171-834 1493

Kathy Webster Bates
East Camaloun Cottage
Fyvi
Turriff
Aberdeenshire AB53 8JY
Scotland
Tel. 01651-891 088

SHEN Therapy
by Richard R. Pavek

SHEN* is an acronym for 'Specific Human Energy Nexus'. It is a physioemotional release therapy entailing a hands-on healing process where the practitioner uses the *qi* (also spelled *ki* or *chi*) energy that flows from the hands to unlock and release trapped emotion from the recipient's body. It is used to accelerate healing after emotional trauma, to assist in emotional growth, and to heal physical conditions that have been caused, at least in part, by trapped, painful emotions as, for instance, in disorders such as anorexia, premenstrual syndrome and post-traumatic stress disorder.

The Development of SHEN

SHEN began in 1977, as a result of an attempt by the author to discover whether the laws of ordinary physics, which govern motion in magnetic fields, hydraulics and weather systems, also applied to the *biofield* (the qi or prana) that surrounds and permeates the human body. Biofield is a term coming into use to replace 'energy field' which has been used incorrectly since it has precise meanings in chemistry and physics. Until that time, most practitioners using hands-on healing methods practised their work entirely from intuition, or internal knowing. Some believed that the biofield coming from their hands had 'intelligence' and knew where to go and what to do without being directed by the practitioner. However, I believed that once the patterns of physics were established and the way unseen energy operated was understood, new and more effective treatment methods could be devised. If the effects noted by healers could be shown to fit the patterns of ordinary physics, it would help encourage physicists and engineers to develop appropriate measuring devices.

All previous attempts at applying scientific methodology to the human energy field had proved inconclusive. Since there were no measuring instruments that could detect or measure the direction of the biofield within the body, I had to rely on the most basic detection device of all, the human hand. I started by detecting when the flow of the biofield passes from one hand through the recipient's body to my other hand and noticing how the recipient responded. Before long I discovered that the

---

*SHEN is the registered service mark of SHEN Therapy Institute, Sausalito, California, USA.

recipient's responses were significantly different when the hand placements were reversed. This effect was reproducible.

For example, when the sending hand is placed low on the recipient's back and the receiving hand is placed higher up on the back and the hands held in place for a few minutes, the recipient will relax into a deep state and when the process is over, feel relaxed and refreshed. However, when the hands are reversed, with the sending hand higher on the spine than the receiving one, the recipient's heart begins to beat faster and the recipient experiences unpleasant sensations and becomes agitated. Clearly, being relaxed and refreshed was health-promoting while being agitated and upset was not. These positive and negative results became my mapping tools.

Mapping of the biofield was a very slow process. It took many observations of hand placement results to be sure that the map was accurate. These observations were confirmed by other practitioners and were checked and rechecked in many ways. As the work progressed, it was noticed that hand placements at certain specific locations on the body resulted in the release of different emotions. It was later discovered that certain physical disorders respond dramatically to treatments that focus on hand placements centred around the physical disorder. It became clear that, properly applied, SHEN breaks deep tensional holding patterns that surround the sites of painful emotions, such as shame, sadness and fear. Breaking these tensions allows the release of debilitating emotions and this allows the return of normal bodily function. With that knowledge, powerful, significant treatments developed for psychosomatic disorders.

The Practice of SHEN

During a SHEN session, the recipient lies fully clothed on a thickly padded table. The practitioner moves around the table, placing hands on the recipient's body in sequential patterns that have been formulated to be appropriate for the particular disorder being treated. Some of the hand placements are on top of the body, some are underneath. Hands are placed lightly, so there is no feeling of pressure but there may be sensations of warmth or tingling. There may be jerks or twitches in the hands and arms or feet and legs of the recipient, as long-term muscular tensions are released. Emotions frequently, but not always, occur during the first session. These emotional releases are unlike the cathartic release of emotions experienced with other forms of therapy; during SHEN the emotions flow out of the emotional centres of the body – principally the heart, upper abdomen and lower abdomen – without any clenching of the fists, banging the table or shouting. The first emotions released are often sadness and grief. Following these emotions are often deeply held, long-forgotten feelings of anger or fear – hidden emotions that may have affected our daily lives without our knowing it. Cleansing the body of these painful emotions allows the basic emotions of joy and strength to emerge and be experienced. Some people report feeling these healthful emotions for the first time since childhood or experience them in richer, deeper ways than before.

Case Study

One long-term migraine sufferer, aged 36, was staying at a chronic pain clinic in a hospital in Fort Worth, Texas. She had suffered frequent attacks for 27 years – since she was nine years old. She had been under conventional treatment for years and recently had been to two other chronic pain clinics seeking relief; one of these clinics specialised in migraines. Nothing had produced any results; she continued to have attacks at least every other week, intense episodes that lasted from three to four days. The psychological evaluations she had been given were not very useful as they only showed a profile common to migraine sufferers – that of a work-oriented perfectionist. After keeping a calendar of her migraines, she had recently realised that the migraines nearly always began on Wednesdays. The day I saw her was Tuesday, so she anticipated one the next day. Many migraine sufferers have episodes that regularly start on the same day of the week because some deeply traumatising emotional event occurred years ago on that day and precipitated the first migraine.

Before beginning a SHEN series with a new person, I always ask a series of questions designed to uncover the emotional state of the person years ago when the trauma began. But after persistent questioning this client could not recall any emotional trauma when she was nine, nothing upsetting in her family, nothing at all out of the ordinary. When I inquired about possible childhood head injuries that might have contributed to the migraine, she said that recently her cheekbone had been broken, but the injury was so minor that the doctor had been able to press the thin bone back in place from inside her mouth. Since the incident had not occurred when the migraines first started, it was ruled out as a causal factor.

I began the SHEN migraine treatment protocol. Soon she relaxed deeply and her breathing became shallower. I then focused the flow from my hands around the portion of the body that is critical during a SHEN migraine session, the region just above the heart. This region contains the big blood vessel from the heart that branches off into the arteries that feed blood to the head and brain. It also contains the baroreceptors – the biological blood pressure regulators – and the vagus nerve, which wraps itself halfway around the big blood vessel at this point and is involved with nausea, which is common during a migraine episode. This is a critical region for migraine sufferers and applying SHEN flows there may often stop the migraines in mid-episode.

As the biofield flow between my hands passed through the big vessel, her breathing deepened and slowed. Her body suddenly visibly relaxed to an even deeper level. This was a significant event; a sudden deepening like this usually occurs when some emotionally charged memory has been touched, at a place far inside the body. It often precipitates a profound release of tension and becomes the turning point in recovery. After a few minutes of deep stillness, she began to return to normal awareness. I went on to finish the session and sat back, waiting for her to regain full consciousness. When she awoke, she remarked on how rested she was but she had no dreams or memories to report.

Later that day I revisited her hospital room to see how she was doing. She excitedly remarked, 'By the way, I just happened to remember that my parents got divorced when I was nine! Do you think that this work will help my nightmares – I've had them since I was very little; I used to crawl into bed with my parents when I had a nightmare.'

It was clear to me that her migraines began when she lost the refuge of her parents' bed. I have learned that revelations like this often indicate that the migraine series is finished and the migraines will not recur. But I did not tell her this; I wanted to wait and see if her usual Wednesday migraine occurred the next day. It did not. She received two or three more SHEN sessions from another therapist during the next week and did not get a migraine that Wednesday, either. However she did casually mention to the therapist that her jaw had been broken by her husband. Until then she had not told anyone that she was married to an abusive man. At the end of the second week she was discharged from the hospital's pain clinic.

Two and a half months later she walked into the clinic to report that she had divorced her husband and that she had not had a migraine in all that time. We lost track of her after two years, but during that period of time she reported no more migraine episodes.

SHEN treatments are tailored to the individual's needs. SHEN practitioners are taught how to assess the recipient's superficial and deeper emotional states and how to plan an individualised treatment series. A series of SHEN treatments is shorter than many types of therapy because SHEN acts rapidly and because emotions in the body are easier to access energetically than through mental activity. Many receiving SHEN have found that a brief series of three or four session restores them to a happier, more energised life. They may not return for additional SHEN until after some future trauma occurs. Others find that once the emotional loosening process has started, deeper, older emotions occasionally drift upwards into consciousness and they decide to continue SHEN to complete the process.

Indications and Contraindications

SHEN can be of considerable benefit for disorders such as anorexia, anxiety attacks, bulimia, chronic pain without organic cause, emotional depression, nightmares, phobias, non-biological sexual dysfunction and emotionally upset bowels and post-traumatic stress disorder. It has been used with great success with children under the age of reason. SHEN should not be given to a psychiatric patient or someone who should be under a psychiatrist's care and supervision unless approved by the recipient's psychiatrist.

SHEN and Other Complementary Therapies

Psychotherapy
Counselling
Postural Integration
Rolfing
Polarity Therapy

SHEN works very well in conjunction with psychotherapy and with all physical bodywork methods. Though it might seem that SHEN is similar to other bodywork therapies such as polarity therapy or Postural Integration, there are marked differences. Polarity therapy is based on a complex mixture of Stone's understanding of several Eastern and Western healing philosophies. SHEN therapy theory is based on the natural laws that apply to all fields in physics. Polarity practice includes applying flows from the hands plus physical pressure on neurological release points and physical pressure while holding different parts of the body. SHEN does not include the use of neurological release points or physical pressure, only the bioflux from the hands. It is applied very differently from polarity therapy – the patterns followed are entirely different as are the hand positions and intent.

Any bodywork process will occasionally tap into bodily held emotions and release them. Often with these systems, the same level of emotion is reached over and over again with no real resolution. SHEN intentionally reaches into the physical body to bring up deeply held painful emotions, expand them and complete them, and then access and bring up the fundamental, beneficial emotions that have been trapped under the painful emotions that have now been removed. SHEN is able to target the individual emotions, not just access them by chance, and bring them to resolution.

As a process of accessing abreaction phenomena, SHEN is far faster than traditional psychotherapy or other talk therapies – and it takes the recipient through the process of emotional release, resolution and growth quickly and with much less trauma.

Research

Clinical case research studies have been gathered for SHEN and major depression,[1] SHEN and migraine[2] and SHEN and menstrual and premenstrual distress.[3] Other studies are in process.

Biography

Richard Pavek was born in Phoenix, Arizona in 1929. He studied many forms of alternative therapies including medical qigong, polarity therapy, Rolfing, homoeopathy, flower essences, massage, Gestalt and Chinese five phase theory. In 1977 he began his research into biofield therapeutics and the effects of qi on health, developing applications such as the treatment of major depression, for chronic pain and to release emotion from the body. In 1989, he collaborated in medical qigong research at the Shanghai College of Traditional Chinese Medicine. He has published many books and papers on SHEN and biofield research studies and gives lectures worldwide. He is currently director of the Biofield Research Institute, carrying out research on the nature of emotion and its effects on physiology and research on physics of the human biofield.

References

1   Beal; Richard Pavek, *SHEN on Major Depression*, study at the Milwaukee County Mental Health Center and the Medical College of Wisconsin, 1985 (unpublished).

2   Richard Pavek, *SHEN Therapy treatment to abort Common Migraine Episodes and end reoccurrence of attacks*, study 1985-89 (unpublished).

3   ———, *Long-term symptom relief of Severe Pre-menstrual Tension following SHEN Therapy treatments*, 1986 (unpublished).

Further Reading

Pavek, Richard R., *Handbook of SHEN*, The SHEN Therapy Institute, Sausalito, CA, 1987.

———, *The Biofield Therapeutics* in: *Alternative Medicine: Expanding Medical Horizons*. A report to the National Institutes of Health on alternative medical systems and practices in the United States. US Government Printing Office, Washington, DC, 1992, p 134-46.

———, *Emotion and the Contractility Factor, A New Model for the Formation of Psychosomatic Disorders*, Featured paper, read at the Founding Conference of the Chinese Society of Behavioral Medicine, Tainjin, P R China, 1988.

———, *Effects of SHEN Qigong on Psychosomatic and Other Physio-emotional Disorders*, Proceedings of the First World Conference for Academic Exchange of Medical Qigong, Beijing, 1988, pp. 150-2.

———, *From 'Stroking' to Modern Biofield Therapeutics: 325 Years of Non-Religious Healing in England, Ireland and Scotland*, Caduceus, August - October, 1995.

———, *Science and Research in Biofield Therapeutics*, Proceedings of the Conference: Examining Research Assumptions in Alternative Medicine, July 11-13, 1994, Bethesda, Maryland.

———; Daily, Terran, *SHEN Physioemotional release therapy: Disruption of the autocontractile pain response*, Occupational Therapy Practice, 1990; 1:3, 53-61.

Resources

Richard R. Pavek, Director
Biofield Research Institute
20 Yellow Ferry Harbor
Sausalito, CA 94965
USA
Tel. (415) 331-3753
Fax. (415) 331-2455

SHEN Physioemotional Therapy
is represented in the UK by:

The SHEN Therapy Centre
26 Inverleith Row
Edinburgh EH3 5QH
Tel/Fax. 0131-551 5091

Shiatsu

by Michael Webster

In shiatsu the body/mind's own healing ability is stimulated by the application of pressure to specific points and areas of the body. These include the specific points of known therapeutic effect called *tsubos* (pronounced 'subos'); *meridians*, which are energetic lines linking together points of similar effect; and points which appear spontaneously along the meridians. Tsubos may be found on the patient or may be absent, and if found, they may alter position or disappear as they are worked on. The pressure in shiatsu is applied with the thumbs, palms, fingers, elbows, forearms and sometimes feet.

The meridian system provides access to the body's energetic system which consists of a universal energy known as *ki* (Japanese) or *chi* (Chinese), also spelled 'qi'. Ki energy affects general quality of health and a shiatsu practitioner uses various forms of diagnosis to gauge the quantities of ki in the meridians, thereby assessing the health of the patient.

As shiatsu is a holistic therapy, treating the whole person on structural, physiological, psychological and spiritual levels, treatments are intended to find the link between cause and effect on all levels of being, thereby addressing the cause of the problem. In shiatsu all aspects of the person are considered to be part of a whole interconnected system, each affecting and being affected by changes in the health and well-being of all the other parts.

Historical Background

Shiatsu has its roots in China but later developed into a Japanese healing art, born of many generations of experience, observation, trial and error, evolving the knowledge that rubbing or pressing a particular place on the body will alleviate pain, soreness, stiffness, headaches, etc. Shiatsu is likely to have been among the very earliest therapies, since rubbing or pressing sore spots is almost a reflex action. Furious rubbing of the outside of the arms when one feels cold is automatic, but, in shiatsu terms, this stimulates the triple heater meridian, which has an effect on temperature control and body heat.

Although it is not known precisely when the information was collated into the form we use today, it is known to predate acupuncture with which it has common roots, and acupuncture is known to have existed prior to 2500 BC. The oldest existing medical text is the Chinese *Nei Ching, the Yellow Emperor's Classic of Internal Medicine,* said to have been written by Huang Ti, the legendary emperor who died in 2898 BC.[1] The Nei Ching makes reference to geographical factors affecting early development of techniques in medicine, and reference is given to the northern areas where treatment in this cold climate comprised mainly acupuncture, herbalism, moxibustion (burning of mugwort on specific points) and massage.

Acupuncture
Traditional Chinese
Medicine

Massage has from the very first been acknowledged as one of the four classical forms of medical treatment. This form of massage was known as *anma* (in Japan) and employed a combination of rubbing and pressing stiff and sore areas. In the seventeenth and eighteenth centuries in Japan, anma became a profession for the blind, as, it was stated, the blind have a particularly sensitive sense of touch. Anma started to become more associated with relaxation and pleasure, although a medical application of massage techniques was retained in the area of pregnancy and childbirth in a form of abdominal massage which has been used for centuries.

Possible evidence that acupuncture developed later than massage and moxibustion comes in the relatively recent discovery of a text dated before the *Nei Ching* in which no points are mentioned, just entire meridians portraying zones of influence needing stimulation by moxibustion. Thus evidence suggests meridians existed before points, the implication being that there were techniques which made use of the knowledge of meridians before acupuncturists began needling specific points.

Chinese medicine was introduced into Japan in the 6th century AD, bringing Buddhism together with Chinese philosophy and culture. Chinese medicine had, by this time, developed concepts which explained the nature of all things and interpreted all aspects of life. Ill health and disease were regarded as a holistic experience, not reduced to a set of symptoms separate from the problem. In Japan this body of knowledge developed further, taking on its own set of characteristics.

Modern Development of Shiatsu

The modern history of shiatsu does not start until the twentieth century when Tamai Tempaku, who had practised anma, *ampuku* and *do-in* (both forms of self-shiatsu), whilst also making considerable studies in Western anatomy, physiology and massage, published in 1919 a work entitled *Shiatsu*. This book brought together the various strands he had been studying and integrated the spiritual dimension of healing into bodywork.

The three most notable of Tempaku's pupils were Serizawa, Masunaga and Namikoshi. These three were to become the most influential figures in the development of modern shiatsu.

Namikoshi had trained in anma and is said to have cured his mother of arthritis using rubbing and pressing techniques. His school, the Japan Shiatsu Institute, was licensed by the Minister of Health and Welfare and shiatsu was recognised as a therapy in its own right. Namikoshi techniques tend to be fairly physical and the approach to treatment tends to be rather Western.

Serizawa was awarded a Doctor of Medicine degree in 1961 in recognition of his research into tsubos and modern scientific methods of proving the existence of the meridians. Serizawa's method is called tsubo therapy.

Masunaga, a doctor of psychology, developed a more energetic approach involving the psychological, emotional and spiritual aspects of energy imbalance using the meridian system (as opposed to tsubos) as a means to diagnose and treat. Masunaga's theory of energy imbalance, known as *kyo-jitsu*, combined with his development of an extended meridian system, beyond but including the traditional meridians, and a system of diagnosis which involves palpation of the abdominal region, gave birth to what is known as Zen shiatsu – a form widely practised in Britain and the USA.

Theoretical Base

At the start of the universe as we know it, all matter that is was already in existence. Matter does not get created or lost. Humankind has explored and gained knowledge of perhaps as little as 1% of that totality and calls it the visible universe. The remaining 99% is known at present by the name of 'dark matter' or universal energy. The only clues to the existence of that 99% are observations of its effects in holding the universe together and of its influence on the 1% of matter of which we are aware. This 99% may be the fundamental underlying energy which interpenetrates all things, known by many names, such as ki, chi or prana.

Quantum physics hypothesises that within the known 1% of matter, at an atomic level everything consists of the same 'stuff' in different quantities. This is held together by vibrating forces, which are subjected to change by the influence of conditions, such as heat, cold, light, etc., which are themselves vibrations.

Humans, who are made up of the same atomic matter, are also subjected to these laws of physics. In addition to being influenced by outer conditions, the inherent energetic pattern of the body systems will affect the functioning of the organism. This energetic pattern will change depending on which different systems in the body or mind are either active or at rest. These changes are recorded by the universal energy, which connects the human body with the rest of the universe. As this energy interpenetrates all other matter, it will carry information to and fro, effecting change all around. It is this mechanism which may explain concepts such as 'thought affects matter', 'the interconnectedness of all life' and the 'holographic universe'.

This natural process of energy exchange is ceaseless. The human organism works continuously to maintain an equilibrium within constant change. This process, in Zen shiatsu terms, is known as kyo-jitsu, referring to the need to balance, energetically, areas of deficiency and excess. Although this is a natural process, problems arise perhaps as a result of lifestyle, stress, shock or poor nutrition when the body is unable to respond to the call to rebalance its energy field. Symptoms of imbalance such as a headache, if not addressed through the cause of the problem, will continue to send out their alarm signal that something is wrong.

The theory of kyo-jitsu and its diagnostic practice indicate the areas requiring attention and the most suitable means of doing this via specific gateways into the energetic system (specific meridians).

In shiatsu, these meridians are influenced though appropriate treatment using pressure, stretching and manipulation. Physiologically the 'traditional' points on each meridian are situated over arteries and/or veins. Therefore shiatsu also affects the vascular system, stimulating it to contribute to the body's rebalancing at a physical level. With this intervention, the organism is freed of its stagnation of energy and is able to undertake its own natural healing process.

The Practice of Shiatsu

Treatment plans differ from one therapist to another; however, there are marked similarities in the basic format used by most. The following treatment plan is based on my own clinical format.

Shiatsu treatment generally takes place on the floor on a futon (padded mattress). If necessary the client can sit in a chair or lie on a bed. Treatments are primarily carried out in prone, supine, side and sitting positions; this varies depending on factors such as pregnancy or structural conditions. However, the major influence is easy access to the areas to be treated, so that a progressive, smooth treatment can be provided. In most forms of shiatsu, treatment is received fully clothed, but the client will be asked to remove shoes, tie, belt, jewelry and anything which may restrict movement. Being able to see the body is not considered a requirement as the practitioner relies on sensitivity of touch.

Before a treatment takes place, a full appraisal of the client's condition and clues as to the possible cause are investigated. Chinese medicine lists four forms of diagnosis – touch, smell, listening and looking – which come into play the moment the client and therapist meet. Observation of attitude, posture, mannerisms, face colour and voice can give indications as to the client's overall condition.

After an introduction and listening to the client's list of symptoms, the therapist may explain the working of shiatsu and what is involved in a treatment. This would include the explanation of shiatsu as an holistic therapy and that the therapist acts as a catalyst in helping the body/mind's own healing process. This requires the involvement of the client. It is a form of partnership. To assist the therapist in understanding the client's problems and how the client functions as an individual, a case history is taken. It is clearly pointed out that all information passing between client and therapist is held in confidence. Having assessed that there are no contraindications to treatment – these may include contagious diseases or anything requiring urgent medical attention – treatment preceded by physical diagnosis can begin.

Once supine, the client will be observed for any physical irregularities not already noted. These may be old injuries, which may have been forgotten, influencing the way a leg lies in comparison to the other leg, for example, or a distorted ribcage (particularly amongst women who have had children as the ribs may have been twisted to one side, displaced by the developing foetus), which may be affecting the function of internal organs. Attitude will also be observed, whether the client appears defensive or open, vulnerable, nervous, guarded, etc. All will have a bearing on the diagnosis and treatment.

Chi Nei Tsang

The therapist may then palpate the diagnostic areas of the abdomen; this is known as *hara diagnosis*. The hara provides extensive information to the shiatsu practitioner and is the equivalent, in diagnostic terms, of the pulses in traditional Chinese acupuncture. The hara is a mirror for all the energies in the body, reflecting both long-term conditions and the acute energy picture, which may change even as the practitioner works on the abdomen. The information obtained will assist in a better understanding of the diagnosis and will indicate the client's state of mind and the areas of the energetic system (meridian system) most requiring treatment.

The therapist may, by this time, have drawn conclusions as to the cause of the problem. This may be presented to the client at an appropriate time during the consultation.

Many treatments commence with work on the back with the client lying face down on the futon. This may take the form of palming and stretching, preparatory work preceding more specific work with thumbs, elbows, etc. This pattern will vary according to the nature of the illness or set of conditions or symptoms. The client is carefully observed throughout the process of treatment, and the hara diagnosis is checked for changes on completion. Depending on the progress, the aim of the treatment and the condition of the client, treatment times may vary from 25 minutes to approximately one hour, although 45 minutes is an average time for most treatments.

Treatments are concluded with a discussion of the diagnosis, an explanation in non-mystical terms and recommendations which may include changes in lifestyle or attitude. Nutritional advice may be offered. These recommendations encourage clients to take responsibility for their own health and not leave it up to the therapist to have a 'magic wand', and take the problem away from them.

Nutritional Therapy

The number of treatments required for each individual is unpredictable, and it is usual for therapists to recommend follow-up treatments from week to week, as they assess the effect of the treatment, any changes that may have taken place and the extent of client involvement in the recommendations given. Clients are free to stop treatments at any time. Many attend on a regular fortnightly or monthly basis as a preventative or maintenance measure.

Clients are usually advised before leaving the treatment room that there may be a reaction to treatment in a small percentage of cases, in the form of nasal secretions or headache the following day; this will pass, usually within a few hours, as such a reaction is part of the healing process and is nothing to worry about.

Osteopathy
Homoeopathy
Chiropractic
Psychotherapy

Shiatsu combines well with osteopathy, homoeopathy, chiropractic, psychotherapy and nutritional therapy. Much depends on the ability, co-operation and communication of the therapists involved, together with the permission of the client for the exchange of relevant information.

Conditions Treated by Shiatsu

Shiatsu therapists deal with the most common problems of everyday life, such as headaches, stress, colds, muscular problems, stiffness and back pain, respiratory, digestive, cardiovascular and reproductive and premenstrual problems. Therapists may be involved with clients in childbirth or those with cancer or patients recovering from strokes. Some may have referrals from the medical profession; patients such as accident victims find benefit from a broad based treatment such as shiatsu.

Shiatsu practitioners are trained to recognise symptoms which require medical attention and will encourage the patient to see their GP if necessary.

Case History

Charlie, 69, a retired farmer, suffered a stroke which left him hemiplegic down the right side and without speech. After eight months in hospital Charlie was sent home with apparently little change in his condition. Iris, Charlie's wife, was informed that nothing more could be done for him, but on her own initiative she determined to try complementary therapies and contacted me.

Prior to Charlie's first appointment, we discussed to what extent Charlie's condition could be improved by shiatsu treatment, if at all. I explained that it was difficult to foresee the degree of improvement that might possibly take place. All I could promise was that I would do my best if Charlie and Iris were willing to give shiatsu a try. When he arrived for the first consultation, Charlie was helped from the car and subsequently wheeled into the clinic accompanied by Iris and his two adult children.

The case history revealed a large number of problems: circulation problems, arthritis, congestion and mucus, and an irregular sleep pattern, which was aggravated by the need to pass water during the night. Charlie's greatly reduced mobility and inability to communicate were causing intense frustration and feelings of isolation, mood swings and an increasing inability to cope with life and the uncertainty of his future. Through the diagnostic assessment, some of the physical conditions could be linked to his emotional state affecting the function of the small intestine in a way which causes peripheral circulation problems, cold hands and feet. The immobility and emotional internalisation were both contributing to congestion and a build-up of mucus. The irregular sleep pattern was in part caused by the frequent need to urinate and anxiety about the uncertainty of his future.

Charlie's treatment would include strong stretches and deep meridian and point work in an attempt to make brain/limb reconnections, and any cross-referencing where possible using the fresh diagnosis taken at each treatment as the vehicle and focal point for the work.

The feedback from the first treatment was that Charlie was feeling more cheerful and there was more movement in his right leg. Also there appeared to be more movement in his right shoulder and his sleep pattern had improved with night visits to the toilet reduced. Although supported, Charlie was able to walk into the clinic for his second appointment.

Six weeks later, Charlie had made significant improvements in mobility and speech and his sleep pattern was fairly stable. Emotionally Charlie had his ups and downs, moving easily between laughter and tears at home and during treatment, and I soon discovered that he liked a good joke, usually at my expense!

The family were involved in assisting Charlie at home by working the flexors and extensors on his limbs manually, and applying pressure to a few shiatsu points I had shown them. This homework was beginning to pay off as warmth and sensitivity started to return to his right hand and the middle finger started to respond.

After four months Charlie was walking unsupported with a stick, and his speech and manual co-ordination had improved. At this point, the improvement was beginning to level out and I decided that a fresh approach was needed. This was discussed with Charlie and Iris and I recommended that Charlie should see an acupuncturist. Charlie decided that he wished to continue with the shiatsu treatment, as well as commencing acupuncture. As had been hoped, the change of approach led to better foot placement and rhythm and although he became more emotional, verbal communication continued to improve.

Over the following months, the balance of the two therapies continued to improve and consolidate Charlie's condition. The close liaison between the acupuncturist and myself allowed us to build on each other's work and select the appropriate treatment for Charlie at any given time. Although shiatsu and acupuncture are different in approach to treatment, we had the same diagnostic 'language', and this particular link was important for smooth communication of information and ideas.

Multidisciplinary
Co-operation

Over the following six months, Charlie continued to make small improvements in speech and mobility; however, the congestion and mucus did not respond well. From the point of view of Chinese diagnosis, it was established fairly early on in the treatment that chesty (metal), damp (spleen) conditions were fairly entrenched.

Ten months after his stroke, Charlie was admitted to hospital with suspected pneumonia and died five days later. The post mortem revealed fluid in one lung and blood clots in both lungs, as well as signs of severe emphysema showing chronic damage to the lung tissue.

In conclusion, Charlie had made a remarkable improvement against all the odds and after he had been advised that nothing more could be done for him. He had regained a degree of independence, had been able to walk unaided and to converse once more. Charlie's right arm had responded only in part to the treatment. However, it had ceased to be cold, stiff and white, and had become warm, flexible and pink with some movement in the middle and index fingers.

There is no question that Charlie's quality of life had improved and that he had regained in some measure his pride and dignity, not only because of the treatment he had received, but also because of his own massive spirit and the continued support and love of a family who just refused to give up on him.

Training

Shiatsu students come from all walks of life. Some students are barely out of college or university before embarking on a training in shiatsu. Others, such as doctors, midwives, nurses and physiotherapists, are coming from the many branches of conventional medicine as the benefits of shiatsu are being realised.

Training in shiatsu may start with an introductory weekend. However, full training takes a minimum of three years, part-time, to obtain a diploma. Although no formal educational qualifications are required, the course is academically demanding and includes not only extensive training in shiatsu but also physiology, anatomy, pathology,

Oriental theory and diagnostic techniques, point location and uses, and also communication and counselling skills. Schools set practical and written work outside of training time and a final assessment will be included at the end of the course although annual assessments are also the norm.

Shiatsu training is a challenging career option, stretching students on all levels of being as they are required to undertake a course of self-discovery through their training and outside pursuits.

The Shiatsu Society and Professional Standards

The Shiatsu Society was set up in 1981 to facilitate communication within the field of shiatsu and to inform the public of the benefits of this natural form of healing. Since then the society has grown to form a focal point for everyone interested in shiatsu, whether teachers, practitioners, students or patients, with members in many countries throughout the world. The Society also fulfils the role of a professional association for teachers and practitioners of shiatsu.

Practitioners registered by the Shiatsu Society, designated by the initials MRSS after their names, have all achieved an approved standard of training as established by the Shiatsu Society assessment panel. All registered practitioners are bound by the Society's code of ethics and have professional indemnity insurance.

Biography

Michael Webster, MRSA, discovered shiatsu through the martial art of jujitsu after a 20 year search for a 'hands on therapy' that would suit him. In 1985 he commenced training with Elaine Liechti, principal teacher of the Glasgow School of Shiatsu. He has also studied with teachers such as Wataru Ohashi and Pauline Sasaki who is considered to be the world's leading exponent of the teachings of Master Masunaga. An 18 month period of training in Orkney with a unique spiritual training group provided insight and practical experience of working with energy. This training provided the basis for his practical workshops on energy, the emphasis being on experiencing.

References

1   Ni Maoshing, *The Yellow Emperor's Classic of Medicine*, an exploratory translation, Shambala, 1995.

Further Reading

Beresford-Cooke, Carola, *Shiatsu Theory and Practice*, Churchill Livingston, 1995.

Dundee, J.; Ghaley, G.; Bell, P F., et al., *P6 acupressure reduces morning sickness*, J R Soc Med, 1988; 34: 4, 171-7.

Jarmey, Chris, *Shiatsu: The Complete Guide*, Thorsons, 1991.

———, *Thorsons Introductory Guide to Shiatsu*, Thorsons, 1992.

Liechti, E., *Shiatsu: Japanese Massage for Health and Fitness*, Element, 1992.

Lundberg, P., *The Book of Shiatsu*, Gaia, 1992.

Matsumoto, Kiiko; Birch, Steven, *Hara Diagnosis – Reflections on the Sea*, Churchill Livingston, 1988.

Namikoshi, Toru, *The Complete Book of Shiatsu Therapy*, Japan Publications, 1981.

Price, H.; Lewith, G.; Williams, C., *Acupressure as an antiemetic in cancer chemotherapy*, Compl Med Research, 1991; 5: 2, 93-4.

Serizawa, Toru, *Tsubo: Vital Points for Oriental Therapy*, Japan Publications, 1992.

Resources

Shiatsu Society
5 Foxcote
Wokingham
Berks RG11 3PG
Tel. 01734-730 836
Fax. 01734-732 752

British School of Shiatsu
6 Erskine Road
London NW3 3AJ
Tel. 0171-483 3776
Fax. 0171-483 3804

The European Shiatsu School
High Banks
Lockeridge
Marlborough
Wilts SN8 4EQ
Tel. 01672-861 362

Glasgow School of Shiatsu
Elaine Liechti MA MRSS
South Hourat Farm
Dalry
Ayrshire KA24 5LA
Tel. 01505-682 889

Sound Therapy

by Lawrence Buchan

Historical Background

The development of sound therapy cannot be attributed to any one source. Its theories and methods have been developed empirically. The pure theory of music and sound was understood by the ancients, but was lost by following generations. Over the past 25 years a resurgence of interest in the healing properties of sound has been evident.

The ancient Egyptians, whose medicine was based on the earlier findings of the Assyrians and Babylonians, used music to cure illness as long ago as 1600 BC.[1] Later the Greeks became the most well-known authority on the subject: Heraclitus (c.550-c.480 BC), Pythagoras (c.570-c.480 BC) and Plato (c. 400 BC). More recently Johannes Kepler (1571-1630) put forward his complex harmonic laws governing the movement of planets,[2] and present-day exponents Hans Kayser, Rudolf Haase, Cousto, Alfred A. Tomatis and Fabien Maman, to name but a few, are considered to be at the forefront of the development of sound therapy.[3]

> *The power of music to heal has been recognised since ancient times, but it is only recently that science has shown an interest in exploring the healing potential of sound. The Sufi master Hazrat Inayat Khan, earlier this century said, 'What makes us feel drawn to music is that our whole being is music; our mind and body...all that is beneath and around us, it is all music.*[4]

Theoretical Background

To understand sound therapy it is essential to realise that everything that exists is vibration. As Pythagoras is reputed to have said, 2500 years ago, 'A stone is frozen music.' Like a fish in water, humankind exists in an ocean of vibration which affects us whether we are aware of it or not. A human being is a mass of resonating frequencies at different stages and states of evolution. This mass of vibration is constantly moving, changing, expanding and contracting. It changes with one's moods and beliefs, the time of day, the seasons and the years.

Sound is vibration. Music is a type of matter that remains in a vibratory state rather than taking on form, but it affects the form of that which it impacts. Experiments were done in the 1930s by a Swiss scientist, Hans Jenny, to demonstrate this. He placed sand on a metal plate and then pulsed sound frequencies through the plate. Each sound caused the sand to vibrate into a particular formation; a different sound caused a different pattern to form.[5]

Colour Therapy

The only difference between the vibrations of sound and the vibrations of colour is the rate of vibration; audible sound resonates in a range of 20 cps to 30,000 cps, while colours vibrate between 400 and 800 trillion cycles per second. But the proportional differences between the seven notes on a scale and the seven colours of the spectrum are the same. Each colour has its corresponding musical note.

'As above, so below' is a basic tenet of ancient wisdom. Plato and Pythagoras, and, later, Kepler outlined the structure of sounds 'above', that is, in the cosmos and the harmony of the planets.[6] Modern astronomy and cosmology are constantly discovering new harmonic relationships far beyond the bounds of this planetary system. The structure of the world 'below' can be understood as genes, cells, DNA, RNA, atoms and elementary particles, which also contain harmonic relationships.

The relationships of the intervals between two or more notes is critical in creating harmony and balance. This relationship of intervals is represented as a ratio. For example, an octave (the interval between the first note of one scale and the first note of the next scale) has a ratio of 2:1, where the octave above vibrates at a frequency twice that of the fundamental note. The fifth (the interval of the first and fifth notes of a scale) has a ratio of 3:2, where the fifth note vibrates three times for every two of the fundamental. The most harmonious ratios are the simplest ones, where the numerator and the denominator are found to be in the range from 1 to 16. These create the healing frequencies needed to procure and bring about a state of well-being.

The body is a manifestation of a harmonic chord. The harmonic interval, that is the relationship between two tones, is of crucial importance in terms of the health of the individual. In order to influence positively the energies of the body, a sound therapist uses intervals that are harmonically relative to one another. The lambdoma matrix[7] is a resource utilised by many sound therapists to determine the harmonic intervals required. The lambdoma matrix is a column of numbers written in the form of the Greek letter lambda, the right leg consisting of whole numbers from one to infinity while the left leg contains the fractions of these same whole numbers. The intervals represented by the ratios in the lambdoma matrix are one way to guarantee affecting any dissonance or discordant sounds within the body.

Sounds can agitate, delight, destroy or heal, as is evidenced by research into the effects of sounds on particular people.[8] When sound is generated to cause multiple vibrations all harmonically equivalent to each other, a complete balancing of a person's energies can result.

There are vibratory rhythms which permeate us and which are us, some so small that they can only be measured in tiny fractions of a cycle per second. The longest and most recently discovered traverse the abyss of outer space, originating beyond our galaxy, and have a frequency of millions of miles between troughs. They are very low and very weak frequencies, but they are almost indistinguishable from the patterns of the human brain. The rhythms that most affect humanity are those of the human body which can be duplicated musically: heartbeat, breathing cycle and brainwave cycles. These are cycles which fall within minutes or seconds and can be shown as beats on a metronome.

The Practice of Sound Therapy

There are many ways to effect healing using sound therapy. A practitioner of sound therapy has a thorough knowledge of the physio/psychological, emotional and spiritual functions of the human body, in particular the acupuncture meridians, the nervous system, the endocrine glands and the major organs.

The vibratory field on which the sound therapist works is energy, which can be referred to as chi, prana or life-force. Vibrational energy transmits morphogenetically through the electromagnetic fields (subtle bodies) into the physical body via the chakras (energy centres).[9] Therefore altering the vibrational energy field affects all levels of the being. If it is considered that each molecule of which an organ or a tissue is composed has its own individual sound pattern, and emits a vibration peculiar to this pattern, a healthy organ will have its molecules working together in harmonious relationship with each other.[10]

In a sound therapy session, the therapist evaluates the words used by the client (sound tone, vowels, consonants) for their musical value or frequency. Clients may be encouraged to express their thoughts in the form of a sung melody – each feeling being expressed in a harmony. In this way the therapist can understand where there is discordance and how to begin the healing process.

Acupuncture

Some of the principles of sound therapy are that all meridian and acupuncture points have their own notes and frequencies, as do the physical organs of the body. The organ notes are the tonics (on the sol-fa scale) of the meridian note to which the organ corresponds in the law of the five elements.[11] A technique in sound therapy is to apply this basic sound, the tonic, to the command point (also known as a horary point) of the meridian. This command point represents the same element as the organ of the meridian. For example, the liver reflects the wood element so the command point will be the wood point, which in this case corresponds to the note F#. This frequency will be generated by a musical or electronic instrument, or the note applied via tuning forks to the specific acupoint in order to disperse, tonify or stimulate the meridian that is out of balance.

Sound therapists do not confine themselves to frequencies established in Western musical notation. They may make use of a specific Greek mode or musical scale (Lydian, Ionian, Aeolian, etc.) to re-establish optimal functioning in the electromagnetic field or chakra. Similarly, Indian modes, known as *ragas*, may be used at specific times to create specific moods. There is a theoretical model for this, for example raga bhupali is a summer raga; raga malkaus is the raga of autumn; raga pilu is a late evening raga and raga asvari is a morning raga.[12]

Tibetan and Mongolian chant masters taught that the human instrument can resonate with basic harmony. Like a wineglass, each person has his or her own fundamental note, but this true note becomes obscured through trauma and conditioning. With overtone chanting, people learn to shape their mouths to produce chords or simultaneous notes, octaves apart, the notes becoming separated out, like colours through a prism. The practice of producing these resonant sounds massages the body's energy centres (chakras) and electromagnetic fields (subtle bodies). It balances the breath and clears the mind. Finding one's own note – one's fundamental note – is a powerful experience in self-discovery and self-healing. Working with a qualified sound therapist can assist people in doing this.

Toning means humming with no melody or under-rhythms. If practised for five minutes every day this balances brain waves, changes skin temperature, releases muscle tension and modifies heartbeat.[13]

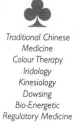

Various forms of diagnosis may be used by a sound therapist. These might include taking Chinese pulses; tongue, face or urine diagnosis; colour tests; iridology; applied kinesiology; dowsing; and ACR (auricular-cardiac reflex), etc. Electronic devices such as AMI, Biotron, Mora or Voll may also be used both in diagnosis and treatment. They measure the difference in energy between two meridian points and can restore harmony and flow. In cases of pain control, serious illness or inherited diseases, it may be more appropriate to use electrostimulation (TENS), laserpuncture, sonopuncture, or magnetic or resonance therapy in conjunction with sound therapy.

Traditional Chinese Medicine
Colour Therapy
Iridology
Kinesiology
Dowsing
Bio-Energetic Regulatory Medicine

The number of sessions required varies depending upon the client and the nature of the presenting illness, which may be physical, emotional, mental, spiritual or a combination of manifestations. Sometimes one or two sessions are sufficient for simple ailments. If the condition is long-standing, then a longer course of treatment may be necessary.

Sound therapy can be used in conjunction with other therapies, especially those of a bioenergetic nature. There is no reason why sound therapy cannot be used as a complementary treatment to allopathic medicine. After a sound therapy session it is recommended that the treatment be given time to take effect before commencing another therapy. Time required for the treatment to take effect varies from patient to patient. One person may experience an immediate benefit while for others it may take several days.

Modern sound therapy is one of the most effective, safe forms of treatment for many physio/psychological, emotional and spiritual conditions. The healing process of any condition can be accelerated through the use of sound therapy. It can also bring relief from suffering caused by a virus, allergy or phobia. It is extremely beneficial in the treatment of premenstrual syndrome, irritable bowel syndrome, high blood pressure, depression, migraine and autoimmune diseases, as well as a host of other presenting complaints.

Acupuncture
Aromatherapy
Reflexology
Homoeopathy

There are very few conditions where sound therapy will not be of benefit. As in acupuncture, aromatherapy, reflexology and homoeopathy, the full effects of the treatment may not be achieved where the patient is intoxicated with nicotine, caffeine, alcohol, etc.

Training

There are various training schools worldwide which offer a high standard of tuition. Sound therapists often have a musical background or are trained in another alternative, complementary or holistic therapy. Some have a natural ability which allows them to distinguish when a person's energies are inharmonious, just by listening to the person's voice.

Research

At present there is an enormous demand and interest in vibrational medicine and in particular sound and music therapies and much research is being done in this field. Fabien Maman[14] is renowned for working with sound to help disintegrate cancerous tumours. Barbara Hero has carried out extensive research into Egyptian musicology and theory, among other things.[15] Don Campbell was able to heal a large aneurysm behind his eye by using the power of his own voice.[16] Alfred Tomatis has had success treating various ailments using his 'electronic ear', which is an auditory apparatus for helping patients train their ears and re-educate their voices.[17] Intensive research has been carried out over many years by Dr Peter Guy Manners who developed a cymatics machine which can detect and correct imbalances throughout the body.[18]

Case Studies

◆ *A 25-year-old man presented with chronic low back pain in the sacrum area. Diagnosis indicated a problem in the bladder and kidney meridians. He was also rejecting the colour red because of strong feelings of being beset by insoluble problems. This was affecting his base chakra (gonads), as well as causing an imbalance in his sixth chakra (pituitary gland). Further questioning revealed that he was having relationship problems. Following two treatments of balancing meridians, in particular the fire and water disharmony, by means of tuning forks and generated frequencies, and clearing disturbed energy around chakras, the patient reported a 70% reduction in the pain he was experiencing. He was then able to discuss and work through the problem with his partner, which was related to control in the home environment. Following the third session he reported that the pain had completely gone and that his relationship had been restored to normal. In fact it was 'better than ever'.*

◆ *A 36-year-old woman presented with Crohn's disease. She had been unable to keep most solid foods down for almost a year and she was two and a half stone below her normal weight. Rather than undergo an exploratory surgical operation, she opted for a duodenal dilation. After the operation she was still unable to eat properly without having an allergic reaction. The sound therapist's diagnosis found an imbalance in the lung, large intestine, stomach and spleen meridians, as well as energy disturbances in three chakras, in particular the crown chakra (pineal gland). Emotionally she had a deep fear of failure and of being criticised, and consequently felt the need to criticise others to feel empowered. Following three sessions of clearing imbalanced energies in related and complementary meridians and chakras using the fundamental note and related frequencies, this client was eating regular meals and had begun to put on weight.*

◆ *A 25-year-old man presented with a collapsed left lung and asthma. It emerged that he harboured guilt for not having fulfilled his emotional commitments. Diagnosis indicated imbalances in the triple warmer, pericardium, lung and large intestine meridians. The young man also presented an energetic disturbance around the throat chakra (thyroid gland). He stated that he sometimes had problems expressing his feelings verbally. Treatment was for the patient to establish a resonance with his fundamental note. It was restored by using singing bowls, instruments, voice, tuning forks and generated frequencies to correct the energetic imbalances. To relieve the symptoms this patient required six sound therapy sessions, and treatment included vitamin and mineral supplementation and the use of flower essences.*

Nutritional Therapy
Flower Essences

Biography

Lawrence Buchan is a bioenergetics practitioner and sound therapist who is interested in the research and application of twenty-first century medicine. He lectures on vibrational medicine at universities and colleges around Europe. His private practice is in Glasgow.

References

1   Joachim Ernst Berendt; Nada Brahma, *The World is Sound, Music and the Landscape of Consciousness*, East West Publications, 1988.

2   Joachim Ernst Berendt, *The Third Ear, On Listening to the World*, Element, 1988.

3   ibid.

4   Michael Diamond, *Returning to Our Natural Rhythm*, Body, Mind, Spirit, Vol 15: 4, 35.

5   David Tame, *The Secret Power of Music*, Destiny Books, Turnstone Press, 1984.

6   Plato in the *Timaeus* and *Harmonia Mundi*.

7   Barbara Hero, *Lambdoma Unveiled, The Theory of Relationships*, Strawberry Hill Farm Studios Press, 1992.

8   Kay Gardner, *Sounding the Inner Landscape*, Caduceus Publications, 1990.

9   Rupert Sheldrake, *A New Science of Life*, Grafton Books, 1983.

10   Peter Guy Manners, *What is Cymatics?*, Bretforton Medical Research Trust, 1986.

11   Dianne Connelly, *Traditional Acupucture: The Law of Five Elements*, The Centre for Traditional Acupuncture Inc., 1979.

12   Brian Lee, *Indian classical music*, an introduction to the tradtion, Caduceus, 1996; 33: 52.

13   Laurel Elizabeth Keyes, *Toning*, De Vorss and Company, 1973.

14   Fabien Maman, *Technique of pure sound: healing mind, body and spirit*, Caduceus, 1988; 5: 5-6.

15   Barbara Hero, op cit.

16   Don Campbell, *Lecture at the Conference 'Songs of Heaven and Earth'*, Findhorn Foundation 1996.

17   Alfred A Tomatis, *The Conscious Ear*, Station Hill Press, 1991.

18   Peter Guy Manners, *What is Cymatics?*, Bretforton Medical Research Trust, 1986.

Further Reading

Berendt, Joachim Ernst, *The Third Ear, On Listening to the World*, Element, 1988.

———; Brahma, Nada, *The World is Sound, Music and the Landscape of Consciousness*, East West Publications, 1988.

Campbell, Don, *Music and Miracles*, Quest Books, 1992.

———, *Music: Physician for Times to Come*, Quest Books, 1991.

———, *The Roar of Silence*, Quest Books, 1989.

Connelly, Dianne, *Traditional Acupuncture: The Law of Five Elements*, The Centre for Traditional Acupuncture Inc., 1979.

Gardner, Kay, *Sounding the Inner Landscape*, Caduceus Publications, 1990.

Gilmore, T; Madaule, P.; Thompson B, (eds), *About the Tomatis Method*, Listening Center Press, 1989.

Hero, Barbara, *Lambdoma Unveiled, The Theory of Relationships*, Strawberry Hill Farm Studios Press, 1992.

Keyes, Laurel Elizabeth, *Toning*, De Vorss and Company, 1973.

Merrit, Stephanie, *Mind Music and Imagery*, Plune Press, 1990.

Sheldrake, Rupert, *A New Science of Life*, Grafton Books, 1983.

Spintge, Ralph, *Music Medicine*, MMB Music, 1992.

Tame, David, *The Secret Power of Music*, Destiny Books, Turnstone Press, 1984.

Tomatis, Alfred A., *The Conscious Ear*, Station Hill Press, 1991.

Resources

The Academy of Sound, Colour and Movement
P O BOX 20505
Boulder, CO 80308 – 3505
USA

Cymatics Bretforton Medical Research Trust (UK)
Bretforton Hall
Nr. Evesham
Worcestershire WR11 5JH

Tomatis International Paris
2 Rue de Palsbourg
75017 Paris
France

The Institute for Research and Study of Bioenergetic Medicine
The Ross Gibson Clinic of Advanced Alternative Medicine
King's Close
264 Bath Street
Glasgow G2 4JP
Scotland

Spiritual Healing

by Robin Robinson

Healing has been practised for thousands of years. The healing gift has always been available to those able naturally or by practice to focus healing energy as a catalyst for physical and emotional change.

Many people discover the talent accidentally or, at some stage in their lives, have a desire to find out about healing and then attempt to develop the talent. Becoming a healer is very much a calling in the traditional sense. Until recently, healers were isolated from one another, known only to the public by word of mouth. Since 1955 a healers' organisation, the National Federation of Spiritual Healers (NFSH) has succeeded in making available training, experience, supervision and certification. It provides a network for practitioners and produces a national directory of healers available to the public. Increasingly doctors are practising healing as part of their professional service or working with healers during a proportion of their clinics or inviting healers to give their service in the doctors' own surgeries. While it is acknowledged by both doctors and researchers that healing is effective, there is nothing tangible, as yet, to give as evidence as to how healing works.[1]

Healing is a therapy which is non-invasive. Whether physical or emotional change is needed, healing is able to help in some way – sometimes dramatically, at other times in more subtle ways, such as assisting a patient in accepting an illness emotionally. Healing may not cure the symptom, but may bring relief in other ways. Other treatment can also be given simultaneously without changing the efficacy of the healing.

Terminology

Healing is also commonly known as 'spiritual healing', 'psychic healing', 'laying on of hands' and in the USA 'Therapeutic Touch', 'psi healing' and 'energetic touch'. 'Faith healing', as spiritual healing is often mistakenly called, requires the faith of the patient, whereas in spiritual healing no faith is required of the patient.

Therapeutic Touch

The Practice of Healing

Each healer develops their own personal style. What healers have in common is that they acknowledge, or believe themselves to be in contact with, the spiritual realms – a source of the divine love, which they channel and which they believe causes the changes in the physical and/or emotional body of the patient. In a healing session the patient will normally sit in a chair or lie on a couch and be asked to relax as much as possible. The patient does not need to believe in spiritual healing, only be willing to open to the possibility that it may help. When the patient is relaxed the healer will intuitively be drawn to place a hand on or near the body and channel energy to the patient. Some healers work in a degree of trance where they enter into a state of altered consciousness, connecting with their source of inspiration. They may contact sources of information available to them, perhaps receiving images or insights regarding the patient's treatment or a particular situation in their lives.[2]

Physiologically what occurs is that the healer's brain wave frequencies between left and right hemispheres become synchronised.[3] Some healers will remain fully conscious, and even chat with their patients. Others may work with several patients at once and after having begun the channelling of healing energy to the patients, will then detach themselves from the healing process. A television programme about healers demonstrated this style of healing and showed patients with rheumatism in a relaxed state sitting on chairs or lying on the floor exercising in a physiotherapeutic way which in normal circumstances would have been impossibly painful. However formal the style, the space in which the healing takes place has an atmosphere of peacefulness created by the healing energy channelled by the healer.

The patients will normally feel increasingly relaxed during treatment and will often say afterwards that they felt sensations in the body, perhaps under or on the skin, or that they experienced visions or light. The full effects of the treatment may not be obvious immediately after one session, although this sometimes is the case. Consecutive treatments will have a cumulative beneficial effect. Apart from the curative effects of healing, patients often feel a greater sense of well-being, for instance increased self-esteem. This aspect of healing is as important as tangible physical or emotional benefits. If this general state of well-being can be maintained, future health is also more assured.

Although adults most commonly receive healing, children, too, can benefit. To work with children the healer must be prepared for the patient's being unable to remain still for an extended period of time.

Research

In the last decade, healing has become increasingly accepted by the medical profession. One of the driving forces of this change in the UK has been Dr Jean

Roberton who has worked in general practice for nearly 30 years. As senior partner of a practice in St Albans, Hertfordshire, she instigated a healing service in normal surgeries and then made an audit of its effects on patients. Although a few objecting patients left the practice, the majority who were offered healing found benefits of a physical or emotional nature. The first group of patients to receive healing included a chronic depressive, a patient with secondary cancer, a patient with chronic asthma and one with recurrent colitis. Two patients were referred by another doctor in the area, with deafness and/or tinnitus. After several healing sessions, their doctor reported, 'There has been a miraculous change in hearing in both these patients, enabling normal conversations to be carried out in the surgery – not possible previously. Both appear to be relaxed and happy whereas before they showed signs of anxiety and tension.' In another referral of a patient with visual problems and ocular hypertension, the patient's GP commented, 'The ophthalmology consultant could not believe his instrument readings five days after the patient's healing session for the vitreous pressure had suddenly gone down from its usual high pressure to normal.' Dr Robertson also audited the progress of other patients with asthma, ME, cellulitis and depression. She commented, 'The partnership of doctors and spiritual healers would seem to be an excellent one. If [our] small project is a true representational prototype of a much wider vision to come, the future seems to hold exciting promises of benefits to patients and lessons to the caring participants.'[4]

According to Dr Daniel Benor, an American psychiatrist researching spiritual healing, over 150 controlled studies into healing have been published.[5] Not all concentrate on the healing effects on humans: experiments have also been designed to study the effects of healing on enzymes, cells, fungi and yeasts, bacteria, sprouting seeds, bean growth, potato yield, plant growth and chick parasites.[6] Dr Benor's analysis is that about half of the studies showed statistically significant results. He also reports many subjective experiences and uncontrolled studies. He believes that healing is an effective therapy. He works as a healer himself nowadays. He describes giving healing by the laying on of hands to a nurse working in the same hospital who had a bad headache. Within a few minutes the headache was gone. Dr Benor writes:

> *I also picked up a mental image of this woman carrying a burden which was much too heavy for her. I shared this with her and she broke into tears. She told me of her struggles in supporting two children as a single parent; having to work extra hours in order to make ends meet; sorting out a relationship with a man who was having legal difficulties; and not having time to meet her own needs. She was very grateful for the healing and for our discussion on reducing the stresses in her life.*[7]

Another interesting case study took place in a clinic in America where a group of people were asked to take part in a double-blind trial. A cut was made on each volunteer's upper arm. Over a period of time and attendance, all were asked to put their arm through a hole in one of the clinic's partitions. They all thought that this was the method by which the wound was being monitored. The wounds of half the group were given healing, the wounds of the other half were not. At the end of the experiment the wounds of 100% of the group given healing had healed more quickly than those of the control group.[8]

Doctors and Healers

A number of doctors who have networked with healers have now formed a link with the NFSH and some have developed the skill of healing and use healing for their patients. Under current NHS rules doctors are allowed to employ healers and some practices can pay them if they wish. A healer working in a doctor's surgery will normally adhere to the code of conduct established by the NHS. Healers have been visiting hospital pain clinics for many years on an informal basis but it is only recently that healing has also been seen by GPs as a means to reduce the cost of patients' medication.

My Personal Practice

Getting to the source of an illness can be very much a part of the effectiveness of healing. Tuning into a 'picture', as Dr Benor did in the example above, of the emotional and/or physical causes of the condition is a powerful remedy.[9] When I first meet a patient I have an impression of how the healing is to proceed and how I need to relate to the patient in order for them to relax. I intuit if they would feel comforted or distressed by touch, whether they would prefer to sit or lie. I enter a state of near meditation. As I form an energetic or intentional link with the patient, ideas, pictures, feelings, colours from the patient become part of my being as I prepare in stillness to approach the patient. I sense where to put my hands and I allow my intuition to tell me for how long before moving to another part of the body.

My understanding is that the energy I channel is focused into the patient's etheric body. The etheric body is an energy blueprint of the physical body. In working on the etheric body, the energy to heal illness is transferred to the physical body. Once this transforming energy has entered the etheric body the patient may receive intuitive information which they can access if they desire.

Patients who are sensitive to the spiritual healing process may have intuitions about diet, life habits or giving themselves time for peacefulness or relaxation. If they follow the intuition which has arrived in their being through healing then they will improve their quality of life and health.

Case Studies

A lady who had suffered with migraine for years had three sessions after which the condition disappeared but a man with a recurring bladder cancer continued treatment for two years before the condition was under control. For both the healing was also about an attitude to themselves, their illness and their lifestyles. They needed to decide for themselves if they had the will to change patterns of behaviour which had resulted in illness. The man with cancer was always angry about the incompetence of others. He also worked in a rubber factory, an environment which has a high incidence of bladder cancer in its work force. The healing sessions introduced a feeling of peace and well-being into his life for the first time. He realised that this peace was what he needed most, but in order to feel peace, he had to become tolerant of others at work which he achieved through meditation. On a physical level, his cancer progressed more slowly while his relationship with his wife, as well as with his colleagues, improved. He became happier, took early retirement and attended to his hobbies. To me this illustrates how healing is able to redirect a lifestyle into health.

Not all healing, I have discovered, results in cure. I have seen many terminally ill patients who will, I know when I see them, die from their disease. In these cases the purpose of healing seems to be about relieving the pain or discomfort in the last stages of their lives and about their coming to terms with their imminent death.

I have never seen a patient who has not said that healing was of some help to them and I know this experience is true for most healers. Sometimes I have seen miraculous changes in patients' health.

Biography

Robin Robinson is a spiritual healer and crystal healer. He is a member of the NFSH and has practised for 12 years in Derbyshire and Moray, Scotland.

References

1   Dan Benor, *Lessons from spiritual healing research and practice*, Subtle Energies, 1993; 3: 1, 73 – 88.

    L Dossey, *Mind, Medicine and the new physics: a time for re-assessment*, Advances, Institute of Advancement of Health, 1988; 5 (1): 57-69.

    J Horgan, *Can Science explain consciousness?*, Scientific American, July 1994; 72-78.

2   R G Jahn, *Out of this aboriginal sensible muchness. Consciousness, information and human health*, J. American Society for Psychical Research, 1995.

3   M Cade; N Coxhead, *The Awakened Mind*, Delacorte Press and Eleanor Friede, 1978.

4   Report by Dr Jean Robertson in the Journal of Alternative and Complementary Medicine, April 1991.

5   Dan J Benor, *Healing Research: Holistic Energy Medicine and Spirituality*, Vol. 1, Helix, 1993.

6   A M Scofield; R D Hodges, *Demonstration of a healing effect in a laboratory using a simple plant model*, J. of Psychical Research 1991; 57: 321-43.

7   Dan J Benor, *Healing Research: Holistic Energy Medicine and Spirituality*, Vol. 1, Helix, Munich 1993, p14.

8   ibid. p214.

9   Michael Dawson, *Healing the Cause*, Findhorn Press, 1994.

Further Reading

Angelo, Jack, *Spiritual Healing*, Element, 1994.

Bek, Lilla with Pullar, Phillipa, *The Seven Levels of Healing*, Rider, 1987.

Benor, Dan, *Healing Research: Holistic Energy Medicine and Spirituality*, Vols 1-4, Helix Verlag, 1993.

———, *Survey of spiritual healing research*, Complementary Medical Research, 4: 9-33.

Beutler, J et al., *Paranormal healing and hypertension*, BMJ, 230: 1491-94.

Borysenko, Joan, *Minding the Body, Mending the Mind*, Simon & Schuster, 1989.

Bradford, Michael, *Hands-On Spiritual Healing*, Findhorn Press, 1994.

Brennan, Barbara Ann, *Hands of Light – A Guide of Healing Through the Human Energy Field*, Bantam, 1990.

Cade, M.; Coxhead, N., *The Awakened Mind*, Delacorte Press and Eleanor Friede, 1978.

Chopra, Deepak, *Quantum Healing*, Bantam, 1989.

Dawson, Michael, *Healing the Cause*, Findhorn Press, 1994.

Furlong, David, *The Complete Healer*, Piatkus, 1995.

Gerber, Richard, *Vibrational Medicine: New Choices for Healing Ourselves*, Bear & Co, 1988.

Hodges, D.; Scofield, T., *The healing effect – complementary medicine's unifying principle?*, The Scientific and Medical Network Review, 1995; 58: 3-7.

Hodgkinson, Liz, *Spiritual Healing*, Piatkus, 1992.

Leskowitz, E., *Spiritual Healing, modern medicine and energy*, Advances, 1993; 9: 4, 50-3.

Levin, J S., *Esoteric v. exoteric explanations for findings linking spirituality and health*, Advances, 1993; 9: 4, 54-6.

Pullar, Phillipa, *Spiritual and Lay Healing*, Penguin, 1988.

Rubik, B., *Energy medicine and the unifying concept of information*, Alternative Therapies, 1995; 1: 1, 55-66.

Young, Alan, *Spiritual Healing – Miracle or Mirage?*, DeVorss, 1991.

Resources

NFSH
Old Manor Farm Studio
Church Street
Sunbury-on-Thames
Middx TW16 6RG
Tel. 01932-783 164/5

(publishes a Healer Referral Directory)

The Confederation of Healing Organisations
The Red & White House
113 High Street
Berkhamsted
Herts HP4 2DJ
Tel. 01442-870 660

The Spiritualist Association of Great Britain
33 Belgrave
London SW1X 8QL
Tel. 0171-235 3351

Stress Management
by Penny Moon

Stress management is not a unified modality as are many other therapies described in this book. Rather it is a conglomerate of different approaches designed to address a specific cause of disease: stress. It is thought that over 80% of illness is stress related. The management of stress is therefore indicated in most conditions of disease. This involves empowering people to help themselves by taking responsibility for their own health.

Self-Responsibility of the Patient

The body is self-regulating and has the capacity to heal on all levels, physical, emotional, mental and spiritual. Stress causes tension which uses up energy, forcing the body to mobilise adrenalin to carry it through specific situations. With energy reserves gone, the immune system is weakened and the body is left vulnerable, increasingly susceptible to bacterial infections and viruses. The negative effects of adrenalin can feed a downward spiral leading to symptoms such as breathlessness, palpitations, stomach disorders, anxiety attacks and loss of memory.

The human body is designed to accommodate a certain level of stress. Stress can serve useful purposes, such as motivating people to find creative ways through problems, thus developing personal strengths and resources. Some people seem able to take more stress than others, some actually seeming to thrive on it. It is in the cases where the individual feels the stresses becoming strains that problems can arise.

Development of the Theories Governing Stress Management

The link between stress and disease was first noted by Sir William Osler in 1910 in relation to angina. In the 1930s, Cannon observed stress in animals and the results of adrenalin release when in extreme danger. Selye (1946) is possibly the best known for having put forward the 'general adaptation syndrome' which describes three stages: the alarm reaction, resistance and exhaustion.[1] Much work has been done since then. Rahe's work involving sports in the USA used a questionnaire which awarded points per life change within the preceding six months. A certain total indicated an increased likelihood of suffering a sports injury the next season.

Cary Cooper's work on stress in occupational health is well documented and focuses on practical ways of managing systemic stress in the workplace.[2] These include options such as better training and working conditions, as well as personal work in time management, assertiveness, individual relaxation techniques and creating a more healthy lifestyle.

In the USA it has been possible for some time to sue places of work for stress-related illness. In 1995 in Britain the first case of a social worker suing a county council for 'burn-out' caused by unacceptable working conditions was successful. Whilst suing is not the most preferable method of effecting change, this trend may catalyse positive change in terms of employers demonstrating care in action and employees making more conscious choices when taking jobs which entail high levels of stress.

Glaser's work on psycho-immunology looks at examination stress in students. This work has gone a long way in tracing the molecular genetic pathways of the mind-gene connections. In 1985 some research suggested that emotional stress can impair the mechanisms of DNA repair in severely distressed mental health patients. Scientific research is constantly coming up with more fascinating details about the exquisite working of human beings and how thought and emotion manifest through the physical body.[3]

The Practice of Stress Management

A variety of things might happen in a stress management session dependent on the training, skills and natural proclivities of the therapist. In most cases, with individuals or in group sessions, there is an element of education, advice on lifestyle, relaxation techniques and breathing exercises. As it is such an individual way, I will illustrate by describing my own practice.

Groupwork

My work in groups is generally in education with teachers and parents. I always include a wide variety of techniques, hoping to provide each person with something that suits them individually that they can take home and practise. This may provide a starter point to the investigation, development and practice of self-knowledge, awareness and preventative health care.

Neuro-Linguistic Programming

The educational part of the session will consider the process of how human beings uniquely perceive and relate to their world. I explain the concept of 'maps of reality' and how each person has their own unique map. The map is not reality, only a guide, and the imposition of one's map (way of looking at the world) on others can lead to conflicts ranging in scale from a family argument to a world war.

The maps are conditioned by genetics, childhood experiences, environment and culture. Using our five senses we create further values and belief systems from what we perceive around us. Being aware of the limitations of the raw material from which the maps are created enables people to become more open to change and influence.

Basic psychological concepts are valuable to increase self-awareness, so I introduce various models of the unconscious put forward by, for example, Freud, Jung, Adler and Assagioli. These basic concepts may provide some insight. For example, if primary needs have not been met, a scar might be left on the psyche which will become a weakness or neurosis during a stress situation in later life. Many people relate to Adler's model based on power, which suggests people use their weaknesses to manipulate others to their will. Assagioli's psychosynthesis model attempts to integrate all parts of the psyche.

Psychological Therapies Psychosynthesis

We then focus on the practical methods of decreasing personal stress, starting with diet, exercise, body language and massage. I demonstrate a deep relaxation technique using breathing exercises. In some groups it is appropriate to introduce simple healing techniques. Visualisation, imaging and some basic neuro-linguistic programming techniques are often useful.

Nutritional Therapy Relaxation Therapy Visualisation

Individual Work

For an individual, six sessions is an average contract. Sometimes one is sufficient. I usually suggest they support the work by attending a yoga class or having aromatherapy sessions, as appropriate to their needs.

Yoga Aromatherapy

The case history taken in the first consultation is very detailed, including medical and psychological history, family patterns, birth details, sleeping patterns, pastimes and hobbies, as well as relationships and diet. A sensitive, client-centred approach when asking these questions helps to build a trusting relationship. From this information, an individual plan, both appropriate and realistic to the client's present position, can be drawn up thus empowering them to begin to take control of their life.

The long-term effects of stress management sessions can be very powerful depending on timing, motivation and readiness of the client to make change. Sometimes nothing seems to happen but a seed is planted which will develop in the client's own time. It is not up to the therapist to impose or force ideas but to respect the client's unconscious in which lies all relevant knowledge for growth. Interpretation and judgement is to be avoided. At all times the endeavour is simply to be with the other person. The process of therapy is both a privilege and learning for the therapist.

Homoeopathy Reflexology Flower Essences Shiatsu Yoga Transcendental Meditation Hypnotherapy

Stress management can be useful in all cases, when used in a way that is relevant and appropriate, and combines well with other therapies, including homoeopathy, reflexology, the Alexander Technique, flower essences, Autogenic Training, shiatsu, yoga, meditation and hypnotherapy.

Training and Research

Psychotherapy
Counselling
Kinesiology
Neuro-Linguistic
Programming
Autogenic Training
Visualisation
Nutritional Therapy

Given the complexity of stress management, practitioners come from many different backgrounds, often having trained in a therapeutic modality, for instance psychotherapy, counselling or hypnotherapy, and combining it with skills acquired through further training such as NLP, Autogenic Training, visualisation, nutrition, kinesiology, etc. They then amalgamate their skills to create an individual approach to managing stress.

So far there has been no regulated training or professional body for stress management practitioners in the UK. As it is not a unified approach, stress management has not been researched as a single topic but there has been a lot of research demonstrating the role of stress in the etiology of illness (through the emerging science of psychoneuroimmunology) and the efficacy of stress reduction in health care.

Case Study

The following is a drastic case which illustrates how a little help can go a long way in normalising a life in crisis. A boy of seven, John, was referred by his school, from which he was about to be expelled, and by social services as he was on the 'at risk' register. His behaviour was wild and aggressive and he had a predilection for setting fires. He had no sense of danger and would produce such behavioural stunts as jumping out of high trees wearing roller skates.

In this case, the mother, Judith, age 28, was very co-operative. In taking her history I uncovered a tragic story of repeated and compounded violence and intervention of social services. Judith's childhood was violent. She spent time in residential care for children with emotional and behavioural difficulties where she was placed by social services after her mother had tried to chop off her hands. One of her brothers has been in prison for arson and her father committed suicide in prison where he was staying after committing murder. At present she lives with her son, daughter (Susan, aged five) and boyfriend who has a 14-year-old son also with emotional behavioural problems. The children's father left about five years ago but still lives in the area. He once tried to drown Judith in the bath when John and Susan were present. He has been in prison and also comes from a violent family. Judith is working nights as a carer and desperately wants to keep her children as well as her new supportive relationship. She is very proud of her home.

She drinks a lot of coffee, eats a lot of chocolate, and suffers from insomnia and anxiety attacks. Judith is well intentioned but struggling as she has felt helpless and desperate for years, not knowing how to control her fury which she is venting in physical violence on her son.

We began by building a trusting relationship and talking about different ways of managing stress. Judith received reflexology treatments, learned visualisation and relaxation techniques and was given homoeopathic first aid. Both she and John were given a specific re-bonding relaxation tape to listen to as well as homework which gave them the opportunity to spend time together in a constructive and creative way.

Very quickly Judith altered her diet and engaged in visualisation exercises as used in psychosynthesis, to increase self-awareness and to retrieve lost aspects of herself.

John's behaviour improved enough to keep him in school. Judith changed her job and is now consistently able to care for John without losing her temper. She has retained her relationship and even taken the children abroad for a week's holiday alone. The anxiety attacks are rare and she is sleeping again.

This is not the end of the story but is certainly a good beginning which hopefully ensures that Judith and her children can mend some of the destructive patterns of the past and have more hope for the future.

Conclusion

Stressful symptoms are caused when too much change occurs in too short a time or long-term chronic problems have drained all the positive resources of the individual. Letting the pressure off gently by any technique appropriate to the person, allowing them to smile, regain their sense of humour and see the pleasures in life can help them relax enough to let the natural healing processes of the body take place. Life then has an opportunity to re-create balance.

Biography

Penny Moon trained as a teacher in 1972 with a Youth Work Diploma. She was interested in yoga and trained to teach in 1979. From 1983 to '87 she trained in psychotherapy, NLP, allergy testing and homoeopathy. She works in private consultancy, in the pain relief unit at Walton Hospital and in St John's Hospice, Clatterbridge.

References

1   H Selye, *The general adaptation syndrome and the diseases of adaptation*, Journal of Clinical Endocrinology, 1946; 6.

2   C L Cooper, *Job Distress*, Bulletin of the Brit Psych Soc, 1986; 39.

3   A R Wyler; T H Holmes; M Masuda, *Magnitude of life events and serious Illness*, Psychosomatic Medicine 1971; 33.

M L Schneider; C L Cop, *Repeated social stress during pregnancy impairs neuromotor development of primate infant*, Journal of Developmental & Behavioural Pediatrics, 1993; 14: 2.

P J Morgans et al., *prenatal malnutrition and development of its brain*, Neuroscience and Biobehavioural Reviews, 1993; 17: 1.

C A Czeisler, *Arousal cycles can reset*, Science, 1986; 233.

R Ader and N Cohen, *Behaviourally conditioned and immuno-suppression*, Psychosomatic Medicine, 1975; 37.

H Benson, *Your innate asset for combating stress*, Harvard Business Review, 1974; 52: 49-60.

K Bowers; P Kelly, *Stress disease, psychotherapy and hypnosis*, Journal of Abnormal Psychology, 1988; 5.

J Dobbin, M Harth, G McCain, R Mark, K Cousin, *Dylokin production and lymphocyte transformation during stress*, Brain Behaviour & Immunity, 1991; 5.

T Field; C Morrow; C Valdeon; S Larson; C Kutin, S Schanberg, *Massage reduces anxiety in children and adolescent psychiatric patients*, Journal of the American Academy of Child – Adolescent Psychiatry, 1993; 31.

R Glover; J Rice; J Shendon; R Fertel; J Stour; C Speicher et al., *Stress related immune suppression: Health implications*, Brain Behaviour & Immunity, 1987; 17: 20.

R & M Green, *Relaxation increases salivary immunoglobulin*, Psychological Reports, 1987.

J Hillhouse; J Kiecott-Glasser; R Glasser, *Stress associated modulation of the immune response in human stress and immunity*, Caldwell, 1991.

S Locke; L Krouss; J Leserman; M Hurst; J Heisel; R Williams, *Life change stress, psychiatric symptoms and natural killer cell activity*, Psychosomatic Medicine 1994; 46.

Further Reading

Bach, Richard, *Illusions*, Pan Books, 1979.

Becker, Robert, *The Body Electric*, Morrow William & Co., 1987.

Cooper, Cary L., *Living with Stress*, Penguin, 1988.

Dilts, Robert, *Strategies of Genius*, Meta Pub., 1994.

Gibran, Kahlil, *The Prophet*, Heinemann Ltd., 1980.

Hanson, Peter, *The Joy of Stress*, Pan, 1998.

Hoff, Benjamin, *Tao of Pooh*, Viking Press, 1983.

Jeans, James, *Physics & Philosophy*, Dover Publications, 1995.

Jensen, Eric, *The Learning Brain*, Turning Point, 1994.

Kaku, Michio, *Hyperspace*, Oxford Paperbacks, 1994.

Lamberg, Lynne, *Bodyrhythms*, Morrow William & Co., 1994.

McKay, Matthew; Davis, Martha; Eshelman Elizabeth, *Relaxation and Stress Workbook*, New Harbinger, 1988.

Mills, Sandra, *Stress Management for the Individual Teacher*, Framework Press Educ., 1995.

Ornstein, Robert, *The Evolution of Consciousness*, Simon & Schuster, 1993.

Rossi, Ernest Lawrence, *The Psychobiology of Mind and Body Healing*, W W Norton, 1994.

Russell, Peter, *The Brain Book*, Routledge, 1980.

Simonton, Carl; Matthews-Simonton, Stephanie; Creighton, James, *Getting Well Again: A Step-by Step Guide to Overcoming Cancer for Patients and Their Families*, Bantam, 1986.

Watson, Lyall, *Supernature*, Hodder & Stoughton, 1986.

Resources

International Stress Management Association
South Bank University
LPSS
103 Borough Roas
London SE1 0AA
Tel. 0171-258 4025

Stress Management in Education:

Teacher Stress
Dr S Mills
Framework Press
St Leonard's House
Lancaster

Research in Complementary Medicine:

Positive Health
6 Alfred Road
Bristol BS3 4LE

Insitute of Complementary Medicine
P O Box 194
London
Tel. 0171-237 5165

Therapeutic Touch

by Jean Sayre-Adams

Therapeutic Touch (TT) is a modern version of one of the oldest of therapies: the use of touch – or near touch – as a means of comfort and healing. The effort to understand how this form of healing works has continued through the centuries and is now at the cutting edge of many modern scientific disciplines such as quantum physics.

When working with TT, practitioners use their hands as the tool for becoming attuned to the energy field of the person they are working with. They assess the field in ways which are as empirical as any other technique. (When people are stressed or at 'dis-ease', their energy field feels disharmonious to the practitioner.) When the assessment is complete, the practitioner then brings balance into the energy field by a process of rebalancing or repatterning. When the repatterning is accomplished and the energy field is in balance, there are various changes in the patient. Patients may manifest a relaxation response or relief from anxiety. There may be an altered perception of pain, sometimes complete relief of pain. An acceleration of wound healing has been observed, and often those who are in the dying process are greatly comforted.[1]

Spiritual Healing
SHEN Therapy

Relaxation Therapy

It is observed that when these improved responses are experienced by patients receiving TT, they are then in the best possible condition to heal themselves. TT practitioners work with the hypothesis that all healing is self-healing and their intention is only to facilitate this.

Case Study

I received an urgent telephone message from the senior staff nurse on one of the adult oncology wards which use and support complementary therapies. The staff nurse is a qualified masseur, one of three who regularly treat the patients, but she had been unable to help the patient this time, and the physiotherapist would not attend without a doctor's referral.

When I arrived, the nurse gave me an update of the situation. It had begun as a simple movement of the head and a 'twinge' that ended in a severe spasm (torticollis). Now approximately two hours since the first movement, the patient was in 'excruciating pain and feeling helpless' as he curled further over the arm of his wheelchair in an effort to relieve it. I knelt in front of him, covered his clenched fists with my hands in greeting and looked into his pain-filled eyes. He was ashen, the fine sweat covering his face and hands making his skin look even more transparent. The pain had rendered him helpless and vulnerable: he was unable to move, read, talk or swallow, and this meant not being able to take oral analgesics. His scalp felt damp and cool on the surface, but by holding his head gently, heat could be felt, mostly on the right (twisted) side.

Standing behind him, I placed my left hand on his forehead and gently and slowly massaged my right hand into the angle of his neck. As I held his head, I became aware of a deep, fine vibration in his neck. I asked him to breathe as slowly as possible and to allow the side of his neck to 'give' as it relaxed. I synchronised my breathing with his, visualising the energy flowing as we breathed out. Gradually, his neck relaxed and the tissues under my hand changed from tense and hot to softer and more even. With an audible sigh, his neck relaxed and he was able to look at me with a straight gaze. He smiled and said, 'I would never have believed it possible if I hadn't experienced it for myself.' Once back on his bed he was made comfortable and I continued to work from head to foot, feeling the energy becoming more uniform in temperature and flow. Each time I returned to his head he would open his eyes and smile, following my hands with his gaze until his eyes closed and stayed closed as he surrendered to a restful, painfree nap.[2]

The Development of Therapeutic Touch

TT was originally developed and introduced to nursing in the early 1970s by Dr Dolores Krieger, professor of nursing at New York University and Dora Kunz who had been born with a unique ability to perceive subtle energies around living beings. Krieger studied the results of research done in Canada on the phenomenon of laying-on of hands by Kunz and other healers, and concluded that they could be relevant within the context of nursing training. After much practice and some fledgling research, Dr Krieger felt it was an inherent human potential that could be learned by anyone with the desire and commitment to help. Krieger also felt TT differed from laying-on of hands in that it has no religious base and faith is not required.

Framework for Therapeutic Touch

In the beginning Krieger took the framework of TT from Eastern philosophical thought. Similarities between Eastern philosophy and Western mysticism and quantum physics have been noted by many mystics and scientists.[3] The East believes in an energy force called *prana*.[4] Prana is seen to sustain life, when in abundance, while its depletion or disruption causes a move from health to disease. TT was believed to be a modality which helped to smooth out disruptions in the human energy field and facilitated the ability of people to participate in their own healing process. In this Eastern framework, illness is seen as a deficit in prana and wellness as an abundance of prana. However, in the past 25 years research has become more sophisticated and the branch of physics known as quantum mechanics has expanded. Nowadays, for their exploration and explanation of TT, most researchers, academics and teachers of TT use the theory devised in a nursing framework by Dr Martha Rogers, called the Science of Unitary Human Beings (SUHB).

Science of Unitary Human Beings (SUHB)

F. Biley has called Rogers's work an 'outrageous nursing theory', the complexity of which is 'difficult to understand', but he suggests that if an attempt is made to try to understand the conceptual framework, readers will begin to realise why Rogers has also been hailed as 'a brilliant nurse theorist' and 'one of the most original thinkers in nursing' without whom it is 'difficult to imagine what nursing would look like today'.

Biley also suggests that this framework provides an alternative to the traditional view of nursing, which could be described as reductionistic, mechanistic and analytic, consisting of 'breaking up thoughts and problems into pieces and arranging these in their logical order'. SUHB has 'guided nursing out of a concrete, static, closed system world view and as a result has challenged many preconceived ideas about nursing and beyond'.[5]

The Application of Holism in Health Care

The 'building blocks' of Rogers's theory include wholeness, openness, unidirectionality, pattern and organisation. The human being is regarded as a unified whole which is more than and different from the sum of its parts. The individual and the environment are continuously exchanging matter and energy with each other, existing within an open order of interconnectedness. The life process unfolds along a space-time continuum which moves in one direction and is irreversible. Individuals are identifiable by a specific pattern and organisation of energy which is unique to them and reflects their innovative wholeness.

Rogers's SUHB appears to have much in common with quantum physics, one of the new disciplines that is beginning to explore some of the complex relationships between people and their environment. There is a paradigm shift from the older mechanical world view of the Newtonian pragmatists to the new perspective of an interconnected holistic universe as envisioned by post-Einsteinian thinkers. Newtonian physics is mechanistic and reductionist; it views the person essentially as a group of body systems interacting in predictable ways. Post-Einsteinian thinking encourages a more holistic view of people; there is not just an interrelationship of body organs, but also an interconnectedness with the energy of the whole universe. Modern physicists see the universe as a dynamic web of interrelated events, none of which functions in isolation.[6]

Bohm wrote of quantum theory:

> *...there has been too little emphasis on what is, in our view, the most fundamentally different new feature of all, i.e. the intimate inter-connectedness of different systems that are not in spatial contact...the parts are seen to be in immediate connection, in which their dynamic relationships depend, in an irreducible way, on the state of the whole system (and indeed on that broader system in which they are contained, extending ultimately and in principle to the entire universe). Thus one is led to a new notion of unbroken wholeness which derides the classical idea of analysability of the world into separately and independently existent parts.* [7]

In simpler language, energy and matter are interchangeable; every living thing in the universe is a pattern of moving energy; and all living things are interconnected and interacting all the time. These ideas require us to move from the concrete to the abstract and challenge almost everything we have been taught about the nature of the universe and reality.

Traditional thinking on the nature of the body relies heavily on the solid and predictable behaviour of atoms, molecules and cells. A quantum physics or SUHB view reveals a very different universe of an enormous interchange of energy; the body not so much a solid, fixed mass, but in constant exchange of energy, internally and externally. It is within this new paradigm that TT researchers are now exploring the reasons why TT works. In the meantime, thousands of TT practitioners worldwide continue to practise it for one very important reason – it seems to work.

Therapeutic Touch in Practice

Case Study I

The following story was recounted to me by one of my students, a nurse who was on night duty in a university teaching hospital:

Transcendental Meditation Yoga

One of my patients was Joan, a 33-year-old woman with leukaemia, whom I had known for over a year. Joan had experienced two remissions but was now in the hospital again with a liver abscess. She had been admitted almost 72 hours before and I was her primary nurse. I identified with Joan in her role as a mother and wife, and greatly admired her courage in the way she approached her physical disease with the use of meditation, yoga and other alternative approaches in her quest towards healing. She had been a wise teacher, not only to me but to many of the oncologists who had treated her.

A good deal of my time had been spent with her for the last eight hours, for in spite of every technique or medication available, Joan was still running a high temperature and was in intense pain – tossing, turning, moaning on her bed, unable to fall asleep. While searching my repertoire for some way in which I could relieve her pain and give her some comfort, I remembered a class in 'Therapeutic Touch' I had taken a few months earlier. It had been interesting, but at the time I hadn't felt I could integrate the technique into my high-tech nursing. In fact, I was a little afraid of the whole idea. But Dolores Krieger's words came back to me: 'Anyone can do TT; anyone can use TT to increase comfort and decrease anxiety'. Joan was beyond judging me, so I did TT with Joan for the next ten minutes. She fell asleep.

Half an hour later, Joan's light went on. As I walked into her room, Joan said sleepily, 'Could you change my wet bedding?' She had been sweating profusely, her temperature had broken and was now 38°C and her pain was completely gone. I was astonished. The next day my clinical supervisor and I went through all her notes to find some other explanation – not only for Joan's pain relief but for the normalisation of her temperature. We did not find it, but over the rest of Joan's hospitalisation, TT administered either by me or her husband to whom I taught it, was used to keep her free of pain and her temperature acceptable (along with the appropriate medications which had not been working before).

I know there could be many explanations for what occurred, but none seem to fit with what happened that night. All I know is it seemed to work. I was able to help someone in need and be confident that I could do no harm in the process.[8]

Case Study II

When I first met Mr J, a 61-year-old farmer, and invited him to come into the treatment room, I had to assist him, his gait was so unsteady. Mr J told me that over the last 15 years his balance had progressively deteriorated to such an extent that, with very few exceptions, he fell every day. Some of the falls had resulted in a broken nose and arm and cuts and bruises of varying severity. He stated that many people thought he was drunk and his walk certainly gave that impression. He said his problems were due to a hereditary disease, that he was not receiving any medication and that his doctors were unable to do anything to help him. Before commencing with TT, I centred myself by visualising an oak tree with its leaves shimmering in a gentle breeze and by inwardly calming myself by taking a few deep breaths. I visualised a universal power of which I became a part. This method is my personal way of centring, which I find effective.

Visualisation

With Mr J lying on his back, I began TT. His initial assessment revealed an overall feeling of coolness in his energy field. As I had not felt any particular energy block or areas of deficit, my intuition led me gently to move towards Mr J's abdominal area and start the rebalancing. I imagined a warm, soothing light encompassing Mr J. I again moved my hands in a head to toe direction to reassess and continued the rebalancing, moving my hands in a continuous, flowing manner. I did this for approximately ten minutes, until a feeling of warmth replaced the coolness. The same feeling of coolness was felt down the spinal column. This too was replaced with warmth after the rebalancing, or repatterning.

During the treatment, Mr J had no sensations but stated, 'Inwardly something is happening,' and wondered if it was possible to feel better immediately. When he left, his gait was unchanged. The following week, he returned and was delighted with how well he had been feeling. He called me the lady with the oil can – his joints were no longer stiff and he had not fallen all week. He was able to negotiate the steps in his house without having to hold onto the doorframe and he could put his shoes on without having to sit down. On the second and third visits there were still areas of coolness in the energy fields around his legs and spinal column. I also recorded small shocks from static when I touched him. A repatterning was done on the third visit and Mr J experienced a 'sensation travelling down my body'. Three weeks later, he had his fourth and final TT treatment. At this time his energy field felt balanced and he had not fallen for six weeks. His unsteady gait was still evident, but was not as exaggerated, and he felt better able to cope. I believe TT improved Mr J's quality of life, enhanced his feeling of well-being and reduced his risk of physical injury through falls.

Research and Practitioners

There are 27 completed doctoral dissertations, 15 post-doctoral researches, and many clinical studies and masters' level theses on the TT process. Krieger began to teach TT to her masters degree students in a programme called 'Frontiers in Nursing' in the early 1970s. There are now thousands of nurses in over 50 countries who have been taught by Krieger or her students. Serious practitioners of TT use a carefully chosen language when speaking about this healing art. This, combined with the extensive research done mostly by nurses in the USA, has made TT part of mainstream nursing practice in the USA. Several thousand health care professionals have been taught in Great Britain over the past ten years, but it is unknown at this time how many or in what capacity these students practise TT. In 1995 a three-module TT programme, leading to a BSc (Honours) degree was accredited by the English National Board through Manchester University. In this programme is a small but strong group of dedicated nurses who are training to become clinical leaders, role models, practitioners and teachers of TT. Some small research has been done and some larger projects are in the planning stage to add to the ongoing good quality research that continues in the USA.

The need for further research is evident, and is reinforced by J. Quinn:

> *The first and perhaps most obvious (need) is the application of TT to a host of real world clinical problems – clinical trials or outcome studies. The second path involves the development of an explanatory model/theory of TT which is validated and refined through the research process.*[10]

Conclusion

A deepening of understanding around Rogers's field theory as well as continued and replicated studies on TT by nurses is still needed. However, the evidence shows that interest in and commitment to TT has grown rapidly among clinicians for essentially one reason – it seems to work.

TT offers an important dimension in healing and caring for many health care professionals. Research so far suggests that it can bring significant benefits to patients, at minimal cost. Some patients are helped and no harmful effects have yet been demonstrated when it is done by practitioners who have been trained by Krieger or her students and who follow the guidelines as set up by the governing bodies of TT.

Biography

Jean Sayre-Adams was a staff nurse for many years, working in the areas of ITU, AIDS and cancer in university hospitals in San Francisco. She successfully integrated TT into her nursing practice for 16 years and has been teaching TT all that time, first in the USA and then for 12 years in Britain. She has a degree in holistic studies and was on the staff of the Alternative Therapies Unit at the University of California from 1978-1985. Living in Britain since 1990, she was founding member and is now director and senior tutor of the Didsbury Trust, and she lectures, writes and serves on many committees whose aims are to empower nurses. She was a founding member of the RCN Complementary Forum.

References

1   Jean Sayre-Adams; Stephen Wright, *Theory & Practice of Therapeutic Touch*, Churchill Livingstone, 1995.

2   ibid.

3   Fritjof Capra, *The Tao of Physics*, Bantam, 1976.

4   also known as *chi, ki,* or *qi.*

5   F. Biley, *The science of unitary human beings: a contempory literature review*, Nursing Practice 1992: 15(4): 23-26.

6   Fritjof Capra, op cit.

7   D Bohm, *Quantum theory as an indication of a new order in physics, implicate and explicate order in physical law*, Foundation of Physics, 3: 139-68.

8   Jean Sayre-Adams; Stephen Wright, *Theory & Practice of Therapeutic Touch*, Churchill Livingstone, 1995.

9   ibid.

10 J. Quinn, *Future directions for therapeutic touch research*, Journal of Holistic Nursing, 1989; 7: 1, 19-25.

Further Reading

Courtenay, A., *Healing Now*, J M Dent, 1991.

Krieger, Dolores, *Accepting Your Power to Heal: Personal Practice of Therapeutic Touch*, Bear & Co, 1993.

———, *Living the Therapeutic Touch: Healing as Lifestyle*, Quest Books, 1988.

Macrae, J., *Therapeutic Touch: A Practical Guide*, Alfred Knopf, 1992.

Sayre-Adams, Jean, *Therapeutic Toouch: research and reality*, Nursing Standard, 1992; 6: 50, 52-4.

———; Wright, Steve, *Theory and Practice of Therapeutic Touch*, Churchill Livingston, 1995.

———, *Therapeutic Touch – principles and practice*, Complementary Therapies in Medicine, 1993; 1: 96-9.

Resources

The Didsbury Trust
Sherborne Cottage
Litton, Nr. Bath BA3 4PS

Cliff Panton
Manchester College of Midwifery & Nursing
Admissions Office, Gateway House
Piccadilly South
Manchester M60 7LP

British Association of Therapeutic Touch (BATT)
Neal Mellon, Membership Secretary
Critical Care Director
Macclesfield District General Hospital
Victoria Road
Macclesfield SK10 3BC

Traditional Chinese Medicine

by Tom Williams

As a system of diagnosis and health care, Chinese medicine has a lineage which can be traced back at least 3000 years and probably further. This unique system is based on the holistic understanding of the universe as outlined in the spiritual insights of Daoism (or Taoism). This system emphasised understanding the place of humanity in the universe as part of the observed processes in the subtle energetics of nature. The Chinese describe the underlying 'life-force' of the universe as *qi* (also spelled *ki* or *chi*) – it is qi which underpins the whole of nature, yet it is impossible to grasp fully the nature of this concept which is neither a physical substance nor simply an energy. Ted Kaptchuk, a well-respected Western practitioner of Chinese medicine, offers what seems to be the nearest thing to a working definition of qi when he describes it as 'matter on the verge of becoming energy, or energy at the point of materialising'.[1] Thus the Chinese view of the universe is one of an exquisite dance in which qi is the choreographer: the physical universe as we see and experience it being the ongoing evolution of this dance. Because qi permeates everything in this universe, it must also be of central importance in the functioning of our physical, psychological, emotional and spiritual being. Qi is the fundamental substance upon which the Chinese build their medical theory and practice.

Shiatsu

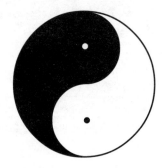

Fig. 1: Taiji symbol

The other key metaphorical concept which is central to the Chinese view of the universe emerges from the observation that the physical world can be seen and understood in terms of complementary and mutually dependent opposites. These opposites are commonly labelled as the yin and the yang aspects of the universe. This is illustrated in the well-known taiji symbol.

Essentially, the taiji represents the whole – the unity of the universe – which can be divided into the two complementary opposites, yin and yang. In keeping with the Chinese emphasis on process rather than physical structure – an idea which is absolutely central to Chinese medicine – yin and yang should be understood as essentially descriptors of the dynamic interactions that underpin all aspects of the physical universe. They are not 'things': they are a system of thinking about the world.

In addition to the concepts of yin and yang, the focus on nature evolved the system of understanding process in terms of the five elements, or phases, of the natural world. These were described as fire, earth, metal, water and wood. Complex models of interactions and correspondences were developed in order to provide a symbolic framework which could be used as a set of guiding principles for understanding the position of human beings in this universal picture.

Chinese medicine is built on these philosophical and conceptual views of the universe, where qi operates at the cusp of the energetic and the physical, promoting the evolution of a dynamic yin and yang interaction which becomes the world – and the body – as we experience it.

History

The principles of Chinese medicine are quite alien to a Western-trained analytical view. The historical evolution of these concepts led to the Chinese medical practitioner being a keen observer of the natural world, where this dynamic energetic interplay was there for all to see. The movement forms of Chinese exercise systems, taiji and qigong, were developed from observing the flowing movements of the animal kingdom and nature. The energetic properties of herbs and other substances were recorded and their therapeutic value understood in terms of the basic principles of the Chinese system. The body was 'mapped' in terms of networks of energetic channels and meridians which disperse the qi throughout the body and it was observed that at certain key points, or energetic vortices, the qi in the channels could be accessed for therapeutic purposes. This knowledge grew and developed in an empirical manner and the practice of acupuncture and therapeutic massage became more refined and sophisticated. Various classic texts regarding acupuncture, moxibustion and herbal medicine were written over the centuries and knowledge and practices were handed down through family groups and evolved into unique and individualistic interpretations of the underlying principles. These laid the foundations for a medical system which was based on a core of accepted principles.

Acupuncture

The growing influence of the Western colonialist powers from the seventeenth century onwards gradually led to the partial retreat of the more traditional views of the universe, under the onslaught of scientific determinism. By the time the communists took power in China in 1949, there was a real tension between the modernist and the traditionalist views. After a fierce debate as to whether or not Chinese medicine was a throwback to an era that they were trying to leave behind, the communist authorities finally accepted this 'medical legacy of the motherland' as a legitimate and valuable part of health care. Thus began the process, which continues in China to this day, of the development of Western and traditional practices in parallel. One of the consequences of the centralisation of the communist system was the first real attempt to draw together the disparate strands of traditional medical theory and practice into a coherent and modern curriculum of Chinese medicine. What has evolved today as Chinese medicine is a relatively recent attempt at producing coherence out of diversity, but at all times the underlying philosophical principles remain true to the basic Daoist view of a dynamic and interactive universe in which we are all crucial components.

Treatment Principles

Taking the view of the body as a dynamic, ever-changing energy system, it can be appreciated that health and well-being are characterised by this system being able to flow and change smoothly in response to the needs of the individual within the environmental context. When something occurs to interrupt or disrupt this dynamic, illness will be the result. The flow of the system is under the control of the life-force – the qi – and the focus of any treatment principle will depend on the qi dynamic of the individual.

The qi of the body can be considered in terms of its complementary opposites – yin qi and yang qi. When a problem arises an imbalance will develop between the yin and yang qi of the body. Essentially, imbalances can result from a problem of excess or a problem of deficiency. The following simple diagrams best illustrate this process:

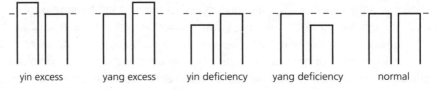

| yin excess | yang excess | yin deficiency | yang deficiency | normal |

Fig. 2: Yin and yang in harmony or disharmony?

The nature of the imbalance, whether it be a deficiency or an excess, will result in certain symptomatic features arising in the individual. The principle of the treatment process – whatever the focus – will be to re-establish the balance between the yin and the yang energies. Where there is a deficiency, it will require to be tonified and where there is an excess it will require to be reduced. This suggests that the approach of Chinese medicine is very simple, but this is most definitely not the case. While it is possible to see all disharmonies in terms of relative excess or deficiency, the reality is a complex mixture of internal and external disharmonies, some affecting channels and some the internal organ systems, some manifesting with heat, some with cold, some resulting from external environmental influences and some resulting from internal emotional processes. Great skill is required of the practitioner to identify the causes of imbalance and correct them using appropriate treatment.

Methods of Treatment

Acupuncture

Almost certainly the most commonly held image of Chinese medicine is that of acupuncture needles being inserted into key locations in the body – often bearing no apparent relationship to the presenting problem, for example a needle being inserted into the foot to treat the problem of a migraine headache. Acupuncture is essentially an energy medicine, not a physical therapy. The effects that are achieved through needling operate at the energetic level of the patient's qi and not at the physical level of the nervous system. By appropriate manipulation, deficient qi can be tonified and excess qi can be reduced and redistributed. By the selection of empirically defined points in the body, specific systemic effects can be achieved, specific organ systems influenced and quite profound physical and emotional changes produced in the individual.

Acupuncture

Moxibustion

Moxibustion is the process whereby a herb called moxa (*Artesima vulgaris*) is burnt either on the skin or over the skin, in order to warm the qi and the blood in the channels. This can have the effect of moving the qi to disperse an excess or of tonifying the qi in the case of a deficiency. Moxibustion can be used on its own or in conjunction with other approaches – especially acupuncture and sometimes cupping.

Cupping

Cupping is a technique that can be especially useful in treating local channel problems. Cups are either of robust round glass or of bamboo construction. A vacuum is created by burning a lighted taper briefly in the cup which is then immediately placed on the skin over the area that has been identified for treatment. The vacuum has the effect of drawing the skin up and moving the qi and blood in the local area. Cupping, for instance, is useful to draw out, from the superficial levels, the effects of 'wind' and 'cold', two of the external causes of disharmony recognised by Chinese medicine.

Herbal Medicine

Alongside acupuncture, Chinese herbs form the other major treatment, working at the internal energetic level of the body. As with acupuncture, herbs are considered as operating at an energetic level, and the selection of herbs chosen for any given formula will reflect the energetics of the herbs themselves, the channel and organ systems of the body that they enter, and the nature of the energetic imbalance that is being treated. It is slightly misleading to use the term 'herb' when talking about Chinese medicine. In addition to flowers, fruits, leaves and roots – the traditional

Herbalism

'herbal' constituents – the Chinese also use minerals and animal parts. There is controversy over the use of substances such as rhino horn and tiger bone. While there is no doubt that such things were used in herbal formulae and are still considered as having important energetic properties, all are readily replaced by ecologically acceptable alternatives which have the same general energetic properties.

In Chinese medicine it would be very unusual for herbs to be used singly and most are combined into formulae which are made up to reflect the energetic nature of the patient's disharmony. Herbs can be given in raw dried form, which are then boiled together to create a decoction to be drunk, in a powdered form, which can also be made into a beverage, or as a tincture, where the herbs are dissolved in alcohol. In addition, many classic herbal formulae are available as readily prepared patent medicines in the form of pills and teas.

Massage

*Massage
Shiatsu*

Massage forms a very important part of the therapeutic repertoire of the Chinese medical practitioner. Various techniques are used to encourage physically the flow of qi and blood through the channels of the body. Acupressure on specific acupoints can also be used to treat specific disharmonies.

Massage and acupressure are often used in concert with other methods, especially with acupuncture and occasionally with qigong healing.

Qigong

One of the fastest-growing areas of Chinese medicine in the West is reflected in the interest in qigong exercises and taiji forms. *Qigong* literally translates from the Chinese as 'energy cultivation' and this gives an impression of the value placed on these exercises by the Chinese. Amongst the oldest records of therapeutics based on the principles of Chinese medicine are examples of breathing, standing and simple moving exercises, which were used to encourage and balance the flow of qi in the body, thus promoting health. It is clear that such exercises were not only used in a preventative manner, but that they were also prescribed to treat specific kinds of illness.

There are literally thousands of qigong exercises and a burgeoning range of books promoting specific approaches. In using qigong it is, above all, important to try and understand that these exercises were developed in an empirical manner – in much the same way as acupuncture and herbal remedies were developed – and that they can offer a powerful tool for energetic self-help which can be used to complement some of the more conventional forms of treatment in the Chinese medicine repertoire.

In addition to qigong exercises, there is a small but growing band of practitioners who use qigong as a direct therapeutic healing technique with patients. This is still controversial, especially in the West, but it is suggested that it is possible for a practitioner with a strong and balanced qi flow system to use it to help balance a weaker and imbalanced qi flow system in the patient.

Chinese Medicine in Practice

A visit to a Chinese medical practitioner is not very different from what would be expected in a Western medical context. Full and thorough assessment precedes the planned intervention, the efficacy of which requires to be monitored, evaluated and altered as necessary in the light of the therapeutic aims and objectives. The difference lies in the nature of the assessment and diagnostic procedures, followed by the selection of appropriate treatment modalities.

Diagnosis

In Chinese medicine, diagnosis consists of gathering information by four means – looking, hearing and smelling, questioning, and touching:

◆ **Looking**
The first thing that the practitioner will do is to observe the patient and note anything about their physical appearance or behaviour that may be of significance. Information will be recorded about body type, movement, colour and condition of the skin and the hair. Very careful note will be taken of the 'geography' of the tongue. The colour, moisture, coating and cracking of the tongue are considered vital indicators of the function of the internal organs of the body, as well as of the general energetic condition of the person.

◆ **Hearing and Smelling**
The practitioner will take note of features such as the sound of the patient's voice and the noise they make when breathing. Characteristic smells and odours from the patient can also give clues about the nature of any possible disharmony, although it is unlikely to find any Western practitioners actively smelling their patients. Second-hand information on the smell of faeces and urine is also usually sought.

◆ **Questioning**
The diagnostic interview will seek to elicit a holistic picture of patients and their condition. This is done by systematically going through a protocol of questions designed to reveal the information the practitioner needs to reach a diagnosis.

◆ **Touching**
In addition to palpating the patient's body in order to assess temperature, moisture and pain, the practitioner also will be particularly interested in the nature and quality of the patient's pulses. Pulse-taking in Chinese medicine goes far beyond the concept understood in Western medicine and there are apocryphal stories of master physicians who are able to diagnose the full range of an individual's energetic disharmonies simply by taking the pulses. The emphasis is on the

quality of the pulse at various positions on each wrist. Chinese medicine recognises some 28 different pulse qualities on three different positions and at three different depths on each wrist. Each position, depth and quality indicates a different aspect of the energetic picture. Pulse-taking is more of an art than anything else and it is a skill that the practitioner will never stop refining.

At the end of the day, the overall diagnostic jigsaw is built up by exploring these four areas. No picture is ever 100% consistent but in conjunction with the practitioner's clinical judgement, it provides the basis for the diagnosis..

Planning a Treatment Programme

At the end of the diagnosis the practitioner will have an understanding of the patient's energetic disharmony in terms of excess or deficient patterns affecting specific organ systems of the body. On the basis of this, certain treatment principles will be identified and a treatment plan developed and agreed with the patient.

In the West today the majority of Chinese medical practitioners will specialise in one of the main modalities, usually acupuncture or herbal medicine. They may also have training in other modalities, especially moxibustion, cupping and massage, but it is uncommon to find practitioners who are also well-versed in all the therapeutic modalities. However, as Chinese medicine becomes more established in the West, it is likely that they will all become available to the patient, even if from several trained and qualified practitioners who work co-operatively.

The nature of the treatment given will vary, but some general principles will apply in each instance.

Acupuncture

◆ **Acupuncture** may be offered, commonly on a weekly basis, although the frequency may be greater early on in a treatment programme and may decrease in the later stages of the programme. The number of treatments required will be wholly dependent on the nature of the disharmony and the energetic profile of the patient; however, it is unusual for a programme to be less than ten treatments for other than minor ailments.

◆ **Moxibustion, cupping and massage** can often be combined with acupuncture treatment.

◆ **Chinese herbs** can be prescribed for periods of up to three or four weeks at a time, although it is vital that the effects of the herbs are regularly monitored and the prescription altered as appropriate. Generally speaking, the effects of herbs are much more specific than acupuncture, and the dose and constituents of the formulae need to be carefully planned in order to avoid undesirable side effects.

◆ **Advice on diet and general lifestyle** may also be given in a manner that is consistent with the general principles of Chinese medicine.

◆ **Specific qigong exercises** may also be used in conjunction with another modality such as acupuncture or herbs.

Generally speaking, Chinese medicine can be used alongside other therapies without any significant problems and in many instances the Chinese approach will serve to support and enhance the benefit of other treatments. The main area where problems arise is with patients on drug regimes. Very often, the energetic nature of Western drugs can pose serious difficulties for the treatment principles of Chinese medicine and where it is not possible for patients to come off drugs, it may be necessary to revise the therapeutic expectations of the Chinese treatments and monitor progress carefully. The biggest problems in this regard tend to occur with major drugs, such as steroids.

However, with this proviso in mind, it is fair to say that Chinese medicine can be practised as an excellent companion to many other forms of therapy.

Conditions Treated by Chinese Medicine

The Chinese system is a comprehensive approach to health care and as such it offers a model of provision which can address the majority of problems that are seen today. However, it also has to be remembered that Chinese medicine, like all other medicines, is not a magical cure-all and there are conditions and patients that will remain resistant to treatment. One of the more fascinating questions in Chinese medicine is not why it works, because it patently does, but why for some patients it does not work, or only works partially. This is not a dilemma unique to Chinese medicine.

A well-trained and professional practitioner will be able to offer reliable advice on treatment effectiveness and which modality is most appropriate in any given condition. For example, it is likely that Chinese herbs would be the treatment of choice with skin conditions, whereas acupuncture may be the treatment of choice in a condition such as a frozen shoulder.

Research

The last ten years or so has seen a tremendous growth in reliable research programmes looking at the effectiveness of Chinese medicine. There are several well-respected academic journals both in China and in the West which are publishing reports of high quality research into acupuncture, Chinese herbal treatments and also, in some instances, qigong therapies.

Acceptance of Chinese medicine within Western medical systems is going to be significantly enhanced with the publication of high quality research and Chinese practitioners are at the forefront of scientific research in complementary therapies.

Training

In China the training in Chinese medicine has the status and facilities associated with any university-level medical training and practitioners undertake a full undergraduate curriculum followed by supervised clinical practice.

In Britain there are several excellent colleges of acupuncture and Chinese herbs, some of which are now offering degree courses ratified by a recognised university. The profession has agreed standards of training in both Chinese medicine and Western medicine and accreditation mechanisms are in place which will allow for legal registration of practitioners. The various different registers that have existed have recently agreed to reconstitute themselves under one registration body, the British Acupuncture Council.

There are also growing opportunities for Western practitioners to undertake clinical experience training in China and the mechanisms are in place for a growing and developing clinical and research base.

Anyone considering going to a practitioner of Chinese medicine should ensure that they are going to a properly trained and accredited clinician with the full backing of the professional register and comprehensive professional indemnity insurance.

Six Cases to Illustrate the Practice of Traditional Chinese Medicine

◆ *Ian complained of sore ears and a general aching which spread over his head and into his shoulders. The pain came on suddenly when he woke up that morning and he had had to take the day off work.*

Ian owned an MG convertible and the previous evening he had been out for a lengthy drive with the top down, despite the fact that the warmth of the day was rapidly being lost in the chill of the evening. This information provided the key to Ian's problem. He was suffering from wind and cold having invaded the channels of the head, neck and face, causing local qi stagnation in the relevant channels and collaterals.

The treatment of choice was acupuncture and the principles of treatment were to expel the wind and cold and to clear the channels. Appropriate acupuncture points were selected and the channels around the ears, which were especially painful, were warmed by using a moxa stick in a pecking motion. The condition was very acute and the acupuncture had an immediate effect. After one treatment the pain was markedly reduced.

◆ *Janet was 60 years old and had been diagnosed as having chronic bronchitis for many years but it had worsened the last winter. She was bringing up copious amounts of thick yellow sputum and was coughing badly. Janet had* smoked between 30 and 40 cigarettes a day since she was a teenager until she stopped five years previously when she had had her first bad attack of bronchitis. She had admitted to still having the odd cigarette. Janet's tongue was red and dry with a thick, sticky yellow coating. Her pulses were weak and slippery, especially on the lung pulse.

The cause and effect here was obvious: Janet had seriously damaged her lung function over an extended period of abuse from smoking. Smoking draws heat into the lungs, consuming the yin fluids and causing lung function to become impaired. Janet was also overweight and lacking energy. It was therefore likely that spleen function was impaired causing damp to build up. Over time the damp transforms into phlegm that obstructed the lungs, which were themselves quite yin deficient.

The diagnosis was phlegm heat in the lungs with associated lung yin deficiency and generalised spleen qi deficiency. The treatment principle was to drain the fire from the lungs, clear the phlegm, stop the cough and tonify the lungs and the spleen.

In this instance acupuncture and herbal treatment were combined. Acupuncture was given to clear the heat and phlegm and to tonify the lungs. A herbal formula was used which would drain phlegm heat from the lungs and at the same time stop the cough and moisten the lungs.

Janet came weekly for six sessions receiving acupuncture treatment each time. The herbal prescription was reviewed and adjusted every two weeks. Her cough improved markedly and the phlegm reduced.

Fifteen months after her initial visit, Janet was much better and generally felt more healthy. It was unlikely that she would ever be free of her lung problem and it would flare up from time to time, but the use of acupuncture and herbs made a marked difference to her condition.

◆ Jim, mid-fifties, in a stressful executive position at work, complained that he felt dizzy and at times thought he was going to pass out completely. He was rather overweight with a red face. He complained of ringing in his ears and occasional headaches. He also had a genital itch. His pulse was rapid and slippery and very full. His tongue was red around the edges with a greasy coating. Throughout the diagnostic interview he was very edgy.

It was likely from the diagnostic information that the dizziness and other 'head' symptoms were caused by phlegm obstructing the orifices in the head. Jim's liver qi was stagnant and over time there had been an imbalance of the yin and yang energies, resulting in the liver yang energy rising to the head taking the phlegm with it. The main principle of treatment here was to subdue the liver yang, promote the smooth flow of qi and clear the phlegm from the orifices.

Treatment was commenced by giving Jim a relaxing acupressure massage. This reduced his edginess and made way for the subsequent treatment to be more effective. This was followed by acupuncture, and a powdered herbal formula was also given to support the treatment. After several treatments Jim said he was feeling much better. Treatment continued for another three weeks by which time he felt that he was able to cope on his own.

◆ *Marie, aged 23, was a primary school teacher. She had suffered from chronic eczema since she was a child. She had been hospitalised and had had numerous steroid preparations, but nothing made much impact on the problem. The eczema was worse on her hands, her arms, her head and her knees. She also had patches on her legs and on her trunk. The skin presented as dry and flaky. It was very itchy and when she scratched, it bled. The worst area was on her hands where the dryness was so bad that the skin cracked and became infected. Marie was a thin, pale young woman. Her tongue was pale and quite dry; her pulse was thin and thready.*

In terms of Chinese medicine, a skin condition like this is seen as resulting from a deficiency of blood allowing wind to invade the channels. The dry, flaky skin, the pale complexion and the tongue and pulse all indicated a blood deficient condition. The itchiness demonstrated the presence of pathogenic wind in the channels. The principle of treatment in Chinese medicine was to clear the wind from the channels, tonify the blood and nourish the skin. While acupuncture may be of some benefit here, the treatment of choice for skin conditions is herbs.

After some initial adjustment to the herbal formula, there was a significant improvement in the condition. After a year of herbs Marie's condition was stable. The skin was much better and her hands were clear. There was the occasional flare-up and Marie retained herbs which she took as soon as there was any problem.

◆ *John had been diagnosed as HIV positive which over the preceeding six months had developed into full blown AIDS. He was receiving orthodox medical treatment. His main complaint was that he had little or no energy, that he could not sleep at night and that he was experiencing night sweats which required him to change the sheets two or three times a night. He was having palpitations and was constantly on edge. John looked thin and emaciated. His skin was dry with lesions on his face and back. His face was red and his tongue was red and peeled with a bright red tip. His pulse was rapid and thready.*

John was presenting with classic signs and symptoms of empty heat resulting from the underlying deficiency of yin energy in the body. The AIDS condition was resulting in the yin fluids being consumed and the body literally 'burning up' from the inside. The empty heat was also affecting the heart yin and this resulted in poor sleep patterns, edginess and palpitations. It was unlikely that Chinese medicine could reverse the AIDS, but there was no reason why the symptoms could not be helped. The principle of treatment was to clear the empty heat, tonify the yin and calm the heart shen.

John was treated twice weekly with acupuncture and then on a weekly basis. After three months of treatment he was sleeping much better, which was increasing his general energy level. He was still having night sweats but their intensity was reduced. John was also encouraged to learn some simple qigong postures and exercises. This he did, attending a class regularly. The condition was far from cured, but John had received some significant benefit from the acupuncture and felt especially that now he was sleeping better, he would be more able to continue to fight his condition in his own way.

◆ *Martha was 76 and suffered from arthritis. She complained of feeling stiff and sore all over, especially in her knee and ankle joints, which were swollen and painful to the touch. She was generally overweight and she complained that her feet and fingers were quite swollen at times. She complained of finding it difficult to keep warm, even when the weather was mild in summer. She also had a problem of chronic diarrhoea. Martha's tongue was pale and wet and her pulse was slow and rather soggy in quality.*

Martha's problem was an example of the invasion of the channels by cold and damp. The invading pathogenic factors tend to lodge in the channels around the joints causing the pain and swelling characteristic of arthritic conditions. Underlying this condition, there was evidence of a generalised yang deficiency. This was characterised by the tendency towards cold, the chronic diarrhoea and the tongue and pulse indicators. Yang deficiency is a common and natural feature of the ageing process.

The principles of treatment in Chinese medicine were to clear the damp and cold from the channels and to tonify the underlying yang energy of the body.

Martha was treated with acupuncture, moxibustion and herbal prescriptions. Cupping was also used on occasions to help try to move the qi around the worst affected areas. After 20 weekly sessions of acupuncture and moxibustion, along with a regular herbal prescription, Martha's condition was much improved. She had more mobility and the swelling was reduced. Martha decided to terminate the acupuncture and related treatments at this stage, but she continued to take herbs for the next six months and her condition remained quite stable.

Biography

Tom Williams took his initial professional training in psychology and he has worked as an educational psychologist since 1979. He is currently the Director of Psychological Services in East Ayrshire. A long-term interest in taiji led him to train in acupuncture at the Northern College of Acupuncture in York. He has subsequently followed this with clinical training in Beijing and a training in Chinese herbal medicine. He is a member of the British Acupuncture Council, a member of the register of Chinese Herbal Medicine and a fellow of the British Psychological Society. He has published books on Chinese medicine and runs a part-time practice in Glasgow.

References

1   Ted Kaptchuk, *Chinese Medicine – The Web That Has No Weaver*, Rider, 1983.

Further Reading

Beinfield, H.; Korngold, E., *Between Heaven & Earth*, Ballantine, 1991.

Kaptchuk, Ted, *Chinese Medicine – The Web That has No Weaver*, Rider, 1983.

Maciocia, Giovanni, *The Foundations of Chinese Medicine*, Churchill Livingstone, 1989.

———, *The Practice of Chinese Medicine*, Churchill Livingstone, 1994.

Takahashi, Masaru; Brown, Stephen, *Qigong for Health: Chinese Traditional Exercise for Cure and Prevention*, Japan Publications, 1986.

Williams, Tom, *Chinese Medicine*, Element, 1995.

———, *The Illustrated Guide to Chinese Medicine*, Element, 1996.

Wiseman, Ellis & Zmiewski, *The Fundamentals of Chinese Medicine*, Paradigm, 1985.

Resources

The Association for Traditional Chinese Medicine
78 Haverstock Hill
London NW3 2BE
Tel. 0171-284 2898

The British Acupuncture Council
Park House
206 – 208 Latimer Road
London W10 6RE
Tel. 0181-964 0222
Fax. 0181-964 0333

The Register of Chinese Herbal Medicine
P O Box 400
Wembley
Middlesex HA9 9NZ
Tel. 0181-904 1357

Feng Shui Network
P O Box 2133
London W1A 1RL
Tel. 0171-935 8935
Fax. 0171-935 9295

Transcendental Meditation

by Marguerite Osborne

Origins of Transcendental Meditation

There are many forms of meditation available, with different places of origin, different methods and different aims. Transcendental Meditation* (TM) is the one which has proved most popular with Westerners. This may be because it is easy to learn, effortless and enjoyable to practise and, in most cases, produces some beneficial results from the very start. It has also been very successfully promoted.

The meditation itself derives from the East, from the Vedic tradition of India, otherwise known as the holy (or 'holistic') tradition. The present revival of the technique stems from Swami Brahmananda Saraswati, who was a much-loved and revered figure in India in the first part of this century. He is the most recent in a long and distinguished line of masters who have taught this form of meditation as an essential part of an integrated life.

What is Meditation

In order to experience full satisfaction in life, the mind, instead of always being turned outwards into activity, sometimes needs to travel within, in order to approach or have some contact with the transcendent, the silent source of thought which lies 'beyond thought'.

Transcendental Meditation is a mental technique known as a mantra meditation. The mantras involved are words, or sounds, to which no particular meaning is attached; they derive from the Vedic tradition. When receiving instruction in the technique a person is given a suitable mantra and taught its correct use. It is perfectly natural to meditate and the student will soon be doing so with great ease. The process is a very ordinary one.

The technique can be learned by anyone, even by children. It does not require any special intellectual abilities or background reading, or even the belief that it will

---

*Transcendental Meditation is a registered trademark.

'work'. It is practised sitting comfortably with closed eyes. No special environment is required; it is possible to meditate in noisy conditions and one can do it as a passenger in a vehicle. No concentration, i.e. holding the mind unwaveringly fixed on an object, is required and no 'thinking about' anything is involved.

The Effects of Meditation

During the actual process of TM the mind automatically travels to finer, more 'subtle' levels of thought and, at the same time, the body is profoundly relaxed. The advantages of this state of 'restful alertness' are experienced not only during meditation but also in daily life. The benefits, which even people new to meditation experience to some degree in the first few days, are at all levels: mental, physical, environmental and spiritual. Meditators tend to feel greater energy, physical as well as mental, and a greater sense of well-being.

Many illnesses are believed to be psychosomatic in origin, resulting from the body's inability to cope with the pace and demands of modern life; these can be referred to as 'stress-induced' illnesses. Practising TM can lead to the alleviation or even the disappearance of such conditions. Good results have been experienced in cases of anxiety, neurosis, hypertension, insomnia, phobias, headache and various breathing diseases (including asthma). More recently TM has been used to help people suffering from ME.

It is quite common for patients taking tranquillisers to find that when they learn TM they need fewer of these, or that they can stop taking them altogether. TM can be useful, too, in helping to break addictions or harmful habits. Smoking, excess drinking, overeating, drug-taking and smaller things such as nail-biting are often to some degree the result of stress. As the meditator becomes more relaxed and more fulfilled, such practices are likely to decrease or cease altogether. There is also an increase in self-esteem, so that meditators are likely to take better care of themselves.

TM has been used in official drug abuse programmes in the USA with some positive results and research studies have shown it can be beneficial in treating alcoholism.[1]

Mental Effects of TM

Those who practise meditation find that their thinking is clearer and that their powers of concentration are improved. Instead of having lots of confusing, undirected 'grasshopper' thoughts, they will have more powerful thoughts leading to some definite action. Because of this, meditators can achieve more things in less time and with less effort than previously and therefore derive more enjoyment from everything they do.

Physical Effects of TM

A great many people in the West have learned TM primarily on account of its well-known good effects on health. It is recommended that one practise the technique for two periods of 20 minutes, morning and early evening, every day. Each meditation gives the body profound rest and relaxation in preparation for dynamic activity. As a result of this physical rest, deep-rooted stresses and tensions can be dissolved. TM may assist preventing illness. There are some health insurance companies (for example Geove in the Netherlands) which offer reduced premiums to people practising TM, under the assumption that they are less likely to fall ill than non-meditators.[2]

Environmental Effects of TM

Practising TM leads to a better rapport with the human environment. Personal relationships, in particular, can be improved. There is a tendency for meditators to feel more harmonious and to experience greater inner peace and fulfilment as a result of practising the technique. As this inner happiness grows, they may find themselves being effortlessly more loving and supportive to the people around them. This can have a ripple effect as other people respond by showing the same qualities in their turn.

New meditators often mention that they have become more tranquil, tolerant, patient and optimistic and have a better sense of humour and a greater ability to laugh at themselves. These traits may increase as they go on with their practice. They may also find themselves more in touch with what they really want out of life, what will be genuinely satisfying for them. Learning the technique can result in beneficial changes of job, interests, friends and lifestyle in general. Meditators can also experience greater self-esteem and greater assertiveness.

Families and other groups where all the members are meditating tend to experience a sense of community and oneness, particularly if they meditate together. It has been claimed – and may be true – that if some 10% of people all over the world were practising TM, there would be a greater likelihood of world peace.

Spiritual Effects of TM

TM is a means of experiencing spiritual values. During the quiet time spent practising TM the mind is turned inwards and identifies with a source of happiness deep within its own nature. This source, being infinite, is itself infinitely satisfying. The ultimate purpose of practising TM is to bring more and more of this infinite spiritual value to our material lives, so that they become meaningful, as we experience inner peace and silence in the rush of everyday life. The result is not a desire to escape from life but an ability to enjoy activity more fully.

Research Experiments on TM

A great deal of scientific research has been carried out on the TM technique and its effects. An impressive collection of research is published in *Scientific Research on the Transcendental Meditation Programme*.[3] One classic study was made at Harvard University by Keith Wallace, PhD, and Herbert Benson, MD, in 1971.[4]

The researchers took a number of people who had learnt the TM technique (some of them quite recently) and monitored them for different factors. During the time they were meditating they showed:

◆ Slower breathing and lower oxygen consumption

◆ Slowing down of the heartbeat

◆ Rapid decline in the concentration of blood lactate (high concentrations of lactate occur in the blood in states of anxiety)

◆ Rapid rise in electrical skin resistance (high electrical skin resistance can be equated with a state of relaxation)

◆ Increase in intensity of alpha waves (again, a sign of a relaxed state)

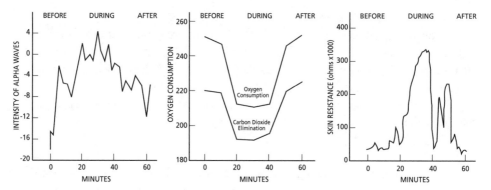

Fig. 1: Some of the physiological effects of TM, recorded before, during and after meditation

As a result of these findings the researchers described TM as 'a highly relaxed though wakeful condition', bearing no resemblance to sleep, hypnosis or trance. They remarked that the wide range of physiological changes noted during TM occur quite spontaneously.

They concluded that the state of reduced metabolism experienced during TM 'may indicate a guidepost to better health'. This conclusion has been borne out both by the subjective experience of many meditators and by further research studies on the physical effects of TM.[5]

My Personal Experience

I learnt TM in 1971 in Devon when I was a teacher in a grammar school. I was hoping it would help me to be less tense in a fairly stressful occupation. My results were dramatic – unusually so. Nervous catarrh and tension headaches cleared up immediately. My mental powers, already acute, improved. I began to feel much more love and empathy for my pupils and therefore found the work more rewarding. Gradually I became more self-confident and independent. The most important thing for me, though, was that the meditation brought a great influx of spirituality into my life. Very soon I had given up my job in order to go abroad and take the TM teacher training course, which in those days was conducted in person by Maharishi Mahesh Yogi, the chief promoter of TM in the West. I taught the technique first in South Devon and afterwards in Yorkshire.

Being a teacher of TM is, I suppose, the most precious thing in my life. I have taught the meditation to nearly a thousand people and have witnessed many miracles of transformation it has brought about. The actual process of teaching also brings great joy and peace and inspiration to me.

In the early days of the TM movement, Maharishi asserted that anyone who practised TM regularly, and especially if they went on residential courses to do even more meditation, would swiftly achieve cosmic consciousness, a state in which all thoughts and actions are spontaneously right and life-supporting. I have practised TM regularly for nearly 25 years and, although it has raised my consciousness to some degree, I realise that I have not attained any particularly high state of consciousness, nor do I expect to by this means.

The benefits to me now are that my meditation practice gives me two welcome periods of quietness in a busy day; these result in my feeling reasonably calm and centred and the afternoon meditation usually infuses me with extra mental and physical energy at a time when I am beginning to flag. TM has had other helpful effects over the years: in such situations as public speaking and public performance, I tend to acquit myself quite well without suffering any 'nerves' beforehand. The same is true of examinations; I have taken a number of these since learning TM and have always had good results. I think practising TM has also kept me fairly healthy over the years, but any claims that it can lead to the reversal of ageing or to 'perfect health' are, from my own experience unsubstantiated.

The TM Movement Today

When I first became a TM teacher the organisation responsible for promoting the meditation was called the Spiritual Regeneration Movement and it professed – rightly, in my opinion – that people who learnt TM would be given some direct experience of the reality at the root of all religions.

The organisation is now known as the World Government of the Age of Enlightenment and has become a cult with His Holiness Maharishi Mahesh Yogi as its leader. It offers many programmes devised by Maharishi. The leaders of the World Government believe and expect all TM teachers to believe that Maharishi's teaching and programmes are 'absolutely complete for every area of life'. In this I have found a personal point of conflict and have felt bound to dissociate myself from the organisation. So I am now an independent teacher of TM.

Learning TM

For those who would like to learn a simple, enjoyable and effective form of meditation, I can recommend the TM technique in every way. Before receiving instruction it is important to realise that the meditation is not something to be done once or twice or every now and then: for the best results you must be prepared to meditate regularly every day. It is also, I think, best not to expect any particular results. I have outlined the sort of effects which the meditation can have but these are not predictable for any one person.

The first step is to go to an introductory talk about TM, which will be followed by an opportunity to put questions and by an enrolment session. When you decide to learn, you have a short interview with the teacher and make appointments for your course of instruction. A fee is charged for this course. Teachers of TM working for Maharishi's organisation charge £490 for a basic course of instruction with three follow-up sessions; reduced prices are available for students but not for the unemployed. Independent teachers of TM advertise locally and charge varying fees. My own are on a sliding scale based on financial status. This scale starts at £40. The suggested fee is one week's gross income.

The course itself (usually taken in a group, although individual instruction is also possible) consists of four meetings with the teacher on four consecutive days. At the first meeting, which lasts about an hour, the student receives personal one-to-one tuition in the technique. They can expect to feel some relaxation immediately and there may be other good results on this first day. Afterwards they will be able to go home and meditate on their own. Each of the three following sessions lasts between one and two hours. At each session vital new information is given, so it is essential to attend them all. Every session includes discussion of the student's experiences and assessment of the experienced benefits so far. If you are learning with a group, these will be group meetings. Once the course is completed the student has all the knowledge required to practise TM alone.

It is essential to be taught by a qualified teacher. I do not know if there are many other people teaching TM independently; it is probably necessary to learn from someone committed to Maharishi and his world view. My own advice in this case would be to learn just the basic meditation and to receive the occasional checking which ensures all is going smoothly, but I would caution against becoming involved with Maharishi's philosophy or with any of the other programmes. It is with this proviso that I give the organisation's address.

Biography

Marguerite Osborne, a graduate in philosophy and English literature, has worked in provincial journalism. For some years she taught English and drama in Devon grammar schools. She has spent six years in Italy and two in Oxford teaching English as a foreign language. A leading interest is ecology and she has worked as a volunteer in reforestation and organic agriculture in Britain, Spain, Italy and Israel. Marguerite has recently moved to Scotland, where she is an Open Community Member of the Findhorn Foundation.

References

1   H Benson; R K Wallace, *Decreased drug dbuse with Transcendental Meditation: a study of 1, 862 subjects, at the Thorndike Memorial Laboratory*, Boston City Hospital, Boston, Mass.

Department of Medicine, Harvard Medical School, Boston, Mass. *Reported in Drug Abuse: Proceedings of the International Conference*, (ed. Chris J. D. Zarafonetis), Lee and Febiger, 1972, p369-76.

Z Lazar; L Farwell; J T Farrow, *The effects of the Transcendental Meditation program on anxiety, drug abuse, cigarette smoking and alcohol consumption in scientific research on the Transcendental Meditation program* (eds D Orme-Johnson; J T Farrow), Collected Papers, Vol 1. Maharishi European Research University Press, 1976.

M Shafii; R A Lavely; B S & R Jaffe, *Meditation and the prevention of alcohol abuse*, Am J Psychiatry, 1975, 132: 942-5.

2   D W Orme-Johnson, *Medical care utilization and the Transcendental Meditation programme*, Psychosomatic Medicine, 1987, 49: 493-07.

3   D Orme-Johnson; J T Farrow (eds) *Scientific Research on the Transcendental Meditation Programme*. Collected papers, Vol. 1. Maharishi European Research University Press, 1976.

4   R K Wallace; H Benson, *The physiology of meditation*, Scientific American, 1972, 226: 84-90.

5   D E Miskiman, *Long-term effects of the Transcendental Meditation program in the treatment of insomnia*, in *Scientific research on the Transcendental Meditation program* (eds D Orme-Johnson J T Farrow), Collected Papers, Vol. 1. Maharishi European Research University Press, 1976.

A F Wilson; R Honsburger; J T Chiu; H S Novey, *Transcendental Meditation and asthma*, Respiration, 1975, 32: 74-80.

K Eppley; A Abrams; J Shear, *Differential effects of relaxation techniques on trait anxiety: a meta-analysis*, J Clinical Psychology, 1989, 45: 957-74.

Further Reading

Benson, Herbert, *The Relaxation Response*, Outlet Books, 1993.

————; Procter, William, *Beyond the Relaxation Response*, Puntam/Berkley Inc., 1984.

Borysenko, Joan, *Minding the Body, Mending the Mind*, Bantam Books, 1988.

Campbell, Anthony, *Seven States of Consciousness. A Vision of Possibilities Suggested by the Teachings of Maharishi Mahesh Yogi*. Gollancz, 1973.

Forem, Jack, *Transcendental Meditation. Maharishi Mahesh Yogi and the Science of Creative Intelligence*, Allen and Unwin, 1974.

Goleman, Daniel, *The Meditative Mind*, JP Tarcher Inc., 1988.

LeShan, L., *How to Meditate*, Thorsons, 1995.

Maharishi Mahesh Yogi, *On the Bhagavad-Gita, A New Translation and Commentary*, Chapters I to VI, Penguin Books, 1969.

————, *The Science of Being and Art of Living*, International SRM Publications 1963, revised 1966.

Orme-Johnson, David; Farrow, John T. (eds) *Scientific Research on the Transcendental Meditation Programme*, Collected Papers. Vol. 1. Maharishi European Research University Press, 1976.

Proto, Louis, *Meditation for Everybody*, Penguin, 1991.

Roth, Robert, *Transcendental Meditation*, Donald I Fine Inc., 1988.

Russell, Peter, *The TM Technique*, Routledge & Kegan Paul, 1976.

Smith, Adrian B (ed), *TM, An Aid to Christian Growth*, Mayhew McCrimmon Ltd., 1983.

Resources

Transcendental Meditation
Freepost
London SW1P 4YY
Freephone 0800-260303

Transformational Self-Healing

by Lee Oldershaw

Over the years I have used my training, skills, interests and abilities to create a synthesis approach to health and healing. At the moment, I call this 'transformational self-healing' and it will develop and transform as time goes on. I believe there are many therapists who work in this fluid and flexible way, and I offer this outline to exemplify a form of healing based on accumulated experience. It is not a cohesive system, but consists of a collaboration of personal experience with the following:

Art Therapy
Spiritual Healing
Twelve Steps
Programme
Visualisation

♦ Mind training and sports/performance-related visualisation during my time as an international-level athlete and coach in the 1970s

♦ Tibetan Buddhist healing and visualisation techniques

♦ Spiritual and attitudinal healing based on the philosophy of *A Course In Miracles*, a workbook for spiritual development[1]

♦ Art and art therapy

♦ Intuitive diagnosis, receiving information intuitively regarding causes of illness

♦ The Twelve Steps programme of recovery for addictive behaviour

Transformational self-healing is a complementary method to bodywork or medical treatment. I have seen this method replace traditional therapy or medical treatment. Because it is simple yet deeply effective, the individual can continue using it at home.

One of the premises with which I work is: 'What you resist persists. What you accept transforms or heals.' This means that the mind (or attitude) is at the root of both sickness and health and that healing will always include changing belief or attitude.

The Practice of Transformational Self-Healing

During sessions, the facilitator helps individuals to access their 'higher self', using the language of intuition, symbols, colours, images, feelings or words which may represent the fundamental cause of the problem on whichever levels it affects them, be it physical, emotional, mental or spiritual. The higher self provides honest and clear symbols about the cause of the problem.

Clients will usually focus on a specific situation, for example an illness or an emotional/physical pattern like addiction or co-dependency. The symptom is often a result of mental or spiritual confusion signalling resistance or denial. It can become the motivation for change.

The first step in the transformative process is to help clients access their higher self simply by asking for an image or symbols to represent the presenting problem. This, when done in a relaxed state, is usually not difficult for people and an image will appear within a few seconds. It is important that they do not censor their mindsbut take the first image received, however unlikely or silly it may appear. The language of symbols is the language of the unconscious mind. No interpretation is given by the facilitator. Usually individuals know the meaning or feeling-level information from their imagery and will talk about it. The facilitator simply helps to encourage this.

Once clients have a clear image, the next step is to ask if they are willing to change or heal this initial image. If so, they ask for help from a power greater than the 'problem' self – a higher mind, God, Buddha, the universe – whatever their belief system can embrace. This is a totally 'receptive' method, never 'directive', which means that each individual observes their own mental images, like watching a video inside the head. The higher self takes over, allowing the initial image or feeling to change to a new symbol that represents the maximum healing which can be fully integrated at that time.

There is usually a perceptible change either in inner imagery or feelings which is experienced physically by the client, either instantly or in the days following a session.

My supposition about what happens is that the higher self 'short circuits' the analytical part of the mind that caused the problem in the first place, by giving it something to observe and interpret. Belief is not a factor in this method. I have worked with cardiac patients who had strong doubts and experienced healing anyway. The higher self bypasses the analytical mind by reprogramming it with new inner imagery.

In most cases, I ask my clients to document this healing by writing or drawing. This helps them measure the changes for themselves, especially if they choose to continue with the facilitator or use the methods at home for continued healing or health maintenance. People find this method quick, easy and graceful, often when traditional psychotherapeutic methods and medical treatment do not seem to be bearing results or seem to be taking too long or when symptoms have recurred. They find that they do not have to recall a painful situation or event to heal, only to access the emotions, feelings or body symptoms that have resulted from it. A secondary result of accessing the intuition through drawing and imagery work is self-discovery, which often incites curiosity, wonder, surprise and expectancy. It gives the power to heal back to the client, building confidence to monitor and change health and well-being in the future. The practitioner is a peer, beginning as a facilitator, but soon becoming an educator or coach, encouraging self-empowerment and use of the tools.

It is a method people can use not only in times of crisis, but for the rest of their lives – for diagnosis, healing, prevention and the enhancement of well-being and the actualisation of potential. Because the client's higher self directs the imagery, this leads naturally to this highest good. People especially appreciate that this method helps them rediscover and validate how their own inner intelligence, or higher self, communicates most naturally to them.

In some cases, emotional release occurs as feelings are acknowledged – anger, grief, sorrow, relief. This release is only a beginning step in the tranformational process and is followed by a healing shift, therefore clients seldom leave a session feeling raw or incomplete.

To integrate what has happened during the session, we discuss what has been learned, what has shifted, what the next steps are, what action can now be taken or not taken. I explain that they may feel vulnerable, powerful, confident or up or down for the next few days as the shift or release which has occurred on a spiritual or psychological level moves through the emotional and physical levels. Often this has begun during the session and the person already feels different or has been able to cry or release through the drawing. Other times the release may be experienced as increased perspiration, elimination of waste, blocked sinuses or weepiness. There may be feelings of freedom, openness, lightness and aliveness. All this is part of the integration.

I then focus on education to enable people to use this method as an ongoing self-healing process, to empower and trust themselves. I emphasise the importance of taking responsibility for their own healing back into their own hands. This also applies to any treatment – orthodox or complementary.

Case History

A boy, 16, had experienced migraines several days each week for seven years. He had seen many specialists with no results. In one session, he identified two consistent areas of pain in his head. Each showed initially as painful images but shifted to images of inner wise teachers. It seems that these inner sources of inspiration and education had been 'knocking' on his head since the age of nine, waiting to be acknowledged. He understood in that session his life purpose and how to access his inner wisdom and intuition and also knew what further university training he needed. The last time I checked, the migraines still had not returned.

Applications of Transformational Self-Healing

These methods can be used in any situation, for example:

◆ for physical symptoms and pain

◆ for situations resulting from trauma, emotional pain, anger or fear

◆ when the client does not want to have to recall or reconstruct a situation in order to heal it. (This may include traumatic incidents that were hidden subconsciously or forgotten and there is fear or horror in re-experiencing their memory)

◆ for addictive behaviour or dependency. (This is a strong complement to any support group or Twelve Steps programme)

◆ for people with high mental or analytical activity (the process bypasses the analytical mind, which caused the problem in the first place)

◆ for people with mental disabilities

◆ for children of four years and older. (The exercises can be turned into games. Because they are based on visual drawing rather than psychological discussion, children can participate fully and heal quickly because their imagination is so powerful. They can heal without understanding the process.)

◆ as preventative maintenance, checking one's own state of health and well-being and correcting when needed

◆ to create spiritual expansion and enhance positive aspects of one's life

The 'Heal Your Heart' Programme

An eight week (16 hour) cardiac programme was sponsored by the Heartbeat Centre Cardiac Rehabilitation Unit of St Andrew's War Memorial Hospital, Brisbane in 1994 and facilitated by myself and Terry Neal, a former cardiac patient, who had demonstrated amazing results, and no longer needed medication.

The participants were six men, between 40 and 70 all of whom had had heart attacks, several with multiple bypasses. The objective of the programme was to encourage them to take responsibility for their long-term health by discovering and healing the fundamental cause of their heart problem in a way that complemented the treatment prescribed by doctors and the exercise and education programme offered at the Heartbeat Centre.

This eight week programme was based on recommendations from Dr Dean Ornish's 'Open Your Heart' programme in the USA. Connecting with others' shared experiences and addressing the fundamental cause in a supportive group has been proven to prevent recurrence of the symptoms and even reverse organic heart disease.[2]

Relaxation Therapy
Visualisation

The programme included facilitated exercises focusing on:

◆ relaxation

◆ directed visualisation to begin to heal the symptoms

◆ receptive visualisation to discover and transform the fundamental cause of the heart problem

◆ life purpose – finding what makes one's heart 'sing'

◆ core beliefs

◆ group support and encouragement to discuss personal progress with:

Nutritional Therapy

> life changes
> diet
> work
> relationships
> beliefs and feelings
> making lifestyle changes to sustain long-term health

Participants' spouses or main support people were invited to the group, knowing that they would also need to make lifestyle changes. The results were increased intimacy; willingness to open and share fears and dreams with others; a sense of brotherhood and of being accepted and understood; honesty about where their passion for life really was and sharing that with their partners; less stress; clarity on what activities created a healthy and enjoyable lifestyle; improved relationships; healing of shame and self-incrimination and realisation that almost all these men expected to die when their fathers had (all had fathers who had died of heart disease). Recognising this last fact led to confidence that they could change their minds, their bodies, their hearts and then enjoy life – that they had choices. One man found that his heart 'reported' to him visually in terms of weather reports so he would know what was upcoming and could respond supportively.

An Example of Similar Work

Gerald Jampolski in the USA has used some of these healing techniques with children dying of cancer, and their families. This work, done in his Attitudinal Healing Centres, has resulted in children beginning to heal themselves and these cases have been well documented.[3] The centre's aim is to support children or young adults who are faced with life-threatening diseases by assisting them with attitudinal healing techniques. There is a strongly spiritual orientation in the centre's approach. The essence of attitudinal healing is the fundamental belief that it is possible to choose peace rather than conflict, love rather than fear.[4] Attitudinal healing involves letting go of the old fear-based patterns and attitudes and discovering that then only love remains. Health is defined as inner peace, and healing is the process of letting go of fear.

The centre offers a wide variety of support programmes, including those targeted at the long-term caregivers and family members of the children or young adults who are dying or who need constant nursing and attention. It also has programmes to assist with bereavement. Workshops and trainings in attitudinal healing are also available, as are videos, books, audiotapes and a quarterly newsletter. The centre will distribute information about other centres worldwide where programmes similar to their own are being run.

Conclusion

I end with a quote from Ornish's book:

> *There are different levels of healing. The further back in the causal chain of events we can address a problem, the more powerful the healing can be. The physical manifestation of the heart problem – the symptom – is addressed by your doctors. But if it is only treated at the physical level, then the patients' improvement is less than it could be and the illness is more likely to recur, either in the same form or in a different one.*

Biography

Lee Oldershaw is a Canadian who has worked with adults' and children's health since 1988 in Canada, USA, Britain and Australia. Prior to that, she coached national-level athletes using the power of imagery as a training tool. Drawing from her skills as a healing facilitator, educator and intuitive diagnostic, she developed and researched a collaboration of philosophies and techniques, which she now calls Transformational Self-Healing. Lee worked at the Findhorn Foundation in Scotland for four years until 1991, then moved to start a private practice in Brisbane, Australia.

References

1   Foundation for Inner Peace, *A Course In Miracles*, Arkana, 1988.
2   Dean Ornish, *Am J Epidem*, 1979; 109: 2, 186-204.
      ———, *Am J Epidem*, 1988; 128: 2, 370-80.
      ———, *Effects of stress management training and dietary changes in ischemic heart disease*, JAMA, 1983; 249: 1, 54-9.
3   Gerald Jampolski, *Love is Letting Go of Fear*, Celestial Arts, 1979.
4   ibid.

Further Reading

Dawson, Michael, *Healing the Cause*, Findhorn Press, 1994.

Foundation for Inner Peace, *A Course In Miracles*, Arkana, 1988.

Glouberman, Dina, *Life Choices and Life Changes Through Image Work*, Unwin Paperbacks, 1989.

Jampolski, Gerald, *Love is Letting Go of Fear*, Celestial Arts, 1979.

McDonald, Kathleen, *How to Meditate – A Practical Guide*, Wisdom Books, 1985.

Rimpoche, Lama Zopa, *Transforming Problems into Happiness*, Wisdom Publications, 1993.

Resources

Center for Attitudinal Healing
19 Main Street
Tiburon
CA 94920
USA
Tel. 415-435 5022

Twelve Steps Programme
by Janice Eddy

Most of us know someone who attends some kind of Twelve Steps recovery group, but we may be unconscious of the fact. The 'anonymous groups' are the best-kept secret, and the fastest-growing and most revolutionary grass-roots movement of the last 60 years. Membership in such a group is generally known only to members themselves and close friends or family. Aside from listings in the telephone directory and at the Citizens' Advice Bureau, groups do not advertise; they must be sought out or learned about through word of mouth. Because of this, not much is known about them and misinformation or even prejudice abounds.

History

Alcoholics Anonymous, the group upon which the others are modelled, dates its beginning from June 1935. In the early 1930s, Carl Jung had as a patient, a wealthy American industrialist and former state senator, Rowland H. Rowland had seen alcohol erode his life and talents, and sought help from Jung in Switzerland. Their work lasted a year, whereupon Rowland, convinced he would never drink again, returned to America, and predictably resumed drinking. He went back to Jung, who advised him that there was nothing further that he or medical science could do for him, and that his case from the standpoint of a medical cure was hopeless. The only avenue open to him, suggested Jung, was to align himself with some group wherein he might be lucky enough to undergo an experience of spiritual awakening.

Rowland involved himself with the Oxford Group, a popular charismatic religious movement active in America and abroad in the 1920s and '30s. Through Rowland, an alcoholic called Bill W. decided to give the Oxford Group a try.

After about six months of activity in the Oxford Group, Bill left New York to go on a business trip to Akron, Ohio, during which the deal fell through. Bill felt in danger of taking a drink. Having understood the power of one 'drunk' helping another, Bill made a number of phone calls to Oxford Group members in the Akron area, asking if they knew of any alcoholics whom he could talk to, to help him safeguard his own relatively new sobriety. He was put in touch with a Dr Bob S., a surgeon who was in danger of losing his practice and reputation to drinking. Bill helped him to sober up and he never ever drank again. The day of Bob's last drink is celebrated as the beginning of AA.

The two men began reaching out to other alcoholics. Bill returned to New York and AA grew both there and in Akron. In 1937 it had forty members; in 1939, a hundred. The 'Big Book', or *Alcoholics Anonymous*, was written by Bill and others in 1939. In 1941, *The Saturday Evening Post*, a popular magazine of the time, published an article on the good work being done by this group, and the small New York AA office received six thousand letters as a result.

Principles and Philosophy

The suggested recovery programme of AA, known as the 'Twelve Steps', which was to touch the lives of so many thousands of people, was based on spiritual principles which are common to many religions and spiritual movements.

They include admission of a problem; surrender of the problem, and one's life, to a power-greater-than-oneself; the taking of a moral inventory of oneself; 'confession', that is, admitting one's faults to oneself, to the 'power greater', and to at least one other person; restitution to those who have been harmed by one's actions; and service in the form of making sure that the message of recovery reaches those who are in need of it. These are not new concepts, but their use in helping people with a common problem to recover has been phenomenal. They may seem simple principles, but they are not necessarily easy to maintain.

In addition to the Steps which are based on the principles above, slogans are used, like 'Live and Let Live', 'First Things First', and 'Just for Today'. Deceptively simple, these reinforce the values and philosophy of the programme. The importance of fellowship, tolerance, humility and gratitude are stressed, as is the concept of staying sober 'One Day at a Time', that is, living in the present moment.

Finally, there are the meetings themselves, and the alchemy which takes place there. The following description is taken from Richard Walker's account of an AA meeting.

> *In a large measure, the meeting is the key to AA's phenomenal and unprecedented success. The meeting is a much more effective persuader and convincer than a book or a pamphlet. It is practically impossible to learn to swim, to drive a car, run a large corporation, or converse fluently in a modern language by reading a book. You have to get into the water, sit behind the wheel... beat your way up the economic ladder, live among foreigners and listen to the music of their inflection and cadence. AA is like that in many respects...The AA member sits in the audience and listens. He is not on the psychiatrist's couch and does not have to say a word. He can admit anything and everything to himself, but he need not tell anyone*

> *in the world about it. At least, not tonight. He may agree with the speaker*
> *or think silently to himself: 'That's bunk...' In his act of agreement or*
> *disagreement, he is beginning to think constructively about alcohol, himself,*
> *and AA. His process of mental recovery is under way.*[1]

Application of the Twelve Steps

In my experience, almost anyone can benefit from attending a Twelve Steps programme. The erroneous myth is that they are for vagrants, old men, those who have lost everything, people without families or friends to support them, 'fallen women', religious fanatics, and variations on these themes. Actually, the Twelve Steps are now being used in at least 30 different kinds of groups, dealing with cancer, depression, phobias, incest, impotence, child abuse, relationship problems and mental health problems; as well as in Narcotics Anonymous, Cocaine Addicts Anonymous, Gamblers Anonymous, Overeaters Anonymous, Sex and Love Addicts Anonymous, etc.

There are also groups to support the families of addicts, who are known as co-addicts and have a recognised personality profile of their own.[2] Although they are generally unaware of it, these people need help which is deeper and longer lasting than symptom relief from the stresses of living with an addict. Examples of such groups are Co-Dependents Anonymous; Adult Children of Alcoholics; Families Anonymous which is for parents of chemically dependent children; Al-Anon for family members and friends of alcoholics; Nar-Anon and Coc-Anon, for family members and friends of drug or cocaine addicts.

In some cases, Twelve Steps involvement can be a substitute for other therapy. However, they are not mutually exclusive and individual sessions can support what happens at AA groups and vice versa. The two primary benefits of Twelve Steps groups are firstly that they are free, and secondly that their members all share a common problem. A therapist who has a good working knowledge of the programme can support attendance of a group by interpreting it for the client, answering questions about it, countering misinformation, exploring resistance and denial and preparing the client to make as full use as possible of the immense amount of support and education which they can find in the group.

Being firmly convinced about the benefits of Twelve Steps programmes, I have, on occasions, refused individual treatment after a time if a client is not willing to accompany therapy with Twelve Steps attendance. My reason is that I cannot do for the client what the group can do. It is amazing how many emotional and physical symptoms clear up when people are able to share on an ongoing basis with others who are seeking recovery from the same addictive problem.

For newly recovering alcoholics, in big cities where many meetings take place each week, the recommendation by professionals working with chemical dependency and by AA members is 90 meetings in 90 days, which provides an excellent foundation for sobriety. In many areas there are few or no meetings, especially of groups like Co-Dependents Anonymous or Adult Children of Alcoholics. It is perfectly possible then for clients to correspond with others with similar problems (by writing first to the main headquarters of the particular group) or to start a group in their area, again by writing away for information on how to do this. The important thing is exposure to the ideas and philosophy of the programme, and to others with the same problem.

Through exposure problems are normalised and hope instilled. Participants are assured that no matter what their problem, others have had them too, and that no matter how great they seem, they can be lessened. Exposure also leads to education about the problem, about recovery from it, and about life and how to relate to people. Increased self-esteem results from knowing that one is not the only one with this problem; from learning to abstain from the addiction 'One Day at a Time'; and from becoming useful to others in a similar predicament. Participants gain spiritual and emotional understanding and growth in an atmosphere of warm fellowship, often punctuated by laughter where friendships form which provide a social life outside of meetings. This can be a new experience for many people formerly isolated by their addictions.

Case Histories

Of the following two case histories, the first concerns a woman who chose not to attend Al-Anon, the second, a woman who did, with predictably beneficial results.

◆ *A 60-year-old woman sought counselling to help her husband of 40 years to stop drinking. For at least 20 of those years his drinking had been heavy and an embarrassment and cause for concern. She listed the distressing ways he behaved and all of the stress-related illnesses she had acquired as a result of living with active alcoholism for so long without support. She had migraines, high blood pressure, and heart disease. And, in addition, she informed me rather self-righteously, she had a stiff neck. 'A stiff neck?' I enquired. 'Yes,' she said, 'a stiff neck from sleeping with a bottle of alcohol under my pillow.' 'Why do you sleep with a bottle of alcohol under your pillow?' I asked. 'Because he drinks up every drop in the house, and when guests come there isn't anything to offer them. Under my pillow is the only place he never looks.'*

Although extreme, these details capture well the extent to which co-dependent spouses can become hooked, until their lives are as completely consumed by the addict's behaviour as the addict is by the drug of their choice. When I suggested to this woman that there was no way in which I could directly influence her husband to stop drinking, but that her life could be immeasurably improved were she to pursue a combination of counselling for herself and Al-Anon, she declined. She was unable to imagine a recovery independent of being able to control her husband's behaviour.

◆ *The other woman was about 30 years old and in the process of divorcing her alcoholic husband. When she came for counselling she was depressed, living with her daughter in her parents' house, and convinced of her unsuitability to take up work of any kind; her self-esteem was very low. Her life was unstructured, except by the needs of her child. She was uncertain of her boundaries, which affected how she dealt with her estranged husband and his access to their child. After a year of both counselling and Al-Anon attendance, this woman was working as a secretary and had moved into her own accommodation with her daughter. Over the next few years she wrote to me occasionally, sharing her successes. She went from strength to strength, and rose to jobs of greater interest and responsibility. She became her own person.*

I strongly recommended Al-Anon in this second case, even though this woman was no longer living with her alcoholic husband, because she came from a family background which was dysfunctional, had married young, and had lived for close to ten years with a practising alcoholic who had intimidated and occasionally hit her. The patterns of such a relationship and the various kinds of wounds sustained in it are best healed by information about what being married to an alcoholic means, with the support of others who are or have been through a similar experience. I have found in many years of professional experience that treatment accompanied by Twelve Steps meetings has a profoundly synergistic effect.

Practice of the Twelve Steps

Attendance at meetings is usually at least weekly, though in early recovery it can be much more frequent. Meetings themselves differ in format depending on the kind of meeting it is and where it is being held. Some meetings discuss a recovery principle or some aspect of *Alcoholics Anonymous*, the main text of the Twelve Steps programme. Others are open sharings and still others have a main speaker who shares his experiences from his own recovery. Telling one's story at a meeting for the first time is a milestone in recovery. Meetings are generally of an hour's duration, often followed by informal time for coffee drinking and fellowship. A sponsorship system exists where newcomers can approach more experienced members and ask if they will be their sponsor. Though styles of sponsoring differ, in general it is suggested that one's sponsor be of the same gender (in heterosexual groups) thus side-stepping the temptation of sexual involvement. Some sponsors stay in touch by telephone; others simply make themselves available for discussion of the Steps, and recovery principles and in any possible crisis.

The programme works through openly acknowledged, mutual vulnerability. The Steps are worded in the plural, meaning 'we are all in the same boat'. Recovery is based on principles, not on the personalities of leaders or members. The fellowship is democratic; everyone, regardless of worldly status, education, race, gender or length of sobriety, is considered to be one drink (pill, gambling episode, etc.) away from their next addictive episode. This shared recognition of limitation is humbling and allows for the possibility of a power-greater-than-self to become involved. Most people experience this process as a relief, and, paradoxically, as ultimately empowering.

The Twelve Steps is a peer programme. What these peers have in common is not their great achievements, virtue or exaltedness; it is their humanness, their struggle, their experience, strength and hope. They share their need of one another as witness, support and friend, and their need of a power greater than themselves. As such, AA or the recovery movement is compatible with all the great religious and spiritual traditions, stressing co-operation, unity through diversity, respect for the individual, humility and service.

Here is Dr Bob's account of the impact his meeting with Bill W. had upon him:

I had read a great deal and talked to everyone who knew, or thought they knew anything about the subject of alcoholism. But this was a man who had experienced many years of frightful drinking, who had had most all the drunkard's experiences known to man... He gave me information about the subject of alcoholism which was undoubtedly helpful. Of far more importance was the fact that he was the first living human with whom I had ever talked, who knew what he was talking about in regard to alcoholism from actual experience. In other words, he talked my language... I spend a great deal of time passing on what I learned to others who want and need it badly. I do it for four reasons: 1. Sense of duty. 2. It is a pleasure. 3. Because in so doing I am paying my debt to the man who took time to pass it on to me. 4. Because every time I do it I take out a little more insurance for myself against a possible slip.[3]

My Personal Involvement

When starting to work in the field of addictions, I routinely recommended AA and Al-Anon to my patients as it was the policy of the hospital rehabilitation programme, and I had heard that these meetings had a better success rate for recovery than any other form of treatment. However, personally I had been influenced by the condescension I had experienced from a colleague who was openly negative about AA. So I felt that if AA had anything to offer, it was certainly only for others in crisis and would have no relevance for me.

It was a full year before I casually attended my first open AA meeting. I was astonished by what I experienced there. Although it was quite some time before I began to grasp the power and subtlety of the Steps, I saw at once how meaningful and inspiring the meetings were for the participants. I continued to attend open meetings because I found them enjoyable, informative and uplifting. Eventually I began going to other Twelve Steps groups which were more directly relevant to issues in my life. At all of these I found people who were coming to grips with often difficult and painful circumstances in a most self-responsible way, growing emotionally and spiritually and able to laugh at themselves in the process. Over time, I applied the Steps to my own life and have come to rely on them as my primary spiritual practice.

Appendix: The Twelve Steps of Alcoholics Anonymous

1 We admitted we were powerless over alcohol – that our lives had become unmanageable.

2 Came to believe that a Power greater than ourselves could restore us to sanity.

3 Made a decision to turn our will and our lives over to the care of God as we understood Him.

4 Made a searching and fearless moral inventory of ourselves.

5 Admitted to God, to ourselves, and to another human being the exact nature of our wrongs.

6 Were entirely ready to have God remove all these defects of character.

7 Humbly asked Him to remove our shortcomings.

8 Made a list of all persons we had harmed, and became willing to make amends to them all.

9 Made direct amends to such people wherever possible, except when to do so would injure them or others.

10 Continued to take personal inventory and when we were wrong promptly admitted it.

11 Sought through prayer and meditation to improve our conscious contact with God as we understood Him, praying only for knowledge of His will for us and the power to carry that out.

12 Having had a spiritual awakening as the result of these steps, we tried to carry this message to alcoholics, and to practise these principles in all our affairs.

Biography

Janice Eddy has a masters degree in counselling psychology, a certification from the State of Illinois as a senior addictions counsellor, and fifteen years of experience working in residential and outpatient treatment. For the past five years she has been in private practice in Scotland. She sees individuals and couples dealing with a wide range of issues, including separation, depression, mid-life crisis, and the empowerment of women. The major part of her training was in chemical dependency, and much of her past and present experience is in working with alcoholics and sex and relationship addicts, as well as with their partners and family members; i. e., the area known as co-dependency. Her familiarity with Twelve Steps fellowships is both personal and professional.

References

1   Richard Walker, *The Seven Points of Alcoholics Anonymous*, Glen Abbey Books, 1989, p35.

2   Timmen L Cermak, *Diagnosing and Treating Co-dependence; a Guide for Professionals who Work with Chemical Dependents, their Spouses and Children*, Johnson Institute Books, 1986.

3   *Alcoholics Anonymous*, Third Edition, A A Sterling Area Services, 1976, pp180-1.

Further Reading

Augustine Fellowship Staff, *Sex and Love Addicts Anonymous*, The Augustine Fellowship, 1986.

Beattie, Melody, *Beyond Codependency*, Harper & Row, 1989.

——, *Codependent No More*, Harper & Row, 1987.

Cermak, Timmen L., *Diagnosing and Treating Co-dependence; a Guide for Professionals who Work with Chemical Dependents, their Spouses and Children*, Johnson Institute Books, 1986.

Covington Stephanie; Beckett, Liana, *Leaving the Enchanted Forest: the Path from Relationship Addiction to Intimacy*, Harper & Row, 1988.

Cruse, Joseph R., *Painful Affairs; Looking for Love through Addiction and Co-dependency*, Health Communications, Inc., 1989.

Diamond, Jed, *Looking for Love in all the Wrong Places, Overcoming Romantic and Sexual Addictions*, Avon Books, 1988.

Fajardo, Roque, *Helping Your Alcoholic Before He or She Hits Bottom*, Crown Publishers, Inc., 1976.

Kurtz, E., *Not-God, a History of Alcoholics Anonymous*, Hazelden, 1979.

Lewis and Williams, *Providing Care for Children of Alcoholics, Clinical and Research Perspecitives*, Health Communications, Inc., 1986.

Maxwell, Ruth, *The Booze Battle*, Balantine Books, 1976.

Norwood, Robin, *Women Who Love too Much*, Arrow Books, 1986.

——, *Letters from Women Who Love too Much; a Closer Look at Relationship Addiction and Recovery*, Arrow Books, 1989.

Pursch, Joseph A., *Sober Alcoholics: Weller than Well*, The Village Voice, 1985.

Twerski, Abraham J., *Addictive Thinking*, Hazelden Foundation, 1990.

Wegschelder, Sharon, *Another Chance, Hope and Health for the Alcoholic Family*, Science and Behaviour Books, 1981.

——, *The Family Trap: No One Escapes from a Chemically Dependent Family*, The Johnson Institute, 1976.

Whitfield, Charles L M D., *Alcoholism, Other Drug Problems & Spirituality; a Transpersonal Approach*, The Resource Group, 1985.

Anon, *Intervention: a Professional's Guide*, The Johnson Institute, Minneapolis 1983.

Anon, *The Bill W – Carl Jung Letters*, ReVISION, The Journal of Consciousness and Change, Heldref Publications, 1987; Vol. 10: 2, 19-21.

Anon, *The 12 Steps, a Way Out; a Working Guide for Adult Children of Alcoholic & Other Dysfunctional Families*, Recovery Publications, 1995.

Resources

An excellent resource in any area in the UK is either the Citizens' Advice Bureau or the Samaritans. They will probably know where meetings are in any area. The following central offices also give information on local meetings.

UK:

Alcoholics Anonymous
P O Box 1
Stonebow House
Stonebow
York YO1 2NJ
Tel. 01904-644026/7/8/9

Narcotics Anonymous
P O Box 704
London SW10 0RP
Tel. 0171-351 6794

Overeaters Anonymous
c/o Manor Gardens Centre
6-9 Manor Gardens
London N7 6LA

Co-dependants Anonymous UK
Ashburnham Community Centre
Tetcott Road
London SW10 0SH
Tel. 0171-376 8191

Al-Anon Family Groups
Great Dover Street
London SE1 4YF
Tel. 0171-403 0888

USA:

A. A. General Service Office
Grand Central Station
New York, NY 10163
Al-Anon Family Group Headquarters
P O Box 862
Midtown Station
New York, N. Y. 10018

Narcotics Anonymous
World Service Office
16155 Wyandotte St
Van Nuys, California 91406
Tel. 818-780 3951

Overeaters Anonymous
World Service Office
2190 190th St
Torrance, California 90504

Co-dependents Anonymous USA
P O Box 33577
Phoenix, Arizona 85067-3577
Tel. 602-277 7991

Adult Children of Alcoholics
Central Service Board
P O Box 3216
Torrance, California 90505

Debtors Anonymous
P O Box 21322
New York NY 10025 – 9992

Emotions Anonymous
P O Box 4245
St Paul
Minnesota 55104

Gamblers Anonymous
P O Box 17173
Los Angeles, California 90017

Visualisation
by David Lawson

Theoretical Background

The visual sense and the continual reference to it within our language and culture is an important component of individual and collective experience. It is a key to how most of us make sense of the world around us, create our understanding of our place within the greater scheme of things and find common ground for communication. This is not to diminish the importance of our other senses but to highlight the significance of vision and visualisation in the process of healing and personal evolution. Even those who are born without sight or who become visually impaired at some time during their lives retain some degree of inner vision and remain steeped in a culture and a language that is full of visual references.

The world of dreams has always taught us much about our inner needs, fears, drives and inspirations. Predictions of future events, scientific breakthroughs, solutions, inventions and transformational leaps of consciousness have often come to light through the dream images of sleep or the daydreams that we experience during our waking hours. Many of these breakthroughs arrive with literal or symbolic visual information that helps us to make sense of them and put them into action.

Historically humankind has been drawn to the visual arts as a way of expressing an abundance of creative energy, making sense of common experience, communicating, informing or instructing. We have done this by making direct visual representations of the world around us and by creating symbols to make sense of inner feelings or concepts. Arts and crafts have been harnessed or adapted for therapeutic purposes and the practice of dream interpretation has spawned many approaches, books and branches of therapy.

In recent times the use of visualisation in itself has been popularised as a method of relaxation, self-healing and self-actualisation. Its purpose is to direct the mind towards images, concepts and ideas that will stimulate changes throughout the entire physical, emotional and energetic system. During a process of relaxation or meditation, specific images are chosen for the participant to picture or conceptualise within their own

Relaxation Therapy
Transcendental
Meditation
Transformational
Self-Healing
Stress Management
Hypnotherapy

mind. A visualisation can be self-directed, guided by a therapist, followed from an audio tape or scripted for friends to guide each other through the required images.

Visualisation essentially works in two ways. First, the images chosen are generally positive and calming, selected for their potential to alter the mood, discharge stress and balance the emotions. The vibrational quality of positive visual images has a tonic effect on the energetic system that supports the natural healing processes of the mind, body and spirit. They send out healthy signals to the whole person rather than the disruptive signals that come with negative, fearful or disturbing images and thought forms. A highly stressed city-dweller visualising beautiful woodland is able to draw from a vocabulary of memories, feelings and images that will help to induce a state of relaxation and create messages of peace and balance.

Second, visualisation works by directing thoughts away from the current illness or problem and towards a desired outcome; creating the mental reality of health first, as a way of supporting the user in creating the physical reality. The theory is that what we think about or picture, we are more likely to create in our bodies and in our lives. It is for this reason that people with cancer have been taught to visualise their immune system taking control and destroying their cancerous cells. Symbols can also be used as documented by the Simontons,[1] who did much research in this area. For example, the cancerous cells are symbolised as cabbages being devoured by rabbits that represent the immune system. In this way, visualisation gives the body a direct message to heal itself.

The Practice of Visualisation

Counselling
Spiritual Healing

Counsellors, healers, doctors or complementary therapists are able to work with visualisation to achieve a number of desired effects with their clients. The use of visualisation can build a good relationship between both parties, giving the client reassurance, hope and trust in the therapies on offer. Health care professionals can guide visualisations whilst undertaking tests and examinations, or prior to procedures that require the client to be as relaxed as possible. In addition, clients can be taught to use visualisation techniques at home between consultations, so that they are working with their therapist as an active partner in the healing process.

Visualisation can be used as part of a regular practice of preventative care and to help in the management of ongoing conditions and symptoms. Picturing ease of mobility in arthritic joints, for instance, can be an important part of a self-care programme that includes an appropriate diet, herbal remedies and carefully chosen medication. It is important to use visualisation as part of a combined approach, where appropriate treatments are used and changes in lifestyle made, as well as visualising our bodies in full and perfect health.

In cases where unresolved issues from the past are inhibiting our present physical, mental or emotional health, visualisation can be used to access old memories or feelings so that we can review them and make new choices about our lives. Sometimes, seemingly innocuous images can bring powerful feelings to the surface to be acknowledged and resolved. The positive, peaceful focus that visualisation induces provides a safe environment for underlying tensions to become visible before they dissolve. The act of visualising health and balance may displace anything that is contributing to a state of imbalance, so that health can be achieved.

Affirmations

Visualisation and all positive thought techniques work directly on the most important relationship of all, the relationship we have with ourselves. How else can we create health and love in our lives if we don not see ourselves as healthy and lovable, and deserving of these things? The use of visualisation is a powerful way of accessing innate abilities and providing a key to positive changes that go beyond the creation of health and well-being and into the realms of personal evolution and spiritual growth. It is sometimes the simplicity of a positive visual image that can provide us with the most profound transformation of consciousness.

There are common frustrations that people may experience when they begin to practise visualisation: some may worry if they are not able to create clear pictures in their minds whilst others find their thoughts moving off at a tangent into ideas and images that do not appear to be directly related. Here are some suggestions to help sustain an ongoing process of effective visualisation.

◆ The ideal environment is a safe, quiet place that is warm and comfortable. Distractions can be minimised by unplugging telephones and ensuring that other people will not interrupt. Music in the background can be used to help relaxation but not if it has lyrics that would fight for attention.

Once the images and techniques are familiar, they can be practised in many situations, for instance while sitting on a bus (but the above scenario is the easiest). They are not to be used while driving a car or in any other situation where concentration is required.

◆ It is important to sit comfortably with the back properly supported. Keeping the arms and legs, hands and feet uncrossed, so that the body is open and receptive. Breathing deeply and slowly throughout the visualisation ensures that the body will remain warm.

◆ Personal images can be used or visualisations that have been found in a book or on a tape. As well as using images that are generally relaxing, such as those drawn from the beauty of the natural world, it is important to tailor images to the specific health needs: picture the body in full health or visualise the fractured bone mending itself rapidly.

◆ It is not important to follow every detail of a visualisation exercise exactly. (It would not be very relaxing to feel that one has to work hard to get all of the details correct and in the right order.) A tape recording can be made in advance using the text from a book.

◆ Some people have a natural ability to think in pictures while for others it comes only with practice. Regardless of how the mind works, the intention is much more important than the ability to get strong visual images. Just holding the concept, the idea or the feeling of the picture in the mind is enough for these techniques to work.

◆ Giving the mind the freedom to play is more beneficial than trying hard to be absolutely accurate. With practice, visualisation becomes easier. With any visualisation exercise it is important to adapt the images to changing needs or special preferences; after a while the imagination automatically extends and enhances them.

Some people will find that their ability to create stronger and clearer images as they visualise will increase with practice whilst others will continue to have only vague images on an occasional basis. Many proceed effectively with visualisation techniques using the concept, the idea or the feeling of the images rather than the images themselves.

Someone who thinks in words rather than in pictures can paint the images in words: 'I am now walking through a beautiful forest with green and yellow birds flying around me and an abundance of flowers and tropical plants on all sides...' A sensual person who is more sensitive to the sound, taste, touch or smell of the environment than to visual images could imagine feeling the ground beneath their feet as they walk, the sound of the bird song, the smell of the flowers and the freshness of the air.

A General Visualisation for Health and Well-Being

Picture yourself looking at your own reflection in a full length mirror. If it helps, you could do this in reality first and then sit or lie down in a comfortable spot, close your eyes and re-create the image in your mind. In your mind's eye, hold the picture or the idea of your reflection. How are you dressed? What is your hair like? What shape would your outline make in silhouette? What is your posture like? What is the look that you have in your eyes?

Colour Therapy

Once you have built the image or concept of your reflection imagine yourself bathed and surrounded with healing light energy. Give the light a colour that you instinctively feel would be healing or protective at this time and imagine every cell of your body drinking in this abundant healing energy.

Picture your clothes dissolving in the light, so that you are completely naked and as you do, imagine all tensions and fears dropping away from you. Visualise every area of your body regenerating and rejuvenating in the light – damaged, diseased, weakened or scarred tissue totally re-creating itself. Your body rediscovers its natural healthy state, full of strength and vitality. See yourself renewed and recharged, physically, mentally, emotionally and spiritually.

To complete this visualisation, picture yourself dressing in a new set of clothing that is more beautiful and more comfortable than anything that you have worn before. Imagine yourself surrounded by a charismatic aura of safety and protection that keeps you magnetic to positive, healthy relationships, situations and environments. Affirm to yourself: 'I see myself in perfect health.'

Biography

David Lawson is an international healer and a teacher of personal development courses who has worked chiefly in the U. K., Ireland, Spain and the USA. He is an authorised facilitator of Louise L. Hay's 'You Can Heal Your Life' study course programme and a therapist offering hands-on healing, counselling, meditational techniques and regression. A leading expert in self-help and self-healing techniques, Lawson is the author of several books.

Further Reading

Achterberg, Jeanne, *Imagery in Healing: Shamanism and Modern Medicine*, Shambhala, 1985.

Borysenko, Joan, *Minding the Body, Mending the Mind*, Simon & Schuster, 1989.

Bresler, D., *Free Yourself from Pain*, The Bresler Centre, 1992.

Bry, A.; Bair, M., *Directing the Movies of the Mind: Visualization for Health and Insight*, Harper & Row, 1978.

Gawain, Shakti, *Creative Visualisation*, Bantam Books, 1978.

———, *Living in the Light*, Whatever Publishing Inc., 1980.

Glouberman, Dina, *Life Choices and Life Changes through Image Work*, Unwin paperbacks, 1989.

Hay, Louise, *You can Heal Your Life*, Hay House/Eden Grove Editions, 1995.

Jaffe, D., *Healing from Within: Psychological Techniques to Help the Mind Heal the Body*, Simon and Schuster, 1988.

Lawson, David, *I See Myself in Perfect Health – Your Essential Guide to Self-Healing*, Thorsons/HarperCollins, 1995.

———, *Principles of Self-healing*, Thorsons/HarperCollins, 1996.

Lerner, Michael, *Choices in Healing – Integrating the Best of Conventional and Complementary Approaches to Cancer*, The MIT Press, 1994.

Millenson, J R., *Mind Matters – Psychological Medicine in Holistic Practice*, Churchill Livingstone, 1995.

Pietroni, Patrick & Christopher, *Innovation in Community Care and Primary Health*, Churchhill Livingstone, 1996, p146-51.

Porter, G.; Norris, P., *Why Me? Harnessing the Healing Power of the Human Spirit*, Stillpoint, 1985.

Roman, S., *Spiritual Growth – Being Your Higher Self*, H J Kramer, 1988.

Rossman, M., *Healing Yourself: A Step-by-Step Program to Better Health Through Imagery*, Walker & Co, 1987.

Schneider, J. et al., *Guided imagery and immune system function in normal subjects: a summary of research findings*, in *Mental imagery*, (ed. R G Kunzendorf), Plenum Press, 1991.

Sheikh, A., *Imagination and Healing*, Baywood, Farmingdale, 1984.

Simonton, Carl; Matthews-Simonton, Stephanie; Creighton, James, *Getting Well Again: A Step-by Step Guide to Overcoming Cancer for Patients and Their Families*, Bantam, 1986.

Singer, J L.; Pope, K S., *The Power of Human Imagination*, Plenum Press, 1978.

Audio Tapes

Lawson, David, *I See Myself in Perfect Health – Volumes I and II – Guided Meditations*, Healing Workshops Press, 1990.

Resources

The Academy for Guided Imagery
P O Box 2070
Mill Valley
CA 94942
USA

The Institute of Transpersonal Psychology
744 San Antonio Road
Palo Alto
CA 94303
USA

Yoga
by Jane Stuart

My Personal Experience

Describing the effect of the practice and influence of yoga, I want to start with my own experience and how it affected my daily life. I was feeling tired, dispirited and slightly ill on a cold winter's day in February, 20 years ago. I was 40 years old, an American living in Scotland in a remote Highland valley, amongst people whose culture and language seemed quite alien to me. Snow beat against the windows of my bedroom and the idea of going for a walk seemed insane. I felt tears of despair welling up as I began to feel sorry for myself.

On the table beside me lay B.K.S. Iyengar's Light on Yoga, a book I had sold hundreds of copies of when I had run a bookshop in London. I used to thumb through it, look at the pictures and wonder how anyone would want to wrap themselves in knots like that. Yehudi Menuhin, a devoted student of B.K.S. was on the advisory board of my shop, and he and devoted students were constantly extolling the virtues and benefits of yoga. I chose not to hear them. As far as I was concerned, yoga seemed a little bizarre and not active enough. I could not imagine how it would get my heart-rate up to desirable aerobic standards. Meanwhile the snow drove harder against my windows.

I picked up the yoga book and started to look through it. I stopped at a picture of an exercise called 'The Bow' and thought, 'Well, I might as well give it a try...' I read Iyengar's instructions and after half an hour of trying this and various other poses, I felt a sense of well-being and elation. So I continued the next day, and the next and the next. I felt surges of well-being as I had experienced in my youth. It was as if someone had handed me the keys to the kingdom where indigestion, aches in my joints, tiredness and depression had been banished, as long as I continued the daily practice.

The weeks went by and my family and friends noticed changes in me. I stood taller, my eyes were brighter and the energy I gave out was almost palpable – I felt myself exuding it. In addition there was a mental change. I could concentrate on jobs which needed doing, I had wells of interest which my practice seemed to release thereby allowing me to express myself with joy and passion. I was hooked.

Finally I sought teachers and became a teacher myself. I practised Iyengar's method for twelve years after which I switched to that of Wanda Scaravelli, after studying with Mary Stewart, her teacher in Britain.

Yoga changed my life and I believe it can change the lives of others. The practice brought me new self-awareness, as well as physical benefits. I began to feel more compassionate towards others and in time found the energy to train as a counsellor for drug addiction and alcohol dependence.

Yoga and Diet

Another influence of yoga on my life was that I changed my diet and became a passionate cook. Yogis believe that food can change consciousness. There are three categories of food: *sattvic* which is pure food – raw milk, butter, fruit, vegetables and grains; *rajasic* which is spicy food with powerful flavours and a stimulating effect on the nervous system, such as meat, fish, eggs and alcohol; and *tamasic* which is impure food – overripe, spoiled or contaminated in some way.

Nutritional Therapy

Obviously the consumption of these foods causes a corresponding state of mind. Tamasic foods cause a gross state of consciousness, rajasic foods cause an intermediate state, while sattvic foods cause a state conducive to a spiritual outlook. If the milk and butter in the sattvic category are made from raw, unpasteurised milk and cream, these foods can be considered alkaline foods. Alkaline foods produce an environment in the body which supports health, and our daily diet would be much more beneficial if we included more alkaline foods, i.e. salads, vegetables and fruits (millet is the only alkaline grain), while moderating our intake of acid-forming foods, such as starches, sugar, meat, fish, eggs, chicken and cheese. An excess of acid foods can cause symptoms such as headaches, insomnia, nausea, depression or arthritis.

As I experimented with diet, I became aware that eating different foods affected both my physical body and my mental attitudes. When I followed the principles of eating sattvic foods, grains and vegetables, combining pulses to make proteins, I found that I could stretch a lot more easily into my practice and I felt much more dynamic and centred. But above all my yoga practice has taught me about flexibility, in relation to diet as well as everything else.

My greatest personal search was for the root causes of my frequent migraines. With practice and research, trial and elimination, I found which foods affected me badly, and learned the asanas or yoga postures which relieved my distress. When I changed to Mary Stewart's way of teaching and learned meditation, my headaches became few and far between, and of far less severity.

Yoga fills my life, from early morning practice to evening meditation. Yoga postures have done for me just what they were designed to do thousands of years ago, which is to bring the body into health and harmony, so that the student can sit still with spine straight to meditate in perfect harmony.

The Practice of Yoga

Yoga can be learned through practice. The daily routine rests with the individual. A teacher and regular classes are guidelines and not to be used in place of the student's consistent work.

Obviously care is needed in choosing a good teacher, one who is experienced and qualified. There are countless schools of yoga and the student is advised to choose carefully among those who pay strict attention to physical alignment and good body mechanics. Yoga is a science as well as an art, so correct guidelines and precise instructions are required for the execution of each asana. Classes on a regular basis are useful to correct any mistakes students may be making on their own. Bad habits in yoga are dangerous and can be repeated over and over again unless corrected by a teacher.

The body is a brilliant piece of architecture in which each bone is balanced and each muscle and tendon is designed to support these bones and to keep the body upright. The foot turned as little out or in as one inch can cause stress and strain the whole way up, from the ankle to the knee, then to the hip, into the spine and the neck. Reserves of energy are used when the body is trying to adjust to these strains and to right itself, and sore backs and knees soon result. The teacher's job is to know how to place those feet exactly in the right position.

From my own experience, I would say that anyone can practise yoga. Age does not matter; neither does size or general state of health. Stiffness need not put off a prospective student, and even those who can hardly stretch into the poses should not be downhearted. Inch by inch, flexibility will increase and the benefits reaped will be experienced on an even greater scale.

Yoga lasts a lifetime. When students start to practise properly, the spine will elongate and they will begin to feel parts of the body they thought they had forgotten, or perhaps even never known existed. Imagine a head poised on a beautifully balanced spine which in turn arises from two legs balanced on feet which are spread with their toes separated to provide a platform for the torso to soar. This is how a body should be.

If, when you wake up in the morning, you open your eyes, close them again and wish you could stay in bed for ever, try this instead: stretch your body, feel yourself growing heavier and heavier, sinking down. Keeping your mind free, drop your jaw and relax your face. You are beginning your practice now. If you grasp this idea the moment you wake up and if you think about the next half hour as being the time you use to arrange your body and mind for the rest of the day, you will learn very quickly to make yoga a part of even the busiest schedule.

To begin with, I learned from a book. I read and practised, for in those days there were no yoga classes in my area. Now no one will have that problem for there are classes even in remote areas. Yoga is recognised, sought after and hailed. In New York there are long waiting lists for classes. The key to vibrant health and the tapping of the organism's enormous reserves of latent energy, yoga has become the discipline of our generation.

My husband is a case in point. When I first started to practise yoga, he wondered what on earth had got into me. One day he hobbled in from the garden, his back twisted like a corkscrew. After four or five remedial poses he got relief from the pain. He wanted to know more and more. The next day I found him practising and now he has hardly missed his half hour daily practice in years. On the weekends he extends it to an hour.

The Role of Yoga in the West

It is known that our physiological processes are within the realm of our conscious control. We can learn 'to play with' our internal organs and systems. We are within sight of turning on and off mental and physical states the way one switches on and off the radio. Yogis have been doing this for centuries before biofeedback verified the results to doubting Westerners. An example is a practice called *tuma*, which is the way to stimulate heat in the body. This was and still is the art of yogis who spend the winter in Tibet in snowy caves at high altitudes wearing nothing but wisps of cloth for warmth. Some of the methods of achieving this state are visualisation, concentration, meditation and breath control.

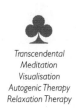

Transcendental Meditation
Visualisation
Autogenic Therapy
Relaxation Therapy

In Scotland where I live, the practice of a few of these techniques has revolutionised my ability to keep warm. I may not live in an igloo, but I am able to control my shivers and increase my circulation in a dramatic way.

People in the West are accused of being self-obsessed, especially in America. In that respect psychology and yoga join hands. The subconscious is a traffic jam and when the snarl is uncovered, steps can be taken to change the damaging behaviour. Yoga practice reveals on a physical level how these snarl ups have translated over the years into stiffness in the body. So in both psychotherapy and yoga one has to look inward in order to free oneself to be more outward, in a balanced way.

Psychotherapy
Bio-Energetic Analysis

Applications

To detail that which can be benefited by yoga would read like a novel, while what cannot at least be improved would be a short story.

Speaking from personal experience, the benefits to my health have been enormous. My flagging endocrine system has been revitalised by inversion poses, headstand and shoulder stand; a low thyroid function was brought up to normal. Abnormally low blood pressure has been equalised and constipation banished for ever. All the women in my family suffer from severe arthritis and when I started yoga my joints were already stiffening. It was difficult to move properly. Now, at 57, I am as limber as most people half my age. When I started practising I drank vast amounts of coffee and craved sugar, no doubt to stimulate my adrenal glands. With time I began to be satisfied with cups of light tea, and a sugar lift is not what I need anymore. Indigestion has been helped and now if I am on one of my frequent trips abroad, I have keys to unlock and banish any discomfort. A few years ago when I was in New York I spent the day at the Metropolitan Museum. After a heavy lunch I was feeling bloated and uncomfortable. I went to the ladies' room, lined myself up against a wall and proceeded to do a yoga pose called 'arda chandrasana' where one stands, balanced on one leg with the other stretched out to the side. A few loud gurgles and I soon felt normal. Several women in the queue said they would like to learn to do that too. They all seemed to suffer from some kind of digestive upset. Before I knew it, I had a yoga class going in the ladies' room. I still receive letters from some of these women who have gone on to study yoga.

Stress Management

One of the greatest areas where yoga can help is in the management and relief of stress. Prevention is even more effective than cure. One claim is that people who practise yoga have 40% fewer illnesses, such as cancer and heart disease. Powerful chemicals are released into the bloodstream during practice and these can alter the physical state of the body, releasing dramatic protective powers.

Pranayama is the science of the breath. Yogis believe that it is the power behind regeneration of every cell in the body. *Prana* means breath and *yama* means stretching, expansion and lengthening. The length of your life is determined by how many breaths you take. Ekken, a seventeenth century mystic writes:

> *If you would foster a calm spirit, first regulate the breath, for when that is under control, the heart will be at peace, but when your breathing is spasmodic, then you will be troubled. Therefore before attempting anything, first regulate your breath in which your temper will be softened and your spirit calmed.*

Using the techniques perfected in yoga to regulate the breath and all other systems in the body will bring vitality and resilience, joy and elation, which can bring about dramatic positive changes in anyone's life. Whatever it was that prompted me to pick up *Light on Yoga* lying on my table all those years ago gave me the answer by chance. I would hope that everyone who reads this will be inspired to take up yoga because each day with a practice, however short, will yield more than a day without it.

Biography

Jane Stuart was born in Kentucky USA and studied in Washington and Montreal, Canada before marrying a Scot and moving to Tahiti where she assisted the Smithsonian Institute in shell collecting. She began studying yoga in 1975 in London under Maxine Tobias in the Iyengar system and began teaching in 1985. In 1986 she met Mary Stewart and began to practise the method of Wanda Scaravelli, and in 1988 began to teach this way of yoga. She teaches in the UK and spends part of the year in the USA.

Further Reading

Eliade, Mircea, *Patanjali and Yoga*, Schocken Books, 1975.

Hutchinson, Ronald, *Yoga – A Way of Life*, Reed, 1974.

Iyengar, B K S., *Light on yoga sutras of Patanjali*, Aquarian Press, 1993.

Iyengar, Geeta S., *Yoga, A Gem for Women*, Timeless Books, 1991.

McCartney, James, *Philosophy and Practice of Yoga*, L Fowler and Co., 1978.

Nagarathna, Dr., *Yoga for Common Ailments*, Gaia Books, 1991.

Rama, Swami, *Lectures on Yoga*, The Himalayan Int. Institute, 1979.

Stewart, Mary, *Yoga over 50*, Simon & Schuster, 1994.

Todd, Mabel Elsworth, *The Thinking Body*, Princeton Book Co., 1980.

Vishnudevananda, Swami, *The Complete Illustrated Book of Yoga*, Harmony Books, 1980.

Resources

Mary Stewart
Flat 0
55 Hans Road
London SW1

British Wheel of Yoga
1 Hamilton Place
Boston Road
Sleaford
Lincs NG34 7ES
Tel. 0529-306 851

The Iyengar Yoga Institute
223A Randolph Avenue
London W9 1NL
Tel. 0171-624 3080

The Yoga Biomedical Trust
P O Box 140
Cambridge CB4 3SY
Tel. 01223-367 301
Fax. 01223-313 587

The Yoga for Health Foundation
Ickwell Bury
Biggleswade
Beds SG18 9EF
Tel. 01767-627 271

Part 3 | Essays

Building Health: The Peckham Experiment

by Lisa Curtice and Douglas Trotter

We doctors are engaged in weary patchwork therapy... Peckham has shown the other way; it has shown how wholeness in human relationships, in family, food and play, means absence of disorder.

— W W Yellowlees

(in a letter to the *Lancet*, 25 March, 1950, on the closure of the Peckham Health Centre)

Our intention was neither to cure nor to prevent disease. It was to find a practical means, based on scientific knowledge, of releasing hitherto unexpressed potentialities of the human organism for living.

— Innes Pearse

(in Introduction to *The Quality of Life*)

The Nature of the Experiment

In 1926 two British doctors, George Scott Williamson and Innes Hope Pearse, began an experiment into the nature of health.[1] They sought to apply biological principles to human society in order to understand the conditions which would enable health to flourish. Their work grew from the insight that health is a positive quality, not defined simply by the absence of disease.[2] They believed that human beings had a natural capacity for health. To seek a deeper understanding of health, the doctors, both research scientists, set up an exploratory social experiment. The question which Scott Williamson asked was, 'What sort of conditions will enable people to be free to make choices that will enrich their own growth and development?' Put another way, how can it become a lifelong habit to make healthy and life-enhancing choices? This chapter describes the Peckham Experiment and reflects upon its qualitative significance for building positive health today.

The Peckham Experiment was a laboratory for the study of family health. It took the form of a family club in a purpose-built centre in Peckham, South London, which ran for a period of eight years between 1935 and 1950 (the building was closed during the war). The Peckham Health Centre provided a unique range of social and leisure facilities, including a swimming pool, a gymnasium, a self-service cafeteria and nurseries.[3] The centre was run according to a philosophy of empowerment for member families.[4] The design of the centre was in itself innovative, being open-plan and full of light.[5] The building, designed by the engineer Owen Williams, had an impressive glass exterior which, when illuminated at night, resembled an ocean-going liner. To members it seemed full of warmth, movement and purposeful activity. The centre was more than a leisure club or community centre because an important part of the life of members was a system of annual health checks and constant, informal health education. The centre did not provide curative medicine, but instead encouraged members to experience positive health and to learn what they could do to attain it.

Peckham was chosen for the site of the Experiment because it was a socially mixed area, neither excessively affluent nor extremely deprived. There was some evidence of social cohesiveness, for example in the number of voluntary groups active in the area. To belong to the Pioneer Health Centre members had to live within the vicinity (pram-pushing distance), pay a small fee, join as a family and have a thorough health check every year. There is evidence that people from all walks of life joined the centre. Housing conditions in pre-war Peckham gave the centre an added appeal. The slipper baths were popular with adults and the children loved the opportunity to learn to swim and the sense of space and freedom as they trampolined or roller-skated. To members, the centre offered not only a place to go and something to do but a sense of belonging. The life of the centre became interwoven with their lives at the deepest level because it played an increasingly indispensable part in major events, particularly the birth of children

How the Experiment Worked

The purpose of establishing the centre was to find out what happened if people could opt to find their own way within a social environment that was sufficiently rich and varied to provide them with opportunities to expand and develop their lives. Scott Williamson aimed to develop an atmosphere in which people at all stages of life had the opportunity to develop friendships, follow new interests and imperceptibly develop healthy habits, for example, in eating and exercise. Choice was fundamental to his plan because he wanted to study the results of people's own decisions in as naturalistic a setting as possible within the constraints of a research experiment.[6] From the innovative self-service equipment which he designed for the cafeteria, to the ticket system by which children got permission from staff to use the facilities to pursue an activity of their choice, the workings of the centre were structured to promote the maximum flexibility and ease so that large numbers of people could use it at the same time. Activities were not prescribed; the aim was to provide space and opportunities for people to engage in the activities of their choice.

Lucy Crocker, the co-author with Innes Pearse of *The Peckham Experiment*,[7] was largely responsible for establishing the social processes in the centre that enabled it to function harmoniously. This did not happen immediately or automatically, but was the result of a period of waiting, watching, listening, learning and responding –

a period of trial and error. For example, initially instructors were employed for various activities, but it was found that this discouraged those who had not yet developed those particular skills, so more emphasis was placed on people learning from each other. The Experiment demonstrated that there was more often a need to remove barriers that created social exclusion than provide yet more structure, even that which was intended to be supportive.

Scott Williamson trained his staff to observe and analyse the patterns of activity amongst members of the centre. Knowledge of the member families and of the patterning of social life within the centre was gained by observation, by taking part in its social life, by systematic recording (for example, of the children's activities) and by talking. This was not a 'pure' scientific experiment in the classic sense, but an exploratory demonstration project that aimed to promote change and learn from it. The significance of everything that was happening was constantly discussed, shared and fed back, not only amongst staff but to members themselves, so that everyone became active participants in the endeavour to understand and nurture health.

On a typical Saturday night before the war, when the centre was at its peak, the whole building would be buzzing with activity. A dance would be taking place in the long room which ran along one side of the building on the first floor. A game of pool might be in progress. In the crèche, the babies would be asleep; elsewhere the older children could make their own entertainment, coming to the cafeteria from time to time to speak to their parents or a staff member. Everywhere there was talk and activity. Whole families might be present but they were not necessarily together all the time; each person had their own things to do, people to see, news to exchange.

Peckham philosophy and practice tried to build a bridge between the home and the outside world. At Peckham it was possible for the parents of young children to continue to have a social life and pursue an interest without feeling that they were neglecting their children for whom they knew adequate provision and opportunities were being made. Young children were not segregated from older children and knew the kinds of things that they did. By the time a child was ready to move from the nursery to playing in the gym, that child would feel at home there and confident enough to join in. Use of the centre followed a pattern dictated by the needs of all the members of the local community, rather than by bureaucratic convenience. Mothers and young children used the centre during the day. Older children joined them after school. Later in the evening teenagers and couples arrived. This arrangement also provided ample opportunity for people to have informal contact with a range of people who were at the same stage of life as themselves.

A key lesson from Peckham then was freedom of access for the community to leisure and social facilities. This freedom was also reflected in the opening hours of the centre which were from 2 p.m. to 10 p.m. and 11 p.m. on Saturdays. Latterly, parents established a school which meant that part of the centre was also used during the mornings. Such an approach meant that people were more readily able to incorporate the use of such facilities into their own family activities and to use them as a natural extension of their own social networks.

The Knowledge and Practice of Family Health

With the expertise of Dr Innes Pearse, care of the growth and development of babies and young children was made central to the life of the centre, contributing to the cohesiveness of the community of members and providing a strong incentive for member families to participate in the ways of living that developed out of their contact with the centre.[8] The observable and evidenced well-being of 'the centre babies' was one of the clearest measures of the centre's success, and it was a tragedy that the closure of the centre prevented the longer-term follow-up of the health of children born and nurtured according to its principles. For couples, advice was given before and after conception and great attention was paid to enhancing nutritional status and general well-being. Breast-feeding was encouraged and the nursery was

Preconceptual Care

used to promote an enlightened and unrestrictive approach to infant and preschool development, the legacy of which may be traced in the preschool play group movement.[9] Less tangibly, but perhaps critically, the centre enhanced the status of parenthood, supporting the confidence of parents-to-be and new parents. A baby arrived into a culture where it was welcomed and the parents continued to be supported through convenient daily contact with other parents and by information on how to approach developmental stages, such as weaning. Moreover, having a

Family Therapy

new baby did not enforce a break with their social contacts as the crèche enabled them to socialise in the evening. Older children were always welcomed and fully catered for in the centre.

Every year members were given a comprehensive health overhaul which had several unique features. First, all family members were seen together. Second, the information and facts were given back and explained to the members themselves and there was as much emphasis on the positive findings – what was right with people – as on problems identified. Lastly people were left free to decide whether they wanted to seek treatment for any problems; this was never imposed and was not provided within the centre itself. The annual health overhauls of all centre members, which were offered in the evenings for working people, combined both scientific and health promotion objectives. Comprehensive screening tests of people's functioning provided data about the health of members and how it changed over time. The results were published, notably in *The Peckham Experiment*, but unfortunately the original records were destroyed in a fire, preventing long term assessment of significant changes in the activity of children and parents. Observational accounts tell of dimensions of health that went beyond what the screening tests could tell, although they may have been reflected in changes in physical status – an increased vitality, enjoyment of life and improved self-confidence.

The holistic approach to family health developed at Peckham is illustrated by the approach to nutrition. The emphasis was on learning through active experience. So, for example, in the cafeteria members became used to organically grown food from a farm in Kent which was run by the centre. Pregnant mothers and families with young children were able to obtain organic milk. Parents took part themselves in preparing the nursery teas. At the farm the families found out how food was grown. Some of them farmed there during the war and afterwards many families spent weekends and camping holidays on the centre farm. The knowledge and experience of any aspect of health at Peckham was imparted informally, through casual chatting in the centre; about food, about child rearing and about any other aspect of daily experience. Health information became a part of the shared experience of members – a natural product of life within the centre.

After the War

During the war, the centre had been closed and used as a munitions factory and the families dispersed. After the war, a group of families successfully clamoured for the centre to be re-opened. It was the subject of huge publicity and visited by people from all over the world. A film was made by Paul de Rotha, on behalf of the Central Office of Information, with the participation of member families, to show the centre's active life. The original building had been financed by large charitable donations and the running costs funded by the research funding and member subscriptions. Now, not only did the building need a lot spending on it, but bombing had destroyed many homes, and the goal, never yet achieved, of making the centre self-funding through member subscriptions, was not attainable.

Despite the inspiration which the Pioneer Health Centre provided to countless visitors, it did not become the model for health centres in the United Kingdom within the new National Health Service. Bevan, the Minster for Health who created the NHS, was inspired by the centre and supportive of it, but continued support for its research, the *raison d'être* of the centre, was rejected by the Medical Research Council, which did not perceive its approach, considered from a statistical basis, as being of scientific value. Scott Williamson chaired a committee on the role of health centres in the new NHS, but his attempt to shape the new health service in a direction that concentrated on the promotion of positive health, in contrast to disease care, was against the trend. Attlee's post-war Labour government's plans for general medical services did not accept Scott Williamson's premise that there should be a clear separation between the cultivation of health and the treatment of disease.

As for the Pioneer Health Centre itself, there were plans in hand to have a doctor from the centre register with the NHS. Unfortunately, in negotiations for a rescue package with the London County Council, it proved impossible to retain both the health and social aspects of the centre. The only option for survival was an unacceptably narrow version of its previous activity, therefore the decision was taken to close. The building itself was sold to the London County Council for use as an adult education centre and survives today, although the purpose of the open plan design has become blurred by dividing walls.

Principles of the Peckham Experiment

The living legacy of Peckham is a knowledge of positive health and of the conditions under which it can flourish. Various fundamental principles emerged from the Experiment:

Health and Wellness as the Focus of Health Care

◆ It was observed that a healthy person displays a quality of spontaneity and ease in the way that he or she responds to a new challenge in life.

◆ Caring for mind and body is important in order that people have the best possible resources available to live life to their full potential.

◆ It is essential that this care is based on self-awareness and on a full understanding of the available options for action.

Self-Responsibility of the Patient

◆ People can be empowered by knowledge of the critical stages of human development, for example birth and ageing. Then, as they travel through life they have the opportunity to grow and mature through these experiences.

◆ An equally important ingredient for the development of health is freedom, more especially the development of a lifetime's habit of feeling free to make choices that reflect a sense of what one really wants to do, rather than following some external pressure.[10]

◆ Lastly, this process of development needs to be supported by contact with social situations and learning opportunities that support a person's growing self-confidence through feedback and the opportunity to expand into new activities when that person feels ready to do so.

The Peckham Experiment also showed how people could learn to take control of their own health in a way that was positive and non-threatening. Fear is a huge barrier to motivation, learning and application. Activities at Peckham were characterised by a sense of fun and self-discovery about health that is almost unimaginable today. Part of the secret at Peckham was that the Pioneer Health Centre provided a context in which people could be given information at a time when they could use it. The informally delivered health-related information was given personally, in a consultation relating to the whole family. It was relevant to the issues that people were concerned about in their lives at that particular time. Health was not abstracted out of ordinary life. Being part of the society of the centre, constantly mingling with the members and being aware of their activities there, the doctors were not speaking from theory about people, nor from screening tests alone, but from experience. People and medical staff knew each other and had a much larger basis of shared knowledge than a family doctor can start from in a two-minute consultation.

A Vision for Today

What if government had chosen to follow a different path over the last 50 years? How might social experiences, and in particular the experiences of families with children, be different? What might be the implications for health and social care systems if Peckham principles had been absorbed into their development ethic?.

The radical vision presented by Peckham entailed the promotion of health being led by primary care with integrated health and social policies at the core of a national strategy that returns responsibility for health to people themselves, supported by national policies to promote the conditions needed for good health. Peckham proposed:

◆ the separation of 'health cultivation' from the treatment of disease; .

◆ the integration of the health and social dimensions of people's experience and qualitative understanding of the significance of social interactions in families and communities for the development of health.

In contrast, the mission of the NHS was to treat the burden of disease. The practice of health and social care became characterised by growing professionalism and fragmentation, and in medical research by the culture of the clinical trial. Peckham advocated the adoption of a norm for health and quality of life that went much further than the absence of disease and for policies much broader than the organisation of medical services, such as a national food policy.

At Peckham there was a positive sense of well-being. The habit of seeing health as a source of pride and confidence is perhaps the greatest missed opportunity of the Peckham legacy. If people were able to feel that they were creating health in their lives as a product of the everyday, rather than as the result of special excursions to the gym or to the doctor, health itself might feel a more comfortable and less threatening idea. How would it feel to be reassured that when we enjoy our work or take a risk for something we value or love our children we are building up our own store of health? Then we might be open to trying to understand how health fits into this picture and how healthy eating, for example, might contribute to these goals.

Peckham teaches that an essential condition for healthy development is personal freedom and the right to choose for oneself. The art of cultivating health can be compared to the skill of a good gardener who prepares the soil and identifies the right conditions for a plant to flourish. Since people are essentially social beings, that soil is made up of social relationships, first in the family and then in the community at large. The medical and disease-based model of health that has dominated the current health care system has been led by experts. Where the experts have all the power, a lay person is bound to feel frustrated and is in danger of becoming dependent and underconfident. Peckham tried to restore to people the confidence to take responsibility for their health.

People have now been trained to depend on a bureaucratic health and welfare system to provide therapy and remedial interventions. This argument should not be seen as supporting those who want to remove the universal safety net the NHS provides for the most vulnerable members of society. The point rather is that a sickness service (health or social) is never a sufficient prescription for the development of health. Western society values health principally through the fear of losing it. People are conscious of dangers to health that seem beyond their control, such as pollution and contaminated food. On the other hand they are told that their own behaviour is responsible for much disease. Peckham encouraged people to take greater control and ownership over their own health and to feel positive about themselves.

The Peckham centre provided for its members a bridge between public space and private leisure, family and community life. This contrasts with the fragmentation of the social life of families dictated by contemporary leisure facilities and social habits. Many sports facilities cater for different ages and abilities at different times. A parent may spend the best part of Saturday morning delivering different children to their different clubs and have no time to relax personally. The danger of privatised leisure is that people lose the confidence to try out new activities; their social life becomes circumscribed and they lose the opportunity to sound out their ideas against the experiences of other people. In other words, they are denied some of the essential resources they need to develop as social beings and therefore to experience health.

Innes Pearse presented radical proposals for the further development and application of Peckham principles: a network of demonstration health centres, based on the Peckham model, with attached gardens to grow organic food and a national food policy to ensure good nutrition for the whole population.[11] The Coventry Experiment of Kenneth Barlow sought to implement that vision between 1944 and 1950.[12] These examples offer a breathtaking glimpse of an alternative route that could have been taken.

Even though there is no longer a single centre where Peckham practice is developed in full, the Pioneer Health Centre continues as a charity, acting as a vehicle for the promotion of Peckham principles. Many projects continue to use and adopt aspects of Peckham ideas and there has been a rising tide of interest since the 1980s in the application of Peckham principles.[13]

Applying the Lessons from Peckham

A wide range of initiatives today continue to find the holistic approach to positive health that was put into practice at Peckham an inspiration for action.[14] The Peckham Experiment has much to offer the development of primary care as it shows how the cultivation of positive health in the community can effectively embrace the aspects of people's life where health develops, such as in parenting and other relationships, leisure and the arts. The development of locality needs assessment, and purchasing and commissioning by general practitioners may provide an opportunity for general practitioners to influence what is available to local communities.

Some of the most exciting projects implementing the Peckham principles today involve the development of links between primary care and leisure centres. Enlarging access to the opportunities to improve health is a key theme in such developments.[15] This strikes an important chord with social care developments, including care in the community, which, in theory at least, aim to make our communities more inclusive, with the most vulnerable no longer excluded by being cared for in isolation. The voluntary sector is often the instigator of innovative community development in health projects which work with the community to identify and meet their needs and attempt to overcome the fragmentation resulting from the statutory division between health and social services. Through the 'Health of the Nation' strategy, national health policy now promotes co-operation to develop imaginative partnership arrangements, 'health alliances' to improve the opportunities for health and the relevance of Peckham to achieving these objectives has gained national recognition.[16]

Opportunities for the Twenty-First Century

Today, many opportunities exist that were not available in the 1940s, to take up and apply the Peckham principles. Health promotion has a much wider focus than health education and, across Europe, public health is adopting a more strategic role. The 'Health for All' movement has shown how other agencies, housing and different branches of local government, can join with each other and with the voluntary sector, to support communities in improving the conditions for good health.[17] Health is a subject of popular concern as people seek connections between mind and body and ways to look after themselves.

The lessons of Peckham need to be heard at this time to reinstil confidence, common sense and enjoyment into the health debate. Peckham was concerned with community building, not just self-development. It attempted to embed concepts of growth and wholeness in the daily lives and practical concerns of ordinary people. The Peckham vision of positive health was not that of a temporary stress remedy resorted to by those with the resources to fund luxurious additions to their lifestyle. Health at Peckham was the natural outcome of choosing a more fulfilling way of life. The vision is for health to be considered everyone's birthright and nurtured as an integral part of supportive and inclusive communities.

Biographies

Lisa Curtice is Chair of Pioneer Health Centre and lecturer at the Nuffield Centre for Community Care Studies, University of Glasgow. She is married with one daughter. She is a social researcher in health who is interested in the evaluation of community-based initiatives in health promotion and the relationship between social participation and health. She is currently researching the development of the alternatives to institutional care in home-based care for frail older people.

Douglas Trotter studied with Dr Scott Williamson and was a member of staff at the Pioneer Health Centre, Peckham. He was a colleague of Kenneth Barlow in the Coventry Experiment. His wife was also a member of the Pioneer Health Centre staff and both were early members of the Soil Association. They have four children and ten grandchildren and are executive members of Pioneer Health Centre Ltd which continues the work of the Peckham Experiment today.

References

1   G S Williamson; I H Pearse, *The Case for Action: A survey of everyday life under modern industrial conditions with special reference to the question of health, 4th edition*, Scottish Academic Press, 1982, first published 1931.

2   G S Williamson; I H Pearse, *Science Synthesis and Sanity: An enquiry into the nature of living by the founders of the Peckham Experiment*, Scottish Academic Press, 1980, first published 1965.

3   I H Pearse; L H Crocker, *The Peckham Experiment: A study of the living structure of society*, Scottish Academic Press, 1985, first published 1943.

4   Scott-Samuel, A (Ed), *Total Participation, Total Health: Reinventing the Peckham Health Centre for the 1990s*, Scottish Academic Press, 1990.

5   J Ashton, *The Peckham Pioneer Health Centre: a reappraisal*, Community Health, 1977; 8: 132.

6   G S Williamson; I H Pearse, *Biologists in Search of Material: An interim report on the work of The Pioneer Health Centre Peckham, 3rd edition*, Scottish Academic Press, 1982, first published 1938.

7   I H Pearse; L H Crocker, *The Peckham Experiment: A study of the living structure of society*, Scottish Academic Press, 1985, first published 1943.

8   I H Pearse, *The Quality of Life: the Peckham approach to human ethology*, Scottish Academic Press, 1979.

9   A Stallibrass, *Child Development and Education – the contribution of the Peckham Experiment*, Nutrition and Health, 1982; 1: 45-52 .

    A Stallibrass, *Bring Me and Also Us: Lessons from the Peckham Experiment*, Scottish Academic Press, 1989.

10 G S Williamson; I H Pearse, *Science Synthesis and Sanity: An enquiry into the nature of living by the founders of the Peckham Experiment*, Scottish Academic Press, 1980.

11 I H Pearse, *Planning for Health, Health and Education*, Broadsheet 14, 3rd edition, PHC Ltd, 1990, first published 1945.

12 K Barlow, *A Home of Their Own*, Faber, 1944.

13 House of Lords, *Unstarred Question: Peckham Health Centre*, Parliamentary Debates (Hansard), Monday 11 April, 1994; 553; 67: col. 1365.

14 A Pepper; L Curtice, *Total Participation, Total Health: Report of a conference at the King's Fund Centre for Health Services Development*, 11th June 1991.

15 B Millar, *The Ballad of the Peckham Health Centre*, Health Service Journal, 19 January 1995: 18-19.

16 K Gaskin, J Vincent, *Co-operating for Health: The potential contribution of the co-operative movement and community well-being centres to Health of the Nation activities*, Centre for Research in Social Policy, University of Technology, Loughborough, 1996.

17 World Health Organisation, *Health for All Targets: The health policy for Europe*, WHO, Copenhagen, 1993.

Further Reading

Ashton, J., *The Peckham Pioneer Health Centre: a reappraisal*, Community Health, 1977; 8: 132.

Barlow, K., *A Home of Their Own*, Faber, 1944.

——, *Recognising Health*, The McCarrison Society, 1988.

Finsbury, I.; Stewart, A B., *Health centres for today*, the Lancet, 1946; March 16, 392-5.

Gaskin, K.; Vincent, J., *Co-operating for Health: The potential contribution of the co-operative movement and community well-being centres to Health of the Nation activities*, Centre for Research in Social Policy, University of Technology, Loughborough, 1996.

Geddes, Lord, *Health, Address delivered at the reopening of the Pioneer Health Centre*, Peckham, March 23, 1946, Joseph Ellis & Sons, 1946.

Lewis, *The Peckham Experiment*, The Times Health Supplement, 1982; February 5, 12-13.

Millar, B., *The Ballad of the Peckham Health Centre*, Health Service Journal, 1995; 19 January: 18-19.

Pearse, I H., *The Peckham Experiment*, Nursing Times, December 9, 1950.

——, *Periodic overhaul of the uncomplaining*, Journal of the Royal College of General Practitioners 1970; 20: 146.

——, *The Quality of Life: the Peckham approach to human ethology*, Scottish Academic Press, 1979.

——, *Planning for Health*, Health and Education, Broadsheet 14, 3rd edition, PHC Ltd., 1990, first published 1945.

——; Crocker L H., *The Peckham Experiment: a study of the living structure of society*, Scottish Academic Press, 1985, first published 1943.

Pepper, A, Curtice, L, *Total Participation, Total Health: Report of a conference at the King's Fund Centre for Health Services Development*, 11th June 1991.

Scott-Samuel, A (ed), *Total Participation, Total Health: Reinventing the Peckham Health Centre for the 1990s*, Scottish Academic Press, 1990.

Stallibrass, A., *Child development and education – the contribution of the Peckham Experiment*, Nutrition and Health, 1982; 1: 45-52.

———, *Being Me and Also Us: Lessons from the Peckham Experiment*, Scottish Academic Press, 1989.

Williamson, G S.; Pearse, I H, *Science Synthesis and Sanity: An enquiry into the nature of living by the founders of the Peckham Experiment, 2nd edition*, Scottish Academic Press, 1980, first published 1965.

———, *The Case for Action: A survey of everyday life under modern industrial conditions with special reference to the question of health*, 4th edition, Scottish Academic Press, 1982, first published 1931.

———, *Biologists in Search of Material: An interim report on the work of The Pioneer Health Centre Peckham, 3rd edition*, Scottish Academic Press, 1982, first published 1938.

Central Office of Information, *The Centre directed by Paul de Rotha*, Central Office of Information, London (film), 1948.

Department of Health, *Health of the Nation*, HMSO, 1992.

House of Lords, *Unstarred Question: Peckham Health Centre, Parliamentary Debates (Hansard)*, 1994; Monday 11 April, 553; 67: col. 1365.

The Pioneer Health Centre Ltd., *Aims and Activities*, PHC Ltd, 1988.

———, *Positive Prospect for Health: Proceedings of a public meeting*, PHC Ltd, 1985.

———, *An Ecological Approach to Health – The Peckham Experiment*, PHC Ltd, 1989, (slide lecture).

———, *Evidence of Health – The Peckham Experiment*, PHC Ltd, 1989, (slide lecture).

———, *A pool of information – the search for positive health: The Pioneer Health Centre, Peckham 1935– 50*, Concord Video and Film Council Ltd, 1993, (video).

World Health Organisation, *Health for All Targets: The health policy for Europe*, WHO, Copenhagen, 1993.

Preconceptual Care
by Cornelia Featherstone

The first and a very important influence on a person's health is the quality of the sperm and ovum at conception. Therefore preconceptual care focuses on the health of the parents prior to conception.

To enter consciously into parenthood with the health of the baby as primary focus is the best start a couple can give their children. This is then followed up with antenatal advice, support and information for a positive experience of the birth. This lays the basis for a fruitful and satisfying relationship with the health care professional, enabling the parents to seek advice on all questions of rearing a healthy child. Particularly in the first few weeks and months, questions regarding breast-feeding, sleep patterns, the weaning process, appropriate stimulation of the child through the developmental stages and, of course, childhood vaccinations can be addressed in a way that empowers the parents and reduces their possible insecurity and anxiety.

The process of their child's growing up poses many challenges for parents, including childhood illnesses and the individuation process. These can be faced more easily when the attending health care professional holds the perspective that the healthy evolution of a person can be trusted and does not generally require interference. This combined with the provision of medical treatment, should it really be necessary, gives the parents the reassurance and safety of a positive and integrated health care system, enabling them to develop trust in the innate wisdom of their child's development and to enhance and nurture their child's unfolding in the best way.

Preconceptual Care – The Foresight Programme

Since 1978 Foresight, a registered charity, has been campaigning on behalf of the importance of preconceptual care. Slowly there is an increased recognition of the need for such a thorough approach to health care. Foresight's aims are:

◆ To secure optimum health and nutritional balance in both parents before conception;

◆ To instigate research aimed at the identification and removal of potential health hazards to the developing baby, especially with regards to the environment;

◆ to present the facts and know-how of preconceptual care, so that prospective parents are motivated to choose to contribute to their family's greater health and happiness.

There are doctors and nutritionists throughout the UK providing Foresight clinics which focus on the aspects of health that can be improved to optimise the outcome of pregnancies.

Nutrition

A wholefood diet, based ideally on organic produce, is the cornerstone of optimum nutrition. The avoidance of food additives and preservatives is crucial. Mineral and vitamin supplements are prescribed according to a hair mineral analysis which gives an eight-week history of the minerals excreted. Testing of body fluids, especially blood and sweat, gives important additional information in specific cases.

Nutritional Therapy

The Poisons of Civilisation

The harmful effects of alcohol and smoking on foetal development have been well documented.[1] Even so-called moderate usage must be suspected of impairing foetal outcome. Therefore Foresight advocates a complete embargo on alcohol for both parents in the four months leading up to the intended conception, and for the mother throughout pregnancy and breast-feeding. Smoking constitutes a health hazard at any time and abstinence is recommended. The use of street drugs is to be avoided. Prescribed drugs are best kept to the absolute minimum.

Pollution

Heavy metal pollution with lead, mercury, cadmium and aluminium have been linked with poor pregnancy outcome, miscarriage and infertility. Copper and selenium are both essential minerals for the body, but are toxic in the case of heavy contamination. Organophosphate contamination has recently become of particular concern as there is mounting evidence of its danger to the foetus. Apart from exposure in farming and through contaminated food, organophosphate contamination can originate from moth-proofing, fire retardants, or lice and flea treatments for pets.

Drinking water is often contaminated with lead, copper, aluminium, and more rarely with mercury and cadmium. Agrochemicals and organophosphates can be found at levels above the EC and WHO norms.

The effects of low-level radiation and electromagnetic pollution have to be held in suspicion and the recommendation is to reduce exposure as much as possible.

Allergies

People suffering from food allergies and malabsorption often have chronic health problems and reduced fertility. Allergy testing, and elimination of the offending foods together with a nutritional supplementation programme often improves the state of health and fertility, as well as birth outcomes.

Infections

Genito-urinary tract infections are implicated in the increase in infertility, miscarriage and perinatal mortality. Thorough testing of both partners for a wide range of infections is crucial to enable appropriate treatment. The incidence of such infections in one Foresight clinic was in 69% of patients.[2]

Natural Family Planning

As the contraceptive pill has been shown to lower the levels of vitamins and essential minerals and the copper IUD can increase levels of copper, couples are recommended to use natural family planning and barrier methods whilst preparing for pregnancy. Foresight asks couples not to conceive during the Foresight programme but to wait usually four months until their state of health had been optimised.

Outcomes

A study was carried out of 367 couples who enrolled in the Foresight programme during 1990–92. The study population was characterised by above average previous difficulties with conception or pregnancy: 37% had suffered infertility for up to 10 years; 38% had histories of one to five previous miscarriages; 3% had a stillborn child; 12% had babies who were small-for-date or had low birth weight. Follow-ups in 1993 showed that 89% of couples had become pregnant since joining the Foresight programme; 327 children were born; there were no multiple pregnancies. All babies were born healthy and were well developed at birth which ocurred from 36 to 41 weeks. The birth weight ranged from 2368 to 4145g (mean 3265g). None of the children was malformed; none needed to be transferred to special baby care units. Of the 204 couples who had experienced infertility previously, 86% had achieved healthy pregnancies.[3]

Conclusion

The Foresight programme lays the foundations for a health-conscious lifestyle which enhances life quality not only for the children to be born, but also for the parents. It also influences society as a whole as it addresses important issues, such as environmental pollution and health hazards in the home and at the work place. By addressing health care from the beginning it influences all aspect of health.

References

1   Tuula E Tuormaa, *The adverse effects of alcohol on reproduction – a review from literature*, Foresight, 1994.

      ——, *The adverse effects of tobacco smoking on reproduction – a review from literature*, Foresight, 1994.

2   Christine P West, *Age and infertility*, BMJ, 1987; 294: 853.

3   Neil Ward, *Preconceptual care and pregnancy outcome*, J Nutr & Environm Med, 1995; 5: 205.

Further Reading

Bradley, Suzanne Gail; Bennet, Nicholas, *Preparation for Pregnancy*, Argyll Publishing, 1995.

Jervis, Norman and Ruth, *The Foresight Wholefood Cookbook for Building Healthy Families*, Roberts Publications, 1984.

For Pregnancy and Birth:

Balskas, Janet; Gordon, Yehudi, *The Encyclopedia of Pregnancy and Birth*, Little, Brown &Co., 1994.

Tiran, Denise; Mack, Sue (eds), *Complementary Therapies for Pregnancy and Childbirth*, Baillière Tindall, 1995.

Natural Family Planning:

Billings, Evelyn, *The Billings Method of Natural Family Planning*, Thorsons, 1988.

Flynn, Anna M; Brooks, Melissa, *A Manual of Natural Family Planning*, George Allen&Unwin, 1984.

Nofziger, Margaret, *A Co-operative Method of Natural Birth Control*, The Book Publishing Co., 1978.

Childhood – the Anthoposophical Viewpoint:

Glas, Norbert, *Conception, Birth & Early Childhood*, Anthroposophic Press, 1983.

Glöckler, Michaela; Goebel, Wolfgang, *A Guide to Child Health*, Floris Books, 1990.

Resources

Foresight
28 The Paddock
Godalming GU7 1XD
Tel. 01483-427 839

AIMS – Association for Improvement
in the Maternity Services
12 Cloudesley Street
London N1 0HU
Tel. 0171-278 5628

Association of Radical Midwives
62 Greetby Hill
Ormskirk
Lancs L39 2DT
Tel. 01695-572 776

The Natural Childbirth Trust (NCT)
Alexandra House
Oldham Terrace
London W3 6NH
Tel. 0181-992 8637

La Leche League (UK)
P O Box 29
West Bridgford
Nottingham NG2 7NP
Tel. 0171-242 1278

Integrating Death into Health Care
by Cornelia Featherstone

The Application of Holism in Health Care

The way a health care system integrates death is indicative of the degree of holism implemented in its principles. In the reductionist world view, death is the ultimate enemy, the annihilation of all that is good and meaningful. The task of medicine within the reductionist paradigm is to prevent death at all costs. This cost may be high for the individual, as well as for society. Individuals may undergo dramatic interventions and possibly mutilation, while society incurs tremendous financial costs through the provision of facilities to cater for every possible eventuality. Doctors in this scenario are the heroic saviours who bring people back from the brink of death. An important emphasis in medical training is to produce experts at combating death. They require skills and an outlook on life which is not easily compatible with those who hold out for improved life quality and self-empowerment.

The Holistic View of Death

Health and Wellness as the Focus of Health Care

The dying process is a crucial element of life. It is an important stage in an individual's development, which can provide great learning and evolution. If the dying process is allowed to unfold in a dignified way, it not only serves the individual but also those witnessing the process. This has been experienced by many people who have been working consciously with the dying process in the hospice movement.

In the last 15 years the perceptions of death and its relevance for life quality have changed. The work which was pioneered by Elisabeth Kübler-Ross, Stephen Levine and others has now become part of a common understanding and value system. However, the actual realisation of these values is not fully in place yet, and it will be some time before it has filtered through all the strata of medical practice.

How these values can be implemented during life-threatening illness or trauma is dependent on the presenting situation. Sometimes decisions have to be taken under great duress and time pressure, as in the case of resuscitation, and it is understandable that doctors and medical staff will tend to actions which prolong life. Reports of people being resuscitated and kept alive on ventilators in a comatose or vegetative state have been material for much media coverage to illustrate the inhumaneness of modern medicine. It is in these situations that the voice of the patient is demanding a change in the procedures.

Advance Directives

Patients are drawing up documents of 'advance directives' or 'living wills' where they state that if terminally ill they do not wish to have their life prolonged by medical interventions.[1] The BMA published a statement that:

> *Common law establishes that an informed refusal of treatment made in advance by an adult who understands the implications of that decision has the same legal power as a contemporaneous refusal.*[2]

The Medical Defence Union advises:

> *...that clinicians should consider advance directives very carefully. When there is no hope of alleviating suffering, or of prolonging life with any appreciable quality, and the situation falls within the full terms of the advance directive, then clinicians should treat an advance directive as the settled wishes of the patient and act upon it if the clinical situation requires it. They should also consider that the patient may have changed his mind since signing the directive and take any evidence of this into account. Clinicians should, however, remember that an advance directive does not give carte blanche and that they should still act within the law. Thus, no advance directive will permit any clinician to commit a positive act for the purpose of ending a patient's life.*[3]

This more detailed advice, set in the medico-legal context, shows that there is still considerable room for debating the right of patients to determine their own care, and that patients need to be very clear with their doctors if they want to ensure that their wishes are being acted upon.

Euthanasia

The discussion regarding euthanasia and the question of whether doctors can assist patients in a death of their choice has been prominent in the medical journals in the last year. Bruce Carlton rightly poses the question 'Will you accept a duty to kill?' – for if there is the right to euthanasia then there is someone who has to assist at the death.[4] A survey amongst doctors showed that the profession is split over this issue: 46% believe that doctors should be legally permitted to actively intervene to end life of a terminally ill patient where the patient, when competent, has made a witnessed request for euthanasia; 44% of doctors said they should not be permitted to do so. Only 37% were themselves actually willing to actively intervene in such a case, whereas 48% would not.[5]

A Personal View

Being German I am acutely aware of the potential abuse of euthanasia. I am not interested in investing even more power in the medical profession. I do not have any answers to this complex issue. I question the ethics of keeping someone alive at all costs and particularly against their expressed will. The concept of improving death quality as an expression of life quality is very compelling for me. As death is an integral part of life, its quality and dignity must be an objective as important for health care professionals as supporting patients to improve their health and life quality.

Death and Spirituality

The process of dying is one of the most obvious points in health care where the question of spiritual values and beliefs is confronted in the practical work with the patient. In many cases, health care professionals are unfortunately not very well prepared through their training to use the full potential of these situations.

The purpose of life, the importance of the soul and the significance of the transpersonal level are all questions patients frequently face in their dying process. If the health care professional is willing to accompany the patient in this process, sharing both questions and beliefs, this can create great rapport between them and with the patient's family, becoming a source of nourishment for all and professional fulfilment for the practitioner. Openness, acceptance and a willingness to trust the innate wisdom of a person's life path are the essential qualities needed for this kind of care.

Fun Death

Laughter Medicine

Dr Patch Adams, an American doctor, clown and social activist goes even further. He advocates fun death and asks his patients what kind of death they want.

> *Do you want a miserable, anxious death, alone in a hospital, with everybody acting as if you are already dead? Or would a fun death be more to your liking? By 'fun' I simply mean whatever that individual considers ideal, within the limits of feasibility.*[6]

He encourages his patients to be fully alive, for instance living with cancer, not dying from it: 'Dying is that process a few minutes before death when the brain is deprived of oxygen; everything else is living.'[7]

Death is an important passage in life which can be created consciously as a celebration and acknowledgment of the life people have led and the bonds they have forged. What a tragedy that this opportunity is missed for the vast majority of people in our society.

Contemporary society is experiencing a major breakdown of family structure. It's time to glue it back together again. The intimacy of planning and creating an intimate death experience would form that kind of event. Let's stop fearing death and transform it into an experience that could bring us closer together as a family. Let's have a fun death.[8]

References

1   *Living Will*, The Natural Death Centre, 1993.

2   BMA, *Code of Practice 1995*.

3   David Bereford, comment from the medico-legal adviser with the MDU, J MDDU, 1995; 11: 2, 29.

4   Bruce Carlton, *Will you accept a duty to kill?*, Med Monitor, 7 Feb 1996; 8.
    Sheila A M McLean, *Making advance medical decisions*, J MDDU, 1995; 11: 2, 28-9.

5   Julie Coulson, *Till death us part?*, BMA News Review, Sept 1996; 23-5.

6   Patch Adams, *Gesundheit*, Healing Arts Press, 1993; 80-4.

7   ibid.

8   ibid.

Further Reading

Albery, Nicholas et al (eds), *The Natural Death Handbook*, Virgin, 1993.

Bradfield, J B, *Green Burial, The 'D-I-Y' Guide to Law and Practice*, Natural Death Centre, 1994.

Duda, Deborah, *Coming Home – A Guide to Dying at Home with Dignity*, Aurora, 1987.

Fremantle, Francesca; Trungpa, Chögyam (eds), *The Tibetan Book of the Dead*, Shambala, 1975.

Gill, Sue; Fox, John, *The Dead Good Funerals Book, Engineers of Imagination*, Ulverston, 1996.

Grof, Stanislav; Halifax, Joan, *The Human Encounter with Death*, Souvenir Press, 1978.

Kübler-Ross, Elizabeth, *On Death and Dying*, Routledge, 1973.

———, *Living with Death and Dying*, Souvenir Press, 1982.

Lee, Elizabeth, *A Good Death – A Guide for Patients and Carers Facing Terminal Illness at Home*, Rosendale Press, 1995.

Levine, Stephen, *Who Dies? – An Investigation on Conscious Living and Conscious Dying*, Gateway Books, 1986.

———, *Healing into Life and Death*, Gateway Books, 1990.

Lorimer, David, *Whole in One – The Near-Death Experience and the Ethic of Interconnectedness*, Arkana, 1990.

Rinpoche, Sogyal, *The Tibetan Book of Living and Dying*, Rider, 1992.

Wilber, Ken, *Grace and Grit*, Shambala, 1992.

A Future Scenario?

by Guy Dauncey

In October 1995, I was asked to write a piece about a possible negative scenario concerning the future of Western health care. Little did I know that what I was writing already existed, and was already known about by medical experts (but not, at that time, by the lay person). In what follows, my fictional scenario is augmented by some notes from a *Panorama* documentary that were posted on the Internet a few months later by Keith Hudson.

The Outbreak, 2004

It was Christmas morning, unbelievably, when the first signs of trouble hit. The Royal Infirmary in Glasgow reported an 'unusual incidence' of streptococcus bacteria which was 'not responding to treatment'. When Hugh McCann from the *Herald* called to speak to someone from the hospital, he was put onto a rather tetchy administrator who muttered something about the 'bloody media' before he put on his official voice, and said 'There is really nothing to worry about – we'll call you if there's a problem. It's just a common bug, we're dealing with them all the time,' and then hung up.

'You can tell he's not been to media training school,' Hugh laughed, and sent a 'patient' round to see what she could dig up. Later that evening, Linda McQuarry called from her cellular inside the hospital. 'It's absolutely nuts in here !' she whispered, clearly afraid someone would overhear her. 'I still can't find out what it is, but they've got six wards completely sealed off; they've cut the phones to those wards, and as far as I can tell they're confiscating everyone's cellulars, saying the signals interfere with open-heart surgery. It's bullshit. As far as I can tell, they're panicking. There's been some kind of an outbreak – they're cleaning and scrubbing absolutely everywhere. The younger nurses are shit-scared. All leave's been cancelled, and they've got heavy security on all the doors – male orderlies, big and important. Whatever it is, it's got me freaked. You never told me it was this kind of assignment. I've got young kids at home, and I want to see them. Got to stop – someone's coming. I'll call later.'

The next morning, the *Herald* ran a deliberately small story on the front page: 'Hospital Sealed Off: Staff Say "**Nothing to Worry About**"'. Within hours, the hospital was surrounded by crowds demanding to know what was happening to the mothers, grannies, children, friends, husbands and wives who were locked inside. The police sealed off all the streets leading to the hospital, and the Secretary of State for Health was forced to go on the air, reassuring the public that while the hospital was having a small problem with an unusually stubborn bacteria, it was nothing that a good dose of the right antibiotic would not soon sort out. Yes, she announced, there had been three deaths, but it was a large hospital full of sick people, and there was nothing abnormal about that.

Inside the hospital, it was entirely another story. 'So what the hell *are* we supposed to tell them?' a senior consultant was shouting. 'That we've got this killer strep bug that is killing one patient in ten that it hits, and we've got nothing on it? That the ****ing bug is basically out of control? And have the patients storming down the doors, carrying the wretched thing all over Glasgow? Don't be mad, man – we've *got* to contain it, even if it means lying through our teeth.'

As fate would have it, no force on earth could have kept the doors sealed. They'd thrown every last antibiotic in the book at it, and it came up laughing. By the end of the second day they had lost 100 patients, and the orderlies guarding the rear entrance had run for it. Their escape was kept secret, but three days later, two other hospitals in town reported outbreaks of the same bacteria.

It was then that the Secretary of State for Health made her historic broadcast. 'I am afraid that I have to announce to the country that the outbreak of strep bacteria in Glasgow's Royal Infirmary is far more serious than anyone had anticipated. So far 323 people have died, and the country has entered its worst public health crisis since the flu epidemic following World War I. The government is taking the unprecedented step of closing *all* hospitals in the country, both public and private. Emergency clinics are being set up in civic centres, as I speak. You might think this an extreme course of action: but in the current situation, we have decided it is the wisest course of action. We must bear immediate pain now to minimise the risk of the infection escaping, and avoid more widespread pain later. All patients will be cared for, and emergency hotlines have been set up for every hospital region in the country. We are in a very unpleasant and difficult situation. Let us share the anxiety, and pray together, in each of our faiths. Our greatest sympathy and love goes to those who have lost loved ones. If we have courage, we will overcome this crisis. Thank you for listening. There will be a fresh announcement in three hours.'

Within medical circles, they had been expecting the outbreak for years. 'It's amazing it took this long,' many doctors and medical scientists agreed. 'The bacteria can evolve far faster than we can invent new antibiotics, and each time we overuse an antibiotic, the bacteria come up with resistant strains. It's a battle we can never hope to win. We've been playing a mug's game for the past 50 years, hoping we could trick nature with science: but nature's far smarter than we are – probably than we ever will be. It takes us seven years to research and develop a new antibiotic. How long does nature need to evolve a resistant strain – a few months? We'd do better if we worked on ways to join her, rather than trying to defeat her.'

For a few days, people behaved with remarkable tranquillity, recalling how their grandparents lived through the war with the bombs falling all around them. By the 3rd of January, however, when people started returning to work after the New Year's break, a handful of people began phoning in sick from work, and overnight, the crisis went from bad to appalling. At first, people improvised every kind of protective mask, but then they simply shut themselves up in their homes. The non-electronic economy ground to a halt, share prices tumbled, and the pound sterling lost 10% in the course of a single day. As the news reported the growing death-toll, radio and TV talk-shows ran phone-ins and the Internet buzzed with connections from all over the world, giving people a lifeline to others – and, as it turned out, to hope.

When desperation fills the air, people open their minds to all sorts of ideas and possibilities they would never normally think about. It didn't take long for people to grasp the science of what was happening; nor did it take long for the voice of conventional medicine, urging patience and trust, to be counteracted by the growing number of alternative practitioners and healers phoning in to explain that it was the immune system that we had to focus on, not the drugs. 'For medical science,' they explained, 'it has always been easier to deal with actual sicknesses, through drugs, than it has been to understand the incredible complexity of the human immune system. But at the end of the day, it is the immune system that protects us and keeps us healthy. When our immune systems are weak, we get sick. When they are strong, we don't. Allowing for some simplification, it's as basic as that.'

As the turn-around took place in people's minds, their attention turned to the variety of alternative remedies that placed their emphasis on strengthening the immune system. Over the Internet, radio, TV and telephone, people discussed the latest thing they had heard about herbalism, homoeopathy, natural healing, diet or group prayer. Remedies such as germanium and probiotics that people had never heard of before became household names. The shares of big drug companies collapsed, and a small centre that taught an ancient Vedic system of pranic healing found itself giving daily tuition over national television. When a Canadian company announced that it was selling biofeedback equipment which enabled people to monitor the health of their own immune systems, its shares were oversubscribed 25 times. Alternative practitioners (who insisted on being called 'complementary') kept reminding people that personal attitude was the single most important component of immune system health, and that love, laughter and touch were the best healers going, but people found it hard to let go of the idea that there might not still be a magic pill or potion. In spite of the obvious risk, people wearing protective masks began to gather outside the home of every healer, herbalist or naturopath whose work was discussed over the Internet, and many had to hire security guards to keep order among the queues, night and day.

At the end of January, the death toll unexpectedly dropped, and within a week no new cases were being reported. The medical authorities reported that 'the outbreak is now under control,' but privately, they had no idea why the bacteria had suddenly lost its will to live. Two months after the outbreak ended, an alternative health magazine ran an interview with a woman living in South London who was a well-known healer, who claimed that she deliberately contracted the bug towards the end of January, and wrestled with it on a psychic level for three days, protected by a circle of spiritual supporters, and that (in her words) she finally defeated it – but the story was never picked up by the mainstream papers or the medical press.

The final death toll was 4,532 people – about the same number as die in road accidents in Britain every year, as one journalist reported – but for the shock that the outbreak generated, the number could have been a hundred times higher. The journalist Linda McQuarry never got home to see her children. She contracted the bug a day after being locked into the hospital, and died a week later.

Looking back with hindsight, it is clear that the outbreak marked a clear turning point in the public's approach to health, sickness and medicine. Immune system analysis is now taught in medical school as a standard diagnostic tool, using a combination of biofeedback and other sensory systems, and private insurance companies refuse to accept clients who are not signed onto a positive health plan, emphasising diet, attitude, clean air and water (raising all sorts of environmental issues), exercise, creativity, social involvement and personal fulfilment. Apologists for the old school of medicine call it 'psychosocialism', but for the insurance companies, it is just sound business.

The chief opposition to the new approach, unexpectedly, has come not from the medical establishment, who understood the problems with antibiotics all too well, but from the scientific community. Well-known scientists refused to accept that vague and unprovable things such as pranic healing or the power of laughter can have any possible validity when compared to the clear world of biological reality, in spite of numerous carefully controlled studies that have demonstrated the validity of the links. In private, they admit that it's not the data that troubles them, but the lack of a binding and unifying theory that will enable them to place the data within a clearly demonstrable new paradigm. Life is tough for the scientists. Like the leaders of the Catholic Church in the sixteenth century, it is hard trying to defend what they consider to be proven and accepted truths when half the country has lost its interest, and is pursuing something new.'

— The End —

All too quickly, reality began to catch up with fiction. Three months after writing this piece, I read some notes on the Internet which had been taken from a BBC TV *Panorama* programme of 15 January 1996, describing a situation currently taking place in Great Britain which bore an uncanny resemblance to my fictional account. The following personal notes were posted on the Internet by Keith Hudson.

The programme was presented by Tom Mangold, whose opening statement was: 'There are bacteria resistant to antibiotics spreading out of control in UK hospitals.'

A young patient, David Chuddley, had a minor low impact accident on his motorbike and fractured his leg. It should have presented no serious medical problem. However, he picked up a deadly infection in hospital which antibiotics could not control and he died within two weeks, age 29.

The main bug at present is called MRSA. It is a mutation of staphylococcus aureus which normally lives harmlessly on the skin. MRSA is resistant to almost all of the present repertoire of antibiotics. There are now many thousands of people carrying the mutated form of the bug. As dead skin is shed in microscopic flakes, MRSA can survive in dry conditions for weeks, capable of infecting others if it gets into skin wounds, the bloodstream, the guts and the lungs.

An old lady went into hospital for a leg amputation. The wound became infected with MRSA. After many weeks, finally using the most powerful antibiotics, doctors healed the wound. When she came home in an ambulance, the lady's daughter saw with shock that the ambulance crew were wearing protective clothing and breathing masks. She was then immediately rung by the hospital and told that her mother was an MRSA carrier and on no account should she circulate within the population. The social services department then rang to tell her that no welfare workers could now visit the the old lady at home for their own protection. She is one of a small but growing number of ex-patients who are now outcasts. When the rest of her family come to visit her, they have to stand yards away. She cannot hug her granddaughters.

One or two other ex-patients were interviewed who, although surviving their brush with MRSA, are also now social lepers. Most hospitals in the UK are now infected with MRSA. All hospitals in London and the South-East are infected. The infection started in Kettering General Hospital a few years ago. Patients with mild complaints started dying. The epidemiologist concerned, Dr Rosamund Cox, tried desperately to stop the spread of infection. The hospital was placed on 'war footing'. Wards closed. All operations stopped. Everything was sprayed with disinfectant. But, as soon as its doors were opened again, MRSA re-entered on the skin of some of the new patients and the hospital was immediately reinfected. In a similar manner, MRSA has spread to almost all hospitals now in the UK. With the big throughput of patients in hospitals, all minor injuries are now in danger of turning into dangerous conditions with 10-15% mortality, and recovered patients are becoming carriers of MRSA.

In the programme nothing was mentioned about MRSA infection in hospitals outside the UK, but it would be a reasonable inference that most hospitals in industrial countries are also infected or will be within the next few years because the same repertoire of antibiotics are used in all hospitals. For a period of a year or two, many hospitals in the UK kept their infection secret – even from the Ministry of Health (in case it affected their funding) – while they tried to cope with it. Dr Gary French, epidemiologist of Guy's Hospital, London, gave evidence to this effect.

The World Health Organisation says officially that MRSA is now an epidemic. MRSA is now beginning to colonise old people's homes in UK and many other places where there are ill people already or where there are many intermixings of people.

Dr Michael Zeckel (US epidemiologist, Eli Lilley Laboratories) said that MRSA produces 48 generations in 24 hours – that is, 2000 times faster than the body can produce defences. MRSA is now resistant to almost all antibiotics except the strongest one or two, such as vancomycin. He says it is only a matter of time before MRSA mutates resistance to this also. There will then be no drug defence to any bacterial infection, however slight it may be to start with. No matter how many resources are thrown into development of new antibiotics, MRSA can mutate more swiftly. 'MRSA will always be two years ahead of our efforts.'

Another scenario may overtake the one above. Bacteria can also transfer their antibiotic resistance to other bacteria. There is now a stomach bug which is resistant to vancomycin. If this were to transfer its resistance to staphylococcus aureus then there will be no cure remaining for MRSA and other bacterial infections. In fact, one or two isolated cases have already occurred. It is called VRE.

The programme showed a baby dying from VRE, face and body covered with lesions and in great pain. His condition is so serious that the medics are about to break all rules hitherto and inject the baby with a new and totally untested antibiotic with the theoretical possibility of overcoming infection but which might itself be lethal.

VRE is resistant to all known antibiotics. Dr. Barry Cookson, head of UK Epidemiological Laboratory Services admitted, 'This is the most serious thing I have ever known or heard about. VRE can almost be described as 'clever'. It is incredible. It is awesome. As soon as a new antibiotic is used, VRE mutates resistance to it. The more new antibiotics that are produced, the more dangerous the situation becomes. It is only a matter of time before VRE infects all hospitals.'

Dr Rosamund Cox said, 'In ten years' time we will look back on the 1980s and 1990s as a glorious time because we still had some antibiotics left that overcame bacterial infections.'

Dr Matthew Scott (a senior UK epidemiologist) said, 'There is no drug on the horizon: only variations of existing antibiotics to which VRE will adapt quickly. VRE is truly the Doomsday Bug.'

To paraphrase: 'Man and medical science can fool all Nature some of the time, and fool some parts of Nature all of the time, but not all Nature all of the time.' The coming few years might be the greatest changing point in man's history.

P.S. By coincidence, I visited my doctor this morning for injections for a visit to Nepal in March. I said to her: 'I watched Panorama last night. I was scared.'

She replied: 'We saw it, too. In this practice, we are all terrified. We have suspected for the last ten years or so that something like VRE might come along. Enjoy your holiday because it might well be the last that it will be safe or sensible to take. Or that you'll be able to take.'

Biographies

Guy Dauncey is an author, futurist, sustainable communities consultant, and author of a forthcoming title *2015: Journey into the Future*. He is a Fellow of the Royal Society for the Arts, and of the Findhorn Foundation.

Keith Hudson is a retired engineer who spends some of his time enriching the Internet with his powerful, relevant mailings.

Further Reading

Applebaum P C., *Antimicrobal resistance in Streptococcus pneumoniae: an overview*, Clin Infect Dis, 1992; 15: 77-83.

Boswell T C.; Nye K J.; Smith E G., *Penicillin- and penicillin-cephalosporin resistant pneumococcal septicaemia*, J Antimicrob Chemotherapy, 1994; 34: 844-5.

Brown D F.; Farrington M.; Warren R E., *Imipenem-resistant Escherichia coli*, Lancet, 1993; 342: 177.

Duckworth G J., *Diagnosis and management of methicillin resistant Staphylococcus aureus infection*, BMJ, 1993; 307: 1049-52.

Friedland I R., *Treatment of pneumococcal infections in the era of increasing penicillin resistance*, Current Opinions in Infectious Diseases, 1995; 8: 213-7.

George R C.; Ball L C.; Cooper P G., *Antibiotic resistant pneumococci in the United Kingdom*, Communicable Disease Report Review, 1992; 2: 37-43.

Horn D L.; Hewlett D Jr.; Peterson S.; Sabido D.; Opal S M., *RISE-resistant tuberculous meningitis in AIDS patient*, Lancet, 1993; 341: 177-8.

Johnson A P.; Speller D C E.; George R C.; Warner M.; Domingue G.; Efstratiou, *Prevalence of antibiotic resistance and serotypes in pneumococci in England and Wales: results of observational surveys in 1990 and 1995*, BMJ, 1996; 312: 1454-6.

Klugman K P., *Activity of teicoplanin and vancomycin against penicillin-resistant pneumococci*, Eur J Clin Microbiol Infect Dis, 1994; 13: 1-2.

Lederberg J., *Infection emergent*, JAMA, 1996; 275(3): 243-5.

Lonks L R.; Medeiros A A., *High rate of erythromycin and clarithromycin resistance among Streptococcus pneumoniae isolates from blood clutures from Providence*, RI, Antimicrob Agents Chemotherapy, 1993; 37: 1742-5.

Panlilio A L.; Culver D H.; Gaynes R P.; Banerjee S.; Henderson T S.; Tolson J S.; Martone W J., *Methicillin-resistant Staphylococcus aureus in U.S. hospitals,1975-1991*. Infection Control & Hospital Epidemiology, 1992; 13(10): 582-6.

Plikaytis B B.; Marden J L.; Crawford J T.; Woodley C L.; Butler W R.; Shinnick T M., *Multiplex PCR assay specific for the multidrug-resistant strain W of Mycobacterium tuberculosis*, Journal of Clinical Microbiology, 1994; 32: 1542-6.

Ridgeway E J.; Allen K D.; Galloway A.; Rigby A.; O'Donoghue M., *Penicillin-resistant pneumococci in a Merseyside hospital*, J Hosp Infect, 1991; 17: 15-23.

Rowe P M., *Preparing for battle against vancomycin resistance*, Lancet, 1996; 347: 252, 1996.

Anonymous, From the Centers for Disease Control and Prevention, *Nosocomial enterococci resistant to vancomycin – United States, 1989-1993*, JAMA, 1993; 270(15): 1796.

Complementary Therapies Principles and Terminology
by Cornelia Featherstone

Giving a comprehensive description of complementary therapies is a challenging task. First of all there are many different therapies – this book lists more than 60. There are at least 20 more disciplines of which I am personally aware that are not represented, and if one considers all the specialised branches, different schools and varying approaches in different countries, several hundred modalities or therapies could be described. No cohesive philosophical framework connects them all. In fact, the theories are at times even diametrically opposed.

However, it is possible to allocate complementary therapies roughly to four categories:

◆ complete systems;

◆ therapeutic modalities;

◆ self-care approaches;

◆ diagnostic methods.

As always, categories can only be an approximation, there will be exceptions and overlaps. The map is not the territory, but it may help to find a way through the maze.

Complete Systems

Homoeopathy
Herbalism
Traditional Chinese
Medicine
Naturopathy

Complete systems, such as homoeopathy, herbalism, traditional Chinese medicine, naturopathy and Ayurvedic medicine have a comprehensive theoretical background and are able to treat most presenting conditions within that system. They very often have their intrinsic explanation for causes of disease and mechanisms for cure and their own unique treatment approaches. A health care system which has evolved in the context of a society's culture, for instance Chinese, Tibetan or Indian, will fall into this category.

To have several complete systems available as a choice for the patient, or better still within a multidisciplinary team, is of great value, as presenting symptoms which form a confusing or unclear picture to one system may make perfect sense within the framework of another.

*Multidisciplinary Co-
operation*

For instance, I had a patient who complained about stomach pain, sore knees and pains in his wrists since the autumn of the previous year when he worked in road construction. Within the Western medical concept I could not come up with a unified diagnosis but would have needed to treat symptomatically three separate conditions. However, to the acupuncturist on the team this created a coherent symptom picture. 'Oh yes,' he said, 'these are all problems of cold and damp invading the channels.' After three acupuncture treatments all symptoms were relieved.

Practitioners of complete systems may not often share the care of one patient. A more likely scenario is that one will refer on a patient whom they have not been able to treat with any effectiveness.

Therapeutic Modalities

*Massage
Reflexology
Sound Therapy
Aromatherapy
SHEN
Postural Integration
Rolfing
Therapeutic Touch
Transformational
Self-Healing*

A large number of treatment approaches have been formulated within the last century. Some are practised more or less as in ancient times, such as massage and reflexology; others have been developed further, like sound therapy or aromatherapy. Some modalities have been created by the founder/s as they evolved their work over many years of clinical experience, often as a result of amalgamation of different approaches. This can be said about SHEN, Rolfing, Postural Integration and Therapeutic Touch.

It is quite common that practitioners will use several therapeutic modalities, creating their own unique practice based on their experience and tailored to the needs of the patients.

*Acupuncture
Traditional Chinese
Medicine*

It is possible to use treatment methods from the complete systems also in this way. For instance, acupuncture can be studied and used without the whole background of traditional Chinese medicine. This commonly takes the form of 'formula acupuncture', which treats a symptom by needling a specific set of points. This can be very effective in certain conditions. However, it is important to acknowledge that this is very different from using traditional Chinese medicine as a health care system.

Self-Care Approaches

*Self-Responsibility
of the Patient
Yoga
Transcendental
Meditation
Shiatsu, Iridology
Holotropic
Breathwork
Relaxation Therapy*

As patients become more involved in their health care, approaches which give them skills to take care of themselves become increasingly important. This may well be the area of greatest expansion in health care in the next century. A great variety of approaches have been adapted from old traditions, such as yoga, meditation and shiatsu. Others have evolved from those original modalities and put in a Western context, such as iridology and Holotropic Breathwork. Another good example is relaxation therapy, which is based on the newest insights of psychoneuroimmunology and with that is anchored within the modern science of medicine.

Nutrition is certainly a growing field, and a confusing one, as so many different theories and prescriptions of 'the right diet' are being suggested that it is impossible to know whether there is one correct way of eating healthily. Some recommendations come from ancient traditions, such as macrobiotics or the dietary prescriptions within traditional Chinese medicine or Ayurvedic medicine. Others are specialised diets formulated for certain conditions (Gerson, Feingold, Hay, etc.).

Nutritional Therapy

Recent decades have brought an array of different self-help and self-healing techniques and it is impossible to keep an overview of all that is on offer as it is steadily expanding. The following is a random sample of that which is available – affirmations; divination with cards, runes, the I Ching and tarot; colours, crystals and gems; visualisation; many different kinds of meditation; voice and sound work; self-hypnosis and subliminal suggestions; self-development and personal growth tools. The effectiveness of these tools varies greatly. In general, they are harmless and bring comfort to the people who use them, as well as a sense of empowerment in doing something for themselves. In some cases this has resulted in dramatic improvement of health and even miracle cures. The more a person is committed to one approach the more benefit is reaped from it. If someone is using them all, and is ever busy to learn the newest technique, there may be danger of an attitude of consumerism towards these approaches which can be counterproductive.

*Affirmations
Colour Therapy
Crystal Healing
Visualisation
Transcendental
Meditation
Sound Therapy
Hypnotherapy
Psychological
Therapies
Co-Counselling
Medical Assistance
Programme*

It is the task of practitioners to educate themselves as to what is available to the patients. This allows them to give advice, to train patients in the simpler techniques, and to offer them support along the way as patients take care of themselves and become increasingly confident in their ability, and therefore independent of the practitioner.

Diagnostic Methods

Many complementary therapies have their own diagnostic system which is used in conjunction with the treatment modalities. Examples are hara diagnosis in shiatsu, and pulse and tongue diagnosis in traditional Chinese medicine. Some methods have been developed which can be used in combination with various treatment modalities. Iridology, muscle testing, Vegatest and hair analysis are, for instance, used by doctors, homoeopaths, herbalists or nutritionists to determine which remedy is most appropriate in the presenting case.

*Shiatsu
Traditional Chinese
Medicine
Iridology
Kinesiology
Bio-Energetic
Regulatory Medicine*

These diagnostic methods may produce results which do not relate to findings by Western medicine. 'Congestion' or 'weakness' of the liver does not necessarily correlate with transaminase levels. However, they can give an explanation for a presenting condition and lead to successful treatment in cases where a GP can only say, 'There is nothing wrong with you – all your blood tests are normal,' even though the patient clearly feels unwell.

Availability of these diagnostic tools in conjunction with those of Western medicine creates more options for finding an explanation for a patient's condition and for devising a successful treatment plan.

Terminology

To describe the different approaches to health care, an array of different terms are used.

Medicine or *discipline* is used for the complete systems of health care such as modern medicine, Chinese medicine or homoeopathy.

Therapies describe specific approaches to treatment, for example cranial-sacral therapy.

Modalities of treatment or approaches to treatment imply that there is a larger concept – holistic health care – with different facets of intervention.

That effort is put into defining the terms used demonstrates the problems which exist. The plethora of terms shows that there is no coherent system which can be subsumed under one single term. There have not been any general agreements which define the terms used, so that everybody understands what is being talked about. It is an indication of the evolving nature of holistic health care. If seen positively, finding a path through the exciting diversity can be an adventure. With consideration and sensitivity, it may be possible to avoid the fragmentation and separation which might be caused by the diverse, ununified language.

Different Terms Are Used to Describe the Work in Health Care

What is known as health care is, in most cases, disease care. Health care professionals today are mainly busy seeing patients whose health is failing and who expect help, and in many cases the 'quick fix', that is, relief of the presenting symptoms as quickly as possible, so that they can get on with their lives. Different terms are used to describe the work and it is useful to take a moment to reflect on their meanings:

To cure – the treatment provided removes the symptoms and the causes of the symptoms, presumably leaving the body in a state of health. In mainstream medicine this is mainly done through drugs, for example eradicating *heliobacter* infection can cure duodenal ulcer. However, homoeopathy uses the term 'cure' as well but in another sense. The 'laws of cure' were formulated by Constantine Hering, a German doctor and homoeopath in the nineteenth century, and describe how a person moves through different stages of symptom presentation as they get cured.

Homoeopathy

To restore – restoring health or the physiological balance is an objective of holistic medicine. The traditional Chinese system refers to this often. Mainstream medicine also restores health, for instance through physiotherapy after injury.

To replace – this is a domain of mainstream medicine. Synthetic products are used to replace the diseased function or organ: hip replacement, hormone replacement, insulin or organ transplants to name just a few. Holistic medicine might debate whether health has actually been improved by these interventions.

To palliate – to relieve symptoms without removing the underlying cause. This applies, for instance, to pain control in cases of cancer.

To heal – this term is more common in the field of holistic health care. As in the definition of health discussed in Part I, this may mean that the presenting symptoms have been relieved never to occur again, or it may be that the patient has integrated a limitation on the physical level in a way that increases their capability, responsibility, autonomy, spontaneity and joy.

Health and Wellness as the Focus of Health Care

Different Terms for the Branches of Medicine

Different terms are used to describe branches of medicine which are not generally part of the curriculum of medical schools.

Alternative medicine was one of the first names given to these disciplines. It is a useful term as it implies the different choices available to the patient. It is only correct, however, if a treatment modality is actually the replacement of another intervention, for example herbs instead of chemical drugs. A disadvantage of the term 'alternative medicine' is historical. It was coined at a time of controversy between mainstream medicine and the newly emerging, though often very old, modalities. It still carries the flavour of exclusiveness, an either/or decision, a sense of two camps rather than of options in a positive health care system.

Most modalities are much more suitably described as *complementary therapies* as they work well side by side with other treatment approaches, be they conventional or unorthodox. I personally prefer the term complementary as it represents the philosophy of multidisciplinary co-operation.

Other terms are used at times, such as *non-conventional* or *unorthodox medicine*. Orthodoxy and convention are definitions within a certain philosophical and cultural context. It is correct to use these terms when we speak about the British health care system – as in that context it is clear what orthodoxy is. To apply these terms in principle to Western medicine is presumptuous as it imposes this paradigm on the rest of the world, despite the fact that modern Western medicine reaches only a minority of the world's population. Globally, the majority of health care is still delivered within the different ancient cultural traditions. Given that these traditions are many thousands of years old, it becomes almost a joke when modern Western medicine is referred to as 'traditional medicine'. Many of the complementary disciplines have come from ancient cultures, such as acupuncture, massage and herbalism, to name just a few. Compared to these, modern medicine has a short history indeed. Medicine as it is taught in medical schools in the UK today is essentially only 50 years old. Most of the major interventions and diagnostic tools have been developed in that time. It would therefore be much more correct to call it *contemporary medicine*.

Sometimes the term *allopathic* is used to describe the mode of drug intervention using substances different from those causing the symptoms. This is in contrast to homoeopathic medicine which uses in high potencies substances that cause the symptoms when taken in undiluted form. The use of allopathic as a word to describe all of modern medicine is an incorrect generalisation.

Offering these thoughts I admit that I myself have been using all the terms mentioned. I, too, am guilty of contributing to the confusion and lack of clarity in language. I have used some of the terms interchangeably, even though my preference is the descriptive way of saying modern, Western or contemporary medicine and referring to the others as complementary therapies or medicine.

Further Reading

Pietroni, P., *Beyond the boundaries: relationship between general practice and complementary medicine*, BMJ, 1992; 305: 564-6.

BMA, *Complementary Medicine – New Approaches to Good Practice*, BMA, Oxford University Press, 1993.

Choosing A Practitioner

by Cornelia Featherstone

To choose a practitioner wisely is important in all areas of health care – orthodox and complementary. The following recommendations can be applied equally in the choice of a dentist or a GP, a massage therapist or a herbalist.

There is no such thing as the one right therapy for any given condition. When the holistic principle – that the patient is being treated, not the symptoms – is applied, then any generalisation like 'acupuncture is for pain treatment' or 'homoeopathy is the best treatment for eczema' is misleading. Even though there are certain conditions which empirically respond well to a particular modality, the right option for one individual may be different than for another. Many considerations determine the choice. Clinical experience of general positive response to one modality is certainly important; local availability is another. For instance if it takes a patient several hours to get to the chiropractor for lower back pain, all benefits from the treatment may be negated by the journey. The patient's personal preference is crucial. If a patient says, 'I just hate needles,' then acupuncture would not be the first choice of treatment.

Above all, it is essential that the patient can establish a relationship with the practitioner which is based on trust and confidence. Patients need to feel confident that they are working with a qualified and experienced practitioner, that they have all the facts to make informed choices and that they feel empowered to say 'no' if they are not receiving the service they want.

Training and Qualification

It is good to know where and how long the practitioner has trained. Was it a full-time or a part-time course? What did the course entail? When did the practitioner qualify? It is impractical to discuss all these details with every practitioner. Ideally their practice leaflet would give that information.

The debate around validation and competence is complex and many different perspectives are being considered.[1] A long list of initials behind a name does not necessarily help to clarify the situation as few people know what the initials stand for. As there are so many different training institutions and qualifications, it is nearly impossible to know all the various curricula and standards of training.

Also, while a good training is an important aspect of professional practice, practitioners with only basic formal training can expand their knowledge and experience through years of practice and postgraduate training, and in the end be experts in their own field.

Registration

In the UK the great majority of complementary therapies have their own professional associations. Some of them have more than one, which complicates matters. Registration with a professional body generally means that practitioners operate under a code of ethics and practice, that they have access to further education in their field – through journals and conferences – as well as to supervision from more experienced members of their organisation. It also assures that in case of a complaint which cannot be settled with the practitioners themselves the patient has access to a formal complaints procedure and will be heard by the professional body of which the practitioner is a member.

Some of the professions are now setting up umbrella organisations for the different associations, which will hopefully reduce the confusion and help to overcome the fragmentation in the complementary field. The following organisations have been founded for that purpose: The General Osteopathic Council, the Council for Acupuncture, the Aromatherapy Organisation Council, the Affiliation of Crystal Healing Organisations, the Confederation of Healing Organisations, the General Chiropractic Council and the Reflexology Therapy Group.

Insurance

Most professional associations provide insurance cover for their members. In other cases, registration with a professional association will be a prerequisite for an insurance company to provide professional indemnity cover for a practitioner. The insurance cover should be up to one million pounds.

The Practice

Following these more formal facts, the practice set-up is another essential source of information. When did the practitioner start to practise? Does the practitioner work full-time or part-time? How many patients do they see each day or week? There are big differences in clinical expertise between someone who is new in practice and someone who has seen 60 patients a day for the last 25 years. It does not necessarily mean that the less busy and less experienced practitioner is not the better one for a particular patient. It may well be that the patient prefers someone who is willing and able to dedicate time and attention to them rather than being seen by a practitioner who can give them only ten minutes and may possibly be jaded from having seen it all many times before.

What is the practice set-up? Does the practitioner work from home and perhaps at flexible times, accommodating the patient's requirements? Or do they work in a professional practice or centre? The BMA recommends the establishment of 'centres of excellence', where practitioners work in a group practice, which ensures a wider spectrum of clinical experience where those who have qualified more recently can benefit from the experience of colleagues who have been practising for years.[2]

Does the practitioner provide house calls where necessary? Are they available out-of-hours? These questions allow patients to assess the level of service they can expect from the practitioner.

Supervision and Peer Support

Does the practitioner have supervision? Technical supervision from a more experienced practitioner of the same discipline will allow them to discuss the details of the application of their modality and thereby improve their expertise. Peer supervision from practitioners with the same level of experience in the same discipline and/or from practitioners from other disciplines gives practitioners opportunities to reflect upon their practice and to refine their professional skills. It also gives them personal support to off-load stress by sharing about difficult cases or situations with patients thus clarifying their own mind and enabling them to enter a future consultation more prepared and free to respond to the patients' needs in an appropriate manner.

Multidisciplinary Co-operation

Limits of Competence

One question is crucial and determines the quality of health care provided. Is the practitioner able to assess the boundaries of their competence? Are they willing to inform patients when they have reached their limit and are they willing to refer patients on? This safeguards patients from treatment that may delay effective help being sought and potentially saves them a lot of money and grievance.

Failing to recognise the limits of competence is the one serious flaw I have personally experienced with complementary practitioners. I have not met any of the charlatans or quacks who are so often mentioned in the media. However, I have met practitioners who were out of their depth and unable to acknowledge that to their patients. This could be for many different reasons: lack of training, lack of supervision, defensiveness, a personal stress situation. Good practitioners guard themselves by establishing either regular supervision or arranged supervision for unclear or difficult situations (personal as well as professional).

Conclusion

The personal relationship with a practitioner is the best guarantee for effectively evaluating their qualification and suitability for a specific situation. This is true for a prospective patient, as well as for health care professionals who want to advise their own patients or co-operate with the practitioner.

Appendix: Index of Professional Qualifications and Abbreviations

This list is not comprehensive but contains many of the abbreviations used to describe qualifications and professional organisations.

AHPP	Association of Humanistic Psychology Practitioners
AIPTI	Association of Independent Professional Therapists International
AIRMT	Associate of the International Register of Manipulative Therapists
AITI	Association of Independent Therapists International
AMA	Anthroposophical Medical Association
AMP	Association of Massage Practitioners
ANLP	Association for NLP
ANM	Association of Natural Medicine
AOC	Aromatherapy Organisations Council
AR	Association of Reflexology
ASK	Association of Systematic Kinesiology
ATA	Associate of Tisserand Aromatherapists
BA	Bachelor of Arts
BA (Hons)	Bachelor of Arts Honours
BAAR	British Acupuncture Association & Register
BAc	Bachelor of Acupuncture
BAC	British Association of Counsellors
BAHA	British Alliance of Healing Associations
BAc	Bachelor of Acupuncture
BAFATT	British Association for Autogenic Training
BALCCH	London College of Classical Homoeopathy
BAMA	British Alternative Medicine Association
BANMA	British Alternative Nutritional Medicine Association
BAThH	British Association of Therapeutical Hypnosis
BAWA	British Association of Western Acupuncture
BCA	British Chiropractic Association
BCh	Bachelor of Surgery
BCHE	British Council of Hypnotherapy Examiners
BCMA	British Complementary Medicine Association
BCNO	British College of Naturopathy and Osteopathy
BCP	British Confederation of Psychotherapists

BDA	British Dietetic Association
BEd	Bachelor of Education
BH (Hons)	Bachelor of Humanities (University of London)
BHMA	British Holistic Medicine Association
BIAT	British Institute of Allergy Therapists
Biod.Phys	Biodynamic Psychiatrist
Bio-MA	Bio-Magnetic Association
BM	Bachelor of Medicine
BMA	British Medical Association
BMAS	British Medical Acupuncture Society (doctors only)
BNA	British Naturopathic Association
BNOA	British Naturopathic and Osteopathic Association
BPS	British Psychological Society
BPsS	British Society of Psychotherapists
BPsS	British Psychological Society
BRA	British Reflexology Association
BRCP	British Register of Complementary Practitioners
BRI	British Register of Iridologists
BRS	British Rebirth Society
BS	Bachelor of Surgery
BSAEN	British Society for Allergy and Environmental Medicine
BSANIM	British Society for Allergy and Nutritional Medicine
BSc	Bachelor of Science
BSc (Hons)	Bachelor of Science Honours
BSD	British Society of Dowsers
BSECH	British Society of Experimental and Clinical Hypnosis
BSENM	British Society of Environmental & Nutritional Medicine
BSI	British Society of Iridologists
BSMDH	British Society of Medical and Dental Hypnosis
BSNM	British Society for Nutritional Medicine
BSO	British School of Osteopathy
BTech	Bachelor of Technology
BWOY	British Wheel of Yoga
CA	Council for Acupuncture
CAc	Certificate of Acupuncture (China)
CBiol	Chartered Biologist
CCAc	Certificate in Chinese Acupressure
CCAM	Council for Complementary and Alternative Medicine
CertEd	Certificate of Education
Cert HS	Certificate in Herbal Studies
ChB	Bachelor of Surgery
CHO	Confederation of Healing Organisations
CHM	Certificate in Herbal Medicine
CHNH	College of Herbs and Natural Healing

CHP	Certificate in Hypnotherapy & Psychotherapy (from the National College of Hypnosis & Psychotherapy)
CHyp	Council of Hypnotherapies
CIA	Colonic International Association
CMH	Council of Master Hypnotists
CO	College of Osteopaths
COA	Cranial Osteopathic Association
CPS	College of Psychic Studies
CQSW	Certificate of Qualification in Social Work
CRAH	Central Register of Advanced Hypnotherapists
CSAS	Chung San Acupuncture Society
CSK	Certificate in Systematic Kinesiology
DA	Diploma in Aromatherapy
DAc	Diploma in Acupuncture (from the College of Traditional Chinese Acupuncture)
DC	Diploma in Chiropractic
DCH	Diploma in Child Health
DCHM	Diploma in Chinese Herbal Medicine
DCM	Diploma in Chinese Medicine
DCN	Diploma in Clinical Nutrition
DHD	Diploma in Dietary Healing
DHM	Diploma in Holistic Medicine
D.Hom	Diploma in Homoeopathy
DHP	Diploma in Hypnotherapy & Psychotherapy (from the National College of Hypnotherapy & Psychotherapy)
DipAc	Diploma in Acupuncture
Dip BWY	British Wheel of Yoga Diploma
Dip C	Diploma in Counselling
DipCNS	Diploma from Centre for Nutritional Studies
DipDTh	Diploma in Dietary Therapy
DipFDZ	Diploma from the Federation of Danish Rcflexologists
Dip Hyp	Diploma in Hypnotherapy
DipIFW	Diploma in International Federation of Reflexologists
DipION	Diploma from Institute for Optimal Nutrition
DipISM	Diploma Institute of Stress Management
DipISPA	Diploma from the International Society of Professional Aromatherapists
DipNut	Diploma in Nutrition
Dip PC	Diploma in Psychic Counselling
Dip Phyt	Diploma in Phytotherapy (herbal medicine)
DipPsych	Diploma in Hypnosis and Psychotherapy
DIrid	Diploma in Iridology
Dip THP	Diploma in Therapeutic Hypnosis & Psychotherapy
DLI	Diploma in Lymphatic Irrigation
DN	Diploma in Nursing

DNM	Diploma in Nutritional Medicine
DO	Diploma in Osteopathy
DRCOG	Diploma from Royal College of Obstetricians & Gynaecologists
DPH	Diploma in Public Health
DPM	Diploma in Psychological Medicine
DrAc	Doctor of Acupuncture (from the British College of Acupuncture)
DSc	Doctor of Science
DSH	Diploma from the School of Homoeopathy
DHD	Dietary Healing Diploma
DThD	Diploma in Dietary Therapy
DTM	Diploma in Therapeutic Massage awarded by London College of Holistic Medicine
EA	Energetics Association
ESO	European School of Osteopathy
FBAcA	Fellow of the British Acupuncture Association
FBM	Foundation of Biological Medicine
FBRA	Fellow of the British Reflexology Association
FFHom	Fellow of the Faculty of Homoeopathy
FHSMS	Fellow of the Henderson School of Manipulative Surgery
FICGT	Fellow of the Institute of Crystal and Gem Therapists
FIH	Fellow of the Indian Institute of Homoeopathy
FIHP	Fellow of the Institute of Hypnosis and Parapsychology
FIMLS	Fellow of Institute of Medical Laboratory Science
FNIMH	Fellow of the National Institute of Medical Herbalists
FRCP	Fellow of the Royal College of Physicians
FRCS	Fellow of the Royal College of Surgeons
FRCPG	Fellow of the Royal College of Physicians, Glasgow
FRH	Fellow of the Register of Herbalists
FTA	Floatation Tank Association
GCRN	General Council and Register of Naturopaths
GCRO	General Council and Register of Osteopaths
GNI	Guild of Naturopathic Iridologists
GOsC	General Osteopathic Council
GP	General Practitioner
HAR	Holistic Association of Reflexologists
HPA	Health Practitioners Association
IACT	International Association of Colour Therapy
IAHP	Inter-Association of Health Care Practitioners
IAPM	International Academy of Preventative Medicine
IAT	Institute of Allergy Therapists
ICAK	Institute of Complementary Applied Kinesiology
ICM	Institute for Complementary Medicine
IFA	International Federation of Aromatherapists
IFADip	Diploma from the International Federation of Aromatherapists

IFR	International Federation of Reflexologists
IMH	Institute of Medical Herbalists
IOB	Institute of Biology
ISPA	International Society of Practising Aromatherapists
ITEC	International Therapy Examination Council
KF	Kinesiology Federation
KFRP	Kinesiology Federation Registered Profession
LCCH	London College of Classical Homoeopathy
LCH	Licentiate of the College of Homoeopathy
LCSP	London & Counties Society of Physiologists
LCSP(Assoc)	Associate of London Counties Society of Physiology
LCSP(BTh)	London & Counties Society of Physiologists (Beauty Therapeutics)
LCSP(DO)	London & Counties Soc. of Physiologists (Osteopathy)
LCSP. Phys	London & Counties Society of Physiologists (Manipulative Therapy)
LDS	Licentiate in Dental Surgery
LGSM	Licentiate of the Guildhall School of Music
LicAc	Licentiate of Acupuncture
LLSA	Licentiate of the London School of Aromatherapy
LNCP	Licentiate Member of the National Council of Psychotherapists & Hypnotherapy Register
LRCP	Licentiate of the Royal College of Physicians
MA	Master of Arts
MAA	Member of the Auricular Therapy Association
MABP	Member of Association of Bodynamic Psychotherapists
MAc	Master of Acupuncture, diploma awarded by College of Traditional Chinese Acupuncture and by the ICOM.
MACH	Member of the Association of Classical Hypnotherapists
MAHPP	Member of the Association of Humanistic Psychoiogy Practitioners
MAPT	Member of the Association of Professional Therapists
MAQCH	Member of the Association of Qualified Curative Hypnotherapists
MAR	Member of the Association of Reflexologists
MAWAc	Member of the Association of Western Acupuncture
MB	Bachelor of Medicine
MBAcA	Member of the British Acupuncture Association
MBBS	Bachelor of Medicine & Surgery
MBCA	Member of the British Chiropractic Association
MBEOA	Member of the British European Osteopathic Association
MBNOA	Member of the British Naturopathic & Osteopathic Association
MBRA	Member of British Reflexology Association
MBRI	Member of the British Register of Iridologists
MBSA	Member of the British School of Acupuncture
MBSAM	Member of the British School of Acupressure
MBSH	Member of the British Society of Hypnotherapists
MBSR	Member of the British School of Reflexology

MC	McTimoney Chiropractor
MCA	McTimoney Chiropractic Association
McC Soc	McCarrison Society
MCH	Member of the College of Homeopathy
MCHNH	Member of the College of Herbs and Natural Healing
MCIA	Member of the Colonic International Association
MCO	Member of the College of Osteopaths
MCOA	Member of the Cranial Osteopath Association
MCROA	Member of the Cranial Osteopathic Association
MCSP	Member of the Chartered Society of Physiotherapists
MCSAcS	Member of the Chung San Acupuncture Society
MD	Doctor of Medicine
MEA	Member of the Energetics Association
MEd	Master of Education
MFG	Member of the Felderkrais Guild
MFHom	Member of the Faculty of Homeopathy
MFPhys	Member of the Faculty Physiatrists
MGO	Member of the Guild of Osteopathy
MH	Master Herbalist
MHMA	Member of the Herbal Medicine Association
MHMA(UK)	Member of the United Kingdom Herbal Medical Association
MHPA	Member of the Health Practitioners Association
MIAC	Member of the Institute of Applied Osteopathy
MIACT	Member of the International Association of Colour Therapists
MIAH	Member of the Institute of Analytical Hypnotherapists
MIAT	Member of the Institute of Allergy Therapists
MICH	Member of the Institute of Curative Hypnotherapists
MIFA	Member of the International Federation of Aromatherapists
MIFR	Member of the International Federation of Reflexologists
MIIR	Member of the International Institute of Reflexology
MIGN(med)	Member of the International Guild of Natural Medicine Practitioners
MIIR	Member of the International Institute of Reflexology
MInstAT	Member of the Institute of Allergy Therapists
MIPC	Member of the Institute of Pure Chiropractic
MIPTI	Member of Independent Professional Therapists International
MIr	Master Iridologist
MIRMT	Member of the Independent Register of Manipulative Therapists
MIROM	Member of the International Register of Oriental Medicine
MISPA	Member of International Society of Professional Aromatherapists
MISPH	Member of the International Society for Professional Hypnosis
MISPT	Member of the International Society of Polarity Therapists
MLCOM	Member of the College of Osteopathic Medicine (doctors only)
MMCA	Member of the McTimoney Chiropractic Association
MNAHP	Member of the National Association of Hypnotists & Psychotherapists

MNCA	Member of the Nutrition Consultants Association
MNCP	Member of the National Council of Psychotherapists & Hypnotherapy
MRad A	Member of the Radionics Association
MNIMH	Member of the National Institute of Medical Herbalists
MNS	Member of the Nutrition Society
MNTOS	Member of the Natural Therapeutic Osteopathic Society
MPhil	Master of Philosophy
MPNLP	NLP Master Practitioner
MRCGP	Member of the Royal College of General Practitioners
MRCHM	Member of the Register of Chinese Herbal Medicine
MRCN	Member of the Register of Clinical Nutritionists
MRCP	Member of the Royal College of Physicians
MRCS	Member of the Royal College of Surgeons
MRH	Member of the Register of Herbalists
MRN	Member of the General Council & Register of Naturopaths
MRO	Member of the Register of Osteopaths
MRS	Member of the Reflexologist Society
MRSH	Member of the Royal Society of Health
MRSS	Member of the Register of the Shiatsu Society
MRTA	Member of the Relaxation Therapy Association
MRTCM	Member of the Register of Traditional Chinese Medicine
MSAAc	Member of the Society of Auricular Acupuncturists
MSAPP	Member of the Society of Advanced Psychotherapy Practitioners
MSBM	Member of the Society of Biophysical Medicine
MSc	Master of Science
MSF	Member of the Smae Institute (Swedish massage & chiropody)
MSHP	Member of the Society of Holistic Practitioners
MSS	Member of the Shiatsu Society
MSTAT	Member of the Society of Teachers of the Alexander Technique
MTAcS	Member of the Traditional Acupuncture Society
MWFH	Member of the World Federation of Hypnotherapists
NCA	Nutrition Consultants Association
NCP	National Council of Psychotherapists
NCRI	National Council and Register of Iridologists
ND	Diploma in Naturopathy
NFSH	National Federation of Spiritual Healers
NHN	Natural Health Network
NHP	Natural Health Practitioner
NIMH	National Institute of Medical Herbalists
NMS	Natural Medicines Society
NRHP	National Register of Hypnotherapists & Psychotherapists
NutCert	Certificate of Nutrition
OHN	Occupational Health Nurse
PGCE	Post Graduate Certificate of Education

PhD	Doctor of Philosophy
RAH	Register of Advanced Hypnotherapists
RATh	Registered Art Therapists
RCCM	Research Council for Complementary Medicine
RCGP	Royal College of General Practitioners
RCHM	Register of Chinese Herbal Medicine
RCT	Registered Colonic Therapist
RCTh	Registered Celloid Therapist
RGN	Registered General Nurse
RIr	Registered Iridologist
RMANM	Registered Member of the Association of Natural Medicines
RMAPC	Registered Member of the Association of Psychic Counseliors
RMN	Registered Mental Nurse
RMTh	Registered Music Therapist
RNT	Register of Nutritional Therapies
RPT	Registered Polarity Therapist
RS	Reflexologists' Society
RSHom	Registered with the Society of Homoeopaths
RTCM	Register of Traditional Chinese Medicine
SAPP	Society of Advanced Psychotherapy Practitioners
SCM	State Certified Midwife
SHL	Society of Homoeopaths Licenciate
SMDH	Society of Medical and Dental Hypnosis
SNC	Society for Nutritional Councellors
SPCertA	Shirley Price Aromatherapy Certificate
SRC	State Registered Chiropodist
SRMTh	State Registered Music Therapist
SRN	State Registered Nurse
SRP	State Registered Physiotherapist
STAT	Society of Teachers of the Alexander Technique
TAS	Traditional Acupuncture Society
TDHA	Tisserand Diploma in Holistic Aromatherapy
UKCP	United Kingdom Council for Psychotherapy
WFH	World Federation of Healers

References

1   George Lewith (ed), *Competence and Validation*, Complementary Therapies in Medicine, 1995; 3: 1, 1-64.

2   BMA, *Complementary Medicine – New Approaches to Good Practice*, BMA, Oxford University Press, 1993.

Further Reading

Heyes, Anne, *Guidelines for Employment of Complementary Therapists in the NHS*, West Yorkshire Health Authority, 1995.

Woodham, Anne, *Health Education Authority Guide to Complementary Medicine and Therapies*, Health Education Authority, 1994.

BMA, *Complementary Medicine – New Approaches to Good Practice*, BMA, Oxford University Press, 1993.

Who Should Practise Complementary Therapies: The Take-Over Debate

by Cornelia Featherstone

Medical Marriage is not the only way forward. One possible option is for techniques from complementary therapies to be subsumed under mainstream medicine. This is put into practice in the 'Münchner Modell', the curriculum for medicine of the Ludwig-Maximillian University in Munich, where complementary therapies are an integral part of training and research.[1] This model has drawn international attention and is being followed with great interest by the medical profession.

In the UK similar trends are establishing themselves in both the medical and the nursing professions. Julian Kenyon, from the Centre for the Study of Complementary Medicine in Southampton, who has for many years been involved in training doctors in acupuncture and bioregulative medicine writes: 'The number of doctors practising complementary medicine is beginning to approach a critical mass. This would allow young doctors to regard complementary medicine as a viable career option.'[2]

In the nursing profession the integration of complementary therapies in the practical work has long since begun. There is a debate whether nurses need further training or whether they can assimilate complementary modalities in short courses. The first leads to an increasing number of postgraduate diploma courses with academic qualifications in complementary therapies. The latter was argued by Fiona Mantle, lecturer in complementary therapies, at a major nursing conference in London in October 1995:

> *4600 hours of nurse education provides a sound foundation for the learning of complementary therapies in short courses, specifically geared to nursing, and would prove to be all that is required for the safe implementation of some therapies into nursing care. In addition to the utilisation of a complete therapy, it will be suggested that specific techniques could be taught to nurses as a normal part of their practical training. Nurses have a long history of borrowing techniques from other disciplines in order to enhance nursing care.*[3]

In a recent Nursing Times survey, 58% of respondents had used complementary therapies in their work, mostly massage and aromatherapy; 88% of those using the therapies had undergone training in them.[4]

In his survey of young doctors, David Reilly found a positive attitude towards complementary therapies in 86%, with 18% already using complementary methods and 70% wanting to train in one or more.[5] Doctors are attending training courses in complementary therapies; a majority attending will train in one or more of the following disciplines: acupuncture, homoeopathy, hypnotherapy and manipulation. The training courses are part-time and last anything from a couple of weekends up to several years.

Acupuncture
Homoeopathy
Hypnotherapy
Manipulation

The foundation courses, which last only a few weekends, are very useful in providing the education doctors require when referring a patient to the relevant specialist. This type of education is encouraged by the BMA.[6] It also exposes doctors to the paradigm of holistic care which considers the whole person – body, mind and spirit – and allows them to use the least invasive intervention possible.

Some of the courses also teach 'active' knowledge which gives doctors another modality in their repertoire. Practised in this way, the modality can be used in a limited fashion and be very effective in certain cases, for instance acupuncture for pain relief. However, there are considerable limitations to the use of a complementary system in this way. To fully utilise the power of the discipline, practitioners need to 'live and breathe' the paradigm on which it is based. To do that they need to have an intensive training and to use the therapy on a daily basis. It can be likened to driving a Rolls Royce in first gear all the time, not having the wherewithal to make use of all the five gears.

Voices in the complementary field point out the dangers of complementary therapies being taken over by modern medicine:

> *As a result of the plethora of research now being undertaken by doctors worldwide it is highly likely that acupuncture will soon become an accepted treatment within the conventional medical setting – but without its Oriental trappings (which most medical acupuncturists dismiss as 'mumbo-jumbo'). Doctors are also likely successfully to campaign for acupuncture to be available only through them – as already happens in most other countries. This could happen within as little as two or three years.*[7]

The same paper talks about 'doctors threatening a take-over'. Words as strong as usurpation are being used in the debate with the full strength of emotional charge this concept can engender.

As Penny Brohn from the Bristol Cancer Help Centre evocatively put it: 'Cherry-picking, splicing and grafting are appropriate in the garden but may be disastrous when applied to medicine.'[8]

Arguments for the Take-Over

The practice of complementary therapies by orthodox health care professionals makes them available on the NHS thereby allowing more people to explore the therapies and receive benefits from them. It raises the profile of these disciplines in the public eye and gives validation to the approaches, opening avenues for further research and development. With increased acceptance more academic training programmes can be established, which will standardise the quality of the education of practitioners, as well as provide the infrastructure and knowledge base for relevant research.

Arguments against the Take-Over

Assimilation of complementary modalities in orthodox medicine threatens to bring a dilution of the knowledge of the complementary therapies as many practitioners will only have a superficial understanding and will not be dedicated to one specific discipline. The holistic approach to care cannot be easily adapted to the care provided within the medical system at present, and the danger is that the holistic qualities will be lost. Some of the most important qualities which patients value when seeing a complementary practitioner are the time spent, the individual approach and the sense of empowerment they feel. These qualities are not automatically preserved when applying a complementary modality as adjunct to orthodox practice.

Unique Situation in the UK

Legislation in other European countries limits the practice of complementary therapies to doctors and paramedical staff. Acupuncture, for instance, is legally restricted to doctors in many countries including France, Italy and Greece. In Germany only 'Heilpraktiker' and doctors are allowed to practise most complementary therapies. Physiotherapists can choose to learn manipulation and psychologists can apply the more unconventional psychotherapeutic therapies. Other than that it is technically illegal for anyone else to practise complementary therapies. This leads to the situation in which most disciplines are practised by practitioners who use many different modalities and often arrive at an amalgamation of approaches which then constitutes their personal practice.

The UK has the unique situation that the majority of complementary therapies are practised by professionals who are almost exclusively working with one modality. They are making this work their professional practice and are furthering the development of that discipline in a focused and dedicated manner.

This is the ideal condition for evolving a discipline to the highest possible level of skill and refining the practice to an art. Education, research methodology and professional standards of practice can be tailored to suit best each therapy. This purity of approach is precious.

Conclusion

Complementary therapies are here to stay. It is important to find ways of integrating them into the present health care systems. This can be achieved through the integration of complementary therapies in primary and secondary care in several ways:

◆ Specialists in complementary therapies provide their services in co-operation with orthodox health care professionals. This can happen in a way similar to that in which hospital specialists are available.

◆ Doctors, nurses and physiotherapists use some modalities in their daily practice as adjuncts to the conventional approaches. This will allow them to become familiar with the holistic approach to care and enable them to refer to specialists in an appropriate manner.

This is the essence of Medical Marriage, which applies the best from both paradigms.

References

1   Dieter Melchert et al., *The university project Münchner Modell for the integration of naturopathy into research and teaching at the Ludwig-Maximilian university Munich*, Complementary Therapies in Medicine, 1994; 2: 147-53.

2   Abstract for talk given at the *Medical Marriage – the new partnership between orthodox and complementary medicine* conference at Findhorn, June 1996.

3   Conference report from *Complementary Therapies – who benefits?*, October 1995.

4   Joanna Trevelyan, *A true complement?*, Nursing Times, 1996; 92: 5.

5   David Taylor Reilly, *Young doctors' views on alternative medicine*, BMJ, 1983; 287: 337-9.

6   BMA, *Complementary Medicine – New Approaches to Good Practice*, Oxford University Press, 1993, p49.

7   Richard Thomas, *The fatal flaw*, JACM, 1995; 13: 5, 18-9.

8   Peter Fisher, Adam Ward, *Complementary medicine in Europe*, BMJ, 1994; 309: 107-10.

Further Reading

Lannoye, Paul, *European report on the status of non-conventional medicine*, The Natural Medicine Society, 1996.

Educating Complementary Therapists
by Mark Kane

The dramatic increase in interest and utilisation of complementary therapies by the public, as well as health professionals, has led to a proliferation of trainings in the various disciplines. Some of the more established professions, such as osteopathy and acupuncture, have started introducing their disciplines into the higher education system, and university degrees are now available. The emerging professions are asking themselves what constitutes an appropriate professional education for a competent practitioner.[1]

This chapter draws attention to some of the difficulties in defining competence to practise:

◆ firstly by considering the basis of the relationship between the patient and the health professional;

◆ secondly by looking at the way expert practitioners relate to the knowledge base of their discipline.

Any effective educational strategy will need to take account of both these areas.

The Purpose of Education

The purpose of professional education in complementary therapies is to produce safe, competent practitioners who understand their discipline and know how to apply its techniques to address their patients' concerns.

A profession enters into a contract with society. In exchange for access to specialist knowledge and expertise, society grants the profession considerable freedom to regulate its own activities, including the evaluation of its own standards and training. There is an underlying assumption that the profession will act for the benefit of the client and society. Patients come to complementary therapists with issues related to health and illness and expect the practitioner to be competent to address these problems. How each profession sees itself acting in relation to these fundamental human experiences will depend upon its specialist body of knowledge and skills. One thing is certain: if suffering is a central part of the experience of illness and often the *raison d'être* of the therapeutic encounter, then the education of the professional needs to be explicitly directed towards its relief.

The educational process required for the different professions will depend upon what each of the professions claims its members are competent to deal with, as well as those areas it sees as outside its remit. How the different professions describe what occurs in a healing encounter will, in some way, shape their beliefs about what the safe, competent professional needs to know. For example, if the shiatsu practitioners see patients in terms of energy balance, it might be argued that biological and psychological knowledge are not particularly important in their education. On the other hand if, as part of their assessment, practitioners consider the psychological or social dimensions of their patients' health, then an appropriate level of education and training in these areas is mandatory. How practitioners describe what is encountered in the patient/therapist interaction and the meaning they attribute to those events will radically alter what is considered appropriate knowledge and competence. This will have implications for curriculum development.

Shiatsu

Changing Notions of the Healing Encounter

What is meant by the term *illness?* Many of the complementary therapies construct their beliefs about health and illness in quite different terms from biotechnical medicine with its predominantly biological approach. What is considered legitimate knowledge and worthy of study will very much depend upon a discipline's beliefs about what happens in health and illness.

New Strategies for Disease Care Health and Wellness as the Focus of Health Care

There has been a sustained critique of orthodox medicine's 'biologisation' of illness.[2] The increasing popularity of complementary therapies can be explained partly by sufferers' dissatisfaction with the disease oriented focus of biotechnical medicine.[3] There is a great deal of rhetoric in complementary therapies about treating the whole person, but what are the features of the whole person and on what basis can practitioners understand and offer treatment for the whole person? Acknowledging the social, psychological and spiritual elements of the illness experience, as well as disease, might form the basis of whole person treatment,[4] and education needs to prepare aspiring professionals to deal with these realms. Complementary therapies' claim to holism will only be sustainable if training takes account of these different dimensions of human experience, because illness breaks down the boundaries between these domains.[5] In osteopathy the focus is upon the structure, but no illness is entirely structural. Patients' feelings, beliefs and expectations impact upon their experience of something as apparently mechanical as a joint strain. Osteopaths do not treat bad backs; rather they treat individuals who have bad backs. Therefore osteopathic education needs to be based upon the social sciences, as well as the biological sciences – educating practitioners to engage with individuals rather than conditions. This is not to suggest that practitioners need to be expert in all domains, but that education and training need to reflect the claims and aspirations of the profession.

Osteopathy

The Professions and Higher Education

A look at the evolving relationship between the professions and the universities may shed some light on the challenges facing complementary therapy educators today. Historically the professionalisation of an occupation has led to closer links with higher education institutions. In the late nineteenth and early twentieth centuries, professions such as medicine increasingly based their educational programmes upon academic propositional knowledge taught at universities.[6] The powerful new science being taught by the universities seemed to offer the answers the medical profession was looking for – effective methods for the treatment of disease. Awed by the precision possible in the basic sciences, such as chemistry and physics and the growing disciplines of microbiology and pathology, medicine prioritised the quantifiable and empirically verifiable. This led to a focus upon disease rather than upon the experience of illness. The outcome of this enchantment with an empirical science has produced a medical education that has prioritised the basic sciences at the expense of humanly relevant care.[7] Patients' satisfaction with complementary therapies is based at least partly upon their experience of being addressed as a person experiencing illness, rather than the repository of a disease that needs curing.[8] Historically, professions seeking higher levels of academic rigour and status have oriented themselves more towards the basic and applied sciences and less to the skills and artistry of day-to-day practice. In this view theory and principles are privileged as 'real knowledge' – empirically testable – whilst practice is only rigorous when it is the application of these theories. This educational model takes no account of the way professionals solve problems in practice.[9]

The Application of Holism in Health Care

Research in Holistic Medicine

In an attempt to seem academically credible, some of the complementary disciplines may feel obliged to increase their academic knowledge base at the expense of what may in fact be their greatest strength – the ability to work within the therapeutic encounter. The relationship between expert practice and the discipline's knowledge base cannot be assumed to be a direct one – clearly defined problems solved by the application of theoretical knowledge. If complementary therapies, with their increasing collaboration with higher education institutions, are to ensure that their educational programmes are not swamped by theoretical, propositional knowledge, they need to consider carefully just what they are educating for and what methods would best facilitate students in becoming competent practitioners.

Educational Strategies to Reflect New Beliefs about Health and Illness

As well as its discipline, specific knowledge and skills, each profession needs to consider what is the relationship between skilled practice and the biological and social sciences. How these are integrated into the curriculum is of crucial importance. Without appropriate consideration, such knowledge becomes merely an add-on that does not inform actual practice. A course in biochemistry for acupuncturists would arguably not help them to become better practitioners. On the other hand, an integrated course in life sciences would attempt to link signs and symptoms relevant in oriental diagnosis to medically significant conditions that might require referral or interprofessional management.

As the professions seek greater credibility and prestige and establish stronger links with higher education, they may be swayed towards the 'hard' sciences and lose the elements most important to their professional practice, simply because what happens within the therapeutic encounter is not well conceptualised and is difficult to assess. The social sciences form an important stream in any health professional education. They can inform understanding of the context in which health, illness and the therapeutic relationship occur, whilst the biological sciences, at minimum, are important to recognise warning signals of conditions requiring medical or other attention, as well as to facilitate communication with patients and other professionals.

Whilst not wishing to assume that current Western views about health and illness are the only valid ones, it would seem naive and inappropriate to ignore the currency given by the wider society to biological and psychological concepts. In a traditional Oriental context it may be appropriate to speak purely in terms of energy balance, but patients in contemporary Western society make sense of their experience through concepts of the physical and emotional body.[10] Practitioners need to be sensitive to the different ways that patients experience illness. These need to be acknowledged in the explanatory models offered to patients.

The Importance of Patients' Beliefs

Beliefs about health held by the different professions vary widely as do the beliefs held by patients. An effective therapeutic relationship depends upon practitioners understanding the needs of patients in patients' own terms. Practitioners of a particular discipline can view their patients' needs through the eyes of that discipline at the expense of the patients' perspective. Doctors may focus on the symptoms of disease, osteopaths upon structural imbalance, acupuncturists and homoeopaths upon the concordance between mental and physical symptoms, each putting together the picture in their own way.[11] Patients also put things together in their own way. Professionals often proceed on the assumption that they already know what their clients want, but as numerous studies have shown this is not always the case.[12]

Osteopathy
Acupuncture
Homoeopathy

The core of the therapeutic encounter is the relationship between the patient and the health professional. Therefore effective communication skills and a study of the dynamics of the therapeutic relationship need to be at the core of each discipline's educational programme, as this constitutes the clinical art. The use of case supervision seminars, coupled with theoretical material on the dynamics of the relationship, would be an important component in a comprehensive professional education and training programme.[13]

Multidisciplinary
Co-operation

Educating for Interprofessional Collaboration

One of the difficulties faced in developing a closer relationship between mainstream and complementary medicine is the absence of a common clinical language.[14] How can complementary practitioners communicate effectively with mainstream practitioners, for the benefit of their patients, without a commonly agreed frame of reference or language? On what basis would general practitioners refer to complementary practitioners? If truly interprofessional work is to take place, an attempt to establish common ground is vital. This should not mean colonisation by the dominant professions – inserting their beliefs about the nature of illness into the framework of another profession – but depends upon an appreciation of the models of practice of other disciplines, where they overlap and an attempt to see their discipline as part of a pluralistic system. A genuinely complementary therapy needs to see its relationship to the whole of health care. If complementary therapists are to be integrated into multidisciplinary teams they will have to face challenges well known in interprofessional work. Power issues around clinical autonomy and access to resources, along with establishing meaningful communication and the logistics of an appropriate and effective referral process, are all potential areas of misunderstanding and conflict.[15]

Setting Standards

Education must be linked to what the professional bodies define as the standards of competence necessary for professional practice. The best interests of patients and society are served when the process of defining standards is on the basis of consultation with user groups and allied professions. This applies whether the standards are set within a voluntary or statutory framework. It is not the place of educational establishments to define safe, competent practice. This responsibility rests with the professional accreditation bodies, whether they be statutory, such as the General Osteopathic Council or voluntary, as the British Acupuncture Council is currently constituted. Educational institutions, such as universities, are not in the business of setting standards of professional competence but in educating towards those standards. A mature profession needs to be able to define its sphere of activity – its area of expertise – and be able to evaluate when candidates are sufficiently competent to call themselves a professional osteopath, herbalist or shiatsu practitioner, as the case may be.

Acupuncture
Osteopathy
Herbalism
Shiatsu

Professional Competence

Aromatherapy
Homoeopathy
Hypnotherapy
Reflexology

There has been considerable interest shown by the complementary therapy professions in the National Vocational Qualification (NVQ) competencies model as a basis for professional qualifications.[16] The UK government, through the Occupational Standards Council, is currently developing competency-based occupational standards for a number of complementary therapies, such as aromatherapy, homoeopathy, hypnotherapy and reflexology. However, this is problematic because the task of defining competencies is also tied up with the task of defining limits. Within disciplines such as homoeopathy, some might respond with the argument that because they work within the 'holistic paradigm', treatment is based upon the pattern presented by the 'whole person', not the recognition of specific conditions. This kind of rhetoric is unhelpful and sidesteps the issue that education and training must reflect the claims made by practitioners.

Because some of the new professions are still forming, they have not yet clearly articulated what they see as their sphere of activity and therefore what competencies might be required for competent practice that is safe and effective. A claim such as: 'We would not treat cancer but we would treat a patient with cancer', skirts around the issue of clinical responsibility. If practitioners are managing patients with serious medical conditions, it is important they can demonstrate adequate training and experience to be competent and safe in these areas. If they are not taking such responsibilities, it is important to define where the boundaries of competence and clinical responsibility lie.

The NVQ approach to defining competencies is based upon a description of the skills and activities performed by a 'competent practitioner'. This principle of a performance-based qualification is sound, giving due emphasis to what is needed in practice. Whilst this is a good counterbalance to theory-based assessment, this latter still has its place, as possession of the discipline's underpinning knowledge is essential to ensure competent practice. However, establishing professional competency is not as simple as outlining the skills that are used in practice or the theory underpinning it. Something more is needed.[17]

The Concept of the Reflective Practitioner

Each profession has a knowledge base to which its practitioners relate. It is sometimes assumed that if students have a good grasp of that knowledge, then they have the ingredients necessary for good professional practice. On this assumption, curricula are developed, to provide students with the appropriate academic knowledge to underpin their future practice. But the relationship between theory and the practice is not a straightforward one, since theory and concepts cannot be applied 'off the shelf'.[18] More than a set of learned skills, professional practice requires the ability to learn from experience and modify or change practice in the light of new knowledge and understanding. This leads to new ways of conceptualising the problems encountered in practice.[19]

Through experience, the practitioner builds up a repertoire that can be called on as a means of understanding. When experienced professionals encounter a new situation in which previously learned knowledge does not fit, they will attempt to reformulate the problem in a new way that will facilitate the finding of a solution. Practitioners need a flexible connection with their knowledge that allows for theory to be generated out of actual problem situations. Learning to think and act like a professional is an

Multidisciplinary Co-operation

important part of any professional education. This ability to process knowledge needs to be given priority without neglecting the contribution of theoretical or practical knowledge.[20]

Courses integrating theory and clinical experience using a problem-solving approach are receiving increasing recognition by clinical disciplines[21] and may offer the most effective educational opportunities for complementary practitioners and help them to become reflective practitioners. If the primary function of initial education is helping students learn how to learn, rather than accumulating vast quantities of information that will be assessed prior to qualification, then educational programmes must be shaped to facilitate this.

Continuing Professional Development

Learning from experience is an important part of professional development. It is commonly understood that completion of a professional training only prepares candidates to begin professional practice. There need to be clearly articulated links between initial qualifications and continuing professional development.

Professionals need to sustain a critical and evaluative attitude towards their practice. The Osteopaths Act of 1993 created provision for compulsory postgraduate education of osteopaths, the idea being that practitioners will need to demonstrate that their education is continually being developed. This could include a preregistration year of supervised practice and update courses in important safety areas, as well as credits being given for courses that expand practitioners' skills or knowledge base. An initiative being developed by the Osteopathic Continuing Professional Development Council is a system of mentoring and peer review. This will enable practitioners to identify their own learning and personal development needs, with support and guidance from other members of the profession. Continuing professional development in some form is essential for any credible complementary therapy profession wanting to ensure the highest standards of practice from its members.

The University of Westminster

The University of Westminster has developed a programme of education in complementary therapies which uphold these aspirations. Undergraduate degrees in complementary therapies include BSc (Hons) Complementary Therapies; BSc (Hons) Traditional Chinese Medicine: Acupuncture; BSc (Hons) Homoeopathy. They are based around a common core or spine of appropriate biomedical and social sciences. There is equal emphasis given to practitioner development, as well as the underlying mechanisms leading to health and illness. These themes are integrated through clinical practice modules. Through the practitioner development modules, students develop skills of reflection and self-appraisal in relation to their interpersonal skills, as well as developing a critical awareness of the influences of social, cultural and political factors on health care provision and on the therapeutic relationship. As students progress up their pathway, these core themes are integrated through actual and constructed clinical pictures. The complexity of the cases and the analysis and evaluation required develop as the student progresses. This culminates with clinically supervised practice, up to a level of competency that will satisfy the appropriate professional accreditation bodies.

Postgraduate courses which support continuing professional development are MSc in Complementary Therapy Studies and MA in Therapeutic Bodywork. These courses take the educational process further by encouraging critical reflection on a range of contextual issues, such as the social, cultural and political dimensions impacting on complementary therapies, as well as comparative studies on the philosophies and principles of the different healing traditions. New models for understanding mind–body interactions are explored, as are the range of research methodologies appropriate for understanding what takes place in a therapeutic encounter.

Conclusion

Complementary therapy education needs to be based upon a clear understanding of what each profession expects its practitioners to be competent in. This would require a grounding in appropriate social and biological sciences, as well as the discipline's specific knowledge. It also needs to have an interprofessional component. The emphasis should be to educate practitioners to be lifelong learners who will reflect upon their practice and have the ability to change or modify their practice in the light of new knowledge and experience. If the focus of the educational process is directed towards final examinations, candidates' learning will be directed toward those examinations. But if it is more desirable that graduates learn how to manage their own learning, how to assess themselves, how to reflect upon their own practice, how to be effective in dealing with the human experience of illness on its own terms, then these qualities need to be built into the curriculum, and the assessment methods used must be valid and reliable in these areas. The challenge for educators in complementary therapies is to provide programmes that are both rigorous academically and relevant to the demands of professional practice.

Biography

Mark Kane is senior lecturer in the academic programme for complementary therapies in Westminster University. He is also a practising osteopath and acupuncurist in the Marylebone Health Centre, London, and a researcher with the British School of Osteopathy.

References

1   S Cant; U Sharma, *Professionalisation of complementary medicine in the United Kingdom*, Complementary Therapies in Medicine 1996; 4: 157-62.

2   G Engels, *The need for a new medical model: a challenge for biomedicine*, Science 1977; 196: 129-36.

    A Klienman; L Eisenberg; B Good, *Culture, illness, and cure: clinical lessons from anthropologic and cross-cultural research*, Annals of Internal Medicine 1978; 88: 251-8.

3   U Sharma, *Complementary Medicine Today: Practitioners and Patients,* Routledge, 1992.

4   E Cassel, *The nature of suffering and the goals of medicine*, The New England Journal of Medicine, 1982; 306: 11, 639-45.

5   S K Toombs, *The Meaning of Illness: A Phenomenological Account of the Different Perspectives of Physician and Patient*, Kluwer Academic Publishers, 1993.

6   M Burrage, *Practitioners, Professors and the State in France, the USA and England.* in S Goodlad (ed), *Education for the Professions: Quis Custodiet?* Society for Research into Higher Education & Nelson, 1984.

     D Schon, *The crisis of professional knowledge and the pursuit of an epistemology of practice*, Journal of Interprofessional Care 1992;6:(1) 49-63.

7   E Cassel, op cit.

8   U Sharma, op cit.

9   D Schon, *The Reflective Practitioner: How Professionals Think in Action*, Basic Books, Harper, 1983.

     M Eraut, *Developing Professional Knowledge and Competence*, Falmer Press, 1994.

10   C Helman, *Culture Health and Illness*, Wright, 1995.

11   ibid.

12   A Klienman; L Eisenberg; B Good, op cit.

     L Hunt; B Jordan; S Irwin, *Views of what's wrong: the role of diagnosis in patients' understanding of their illness experience.* Social Science in Medicine 1989; 28: (9)945-56.

13   E Balint; M Courtnay; A Elder et al, *The Doctor, the Patient and the Group: Balint Revisited*, Routledge, 1993.

14   D Peters, *Perspectives from general practice: skilled doctors or imported complementary practitioners*, Complementary Therapies in Medicine 1995; 3: 32-6.

15   P Reason, *Power and conflict in multidisciplinary collaboration*, Complementary Medicine Reseach 1991; 5: 144-50.

16   GCRO, *Competencies Required for Osteopathic Practice*, General Council and Register of Osteopaths, 1993.

17   R Barnett, *The Limits of Competence: Knowledge, Higher Education and Society*, Society for Research into Higher Education & Open University Press, 1994.

18   M Eraut, op cit., p100-22.

19   D Schon, *Educating the Reflective Practitioner*, Jossey Bass, 1987.

20   M Eraut, op cit.

21   S Lowry, *Medical Education*, BMJ Publishing, 1993.

     D Boud; G Feletti (eds), *The Challenge of Problem Based Learning*, Kogan Page, 1991.

Further Reading

Balint E.; Courtnay M; Elder A et al, *The Doctor, the Patient and the Group: Balint Revisited*, Routledge, 1993.

Barnett R., *The Limits of Competence: Knowledge, Higher Education and Society*, Society for Research into Higher Education & Open University Press, 1994.

Boud D.; Feletti G (eds), *The Challenge of Problem Based Learning*, Kogan Page, 1991.

Burrage M., *Practitioners, Professors and the State in France, the USA and England.* in Goodlad S (ed), *Education for the Professions: Quis Custodiet?* Society for Research into Higher Education & Nelson, 1984.

Cant S & Sharma U., *Professionalisation of Complementary Medicine in the United Kingdom*, Complementary Therapies in Medicine 1996; 4: 157-62.

Cassel E., *The Nature of Suffering and the Goals of Medicine*, The New England Journal of Medicine, 1982; 306: 11,639-45.

Engels G., *The Need for a New Medical Model: A Challenge for Biomedicine*, Science 1977; 196: 129-36.

Eraut M., *Developing Professional Knowledge and Competence*, Falmer Press, 1994.

Helman C., *Communication in primary care: the role of patient and practitioner explanatory models*, Social Science in Medicine, 1985; 20: (9), 923-31.

———, *Culture Health and Illness*, Wright, 1995.

Hunt L.; Jordan B.; Irwin S., *Views of what's wrong: the role of diagnosis in patients' understanding of their illness experience*, Social Science in Medicine 1989;2 8: (9)945-56.

Klienman A.; Eisenberg L; Good B, *Culture, illness, and cure: clinical lessons from anthropologic and cross-cultural research*, Annals of Internal Medicine 1978; 88: 251-8.

Lowry S., *Medical Education*, BMJ Publishing, 1993.

Peters D., *Perspectives from general practice: skilled doctors or imported complementary practitioners*, Complementary Therapies in Medicine 1995; 3: 32-6.

Reason P., *Power and conflict in multidisciplinary collaboration*, Complementary Medicine Reseach 1991; 5: 144-50.

Sharma U., *Complementary Medicine Today: Practitioners and Patients*, Routledge, 1992.

Schon D., *The Reflective Practitioner: How Professionals Think in Action*, Basic Books, Harper, 1983.

———, *The crisis of professional knowledge and the pursuit of an epistimology of practice*, Journal of Interprofessional Care 1992; 6: (1) 49-63.

———, *Educating the Reflective Practitioner*, Jossey Bass, 1987.

Toombs S.K., *The Meaning of Illness: A Phenomenological Account of the Different Perspectives of Physician and Patient*, Kluwer Academic Publishers, 1993.

Usher R.; Bryant I., *Re-examining the Theory-Practice Relationship in Continuing Professional Education*, Studies in Higher Education 1987; 12: (2)201-12

GCRO, *Competencies Required for Osteopathic Practice*, General Council and Register of Osteopaths, 1993.

Research in Holistic Medicine

by Mike Fitter

Many holistic practitioners view research into medicine as deriving from the paradigm of reductionist science, and therefore to be incompatible with the practice of holistic medicine. There is indeed considerable justification for this conclusion. There are many examples of research which has applied reductionist methods with unfortunate and alienating consequences. One study, the reporting of which had a significant impact on me as a researcher working for the Medical Research Council, was the evaluation of the Bristol Cancer Help Centre.[1] The study reported, with much publicity, that women with breast cancer who went to the Bristol Centre were twice as likely to die as women who did not. Even though the findings were later retracted (the data had been analysed inappropriately), the damage had been done. In retrospect, the people who had invited in the medical researchers realised that, because they had so little research experience themselves, they had been forced to trust the researchers blindly.

The lesson from the Bristol experience, for me, is that practitioners need to have an understanding of research and its methods so that they can either conduct their own research as practitioner-researchers or work in equal partnership with professional researchers. A consequence of the Bristol experience for me was to refocus my skills and experience towards working in close collaboration with holistic practitioners, to learn from them what they need from research, and to develop an approach to health care research that could both support the work of holistic practitioners and build bridges with the world of medical science.

Most importantly, I believe that the development of skilled practice ought to have a research focus, because it requires practitioners to be reflective about what it is they do, and thereby learn from experience. Therefore research should be an integral part of holistic medicine – reflection and practice intertwined. Research need not involve a paradigm which does not do justice to holism; holistic practitioners need to reclaim research as a way of developing themselves creatively 'on the job' and, as such, research should be integral to 'being professionally alive'.

The Present Situation of Research into Holistic Medicine

In my observation, holistic practitioners who have worked with medical science have experienced a kind of 'cultural imperialism', whereby they have provided the data, while medical researchers have set the agenda (by assuming that they were the experts in research and its methods and that holistic practitioners were usually well intentioned, but uninformed, naive and overly idealistic).

I have concluded that research is seen by some holistic practitioners as a 'necessary evil', which cannot be ignored because people with power are insisting on it, but which must be treated with caution. Others seemed to regard it as an 'outright evil', having nothing to do with it.

Richard Thomas, in a recent article, castigated the complementary medicine professions for having so little interest in research.[2] He made a damning attack on osteopathy, acupuncture and homoeopathy in particular. His point is that there will be a take-over of complementary therapies by conventional doctors who, as a profession, are active in research. He sees the very survival of the holistic practice of these therapies as depending on the creation of a substantial research base – and by this he means 'proper' clinical trials. Although I disagree with some of Thomas's specific views on what sort of research is needed, and feel that now is the time to give support, not undermine, his harsh assessment does have some justification.

Who Should Practise Complementary Therapies Osteopathy Acupuncture Homoeopathy

Another writer on the subject, Volker Scheid, offers insight into the cultural and political processes in which we are embroiled.[3] He identifies ways that powerful individuals and institutions, who embody the 'dominant culture', may respond when they feel challenged (and threatened) by 'alternative systems of knowledge'. In Scheid's view, there are three specific options that people who wish to maintain the dominant cultural view may adopt:

◆ *Annihilation.* The most directly attacking option to prevent an alternative system of knowledge becoming established is to attempt to annihilate its practitioners. This is akin to 'ethnic cleansing' in which all practitioners associated with the alternative way are killed or otherwise suppressed. An example of this option in the history of the West is the suppression of the witch-healer.[4] It should be recognised that the traditional healer did not represent an emerging system of knowledge, but a traditional one that was already established but was overrun by what became modern scientific (and predominantly male) medicine. Perhaps the fact that the witch-healers were well established explains why such violent methods of suppression were used.

◆ *Systematic exclusion.* This option is akin to apartheid. A non-dominant system of knowledge is systematically excluded and maintained in an inferior and less influential position. When this path is followed there can be periods of relatively peaceful co-existence as practitioners of each system practise in isolation, interspersed with 'skirmishes' as boundaries are crossed; for example, when alternative therapists make claims for their therapy which directly challenge the conventional approach or when the medical profession acts firmly to place the alternative system back into its inferior position – an intention that can be seen to underlie the British Medical Association's first report on alternative medicine.[5]

◆ *Assimilation.* This option is akin to the 'melting pot' into which many diverse ethnic groups merged to form the currently dominant culture of the United States of America. The consequence for alternative systems of knowledge is that they have some influence as the dominant culture adapts to absorb them. But the cost is that as the different system is assimilated it loses many of its essential characteristics – usually its more radical aspects – as it is absorbed into the dominant worldview.

There are clear signs that the latter is currently happening with complementary/ alternative medicine. Specifically, there are now several projects in which the NHS is contracting with practitioners to provide complementary therapy services to NHS patients. There appears to be a trend emerging that there are changes to the therapies as they are incorporated into the NHS context. In concrete terms, practitioners are under pressure to give shorter consultations and to provide fewer treatment sessions per patient. Less tangibly, the NHS purchasers see themselves as contracting with practitioners who will supply specific techniques, for example the insertion of acupuncture needles in locations according to a symptom-treatment correspondence. This focus on technique fails to recognise other key aspects of the therapeutic process that a holistic practitioner would regard as essential.[6]

In parts of Europe today, for example France and Italy, it is difficult for many alternative therapies to be practised legally, unless carried out by a medically qualified doctor. This could be seen as an attempt to annihilate non-medically qualified practitioners and to assimilate the therapy into conventional medicine by allowing only doctors to practise it.

Scheid identifies a further possibility, that a new and genuinely different discourse may emerge from the meeting of two traditions. I refer to this as the 'integration' option.

◆ *Integration.* This involves the creative integration of diverse systems of knowledge. For this to occur, and thus to avoid regression to any of the other three options, requires that the alternative and non-dominant system engages in the discourse from a firm base. I regard this path as the one holistic medicine needs to tread, with skill and determination. Yet, it will be easy to get sidetracked into reactive counter-attacks; and some will be tempted to 'hole up' in a safe place, away from the mainstream gaze. Others will spot opportunities in the mainstream and too readily let go of some of the defining principles of their practice. However, each of these deviations will lead to the alternative system being overrun eventually.

For holistic practitioners, the path of integration means being clear about the essential and defining characteristics of their approach and their therapy; having a well-grounded research base from which innovations can develop; and engaging in constructive discourse with those representing the dominant worldview.

To summarise, if it is to survive and to thrive in our culture, holistic medicine needs to develop from within as a process of reflective practice and also to direct its gaze outwards and engage with conventional doctors, with health service purchasers, and with the public. Research has an important role to play in both the 'inner' and the 'outer' directed activities. Clearly identified research activity is the one thing that is currently conspicuously lacking from most holistic medical practice. This needs to change.

Obstacles to Conducting Good Quality Research

Historically, holistic practitioners have been reluctant to submit their work for evaluation by people they have regarded as potentially hostile; yet they have not had the skills or resources to scientifically evaluate the therapies themselves. Likewise, doctors and medical researchers in the past have not generally been open to working in collaboration with complementary therapists.

The situation has now changed significantly. Of particular importance, the second BMA report on complementary medicine acknowledged that complementary therapies were now a significant part of many people's health care and therefore recommended that each therapy should be properly regulated; it also argued for good quality research and the setting up of systems of audit.[7] This is now beginning to happen. For example, the five major complementary therapies – acupuncture, chiropractic, homoeopathy, medical herbalism and osteopathy – have each established their own research programmes. In a survey of over one thousand UK acupuncturists registered under the Council for Acupuncture (now the British Acupuncture Council), it was found that there were two main reasons that practitioners were interested in research – to aid their professional learning and development and to demonstrate and promote the benefits of acupuncture.[8] These reasons reflect the 'inner' and the 'outer' focuses identified previously as essential for development.

Acupuncture
Chiropractic
Homoeopathy
Herbalism
Osteopathy

Another obstacle has been a dispute over appropriate methodology. The orthodox medical view has been that the only truly valid way of evaluating the usefulness of a therapy is to carry out the classic 'randomised controlled trial' (RCT), any other research design being regarded as inferior to this 'gold standard' of research methods. This view has been challenged by holistic practitioners and researchers, in particular because the classic RCT design constrains therapists to practise in a standardised way during a trial, thus preventing them from providing what they would regard as the best treatment for their patients.

However, opinions are beginning to change in mainstream medical research with growing recognition of the need for a variety of research methods, there being no single best method.[9]

A third obstacle to good quality research has been lack of funding – 'outer-focused' research can be very time-consuming and expensive. This continues to be a problem. Although there is a significant growth in collaborative studies between medical researchers and holistic practitioners, there is still relatively little funding because the Department of Health and the Medical Research Council do not regard it as a priority area for funding. However, the Labour Party has published a policy document proposing a strategy of research and development linked to support for statutory regulation.[10]

The NHS and Evidence Based Purchasing

An important development, which is refocusing research efforts, is the initiative by the Department of Health to promote evidence based purchasing. The result is that Health Authorities in the UK now have a policy requiring scientific evidence of effectiveness before they will fund new forms of treatment. This is clearly relevant to the uptake of complementary/alternative therapies since there is now a new hoop through which these therapies must jump. It is interesting to note that the majority of conventional therapies currently used in the NHS have not passed through this hoop, and there are indications that some would not stand up to the scrutiny of these new guidelines. However, because they are used routinely, their effectiveness is rarely questioned and it is not, for example, generally being suggested that they should be withdrawn until proved effective. Thus, there is a sense of complementary/alternative therapies being introduced onto an unlevel playing field.

However, these new standards are not necessarily undesirable, provided they are applied evenly, because there is considerable confidence amongst holistic practitioners that their therapies are effective, and would be cost effective if compared over the longer term with conventional treatments.

Linked to the evidence based purchasing initiative, the Department of Health's Research and Development Directorate has created a national programme to fund research that will produce the evidence on effectiveness. This will increase the likelihood that research findings get acted upon. Unfortunately, the resulting guidelines and invitations to tender for research projects make virtually no reference to complementary/alternative therapies, though there are many clinical conditions prioritised in the programme where complementary/alternative therapies may be of benefit. The door is marked, but it is not yet open.

Appropriate Research Methods

'Inner' focused research is about self development and requires the practitioner to be an active participant. 'Outer' focused research has other beneficiaries, 'stakeholders' who stand to benefit from its results, but who do not necessarily actively participate in the action. Research studies may have several different 'stakeholder groups' with an interest in the outcome and may have both an 'inner' and 'outer' focus. It is important that practitioners and researchers are clear about why specific types of research are necessary and who are the 'stakeholders' interested in the results.

For inner-focused research ('improve it'), the reflective practice, the primary stakeholders are the practitioners themselves. Their aim is self-development, improving their professional practice, thus providing a better service to their clients and increasing their own job satisfaction.

For outer-focused research ('prove it'), an important aim is to demonstrate convincingly that the therapy is of value to a population of users and potential users. Thus the stakeholders are the users themselves, the purchasers of the therapy (such as NHS health authority purchasers or insurance company purchasers) and medical practitioners (GPs who need evidence to decide whether to make referrals for specific therapies). The potential value of a therapy has several aspects: it includes the effectiveness for specific clinical conditions, the safety (that is, an assessment of potential risk), the cost of providing the therapy (including negative costs, that is, associated savings that may arise if a treatment is effective), and the users' (client/ patient) satisfaction with the service.

An important question put by Reilly is, 'What evidence is necessary to demonstrate benefit to stakeholders?'[11] He argues that here is a need to develop an 'evidence profile' for each therapy. For example:

Is it effective when examined scientifically?
Is it effective when applied clinically?
Is it clinically relevant?
Is it able to be integrated with orthodox approaches?
Is it safe?
Is it cost effective?
Is it in demand by patients?
Is it in demand by doctors?
Is it in demand by purchasers?

Table 1: Evidence profile for homoeopathy

He concludes that systematic evidence of a beneficial outcome is most important, with cost-effectiveness and patient satisfaction surfacing as emerging priorities for the medical profession. Personal experience (or the experience of a colleague) is also very influential to doctors' and purchasers' decisions.

How should this evidence be collected? Or, what research strategy is necessary to develop and promote holistic medicine and to maximise the opportunity for it to play a key role in twenty-first century health care? As holistic medicine does not lend itself to the classic RCT, research methods are needed which ensure:

◆ the holistic principles of the therapy are not compromised by the research method;

◆ users' (patients') preferences for therapies are taken into account;

◆ practitioners are free to give treatment, without constraint, individualised to the needs of each patient;

◆ every opportunity is taken to maximise the quality of the patient–practitioner relationship;

◆ the assessment of the 'outcome' of treatment takes a broad view of potential benefit and includes changes in lifestyle, health beliefs and quality of life, as well as alleviation of the symptoms of illness.

A key aspect of the research strategy should be to build up, within each complementary medicine profession, a community of practitioner–researchers, that is, practitioners who have training in research methods, who can carry out their own research studies (both 'inner' and 'outer' focused), who can 'hold their own' in dialogue with orthodox medical researchers, and play a full part in collaborative research projects.

The following methods will play an essential role within a holistic research strategy:

Literature Reviews (primarily 'outer' focus)

Despite the commonly accepted view that there has been little research evaluating holistic therapies, there are a considerable number of published studies that have usually been conducted in isolation from a research strategy and on a meagre budget. Nevertheless, there are thousands of papers and articles of mixed quality and an obvious starting point for a research strategy is to review what exists on specific topics (for example the results that have been obtained using a particular therapy for a specific health problem).

The British Library publishes a database of publications on complementary medicine (AMED) which is updated monthly and contains over 25,000 entries. The Research Council for Complementary Medicine provides a database search service (CISCOM), which can be used to find the better quality research papers on specific topics, drawn from a range of published sources. The Acupuncture Research Resource Centre in York provides a support service to acupuncturists and others, carrying out searches of complementary and conventional medicine databases on request and providing briefing papers for the profession.

The Nuffield Institute for Health in Leeds has recently published two reports, one on searching the literature on the efficacy and effectiveness of complementary therapies[12] and the other on reviewing the state of the evidence that arises from this literature.[13]

Cost-Effectiveness Studies (primarily 'outer' focus)

This type of study is the most appropriate for answering the question, 'How should we spend limited resources in the best interests of the population of users and potential users?' It is therefore the key question that faces NHS purchasers.[14] The question focuses on needs of a population or group, rather than individual cases and requires a methodology somewhat different from the 'classic RCT' which was developed to answer the question, 'What treatment should I offer my patient with this condition?' Thus, somewhat paradoxically, the methodology that enables practitioners to practise holistically without being constrained by the research design is the one that focuses on population needs. This is because, in effect, it draws a 'box' around the therapeutic process and leaves the 'inside' completely untouched. Thus, it has been called the 'black box' methodology, because it does not attempt to examine or influence what happens 'inside', but focuses on the 'outer' conditions – what are the outcomes of the service, what does it cost to provide it, are there any associated (side) effects?

This twin-track methodology is described more fully in a paper which outlines a study at the Foundation for Traditional Chinese Medicine to evaluate the cost effectiveness of an acupuncture service for people with low back pain.[15] It also reports the results of the initial feasibility study. The twin track approach is illustrated in the diagram below.

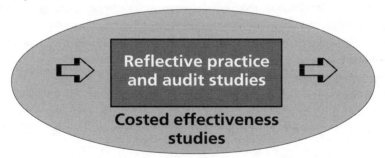

Fig. 1: Twin track approach

Reflective Practice (individual and peer review of clinical practice using clinical case studies – primarily 'inner' focus)

These are the studies that take place 'inside the black box'. They are designed to inform the practitioners, to help them gain insight about their practice and to make improvements where indicated. Schon has written about the process of being a reflective practitioner, which he calls 'reflection in action'.[16] It is interesting that in the West we need to be reminded to link theory and practice, that one informs the other. In Chinese medicine, the separation never occurred and reflective practice would therefore be regarded as obvious and natural, although Chinese practitioners would not share the need we have to be consistent or systematic in our research.[17] It is only by examining our daily practice that we can identify patterns, notice when we are surprised by something a client says, highlight aspects of our work that merit attention, target changes that are needed, and implement an intervention that will make the necessary difference. Finally, we need to review the consequences of our intervention and learn the appropriate lesson.

Multidisciplinary Co-operation

Beyond personal reflective practice, reflection can occur through discussion and examination of individual case studies in peer groups and, further still, in the systematic review of particular difficulties that face the profession. Research can be carried out by individuals, as part of their normal daily practice, but is usually more effective, and more satisfying, if done within a peer review process, because this requires the learning to be made explicit and offers the benefits of shared insight and learning.[18]

Service Monitoring and Audit Studies ('inner' and 'outer' foci)

These involve a more systematic and quantitative research design than reflective practice. They can be developed from clinical case studies as a specific question emerges that requires more systematic data to be collected to provide an answer. For example, a group of practitioners may ask, 'What are the main reasons (clinical problems) that our clients come to us and how many treatment sessions do we give, on average, for each type of clinical problem?' If an aim of the study is to review the information that has been collected and then make a decision to change the method of practice on the basis of that information, then it is known as an audit study. For example, a practitioner may review the source of referral of their clients and learn that there are some GPs who very seldom refer. They may then decide to investigate why and then promote their service more with some of these GPs. The focus of these studies can be simultaneously in two directions, 'inner' for self-development (of the individual or a group practice), and 'outer' for the benefit of the wider profession or to provide information to potential purchasers or referrers.

The Foundation for Traditional Chinese Medicine, for whom I am currently working as a researcher, promotes within the acupuncture profession the use of audit to raise standards of practice and care. Based on an initial survey of the needs of acupuncturists,[19] a training course in research methods including audit was organised in 1994. To consolidate the learning process, a group of eight acupuncturists from this training course undertook a multi-centre audit project with the support of a research award from the Research Council for Complementary Medicine. These collaborating practitioners identified characteristics of patients they treated (age, gender, type of presenting condition, its severity and duration) and the outcomes of treatment over time for up to ten treatment sessions.

The results detailed in the final report revealed that two-thirds of patients were female, that patients had slightly poorer health than those visiting a GP, that nearly 60% had had their problem for more than two years, and that nearly half were presenting with musculo-skeletal conditions. The study also gave some tentative indications on the number of treatments that are most beneficial, depending on the patient's characteristics and situation, though further research is required before any firm conclusions can be drawn.

A number of lessons arose from this audit work that should guide further studies in this area. These include a need to develop explicit criteria for terminating a course of treatment. Also a new measure of outcome is needed to assess the changes that take place in health, understanding and lifestyle that could contribute to prevention and reduce likelihood of further ill health. Further studies need to be designed at two levels: basic audit studies that are introduced to a wider range of practitioners and more advanced studies that could address more specific issues in greater depth.

Further reading on research design and methods can be found in Robert Yin's book on case study research.[20]

Organisational Case Studies ('inner' and 'outer' foci)

To provide an effective service requires more than good clinical skills in the consulting room. The service needs to be located in an 'organisational system' that is well designed. This is particularly important when holistic practitioners move from private practice to working in the NHS. There are many examples of practitioners being frustrated and dissatisfied because they are expected to work in unsatisfactory conditions or patients are referred inappropriately because referring doctors do not have a clear understanding of the types of patient the practitioner can most help.

Organisational studies are needed of how complementary services can be best integrated with conventional services, and different organisational models need to be assessed. For example, the GP is usually regarded as the 'gatekeeper' to all other health services; is this also the best model for providing complementary therapies? The organisational model used at the Marylebone Health Centre, in which GPs and complementary therapists work together in a single organisation, has been studied in depth and interesting results have been published.[21]

The focus for organisational studies is both 'inner', to enable the organisation and its practitioners to discover the best ways of working together, and 'outer' to share this learning with others and, often very importantly, to demonstrate to potential funders that a particular organisational model will deliver an effective service.

At the Foundation for Traditional Chinese Medicine, in the pursuit of our goal of making acupuncture more available on the NHS, we are interested in promoting effective collaboration between acupuncturists and GPs. To this end, we are undertaking a small action-research case study to explore the process of establishing an acupuncture service within a general medical practice. Our aims are to help evaluate the benefits to patients and GPs and identify the most effective ways of developing collaborative working and an integrated service. Over a twelve month period, the acupuncturist is monitoring her case work using some standard outcome measures, and we are assisting with exploring with the acupuncturist and the doctors how the acupuncture service is 'fitting in' to the general medical practice.

User Focus Groups and Surveys ('outer' and 'inner' foci)

All health practitioners recognise that their raison d'être is to serve their patients. Some, sometimes at least, think they know best what their patients need. This may or may not be true. However, it is important to seek the view of the client group, particularly when innovative ideas are being tested. This clearly happens on a one-to-one basis within the confidentiality of the consultation. But sometimes more is needed. Often there is a need to demonstrate to 'others' (for example purchasers) that the clients are satisfied with the service, or there may be specific questions about whether some clients would prefer the service to be organised in a different way. Surveys using questionnaires are the usual way of obtaining such information from a wide sample of users. This can be an effective method provided the questions asked are well conceived and are valid from the user's perspective. Focus groups, in which a group of clients sit together with a facilitator and share their views about the service, are usually the best way for the practitioner and the researcher to understand the client's perspective and to help formulate questions to put in a questionnaire.

Thus, although focus groups and surveys are usually motivated by an 'outer' focus, there can be considerable learning for the practitioner about their patients' experience. Things are likely to be revealed in a group that would not emerge in a one-to-one consultation, where the client may be somewhat inhibited or narrowly focused. Often new ideas emerge from the energy created by the group process.[22]

Resourcing and Supporting Research

The Research Council for Complementary Medicine was set up in 1983 to promote and support research within complementary medicine and to inform and advise health professionals on published research relating to the efficacy and safety of complementary medicine. It provides an information service on published scientific studies, organises colloquia on specific topics, for example 'Purchasing Complementary Medicine', and from time to time organises conferences on current research.

A priority for the Foundation for Traditional Chinese Medicine has been the provision of resources and information on research into acupuncture, and making them available to acupuncturists, medical practitioners and the general public. The Foundation also has a commitment to encouraging collaboration between orthodox and complementary practitioners as part of its larger goal of bringing acupuncture more centrally into the nation's system of health care. This work is being carried out in close association with the Acupuncture Research Resource Centre, the first national resource centre for acupuncture research. It is jointly managed by the British Acupuncture Council and the Foundation. Its aims include the provision of good quality information, such as literature searches from the British Library's AMED complementary medicine database, from MEDLINE and other international databases, and its own developing database on traditional Chinese medicine. The information is made available to people working in the field of acupuncture research, whether within the profession, or more widely to the media, doctors, policy makers, health and educational institutions and the general public. The centre also maintains a directory of acupuncturists working in research, and organises an annual symposium focusing on the state of the art in acupuncture research.

With the recent dramatic development of the Internet (the international computer network), which has been largely due to the introduction of the World Wide Web, the Foundation established an Acupuncture Home Page in May 1995. This is a World Wide Web information resource that reaches people worldwide. It contains information on acupuncture, on conditions that acupuncture treats, on how to find a practitioner, and on where to train. It also describes many key organisations in the field, including the British Acupuncture Council, the British Acupuncture Accreditation Board and the Research Council for Complementary Medicine. It is currently being logged on to by around 300 people a week from around the world.

While the Foundation for Traditional Chinese Medicine will continue to have a practice-based orientation in its research activity, plans for the future include a broadening out of our focus from what has been primarily practitioner-centred to a twin focus that is both practitioner-centred and user-centred. Initial research is being expanded by including the patient's experience of acupuncture into the studies.

Conclusion

After a rather slow start for research into holistic therapies, much is now beginning to happen. In approach and method new ground is being broken, fuelled by the passion and commitment to an holistic approach in health care.

My strongest motivation is the belief that research into holistic medicine has the potential to influence the development of conventional medical research in significant and valuable ways. Helping it turn itself around from the direction in which it originally set off, that of understanding the human being by reducing everything to its component parts, towards a recognition that to understand health and healing processes we need to attend to the integration of body, mind and spirit.

Biography

Mike Fitter is the research director for the Foundation for Traditional Chinese Medicine since 1993 and founding member of the Acupuncture Research Resource Centre. He is a chartered psychologist and was a researcher for the Medical Research Council for 19 years.

Acknowledgements

The ideas expressed in this chapter and the work described has benefited immensely from the support of my colleagues Alison Gould, Hugh MacPherson, Mark Lankshear and Richard Blackwell.

References

1   F S Baganal et al., *Survival of patients with breast cancer attending Bristol Cancer Help Centre*, Lancet, 1990; 336: 1185-8.

2   Richard Thomas, *The fatal flaw*, International Journal of Alternative and Complementary Medicine, May 1995, 18-19.

3   V Scheid, *Orientalism revisited: reflections on scholarship, research, and professionalisation*, European Journal of Oriental Medicine, 1993; 1: 2, 23-33.

4   B Ehrenreich; D English, *Witches, Midwives, and Nurses: A History of Women Healers*, The Feminist Press, 1973.

5   British Medical Association, *Alternative Therapy*, BMA Publications, 1986.

6   Research Council for Complementary Medicine, *Purchasing Complementary Medicine, Report on the Colloquium held at the Royal London Homoeopathic Hospital*, 10 April 1995.

7   British Medical Association, *Complementary Medicine: New Approaches to Good Practice*, BMA Publications, 1993.

8   M Fitter; R Blackwell, *Are acupuncturists interested in research?: a survey of CFA acupuncturists in the UK*, European Journal of Oriental Medicine, 1993; 1: 2, 44-7.

9   M Fitter; K Thomas, *Evaluating Complementary therapies for use in the NHS: horses for courses*, Complementary Therapies in Medicine, 1996.

10   D Primarolo, *Complementary therapies within the NHS: facilitation not prescription*, The Labour Party, London, 1994.

11   D Reilly, *Building a new future for homoeopathy and integrated care: the 1995 portfolio*, The Academic Departments, Glasgow Homoeopathic Hospital, Scotland, 1995.

12   A F Long; A Brettle; G Mercer, *Searching the literature on the efficacy and effectiveness of complementary therapies, A report by the Yorkshire Collaborating Centre for Health Service Research*, Nuffield Institute for Health, University of Leeds, 1995.

13   A F Long; G Mercer, *Reviewing the state of the evidence on efficacy and effectiveness of complementary therapies, A report by the Yorkshire Collaborating Centre for Health Service Research*, Nuffield Institute for Health, University of Leeds, 1995.

14   M Fitter; K Thomas, *Evaluating Complementary Therapies for use in the NHS: horses for courses*, Complementary Therapies in Medicine, 1996.

15   M Fitter; H MacPherson, *An audit of case studies of low back pain: a feasibility study for a controlled trial*, European Journal of Oriental Medicine, 1995; 1: 5, 46-55.

16   D Schon, *The Reflective Practitioner*, Basic Books, 1983.

17   V Scheid, *Home and away: In search of Chinese medicine*, European Journal of Oriental Medicine, 1994; 1: 4, 14-9.

18   P Reason (ed.), *Participation in Human Inquiry*, Sage Publications, 1994.

19   M Fitter; R Blackwell, *Are acupuncturists interested in research?: a survey of CFA acupuncturists in the UK*, European Journal of Oriental Medicine, 1993; 1: 2, 44-7.

20   P Luty; H MacPherson; M Fitter, *Clinical audit of treatment with acupuncture: patient profile and variations in outcome, Final Report*, Foundation for Traditional Chinese Medicine, York, 1995.

21   P Reason; H D Chase et al., *Towards a clinical framework for collaboration between general and complementary practitioners*, Journal of the Royal Society of Medicine, 1992; 86: 161-4.

22   R A Krueger, *Focus Groups: a practical guide for applied research (2nd edition)*, Sage Publications, 1994.

       J Kitzinger, Introducing focus groups, BMJ, 1995; 311: 299-302.

       A Fink, The Survey Kit (in 9 volumes), Sage Publications, 1995.

Further Reading

Birch, S., *Letter to the editor*, Journal of Alternative and Complementary Medicine, 1995; 1: 3, 221-2.

Cassidy, C M., *Social science theory and methods in the study of alternative and complementary medicine*, Journal of Alternative and Complementary Medicine, 1995; 1: 1, 19-40.

Reason P (ed), *Participation in Human Enquiry*, Sage Publications, 1994.

Stake R., *The Art of Case Study Research*, Sage Publications, 1995.

Yin R K., *Case Study Research: Design and Methods (2nd edition)*, Sage Publications, 1994.

Resources

Research Council for Complementary Medicine (RCCM)
60 Great Ormond Street
London WC1N 3JF
Tel. 0171-833 8897
Fax. 0171-278 7412

Acupuncture Research Resource Centre (ARRC)
122a Acomb Road
York
YO2 4EY
Tel. 01904-781630
Fax. 01904-782991
http://www.demon.co.uk/acupuncture/

Natural Therapies Database UK
47 Ashby Ave
Chessington
Surrey KT9 8BT
Tel/Fax. 0181-391 0150

Complementary Medicine and the Law
by Julie Stone

The growth of complementary medicine over the past decade has been accompanied by calls for greater regulation. To date, discussions on regulation have confined themselves to the parameters set by orthodox medicine, and as a result, critical issues which need to be more publicly aired may have been overlooked. The legal and regulatory mechanisms which govern orthodox medicine are not an appropriate model for the regulation of most complementary therapies. In short, the patient – centred, holistic approach central to the theory and practice of many complementary therapies presents a unique problem for the law: the highly individualised, more intuitive, whole-person approach of complementary medicine is not amenable to the quantification and certainty required to establish that someone has acted unlawfully. Only by implementing a more dynamic form of ethics – directed regulation can the consumer be protected without sacrificing the unique contribution that complementary medicine has to make.[1]

Aims of Regulation

Most people assume, somewhat uncritically, that consumer protection is the sole aim of regulation. A closer examination of the history of the regulation of the medical profession indicates that professional self-interest is also a highly persuasive factor in seeking formal regulation, with a view to establishing a strong professional base and creating an occupational monopoly. Rejecting blatant self-interest as a suitable justification for the pursuit of statutory regulation, what should the central aims of regulating complementary medicine be?

The Promotion of High, Uniform Standards of Practice

Educating Complementary Therapists

Consumers are best served by ensuring that all practitioners are able to practise the skills of their particular therapy in a safe and competent manner. A high standard of training is of the utmost importance. Some system of licensing or registration is thought to be the best way of achieving this, so that all therapists who use a particular title have received appropriate education and have demonstrated an ability to apply their therapeutic skills in practice. But whilst some therapies have the sort of knowledge base which can be taught and tested by means of formal written examinations, others may equally rely on the demonstration of various practical skills, whilst others depend almost entirely on non-measurable, intuitive healing skills. Certainly, the starting point for any therapy is to define what its required competencies are, and to proceed to develop methods of imparting those skills and measuring them.

Ability to Identify Competent Practitioners

Having ensured that practitioners are suitably 'qualified', patients must then be able to identify an appropriate practitioner for their needs. Also, to the extent that doctors wish to recommend, employ or refer to complementary therapists, they will need assurance that therapists are competent. Most therapies have a register to enable the public to choose from appropriately qualified practitioners. Many therapies are still fragmented and may have several registering bodies. Obviously, the more united a therapy becomes, and the fewer registers a patient has to consult, the better. Most patients will assume, quite legitimately, that provided practitioners are registered, their bona fides is guaranteed. Unfortunately, this may not be the case, given that each registering body will claim to ensure high standards.

Means of Ensuring Accountability

The concomitant of high standards of practice is having mechanisms to ensure that professional standards are enforced. Whilst one might hope that education alone will protect patients from harm, this cannot be guaranteed. No practitioner is perfect and mistakes will occur in any occupation. Whilst some mistakes may be excusable, others may require action to be taken against the practitioner. Disciplinary procedures must be sufficiently flexible to take account of the seriousness of the complaint, and must be able to respond appropriately. In order to protect the public, disciplinary mechanisms must be both accessible and visible and must be capable of responding to complainants in a meaningful way.

Existing Controls over Complementary Medicine

Common Law Freedom to Practice

Complementary therapists in the UK, unlike the situation in other jurisdictions, enjoy a common law freedom to practise. Whereas the practice of complementary therapies is limited elsewhere to registered medical practitioners,[2] currently anyone may set up as a therapist and offer services directly to the public. Provided therapists do not use protected titles when they are not entitled to do so, or make claims to be able to cure certain medical conditions, there are no specific legal restraints on the right to practise.

Until the Osteopaths Act 1993 and Chiropractors Act 1994 are fully in force, all complementary therapies are subject to varying degrees of voluntary self–regulation.

This ranges from highly formalised regulation at one end, to virtually no regulation at the other.

Complementary therapists and the courts

Alongside self-regulation, all complementary therapists are subject to the common law, that is law made by judges. This is the case regardless of whether they are statutorily or voluntarily regulated. Common law divides into the civil law, which mostly relates to actions brought by one individual against another, and criminal law, which involves the prosecution of an individual by the State. Most legal actions against practitioners will be civil actions for negligence.

Why the common law cannot respond to complementary medicine

Despite the huge increase in medical negligence claims over the last decade, this has not been matched by a corresponding increase in claims against complementary therapists. Although there is a marked increase in the number of complaints to disciplinary bodies, this bears no relation to the huge increase in usage of many therapies. Why are there so few complaints? It is unlikely that this is because all complementary therapists are exemplary. One obvious answer is that most therapies are not inherently harmful. This, however, is too simplistic an explanation as all therapeutic interventions are capable of causing harm of some level. The lack of complaints is more likely to reflect the inadequacy or visibility of grievance procedures at both a professional and a pan–professional level, than an absence of complaints.

But why, in an era of greater litigiousness and increased consumer expectations, are more complementary practitioners not being sued? The more plausible explanation is that existing legal structures cannot be applied in their existing form to the complementary therapeutic relationship. This is because the common law of negligence is determined utterly by reference to the doctor/patient relationship. This is not an appropriate basis for holistic relationships which are characterised by three vital features:

◆ *The highly individualised nature of the therapy.* In law, the court judges a practitioner's conduct according to an objective standard of reasonableness. Such a standard cannot readily be applied to therapies which are highly individualised, subjective and intuitive. Equally, the problems of proof which beset 'scientific' research apply no less to establishing negligence. If there is no way of proving that a therapy is capable of causing a specific effect, it may be equally impossible for legal purposes to demonstrate with the requisite degree of certainty, i.e. proof on a balance of probabilities, that the therapy caused the alleged harm.

◆ *The wrong sort of harm.* Even if harm can be established, the sorts of harm that most therapies are likely to produce are emotional, rather than physical. Generally speaking, the law, reliant once again on a medicalised model of harm, is ill-equipped to compensate for harms other than physical harm. Unless a plaintiff can establish that they have suffered a recognisable psychiatric disorder, the law of negligence cannot respond. The emotional harm that could derive from an abusive therapeutic relationship would rarely fit within the existing framework of the law.

◆ *The need for patients to exercise self-responsibility.* Many complementary therapies depend on a higher degree of patient participation than orthodox medicine, and an understanding that the patient will agree to take responsibility for their own health. The law places all of the legal responsibilities on the practitioner and none on the patient, as the professional health carer is presumed to have expert knowledge and thus power which the patient does not possess. This may be appropriate in highly technical, skill-based therapies such as acupuncture and homoeopathy, but it is an unhelpful and disempowering model for most patient – centred, holistic therapies. Patients would be better served by a contractual model in which both sides of the relationship have expectations and responsibilities.

Self-Responsibility of the Patient

Acupuncture Homoeopathy

Is Statutory Regulation the Way Forward?

A number of major therapies are actively considering statutory regulation. What precisely is it that therapies think that they stand to gain from statutory, as opposed to better voluntary, self-regulation? Anticipated benefits may include:

◆ The ability to achieve higher standards and greater accountability through a system of statutory registration;

◆ The medical profession's respect, together with a greater willingness to refer patients to complementary therapists;

◆ Improved prospects of integration within the NHS;

◆ Enhanced public status.

Notwithstanding the advantages of a protected title, other perceived benefits are probably illusory. Statutory regulation has a number of disadvantages for complementary therapists. It is extremely expensive to administer, it may ossify therapies and stifle their therapeutic development, and most importantly of all, it cannot guarantee high standards of practice. The threat of criminal sanctions should not be the impetus for working towards high standards. In any event, statutory regulation is unlikely to be granted to therapies which are unable or unwilling to demonstrate their effectiveness in scientific terms. Currently this excludes most therapies. Even if statutory regulation were feasible, smaller therapies would do far better to put their resources towards improving and developing internal standards of competence.

Greater integration will be influenced as much by economic factors as therapeutic efficacy. In an increasingly evidence-based NHS, it is questionable whether purchasers would contract for therapies for which efficacy has not been established in scientific terms. The approval or disapproval of the medical profession is of diminishing significance since the introduction of the NHS reforms, which allow purchasing decisions to be more responsive to consumer demand. Besides, do therapies really want medical approval if it is only achievable at the cost of the unique holistic perspective? As to the respect of the public, this must be earned through high standards of practice, openness and professional accountability. As M. Stacey points out: 'State recognition does not automatically confer the same status and power upon all professions who achieve it.'[3]

Ethics-Led Regulation

Rather, practitioners must look to ethics-led regulation in which high standards, rather than professional power, are the driving force. This strong ethical basis must be instilled during education and training, and be ongoing when the practitioner is actually in practice. Such an ethical awareness must equip them with the necessary tools to uphold the principles of respect for autonomy, the duty to help and not harm patients, and justice and fairness. Ethical practice requires a commitment to the following:

◆ the acquisition, based on appropriate assessment, of both technical and humanistic skills;

◆ recognition by therapists of their limits of competence;

◆ steps taken to ensure the safety of therapies;

◆ protection for patients against exaggerated or false claims;

◆ protection for patients from unqualified practitioners;

◆ respect for patients' autonomy, in particular by obtaining the patient's consent, and respecting the patient's confidentiality;

◆ clear and effective grievance procedures which provide a means of redress when harm is suffered; and

◆ effective disciplinary structures.

Conclusion

As the common law is incapable, at present, of responding to the holistic relationship, new approaches to regulation must be sought. Building on existing self-regulatory structures, a dynamic ethics-led approach should be fostered. As new therapeutic paradigms emerge, so complementary therapists should stop aspiring to a medicalised model of regulation, and create instead new ethics-led paradigms of regulation in which self-responsibility on the part of both the practitioner and the patient are given their due weight.

Biography

Julie Stone is a lawyer and university lecturer. She is co-author of the book *Complementary Therapies and the Law*.

References

1   J Stone; J Matthews, *Complementary Medicine and the Law*, Oxford University Press, 1996.

2   P Fisher; A Ward, *Complementary medicine in Europe*, BMJ, 1994; 309: 107-8.

3   M Stacey, *Therapeutic Collective Responsibility*, In S Budd; U Sharma, *The Healing Bond*, Routledge, 1994.

Further Reading

Budd S.; Sharma U., *The Healing Bond*, Routledge, 1994.

Fisher P.; Ward A., *Complementary Medicine in Europe*, BMJ, 1994; 309: 107-8.

Jenkins, Peter, *Counselling, Psychotherapy and the Law*, Sage Publications, 1996.

Stone J.; Matthews J., *Complementary Medicine and the Law*, Oxford University Press, 1996.

Index

This index lists illnesses mentioned in the text. This does not constitute recommendations for treatment but rather illustrates the use of the various therapeutic disciplines. In holistic health care the whole person is being treated and not just the presenting symptom. Therefore a consultation with a trained practitioner is advised.

A

Abrams, Albert 427
Ackerman, Nathan 224
acne 261
acupressure 70
acupuncture **69**, 511
addictions 74, 203, 226, 257, 278, 350, 360, 385, 404, 522, 534
Adler, Alfred 403
affirmations **79**, 125
AIDS 83, 113, 368, 404, 519
Alcoholics Anonymous 406, 534
Alexander, F. M. 86, 232
Alexander Technique **86**
allergies 113, 360, 370, 427, 439
Altmaier, M 116
amenorrhoea 303
Angerer, Joseph 302
animals 152, 289, 379, 429, 447
Ankmahor 437
anorexia nervosa 113, 131, 224, 466, 469
anthroposophical medicine **94**
anxiety 122, 175, 296, 360, 385, 450, 469, 522
aromatherapy **100**, 584
art therapy **112**
arthritis 167, 173, 176, 258, 296, 345, 374, 519
artistic therapy 96, 112
Assagioli, Roberto 406, 410
asthma 74, 113, 122, 129, 173, 183, 203, 226, 260, 296, 365, 427, 450, 487, 522
attention deficit 364, 450
audit studies 622
auric field 203
Autogenic Training **119**
autoimmune diseases 486
autonomic nervous system 169, 182, 452
autotoxicity 165
Avicenna 100, 323
ayurvedic medicine 394, 583

B

Bach, Edward 240
back pain 91, 121, 129, 145, 149, 265, 324, 374, 477, 486

Bandler, Richard 354
Barlow, Kenneth 564
Bayly, Doreen 437
behavioural medicine 450
behavioural therapy 188, 404, 417
Bennett, Terence 310
Benor, Daniel 491
Benson, Herbert 451, 524
bereavement 191, 278
bio-energetic regulatory medicine **134**
bioenergetic analysis **127**
birth 266, 274, 432
birth trauma 197, 381
Blake Lucas, Winafred 385
body armour 129, 397
body language 215
bodywork 397
Bohm, David 172
Boszormenyi-Nagy, Ivan 224
Bowen, Murray 224
Brahmananda Saraswati, Swami 521
Braid, James 294
brain waves 204
breath 272, 453, 552
brittle bones 268
bronchitis 260, 516
BSE 365
burns 106, 260

C

Campbell, Don 486
cancer 83, 96, 113, 129, 166, 184, 226, 256, 327, 345, 364, 367, 370, 404, 450, 477, 492, 532
candida 167, 369
Cannon, Alexander 383
Cannon, Walter 451, 495
cardiovascular disease 258, 367, 477
Carruthers, Malcolm 120
case conferences 55
catharsis 161, 275
cerebral palsy 202
chakras 104, 175, 202, 241, 484
chanting 485
Chapman's reflexes 307
chi *see under* qi

Chi Nei Tsang **142**
chicken pox 109
childbirth 107, 477
children with special needs 215
chiropractic **147**
choosing a practitioner **589**
chronic fatigue 145, 268
co-counselling **158**
colds 107, 109, 176, 258, 477
colic 197, 381
colitis 113, 167, 369, 450
Collins, F. W. 302
colonic irrigation (Hydrotherapy) **165**
colour therapy **172**
common law 629
communication 225
communication skills 354, 607
community centre 223
competence 591, 604
complex homoeopathy **180**, 284
compulsions 360, 417
constipation 166, 262, 324
Cooper, Cary 496
cost-effectiveness studies 621
Coué, Emile 80
coughs 260
counselling 160, **186**, 246, 419
Cousins, Norman 315
cranial osteopathy 195
cranio-sacral therapy **195**
creativity 278
Creutzfeldt-Jacob Disease 365
crisis 409, 421
Crocker, Lucy 558
Crohn's disease 487
crystal healing 201
cupping 511
Cyriax, James 379

D

death 191, 226, 432, **572**
Deck, Josef 302
defensive medicine 23
Delawarr, George 427
dental work 197, 381, 265
dentistry, holistic **265**